**1985**
**YEAR BOOK OF**
**NEUROLOGY AND**
**NEUROSURGERY®**

# THE 1985 YEAR BOOKS

The YEAR BOOK series provides in condensed form the essence of the best of the recent international literature in medicine and the allied health professions. The material is selected by distinguished editors who critically review more than 500,000 journal articles each year.

**Anesthesia:** Drs. Miller, Kirby, Ostheimer, Saidman, and Stoelting

**Cancer:** Drs. Hickey, Clark, and Cumley

**Cardiology:** Drs. Harvey, Kirkendall, Kirklin, Nadas, Resnekov, and Sonnenblick

**Critical Care Medicine:** Drs. Rogers, Booth, Dean, Gioia, McPherson, Michael, and Traystman

**Dentistry:** Drs. Cohen, Hendler, Johnson, Jordan, Moyers, Robinson, and Silverman

**Dermatology:** Drs. Sober and Fitzpatrick

**Diagnostic Radiology:** Drs. Bragg, Keats, Kieffer, Kirkpatrick, Koehler, Sorenson, and White

**Digestive Diseases:** Drs. Greenberger and Moody

**Drug Therapy:** Drs. Hollister and Lasagna

**Emergency Medicine:** Dr. Wagner

**Endocrinology:** Drs. Schwartz and Ryan

**Family Practice:** Dr. Rakel

**Hand Surgery:** Drs. Dobyns and Chase

**Infectious Diseases:** Drs. Wolff, Gorbach, Keusch, Klempner, and Snydman

**Medicine:** Drs. Rogers, Des Prez, Cline, Braunwald, Greenberger, Bondy, Epstein, and Malawista

**Neurology and Neurosurgery:** Drs. DeJong, Sugar, and Currier

**Nuclear Medicine:** Drs. Hoffer, Gore, Gottschalk, Sostman, and Zaret

**Obstetrics and Gynecology:** Drs. Pitkin and Zlatnik

**Ophthalmology:** Dr. Ernest

**Orthopedics:** Dr. Coventry

**Otolaryngology:** Drs. Paparella and Bailey

**Pathology and Clinical Pathology:** Dr. Brinkhous

**Pediatrics:** Drs. Oski and Stockman

**Plastic and Reconstructive Surgery:** Drs. McCoy, Brauer, Haynes, Hoehn, Miller, and Whitaker

**Podiatric Medicine and Surgery:** Dr. Jay

**Psychiatry and Applied Mental Health:** Drs. Freedman, Lourie, Meltzer, Nemiah, Talbott, and Weiner

**Sports Medicine:** Drs. Krakauer, Shephard, and Torg, Col. Anderson, and Mr. George

**Surgery:** Drs. Schwartz, Najarian, Peacock, Shires, Spencer, and Thompson

**Urology:** Drs. Gillenwater and Howards

1985

# The Year Book of NEUROLOGY AND NEUROSURGERY®

*"Published without interruption since 1902"*

## Neurology

Edited by

**Russell N. DeJong, M.D.**
*Professor Emeritus of Neurology,*
*The University of Michigan Medical School*

**Robert D. Currier, M.D.**
*Professor and Chairman, Department of Neurology, University of Mississippi*
*Medical Center, Jackson*

## Neurosurgery

Edited by

**Oscar Sugar, M.D.**
*Professor Emeritus and former Head of the Department of Neurosurgery,*
*University of Illinois Abraham Lincoln School of Medicine*

**Year Book Medical Publishers, Inc.**
**Chicago**

International Standard Book Number: 0–8151–2407–4

International Standard Serial Number: 0513–5117

The editor for this book was Joan David, and the production manager was H. E. Nielsen. The managing editor for the YEAR BOOK series is Caroline Scoulas.

# Table of Contents

The material covered in this volume represents literature reviewed up to April 1984.

# Journals Represented

Acta Neurochirurgica
Acta Neurologica Scandinavica
American Journal of Diseases of Children
American Journal of Gastroenterology
American Journal of Medicine
American Journal of Neuroradiology
American Journal of Psychiatry
American Journal of Roentgenology
American Journal of Surgery
Anesthesia and Analgesia
Anesthesiology
Annales de Radiologie
Annals of Internal Medicine
Annals of Neurology
Archives of Disease in Childhood
Archives of Internal Medicine
Archives of Neurology
Archives of Otolaryngology
Archives of Physical Medicine and Rehabilitation
Archives of Surgery
Brain
British Journal of Psychiatry
British Journal of Surgery
British Journal of Venereal Diseases
British Medical Journal
Canadian Journal of Neurological Sciences
Cancer
Child's Brain
Clinical Radiology
Contemporary Surgery
Deutsche Medizinische Wochenschrift
Developmental Medicine and Child Neurology
Diagnostic Imaging
European Neurology
European Urology
Headache
International Surgery
Journal of the American Geriatrics Society
Journal of the American Medical Association
Journal of Bone and Joint Surgery (American vol.)
Journal of Bone and Joint Surgery (British vol.)
Journal of Computer Assisted Tomography
Journal of Medical Genetics
Journal of Neurogenetics

Journal of Neurological Sciences
Journal of Neurology, Neurosurgery and Psychiatry
Journal of Neurosurgery
Journal of Occupational Medicine
Journal of Pediatric Surgery
Journal of Pediatrics
Journal of Pharmacology and Experimental Therapeutics
Journal of Thoracic and Cardiovascular Surgery
Journal of Trauma
Journal of Urology
Klinische Monatsblatter fur Augenheilkunde
Lancet
Laryngoscope
Mayo Clinic Proceedings
Medical Imaging
Medical Journal of Australia
Medicine
Nature
Neurochirurgia
Neurochirurgie
Neurology Medicine Chir. (Tokyo)
Neurology
Neuropediatrics
Neuroradiology
Neurosurgery
New England Journal of Medicine
Pediatrics
Physical Therapy
Postgraduate Medicine
Practitioner
Presse Medicale
Radiology
Revue Neurologique
ROFO: Fortschritte auf dem Gebiete der Rontgenstrahlen und der
    Nuklearmedizin
Southern Medical Journal
Spine
Stroke
Surgery
Surgery, Gynecology and Obstetrics
Surgical Neurology
Therapeutic Drug Monitoring
Zeitschrift fur Kinderchirurgie
Zentralblatt fur Neurochirurgie

# Publisher's Preface

Publication of the 1985 YEAR BOOKS marks the eighty-fifth anniversary of the original PRACTICAL MEDICINE YEAR BOOKS. To mark this milestone, the YEAR BOOKS are being issued with a more contemporary cover design, and the format for the contents has been modified to identify the article titles, authors' names, and journal citations more readily. The substance of the YEAR BOOK—the abstracts of scholarly articles with substantive editorial comments—is unchanged. What is new is the isolation of the reference information as a discrete block of copy. Other, less visible changes will continue to be made as we strive to make the YEAR BOOKS the very best they can be.

The YEAR BOOK OF NEUROLOGY AND NEUROSURGERY is a proud member of the original series of PRACTICAL MEDICINE YEAR BOOKS. In 1901, neurology was covered in the YEAR BOOK OF SKIN, VENEREAL, NERVOUS, AND MENTAL DISEASES. The book was titled YEAR BOOK OF NEUROLOGY, PSYCHIATRY, AND ENDOCRINOLOGY from 1934 through 1944, and it became the YEAR BOOK OF NEUROLOGY, PSYCHIATRY, AND NEUROSURGERY in 1945. From 1969 onward, the YEAR BOOK OF NEUROLOGY AND NEUROSURGERY has been a separate entity.

The year 1985 marks another special anniversary: It is the thirtieth year of Dr. Oscar Sugar's editorship of the Neurosurgery section and, sadly, his last. Dr. Sugar's scholarly editorials will be missed by his legions of faithful readers even as his charming wit and much-appreciated cooperation will be missed by the staff of Year Book Medical Publishers.

We are proud to hail the longevity of this important member of the YEAR BOOK series.

11

# NEUROLOGY

---

RUSSELL N. DeJONG, M.D.
ROBERT D. CURRIER, M.D.

# Introduction

## Alzheimer's Disease

Alzheimer's disease—a progressive dementing disorder of as yet unknown etiology and a condition that can be diagnosed positively only by postmortem examination—is being diagnosed and discussed with increasing frequency and has received much attention and support in recent years.

First described by Alois Alzheimer in 1904, it was originally believed to be solely a disorder of the presenile period (fifties and late forties), similar clinically, but a different disease from senile dementia. Neuropathologic, neurochemical, and related studies have shown, however, that the two disorders are probably identical, although some investigators prefer to call the disease when it affects people in the senile period *senile dementia, Alzheimer type* (SDAT) (Terry and Katzman: *Ann. Neurol.* 14:497–506, 1983). It is said that the disease affects about 1,500,000 Americans over 65 years of age and another 100,000 persons in their forties and fifties.

Interest in the disease stimulated the development of a recent conference entitled "Alzheimer's Disease: Toward Clinical Management," held at the Annenberg Center for Health Sciences at Eisenhower Medical Center in Palm Springs, California, and attended by neurologists, psychiatrists, gerontologists, and psychologists, as well as laboratory investigators in many fields, social workers, family therapists, and others. The clinicians stressed the need for accurate diagnostic criteria as well as preventive and therapeutic progress. Basic investigators stressed the need for etiologic information, studies of genetic and environmental factors and related phenomena, while social workers stressed endeavors to help patients and their families to endure the irreversible: the progression of the illness.

Many investigators believe that the cause of the disease is a neurochemical process that destroys cholinergic neurons, causing a deficiency of acetylcholine (*Med. Res. Rev.* 3:221–236, 1983). Both choline acetyltransferase and acetylcholinesterase are greatly reduced in the cerebral cortex of persons with Alzheimer's disease. The disorder appears to be a genetic one, and the pattern of inheritance suggests the presence of a single abnormal gene. The situation in affected families resembles that in families affected by Huntington's chorea, and the recent success in finding a genetic marker for the latter disease (Gusella et al.: *Nature* 306:234–238, 1983) gives some hope for Alzheimer's disease also. Perhaps the most significant approach to therapy at the present time is the attempt to overcome the cholinergic deficit in the brains of patients with Alzheimer's disease. However, acetylcholine precursors (choline and phosphatidylcholine (lecithin) have not proved to be of help.

Other possible etiologies for the disease are, however, still under consideration. A viral relationship has not been ruled out. Some resemblance both clinically and pathologically between Alzheimer's disease and the spongiform encephalopathies (kuru and Creutzfeldt-Jakob disease) emphasizes the need for further consideration of an unconventional virus as the pathogenetic agent. Antiviral measures such as the use of interferon are being tried in therapy. The presence pathologically of neurofibrillary tangles and senile plaques typical of Alzheimer's disease in the brains of older patients (age 35 and over) with Down's syndrome have led some investigators to suspect that abnormalities of chromosome 21, which are responsible for Down's syndrome, may in some ways be implicated in the development of Alzheimer's disease (Heyman et al.: *Ann. Neurol.* 14:504–509, 1983). The pathologic association of aluminum accumulation in the brains of patients with Alzheimer's disease still merits further investigation, although the possible role of aluminum in the development of the disorder is disputed. Aluminum chelation therapy, however, is being evaluated. Gangliosides have been reported to produce increased sprouting and re-generation of injured nerve cells, and administration of them to patients with Alzheimer's disease is undergoing clinical trials. The finding of an excess of autoimmune disorders in families of persons with Alzheimer's disease and the presence of immunoglobulins in the senile plaques in the brains of subjects with this disease have led to the suggestion that autoimmune dysfunction may be a factor in the development of this type of dementia.

Recent announcement of the forthcoming publication of the book *Alzheimer's Disease: The Standard Reference,* edited by Barry Reisberg of the New York University Medical Center (New York, The Free Press, 1984) brings us an overview of current concepts of Alzheimer's disease, senile dementia, and age-associated cognitive decline. Chapters by large numbers of authors discuss the differential diagnosis, clinical features, pathologic alterations, neurochemistry, epidemiologic and genetic factors, and pharmacologic investigations in Alzheimer's disease as well as the psychotherapeutic approaches to the management of patients and their families. Another recent book, *Dementia: A Practical Guide to Alzheimer's Disease and Related Illnesses,* by L. L. Hestan and J. White (New York, W. H. Freeman Co., 1983), gives much helpful information. Two standard references are *Alzheimer's Disease: Senile Dementia and Related Disorders* (Katzman, Terry, and Bick [eds.], New York, Raven Press, 1978) and *The Neurology of Aging, Contemporary Neurology,* vol. 22 (Katzman and Terry [eds.], Philadelphia, F. A. Davis Co., 1983).

*Coming of a New Age*

In his timely and thought-provoking article, "Recombinant DNA and Neurologic Disease: The Coming of a New Age" (*Neurology* 33:622–625, 1983), Roger N. Rosenberg states, "The evolution in molecular biology begun by Watson and Crick in defining the structure of DNA and by Nirenberg in deciphering the genetic code has clearly entered the arena of neurobiology and clinical neurology." He concludes as follows: "Molecular biology has found the brain a fertile milieu. Neurologists will soon become familiar with and grow to rely on DNA hybridization patterns in evaluating patients with genetic and metabolic disorders and, it is hoped, be able to apply specific gene therapy to their patients." Lewis P. Rowland, in the Robert Wartenberg Lecture entitled "Molecular Genetics, Pseudo-genetics and Clinical Neurology" given at the annual meeting of the American Academy of Neurology in San Diego in April 1983 (*Neurology* 33:1179–1195, 1983) discusses the biochemical genetics of neurology, especially in relation to neuromuscular disorders, and makes a plea for sophisticated clinical investigations to identify and study these aspects of neurology. The finding of the chromosomal localization of the Huntington's chorea gene by using recombinant DNA technology to identify a primary defect is a discovery that may ultimately lead to the development of therapeutic possibilities and is the first important milestone in this new and significant field of investigation (Gusella et al.: *Nature* 306:234–235, 1983).

*New Books*

Neurologists and neuroscientists have become extremely prolific in the production of scientific publications during recent years. This is true not only in contributions to the current journal publications (both the number of journals and the number of articles, basic as well as clinical, in these journals) but in the number of books on neuroscience-related subjects produced by the many medical publishing companies. There are too many of these for one to review them in this brief Introduction, or even to just list them. A few significant ones, however, may be mentioned.

*The Clinical Neurosciences*, a five-volume publication (London, Churchill Livingstone Inc., 1983), is edited by Roger N. Rosenberg, Professor of Neurology and Physiology, and Chairman of the Department of Neurology at the University of Texas Health Science Center, Southwestern Medical School, Dallas. The individual volumes deal with Neurology, Neurosurgery, Neuropathology, Neuroradiology, and Neurobiology. The work is comprehensive in depth, scope, and detail and in its integration of these key disciplines.

*Multiple Sclerosis: Pathology, Diagnosis and Management* (Baltimore, Williams and Wilkins, 1983) is edited by J. F. Hallpike, Department of Neurology, Royal Adelaide Hospital, Adelaide, Australia; C. W. M. Adams, Department of Pathology, Guy's Hospital Medical School, London, England; and W. W. Tourtellotte, Neurology Service, Veterans Administration Wadsworth Hospital Center, and Department of Neurology, School of Medicine, University of California, Los Angeles. It deals with the clinical aspects, pathology, epidemiology, and genetics of multiple sclerosis and discusses various etiologic considerations and the comprehensive management of the patient.

Another important contribution on multiple sclerosis should also be mentioned: *Multiple Sclerosis: A Guide for Patients and Their Families*, edited by Labe C. Scheinberg, Professor of Neurology and Rehabilitation Medicine, Albert Einstein College of Medicine, Bronx, New York (New York, Raven Press, 1983). This is a valuable guide both for patients with multiple sclerosis and for their families, who also must live with the disease. A group of experts in neurology, psychiatry, rehabilitation medicine, law, and other fields have contributed to it. In addition to medical issues, the book addresses social concerns such as sexuality, social adaptation, vocational alternatives, disability benefits, and available community services. It will be welcomed by patients, family members, professionals, and everyone dealing with the disease.

RUSSELL N. DEJONG, M.D.

# Introductory Remarks

I am looking out the window to the south at a jetliner ascending into and through the clouds toward Dallas, and I am thinking of the thousands of nonoccurring errors that enable it to fly. People make errors; every error and accident is somebody's—they don't just happen. One particular group of people, politicians, evidently believe in never admitting error, at least they never are observed doing so. Perhaps editors should do likewise, else they get the axe. On the other hand, the *Oxford Book of Quotations* credits C. P. Scott with saying, "Comment is free but facts are sacred." Therefore we will accept the risk and with only moderate hesitation point out an error or two from the 1984 YEAR BOOK OF NEUROLOGY AND NEUROSURGERY.

The first error is mine and mine alone. Dr. L. J. Endtz of The Netherlands notes that Bousser et al., in their article on the aspirin treatment of stroke (1984 YEAR BOOK, p. 55), used a daily dose of 1 gm and not 330 mg as was stated in our editorial comment. After receiving Dr. Endtz's kind letter, I went back to the original article and under "methods" read it again and again misread it. Only on what was probably the fifth reading and knowing that I had to be wrong did I notice that above the listed dosages the phrase "each given three times daily" appeared. So we hope the reader will forgive but not forget. That study, therefore, does not lend support to the thought that 330 mg of aspirin is better than 1,000 mg per day.

A comment on page 71 contains a mistake that should be mystifying to the reader. The abbreviation ALS, when it reached the printer's hands, became Advanced Life Support. The printer or copy reader is not alone with that error. The abbreviation is becoming more associated with advanced life support than with amyotrophic lateral sclerosis in the medical student's lexicon.

On page 141, I had hoped to define heritability. My explanation evidently was too awkward and was altered between pen and press. I now will attempt it again. Each and every disease results from the sum of its environmental and hereditary causative factors. The heritability of a particular disease is that percentage of the total factors that is hereditary. We will see how that one comes out. The Year Book staff also insisted on changing "sedimentation rate" to "rate of sedimentation," which although strange to the medical ear, at least is understandable.

I agree with C. P. Scott. Facts are sacred and comment is free. I suppose this could be called the credo of scientific democracy. Or perhaps that should read "the democracy of science." It is puzzling that letters to the editor implying error or erroneous thinking on an author's part are never followed by an author's admission of error. And I mean never. Instead we read what is usually a slightly condescending comment implying that the complaining letter writer is a bit slow on the uptake or has not read the article correctly. I hope some day to read an author's reply that says "Yes, by George, we were wrong." Perhaps that is too much to hope for.

I understand the circulation of the YEAR BOOK is considerable. Why have we had no more complaining correspondence? Do you all imagine that when you read some obscure note that you are the dumb one and not me? Matthew Menken does write that our coverage of society's relationship to the neurologist, the care of chronic neurologic disease, and the need for neurologists is deficient, and he intimates that I could stand a cram course on those areas. No doubt true.

Probably the biggest news in neurology this past year is the location of the Huntington's chorea gene locus on the fourth chromosome (Gusella et al.: *Nature* 306:234–238, 1983). I am really not sure how it was done. It has been explained three or possibly four times, and I am just beginning to see a glimmer. Of course understanding how linkage differs from association in our HLA ataxia work took me a while, and that is a much simpler situation.

The business of testing young people for an unwanted dominant disease is not altogether pleasant. Recently an 18-year-old man killed himself some six months after we had counseled him about his status regarding linkage for a hereditary disorder. He seemed to take it all right at the time, and his family denies that there was any relationship; it still causes us to reassess our position. One's logical belief in eugenics can be shaken even though it seems likely that with valid predictors many of the hereditary diseases could be nearly eliminated by selective childbearing choices on the part of those counseled.

Tyler and Harper, in an interesting study in Wales, reported that although "the majority of those at risk for Huntington's found genetic counseling helpful, they did not necessarily wish to alter their childbearing plans in consequence" (*J. Med. Genet.* 20:179–188, 1983). An attitude that I expect will change when the ability to predict more accurately improves. Roses et al., review recombinant DNA strategies in genetic neurologic diseases (*Muscle Nerve* 6:339–355, 1983). This is a look into the future. The next step of course, after finding and characterizing the gene, would be the identification of a method to alter its manifestation. At that time—and how long in the future will this be?—we can expect to prevent with appropriate therapy the manifestation of a genetic disease. Will it be as long as the gap between the discovery of bacilli and antibiotic therapy? That would not surprise me.

On the subject of genes, Haase et al., review the situation in the attempts to find intracellular viral products in neurologic diseases (*Ann. Neurol.* 13:119–121, 1983). This is an extremely pertinent area, since possibly more than one of our remaining puzzles—Parkinson's disease and amyotrophic lateral sclerosis to name the two most prominent—may be the results of a hidden viral change in cells. Waksman, one of the coauthors, then goes on to educate us on immunity and the nervous system (*Ann. Neurol.* 13:587–591, 1983).

The journal *Brain* is always good reading, and I particularly enjoyed the summary by Phillips et al. "Localization of Function in the Cerebral Cortex" (*Brain* 107:327–361, 1984). If you have an hour or two on an undisturbed evening and are interested in how the cerebral cortex might, after all, work, I recommend this. It is a superb summary, appearing three years later, of a meeting on the function of the cerebral cortex that was held in 1981 to commemorate the centennial of a similar meeting in London in 1881 during which the confrontation and argument on brain area specificity between David Ferrier and Friedrich L. Goltz took place. Our congratulations go to the guarantors and editors of *Brain* who both sponsored the meeting and published the summary.

Prusiner gives his speculations about prions, amyloid, and Alzheimer's disease in a recent note (*N. Engl. J. Med.* 310:661–663, 1984). Similarly, Toole and Toole, experts in another field, give us their feelings on federal funding for research in stroke and trauma, pointing out that the average expenditure in the United States for stroke and trauma research is less than the cost of one jet plane (*Stroke* 15:168–173, 1984). Ah yes, you say, but a jet plane is a monument of technical achievement and a very valuable thing to have. But subject to quick write-off. I recall a Canadian pilot (now a psychiatrist) telling me that he had accounted for two planes in his career: both of them Spitfires in Canada while he was attempting landings. Similarly in the early days of rocketry in this country, a peace-minded friend was fond of commenting every time the United States shot one in the air, "ah, there goes a university."

Speaking of experts, Gazzaniga summarized his knowledge of right hemisphere language following brain bisection (*Am. Psychol.* 38:525–527, 1983), and a summary review of the neuropathology of schizophrenia is given by Weinberger et al. (*Schizophr. Bull.* 9:193–211, 1983).

A word needs to be spoken on three who have died. Two or three years ago the American Academy of Neurology put on its first history section, and I was fortunate to have been one of the chairmen. During the session, both Morris Bender and Paul Yakovlev commented on papers presented. We had no recorder at the session, nor did we take down their pertinent, intelligent, and humorous comments. Both of those men were all of those things. Obituaries are in current journals (Cohen B.: "Obituary—Morris P. Bender, 1905–1983." *Ann. Neurol.* 14:208–209, 1983; Kemper T.: "Paul Ivan Yakovlev, 1894–1983." *Arch. Neurol.* 41:536–540, 1984). Douglas Buchanan is gone. He was *the* trainer of pediatric neurologists in America for many years. The way to become a child neurologist in the United States 30 or 40 years ago was to do pediatrics, then do neurology, and then wait your turn to become one of Buchanan's men for a year. Manuel Gomez comments about that lovely little Scot:

> Dr. Douglas Buchanan, Emeritus Professor of Neurology of the Pritzker School of Medicine of the University of Chicago, died in Chicago, May 11, 1983. He had been born in Glasgow on January 14, 1901, attended the University of Glasgow; Trinity College, Cambridge; La Sorbonne, Paris, and was a House Officer of the National Hospital for Neurological Diseases at Queen Square, London.
>
> Dr. Buchanan joined the University of Chicago in 1932 and was the Childrens Neurologist for almost 50 years. He was self-trained in a speciality that did not exist and he helped to create. Most important is that Dr. Buchanan became, to hundreds of medical students, residents and colleagues, the example of what a physician ought to be. He probably would have preferred to be remembered more as a good physician than a great neurologist.

Neurology will miss all three. And just now we read that James Purdon Martin has died (*Lancet* 1:1135–1136, 1984). One couldn't help liking that man. If he *said* something, it *was* true.

Finally, two supplements to the *Acta Neurologica Scandinavica* deserve a note because of their completeness. The first is Sillanpää's epidemiologic study on the social functioning and seizure status of young adults with childhood epilepsy (Suppl. 96, 1983), and the second is Iivanainen's comment on current therapy in epilepsy (Suppl. 97, 1983). For those with an interest in scanning, the *Annals of Neurology* carries an entire supplement (to volume 15, 1984) on research issues in positron emission tomography.

ROBERT D. CURRIER, M.D.

# 1 Diagnosis of Neurologic Disorders

**A Comparison of Digital Subtraction Angiography and Noninvasive Testing in Diagnosis of Cerebrovascular Disease**
Richard F. Kempczinski, Gary W. Wood, Yacov Berlatzky, and William H. Pearce (Univ. of Cincinnati)
Am. J. Surg. 146:203–207, August 1983                    1–1

Noninvasive cerebrovascular testing was performed on 477 patients, and digital subtraction angiograms were obtained on 1,892 patients during an 18-month period. Standard cerebral arteriography was subsequently performed in some cases: results of noninvasive cerebrovascular testing plus arteriography were available for 203 carotid arteries; noninvasive testing, digital subtraction, and arteriography could be compared in 65 carotid arteries (34 patients). Mean patient age was 61 years (range, 12–96 years); 48% of the patients were male. Noninvasive cerebrovascular testing included ocular pneumoplethysmography, periorbital Doppler survey or ophthalmosonometry, and carotid phonoangiography; final diagnosis was by ocular pneumoplethysmography. Intravenous digital subtraction angiography was performed using a Philips system in serial mode for carotid studies; five separate contrast injections were sometimes required for a single study. Standard cerebrovascular arteriography performed on all patients included both biplanar arch and selective carotid injections. A 50% or greater narrowing of the carotid artery, as seen on an arteriogram, was considered a positive test result.

The data were analyzed using noninvasive cerebrovascular testing alone, digital subtraction angiography alone, and both methods for comparison. In the subgroup of 203 carotid arteries for which both noninvasive tests and angiography were available, noninvasive cerebrovascular tests had a sensitivity of 85%, 96% specificity, 92% positive predictive value, 93% negative predictive value, and 93% overall accuracy. In 500 digital subtraction angiograms analyzed separately, stenosis of the internal carotid artery was determined with 93% sensitivity, 94% specificity, 88% positive predictive value, 97% negative predictive value, and overall accuracy of 94%. In the group of 65 carotid arteries (34 patients) for which noninvasive tests, digital subtraction angiography, and arteriography were all available, results of 4 (6%) of the arteries studied digitally were uninterpretable. When noninvasive tests and digital subtraction were compared in the same patients, the results were virtually identical (table). However, four significant lesions of the internal carotid siphon were not identified by digital subtraction but were detected by noninvasive tests and confirmed on ar-

23

---

RESULTS OF 65 NONINVASIVE CEREBROVASCULAR
TESTS VERSUS 61 DIGITAL SUBTRACTION
ANGIOGRAMS COMPARED WITH ARTERIOGRAPHY

|  | NCVT | DSA |
|---|---|---|
| Sensitivity | 81% | 84% |
| Specificity | 95% | 92% |
| Predictive Value |  |  |
| Positive | 92% | 88% |
| Negative | 88% | 89% |
| Overall Accuracy | 89% | 89% |
| Arteriographic findings |  |  |
| Stenosis >50% |  |  |
| Positive test result | 22 | 21 |
| Negative test result | 5 | 4 |
| Stenosis <50% |  |  |
| Positive test result | 2 | 3 |
| Negative test result | 36 | 33 |

(Courtesy of Kempczinski, R.F., et al.: Am. J. Surg. 146:203–207, August 1983.)

---

teriography (arguably reducing digital subtraction angiography to 72% sensitivity).

In patients with hemispheric cerebral ischemia, noninvasive tests were neither necessary nor cost-effective. Digital subtraction angiography often provided diagnostic information in such cases if the intracranial circulation was well-defined and the extracranial lesion matched the patients' symptoms. Noninvasive cerebrovascular testing was the safest and most cost-effective technique for screening patients who had asymptomatic bruits or atypical, nonhemispheric symptoms, or who had undergone carotid endarterectomy. If the noninvasive test result was positive or equivocal, digital subtraction angiography was performed to localize the lesion and exclude carotid occlusion.

▶ We do just about as the authors did, that is, use the noninvasive testing as a screening procedure and go to digital subtraction angiography if something shows up. In this series both the noninvasive tests and the subtraction angiogram had exactly the same overall accuracy: 89%. Yet clinicians would probably agree that the angiogram gives a better picture of what is going on.

The neurotoxicity of radiological contrast agents is reviewed by Junck and Marshall (*Ann. Neurol.* 13:469–484, 1983), who feel the toxicity of angiography represents a direct effect of the contrast agent on the brain or spinal cord, which may be partly due to opening of the blood-brain barrier by an osmotic effect.—R.D.C.

---

**Enhancing Mass on CT: Neoplasm or Recent Infarction?**
Joseph C. Masdeu (Loyola Univ., Maywood, Ill.)
Neurology (Cleve.) 33:836–840, July 1983                                    1–2

Neither mass effect nor contrast enhancement on computed tomography (CT) identifies a cerebral lesion as a neoplasm. The author examined the specificity of other findings in CT studies of 100 patients who had histologically confirmed supratentorial infarcts or tumors. Thirty-five patients had recent infarcts larger than 2 cm in their longest diameter, and 65 had gliomas or metastatic tumors. Seventeen patients with infarcts were examined within five days of the stroke. The CT appearance of white matter edema is shown in Figure 1–1.

The presence of white matter edema favored a tumor by 5 to 1. In all five infarcts with white matter edema, the outline of the cortical ribbon was enhanced. Enhancement restricted to the cortex was uncommon in

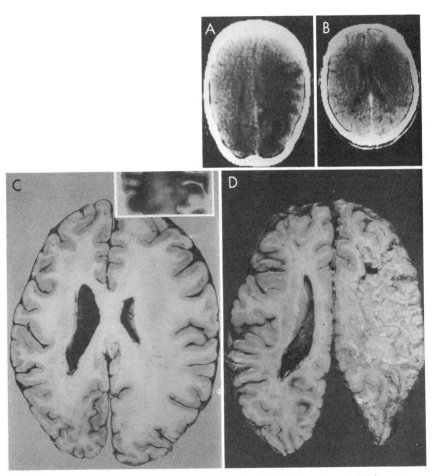

**Fig 1–1.**—Comparison of tumor edema (white matter edema) with infarct edema. **A,** CT shows tumor edema sparing the cortical ribbon. **B,** in recent infarct, CT shows edema involving the cortical ribbon, reaching the inner table. **C,** pathologic specimen with white matter edema staining pale with Luxol fast blue *(insert)*. The cortex was spared. **D,** infarction involving the cortex and white matter. (Courtesy of Masdeu, J.C.: Neurology (Cleve.) 33:836–840, July 1983.)

tumor patients. Histologic studies showed vasogenic edema sparing the cortex and subcortical arcuate fibers when tumor was present. In infarcts, areas of decreased attenuation represented necrosis of the cortex and underlying white matter. The finding of cortical ribbon enhancement made infarction 6 times more likely than glioma and 11 times more likely than metastasis. Only the cortical ribbon had a marked hemorrhagic component on histologic study. Follow-up CT in surviving patients showed an area of lucency where the cortex had previously been enhanced. A pattern of thalamic sparing was evident in 11 of 29 infarcts in the distribution of the middle cerebral artery.

When CT is done within five days after a stroke, a low-density area involving the cortex as well as the white matter suggests the ischemic nature of the lesion. In large ischemic lesions, however, the thalamus is spared. Later, the cortical ribbon usually enhances, contrasting with the nodular or ringlike enhancement associated with tumors. When cortical ribbon enhancement subsides, a mass effect is no longer present, making the diagnosis of tumor unlikely. More refined CT methods or nuclear magnetic resonance imaging may make it still easier to distinguish recent infarcts from tumors.

▶ On computed tomography neither the presence of a mass effect nor enhancement by the use of contrast material differentiates between the presence of a tumor or a recent infarct. These authors, however, note the specificity of three helpful signs in making such a differential diagnosis: white matter edema outlining the uninvolved cortex is less frequent in infarcts; enhancement of the cortical ribbon is more frequent in infarcts; selective sparing of the thalamus occurs more frequently in infarcts.—R.N.D.J.

---

**The Relation of Cerebral Vasospasm to the Extent and Location of Subarachnoid Blood Visualized by CT Scan: A Prospective Study**
J. P. Kistler, R. M. Crowell, K. R. Davis, R. Heros, R. G. Ojemann, T. Zervas, and C. M. Fisher (Harvard Med. School)
Neurology (Cleve.) 33:424–436, April 1983                                    1–3

---

Cerebral vasospasm after subarachnoid bleeding remains the single chief cause of delayed morbidity in patients with a ruptured saccular aneurysm, although only about a third of these patients are affected. A close correlation was noted between severe vasospasm and the presence of subarachnoid clots at certain sites. The authors undertook a prospective study of 41 patients seen within a week of subarachnoid hemorrhage from a ruptured saccular aneurysm in an attempt to predict the occurrence of delayed symptomatic cerebral vasospasm. The CT studies were interpreted before angiograms were obtained. Sequential scanning of slices with a thickness of 8 mm permitted measurement of the horizontal thickness and length of the vertical layers of blood.

Twenty-two patients had subarachnoid clots larger than 3 × 5 mm or layers of blood more than 1 mm thick. Severe vasospasm was correctly predicted and localized in 20 of these patients. The absence of severe vasospasm was correctly predicted in 14 of 19 patients who had no blood, diffuse blood, or blood outside the subarachnoid space. All of the false-positive and false-negative results could be attributed to inadequacies of CT technique.

The extent and location of blood in the subarachnoid space influence the severity and location of cerebral vasospasm in patients having subarachnoid bleeding from rupture of a saccular aneurysm. The use of CT allows identification of most patients at risk of developing symptomatic cerebral vasospasm and allows more accurate assessment of preventive measures. Removal of blood in the first 48 hours may be effective in preventing vasospasm in some cases, but frequently there is clotted blood in the cisterns on both sides of the brain, and aneurysmal clipping with washout of blood at the surgical site would not be expected to prevent vasospasm at a remote site.

▶ These data indicate that the extent and location of blood in the subarachnoid space following aneurysmal rupture determines the severity and location of cerebral vasospasm and that patients in jeopardy of developing symptomatic vasospasm can now be identified. Early preventive measures may now be assessed more accurately.—R.N.D.J.

---

**The Ventricular System in Chronic Schizophrenic Patients: Controlled Computed Tomography Study**
Anand K. Pandurangi, Mantosh J. Dewan, Seungho Howard Lee, Tarakad Ramachandran, Benjamin F. Levy, Michael Boucher, Allan Yozawitz, and Leslie Major (SUNY, Upstate Med. Center, Syracuse)
Br. J. Psychiatry 144:172–176, February 1983                    1–4

---

There is considerable evidence from computed tomography (CT) of ventricular enlargement in patients with chronic schizophrenia, but most studies have focused on a single ventricle. The authors assessed the entire ventricular system in 23 men with chronic schizophrenia, aged 20–40 years, and in 23 control subjects of similar age. The schizophrenics had not been institutionalized for long periods and had not received electroconvulsive therapy, but all had received neuroleptics. None had a history of alcoholism or drug abuse. All the controls had normal CT findings.

The schizophrenics had significantly larger third and fourth ventricles than the controls, and they also had bilateral widening of the sylvian fissures. The ventricle-brain ratio was insignificantly greater in the schizophrenic group; only three patients had a ratio more than 2 SD above the control mean. Five patients had findings of cortical atrophy, but mean sulcal measures did not differ significantly in the two groups. None of the findings correlated significantly with age or duration of illness. Measures of the third, fourth, and lateral ventricles did not correlate significantly with one another.

These findings could support the view of a disturbance of cerebrospinal fluid flow akin to normal-pressure hydrocephalus in schizophrenics, but many factors argue against such a disorder. Atrophy is also an unlikely explanation for the ventriculomegaly observed in schizophrenics. The identification of homogeneous subgroups of patients from analysis of the CT findings should be helpful.

▶ The authors have added their findings to the increasing argument in this area. They find the deeper ventricles are enlarged significantly in schizophrenia and wonder about a spinal fluid flow problem, which seems unlikely but possible.—R.D.C.

---

**A Reconsideration of the Relation of Ventricular Enlargement to Duration of Illness in Schizophrenia**
Bryan T. Woods and Jane Wolf
Am. J. Psychiatry 140:1564–1570, December 1983                                       1–5

Studies on ventricular size in schizophrenics have given conflicting results. Younger patients with chronic schizophrenia were found to have a

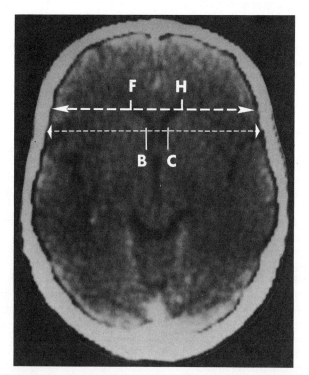

Fig 1–2.—Frontal horn and bicaudate indices determined by (1) dividing width of frontal horn span *(FH)* by width of hemispheres at same level and (2) dividing ventricular widths between caudate nuclei *(BC)* by widths of hemispheres at same level. (Courtesy of Woods, B.T., and Wolf, J.: Am. J. Psychiatry 140:1564–1570, December 1983.)

slight but significant enlargement of the cerebral ventricles. Information was reviewed on 19 young, hospitalized patients who received the diagnosis of schizophrenia between 1976 and 1979, and 29 nonpsychiatrically ill controls of the same mean age (23.5 years). Ventricular size was determined by using the bicaudate index and the frontal horn index (Fig 1–2). Most of the schizophrenics were males, but sex did not influence the computed tomographic findings.

The mean bicaudate ratio of schizophrenics was significantly greater than that of controls. The frontal horn ratio was also greater in the schizophrenic group, but not significantly so. All the patients had received neuroleptics, and three had had electroconvulsive therapy. All had essentially normal neurologic findings. None of the patients showed reversal of cerebral asymmetry. Three patients had a history of substantial brain injury, but the findings were unchanged when these patients were excluded.

There appears to be a direct relation between size of the cerebral ventricles and duration of schizophrenic illness. Conflicting results of different studies can be reconciled by postulating that both clinical schizophrenia and ventricular enlargement are overt signs of an underlying neuronal degeneration that is hereditary and progressive. The genetic component may be a progressive neuronal degenerative process that predisposes to schizophrenia by involving certain critical neural structures and incidentally results in progressive ventricular enlargement from tissue loss. The threshold for the development of clinical schizophrenia might be reached before ventricular enlargement is detectable, so that enlargement is not necessarily apparent in young patients with a short duration of illness.

▶ The duration of the schizophrenia is directly related to the amount of atrophy shown by computed tomographic scan.—R.D.C.

---

**Serial Nuclear Magnetic Resonance (NMR) Imaging in Patients With Cerebral Infarction**

Jorma T. Sipponen, Markku Kaste, Leena Ketonen, Raimo E. Sepponen, Kalevi Katevuo, and Arto Sivula (Univ. of Helsinki)
J. Comput. Assist. Tomogr. 7:585–589, August 1983                    1–6

---

The pathogenesis of ischemic brain infarction is incompletely understood. Findings on serial NMR imaging were compared with those of computed tomography (CT) in seven patients with supratentorial cerebral infarction, followed for as long as two months after the acute onset of stroke. The five men and two women were aged 37–56 years. All had major neurologic deficits due to ischemic infarction. The clinical diagnosis was confirmed by CT in all cases. Both saturation-recovery (SR) and proton density (PD) imaging sequences were used. Six patients had successive NMR studies. Four patients were initially evaluated within 24 hours of the onset of symptoms. A total of 19 NMR imaging studies were carried out.

The infarcted area was clearly demonstrated in early NMR images in

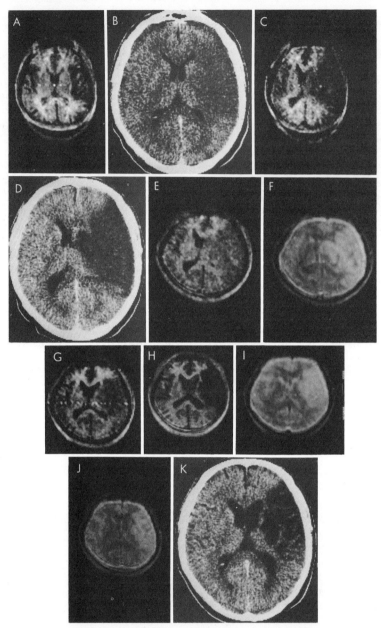

**Fig 1–3.**—Serial NMR and CT studies of man, 43, with infarction in territory of left middle cerebral artery. Saturation-recovery (**A**) and noncontrast CT (**B**) images 12 hours after onset of symptoms; in NMR image, infarcted area is already clearly outlined. Progression of lesion is documented in SR (**C**) and noncontrast CT (**D**) images at three days. Mass effect with midline shift is still evident in SR (**E**) and PD (**F**) NMR images at seven days; SR (**G**) and PD (**H**) images at 14 days; and SR (**I**), PD (**J**), and noncontrast CT (**K**) images at six weeks: infarcted area is more restricted and mass effect is diminished at two weeks, whereas at six weeks, lesion is even more demarcated. In images I and J, 16-level gray scale and, in other images, 256-level gray scale was used. This case offers sequential follow-up assessment of ischemic stroke, from its initial phase to its completion. (Courtesy of Sipponen, J.T., et al.: J. Comput. Assist. Tomogr. 7:585–589, August 1983.)

all four patients studied within 24 hours of the onset. A triangular or square region with decreased signal intensity in SR images was observed. In most cases the infarcted area appeared bright in PD images. Findings were similar at later stages. The NMR and CT findings in one patient are contrasted in Figure 1–3. The involved region became larger over the first week, whereas after two weeks the area of damage was more restricted in both the NMR and the CT images, and the mass effect was less evident. On follow-up of three patients for as long as two months after stroke, both NMR imaging sequences demonstrated sharp margins without mass effect.

Nuclear magnetic resonance imaging provides a new approach to the early diagnosis of ischemic brain infarction. No ionizing radiation is delivered, but the data acquisition time at present is fairly long, and motion artifacts may be a problem with critically ill and uncooperative patients. The technique may also be of value in elucidating the pathophysiology of early cerebral ischemia.

▶ Nuclear magnetic resonance imaging provides a new approach to the early diagnosis of ischemic brain infarction. Also, it aids in elucidating some aspects of the pathophysiology of ischemic stroke in man.—R.N.D.J.

---

**Nuclear Magnetic Resonance Evaluation of Stroke: A Preliminary Report**
R. Nick Bryan, M. Robert Willcott, Nicholas J. Schneiders, Joseph J. Ford, and Howard S. Derman (Baylor College of Medicine)
Radiology 149:189–192, October 1983                                   1–7

---

The authors report the results of nuclear magnetic resonance (NMR) pulse sequence evaluation in nine patients with acute and subacute stroke. Scanning was performed with a Bruker Instruments 6-MHz proton scanner with 7-mm section thickness using a selective excitation technique for section selection and a modified Carr-Purcell-Meiboom-Gill (CPMG) spin-echo pulse sequence for signal detection.

Scanning with NMR demonstrated all nine strokes, eight of which were also seen by computed tomography (CT) (Fig 1–4). In no case were the lesions better demonstrated by CT than by NMR. All of the strokes demonstrated by NMR had a common appearance, suggesting similar changes in spin density (SD) and transverse relaxation time $(T_2)$. The early spin-echo images of the ischemic area had a diminished signal intensity, most likely suggesting a prolonged longitudinal relaxation time $(T_1)$. The calculated SD also showed diminished signal intensity compared with that in normal brain tissue; this was probably related to the timing of the original 90-degree pulse and interprojection period, rather than to an actual decrease in hydrogen concentration. The decreased signal intensity indicated a residual $T_1$ component in the SD images, rather than a diminution in SD from a lower proton concentration. On the later spin-echo images, the signal intensity from ischemic regions was increased compared with that in normal brain tissue. This was reflected in prolonged $T_2$ values in the

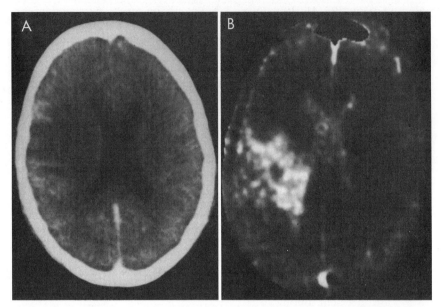

**Fig 1–4.—A**, after administration of contrast fluid, computed tomographic scan angled 20 degrees to the orbitomeatal line shows lucent lesion in patient with right middle cerebral artery stroke four days after onset. **B**, in same patient, calculated $T_2$ image reveals markedly prolonged $T_2$ in the ischemic region. (Courtesy of Bryan, R.N., et al.: Radiology 149:189–192, October 1983.)

calculated $T_2$ images; $T_2$ increased from an average of 48 ± 7 msec to 126 ± 17 msec. In addition to these changes, NMR scanning also demonstrated the associated gross mass effects of stroke, with compression of the adjacent sulci and ventricles. These preliminary findings suggest that NMR scanning in patients with acute stroke may be of clinical value and that the $T_2$ component of the NMR signal is most important.

▶ It appears that NMR scanning is slightly more sensitive than CT scanning for strokes, which is welcome news but hardly enough to convince the local legislature of the need for funding of an NMR scanner this year. Brant-Zawadzki et al. (AJR 140:847–854, 1983) compared CT and NMR in several diseases, including stroke, and came to about the same conclusion: NMR was equal to or slightly more sensitive than CT. A nice review on "the advance of NMR" recently appeared in The Lancet (1:21–23, 1984) with a look into the future of the technique. There is also available a recent comparison of CT and positron emission tomographic scanning of strokes (Baron et al.: AJNR 4:536–540, 1983).—R.D.C.

---

**Patchy, Periventricular White Matter Lesions in the Elderly: A Common Observation During NMR Imaging**
William G. Bradley, Jr., Victor Waluch, Michael Brant-Zawadzki, Richard A. Yadley, and R. Robert Wycoff (Pasadena, Calif.)

Med. Imaging 1:35–41, January 1984                                    1–8

Spin echo nuclear magnetic resonance (NMR) imaging is a sensitive means of detecting demyelinated lesions. The authors frequently observed patchy, periventricular, long-$T_2$ lesions in elderly persons, resembling the lesions of multiple sclerosis seen in younger patients. Nuclear magnetic resonance images of the brain were obtained from 20 consecutive patients older than 60 years of age with no evidence of brain tumor. Multiple-slice spin-echo acquisition, using a two-dimensional Fourier transform technique, provided 20 parallel slices through the brain at 1-cm intervals. Two images were generated for each slice with echo delay times (TE) of 28 and 56 msec.

Six patients (30%) had evidence of periventricular abnormality. Lacunar infarction and ventricular dilatation due to atrophy were also seen. Four of the six patients with NMR evidence of periventricular white matter disease also had computed tomographic (CT) abnormalities, but these were much less obvious. The average age of these patients was 82 years, compared with 68 for those without periventricular abnormality. Significantly more of the former had a history of mild hypertension and transient ischemia or stroke. Cardiac disease and emotional lability or dementia were also more frequent among the patients with periventricular abnormality. Lacunar infarcts were more frequent in these patients, but no significant difference in the incidence of ventricular dilatation was found between the two groups.

The histories and NMR appearances suggest that the patchy, periventricular lesions seen in elderly patients represent subcortical arteriosclerotic encephalopathy. It may be a mild form of Binswanger's disease, previously considered to be a rare cause of dementia. Nuclear magnetic resonance imaging is more sensitive than CT in detecting this entity. Early diagnosis may provide a greater incentive to control hypertension as a treatable cause of dementia.

▶ Well, I guess I will finally have to believe in Binswanger's disease although the relation of this disorder to his original description is remote. Nevertheless it does seem a real entity occasionally seen on CT scan, and we will probably get more reports of its clinical characteristics. It may then be classified as one of the discoverable causes of dementia. Why hasn't this disorder been outlined by our neuropathologic confreres? I stand ready to be battered by responses.—R.D.C.

---

**The Seriously Uninjured Hand: Weakness of Grip**
Harold M. Stokes
J. Occup. Med. 25:683–684, September 1983                            1–9

---

Loss of grip force is a rateable factor in determining permanent disability by compensation boards in some states, but malingerers or patients with psychological disability can voluntarily record lower grip measurements in a presumably injured hand. A sealed hydraulic dynamometer was used for objective documentation of voluntarily reduced grip strength. The patient is unable to observe the distance that he moves the handle he grasps. Grip force is measured at each of five handle positions, first in the normal hand and then in the presumably abnormal one. The patient who is trying to show a weak grip will apply the same minimal pressure at each position, resulting in a straight-line graph. A slightly skewed bell curve is observed when true weakness of grip is present.

The curve produced by this method constitutes objective evidence that the patient did or did not cooperate with the test by applying maximal pressure at each position as instructed. Real loss of grip can be established in this way, and subjective or argumentative statements relating to the patient's cooperativeness are avoided.

▶ This looks like a good way to confirm feigned grip weakness. It can be done with the usual dynamometer. The author also points out that the graph method of displaying the results with a flat line indicating the same grip strength for different handle positions is important in convincing others. The dial should not be visible to the patient.—R.D.C.

---

### Overuse of Evoked Potentials: Caution

Andrew Eisen (Univ. of British Columbia) and Roger Q. Cracco (SUNY, Downstate Med. Center, Brooklyn, N.Y.)
Neurology (Cleve.) 33:618–620, May 1983                                         1–10

The authors discuss the possibility of overusing the various evoked potential (EP) methods that are applied increasingly. Visual EPs can reveal subtle or subclinical pathologic involvement of the optic nerve and chiasm. Brain stem auditory EPs aid in localizing posterior lesions in a region that is resolved with difficulty by computed tomography (CT); these studies are particularly helpful in evaluating patients with acoustic neuromas and brain stem gliomas. Somatosensory EPs are used to screen the central sensory paths and evaluate proximal parts of the peripheral sensory nervous system. The various EP studies are used most widely to evaluate possible multiple sclerosis. They also are helpful in making a prognosis for comatose patients and in distinguishing toxic or metabolic causes of coma from irreversible structural causes. The tests are used to monitor surgical patients for neuronal dysfunction, although what constitutes significant abnormality remains to be precisely defined.

It is probably an oversimplification to ascribe a given EP component to a specific neural source. False results in EP tests may arise from the examiner's lack of experience in recording and interpretation. The tests probably are being overused in many clinical laboratories. Indications have not been clearly defined, and there is a general increase in reliance on laboratory procedures and a reduced emphasis on clinical evaluation. Less comprehensive testing than what is often done may suffice to identify clinically occult lesions in patients with multiple sclerosis. There is relatively little need for EP testing when a given sensory system is clinically involved or when clinically definite multiple sclerosis is present. Evoked potentials should be recorded only if there is a reasonable possibility that new and relevant information will be obtained that can influence patient management.

▶ Evoked potentials are often of great help in both research and differential diagnosis, but they are expensive and time consuming. These investigators express the belief that they should be obtained only when there is a reasonable possibility that information relevant to the management of the patient will be obtained.—R.N.D.J.

# 2 Behavioral Neurology and Cortical Function

**Developmental Learning Disabilities of the Right Hemisphere: Emotional, Interpersonal, and Cognitive Components**
Sandra Weintraub and M.-Marsel Mesulam (Harvard Med. School)
Arch. Neurol. 40:463–468, August 1983                                    2–1

Damage to the right side of the brain in adulthood produces profound changes in functions dependent on visuospatial skills, directed attention, modulation of affect, and paralinguistic aspects of communication. Difficulty in acquiring these functions may reflect underlying early injury. The authors encountered 14 patients who had a behavioral syndrome starting in early life and who were characterized by emotional and interpersonal difficulties, shyness, visuospatial disturbances, and inadequate paralinguistic communicative abilities.

Two patients were born with left-sided infantile hemiplegia. Three had a history of perinatal stress, and five had early onset of a seizure disorder. Two patients had a family history of seizures. All the patients had at least average intellectual capacity, but all had had academic failures, especially in arithmetic. The neurologic and neuropsychological findings were consistent with right hemispheric dysfunction. "Soft" neurologic signs were fairly frequent. The patients did poorly on memory tasks requiring the processing, storage, and retrieval of visual, nonverbal information. Most of the patients avoided eye contact and lacked the gestures that normally accompany speech. Many could not convey their feelings, but there was no indication of lack of affect. Eight patients reported chronic depression. All patients but one described themselves as "loners." All but two had been unable to make lasting peer relations, and they acknowledged considerable discomfort in one-to-one interactions.

Right hemispheric damage that is inherited or acquired in early life apparently can produce chronic emotional difficulties, disordered interpersonal skills, and poor visuospatial abilities. Traditional treatments may be ineffective. An approach similar to that used in treating persons with dyslexia may be more helpful.

▶ It has long been known that the right cerebral hemisphere is important in visuospatial relationships, but its functions in emotional and interpersonal relationships has not been recognized. Patients with disease causing disabilities in these latter spheres need more than guidance for therapy, and they often require specific remedial strategies. As Martha Denckla says, "There is need for more work on the neurologic basis of social competence" (*Arch. Neurol.* 40:461–462, 1983).—R.N.D.J.

### Prognosis for Improved Verbal Communication in Aphasic Stroke Patients
Robert C. Marshall and David S. Phillips (Oregon Health Sciences Univ.)
Arch. Phys. Med. Rehabil. 64:597–600, December 1983          2–2

The many factors that help determine recovery from aphasia make it difficult to formulate a prognosis in individual patients. The role of 10 selected prognostic variables was examined in relation to recovery of verbal communication in a series of 80 aphasic men with a single left hemispheric stroke of thrombotic or embolic origin. Their mean age was 56.5 years. All were right-handed and had at least an eighth-grade education. The Porch Index of Communication Ability was administered one to six months after the stroke and before a program of speech and language therapy was begun. Individual treatment was given for at least two months, usually two to five times per week, with the goal of ameliorating specific deficits.

Thirty-four men frequently used meaningful sentences of five or more words and produced many multiple-sentence comments with no more than minor hesitancies or misarticulations after treatment. The other 46 were considered to have poor terminal speech performance (TSP). Comparable numbers of patients in the two groups were fluent aphasics and were working at the time of stroke. More than 40% of both groups were in good general health. Terminal speech performance could be discriminated 86% of the time using the variables of initial severity of aphasia, time after stroke, auditory comprehension ability, age, speech fluency, and general health. The predictive value of these factors was 91% in the patients with good TSP and 83% in those with poor TSP.

Younger patients with a first thromboembolic stroke who are in better general health are more likely to regain verbal communication. They also are likely to have less severe aphasia, to have good auditory comprehension, and to be fluent speakers. The significant predictive factors can be assessed reliably a month after stroke. Treatment intensity may prove to be a prognostic factor if a more inclusive or functionally based measure of communicative skill were used as the dependent variable.

▶ These are all sensible predictors of recovery from aphasia. And as we go to press comes the news in *The Lancet* of a randomized controlled trial of speech therapy for aphasia—there was no apparent difference in the outcome for the treated and untreated groups (Lincoln et al.: *Lancet* 1:1197–1200, 1984). The speech therapy was two one-hour sessions per week.—R.D.C.

---

### The Characterization of an Amnesic Syndrome Following Hypoxic Ischemic Injury
Bruce T. Volpe (Cornell Univ.) and William Hirst (Princeton Univ.)
Arch. Neurol. 40:436–440, July 1983          2–3

A wide range of focal and diffuse injuries can cause amnesic syndromes. Memory deficits were studied in a patient with hypoxic ischemic injury and coma after cardiac arrest. Criteria were derived from experimental studies of classic amnesic syndromes. Data on two patients with amnesia that followed hypoxic ischemic injury whose initial courses were complicated by focal brain injury were also analyzed. The amnesias associated with alcoholic Korsakoff syndrome, herpes encephalitis, and temporal lobe resection are characterized by intact short-term memory, poor free recall, less depressed recognition ability, some responsiveness to retrieval cues, and increased susceptibility to interference. The first patient had deficits in acquiring and retaining new information despite a normal sensorium and adequate intellectual function. He was frustrated by his limited mnemonic capabilities, but relatives reported the return of some aspects of his previous personality. In the patients with focal brain damage, it is unlikely that this injury caused the amnesia.

Studies of hypoxic ischemic injury after sudden cardiac or respiratory arrest have shown severe neuronal destruction in the hippocampus and anterior thalamus and diffuse cortical damage. An alternative pathophysiologic scheme is based on specific biochemical abnormalities associated with behavioral deficits. The cholinergic system appears to be particularly vulnerable to hypoxia. The metabolism of several neurotransmitter systems is oxygen dependent, and acetylcholine synthesis may be impaired even under relatively mild hypoxic conditions. Cholinergic impairment has been related to decreases in memory performance in human subjects, and the amnesia associated with hypoxic ischemic injury may be related to a cholinergic deficit.

▶ The amnesic syndrome following hypoxic ischemic brain injury is a common hospital occurrence and often develops after cardiac or respiratory arrest. It has neuropsychological characteristic features, which differ from those of Korsakoff's syndrome in that there is no disorientation and no confabulation.— R.N.D.J.

---

**The Function of Dream Sleep**
Francis Crick and Graeme Mitchison (The Salk Inst., La Jolla, Calif.)
Nature 304:111–114, July 1983                                          2–4

---

The authors discuss the cerebral cortex and associated neuronal networks and the differences between rapid eye movement (REM) and non-REM sleep, and they propose a new explanation for the function of REM sleep. The theory is based on the assumption that the cerebral cortex and certain associated subcortical structures in viviparous mammals can be regarded as a network of interconnected cells that can support a considerable variety of modes of mutual excitation. This system is likely to be subject to unwanted or "parasitic" modes of behavior that arise as the system is disturbed by growth of the brain or by modifications produced by experience. Theoretically, these modes are detected and suppressed by a special mechanism that operates during REM sleep and that, in effect, is a reverse learning mechanism, which is not the same as normal forgetting.

Evidence suggests that in REM sleep the brain is isolated from normal input and output channels and that it is very active, responding to rather nonspecific signals from the brain stem that are reflected in the unconscious equivalent of dreaming, which only reaches normal consciousness if the sleeper awakens. The proposed mechanism is based on the more or less random stimulation of the forebrain by the brain stem, which tends to excite the "parasitic" modes of brain activity, especially those that are likely to be set off by random noise rather than by highly structured specific signals. Thus, the reverse learning mechanism modifies the cortex so that the particular activity is less likely in the future. In short, humans unlearn their unconscious dreams in REM sleep.

If correct, the proposed mechanism could help in understanding the evolution of the neocortex in mammals. It is postulated that without REM dreams, evolution could not have produced the highly refined human neocortex. The possibility that some forms of schizophrenia may be caused by a defect in the reverse learning process should not be disregarded.

▶ Crick and Mitchison's idea about the function of dream sleep is truly delightful, and I propose to believe in it. However, Shakespeare beat them to it by four centuries: " 'Sleep no more! Macbeth does murder sleep!' the innocent sleep, sleep that knits up the ravel'd sleave of care."—R.D.C.

---

**A Case of Being Scared to Death**
Paul L. Schraeder, Raymond Pontzer, and Toby R. Engel (Med. College of Pennsylvania)
Arch. Intern. Med. 143:1793–1794, September 1983                    2–5

---

Vasovagal syncope is common in young persons, but concomitant generalized seizures are unusual. The authors describe a healthy young adult whose seizures resulted from asystole induced by the mental imaging of human pain.

Man, 21, experienced a generalized tonic-clonic seizure after rhythmic contractions of the right arm developed just after he heard graphic descriptions of torture. Several previous episodes of loss of consciousness were reported, including some associated with bleeding from a cut and with hearing descriptions of unpleasant experiences. Lightheadedness was reported as the blood pressure was being recorded. During EEG recording while the same seizure-provoking text was read to the patient, bradycardia and then asystole developed, followed by electrocerebral silence (Fig 2–1). A tonic seizure that began without focal onset was followed by generalized tonic-clonic seizure activity. The patient was momentarily confused after regaining consciousness and felt fatigued for 30 minutes. Findings on subsequent ECG were normal, but ECG monitoring showed episodes of progressive sinus bradycardia and PR prolongation with Mobitz I second-degree atrioventricular block. Atrial extrastimulation and atrial overdrive pacing produced normal findings even during carotid sinus massage and unsuccessful attempts to frighten the patient with blood. A permanent ventricular pacemaker was implanted. The patient was asymptomatic during one year of follow-up. Monitoring the patient's sister and father showed only unifocal premature ventricular contractions.

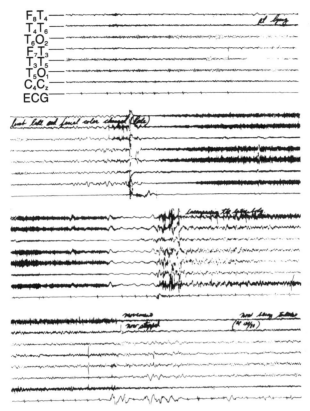

Fig 2–1.—Four panels of electroencephalography (EEG) represent 75 seconds of continuous recording. Top three channels represent recordings from the right temporal region. The fourth, fifth, and sixth channels represent direct recordings from the left temporal region. The seventh channel records the right central region, and the eighth channel is lead II ECG. Bradycardia developed, progressing to asystole as patient listened to descriptions of torture. After 13 seconds of asystole (**center top**), the EEG signal slows and becomes silent; at 15 seconds of asystole, a muscle artifact associated with seizure is seen, lasting for 30 seconds (**center bottom**). After 25 seconds of asystole, cardiac activity returns, with 35 more seconds required before alpha rhythm is reestablished (**bottom**). (Courtesy of Schraeder, P.L., et al.: Arch. Intern. Med. 143:1793–1794, September 1983; copyright 1983, American Medical Association.)

A connection between emotion and sudden death has long been recognized, and abnormal cardiac sympathetic responses appear to be an important factor. Vagally induced cessation of cardiac action can precipitate sudden death in man. Marked asystole and electrocerebral silence can be induced voluntarily. A detailed history of the events associated with apparently typical seizures is important.

▶ The observations in this interesting case report give further support to the concept that mentally mediated vagotonic mechanisms may result in cardiac arrest. This case also demonstrates the advantages of reproducing the circumstances associated with an unexplained loss of consciousness while monitoring both the electroencephalogram and the electrocardiogram.—R.N.D.J.

### Alexia Without Agraphia in a Composer

Tedd Judd, Howard Gardner, and Norman Geschwind
Brain 106:435–457, June 1983

2–6

Man, 77, a right-handed composer-conductor in previously excellent health, was conducting an orchestra when he felt as if he had been "hit in the head." The next day he was admitted to Massachusetts General Hospital with unintelligible speech and faltering gait. The patient had right homonymous hemianopia; corrected visual acuity was ⅕ normal at 2 ft; range of eye movements was full, but optokinetic nystagmus was markedly diminished with targets moving to the patient's left. Lumbar puncture revealed yellow-pink cerebrospinal fluid. Skull x-ray films were normal, but a computed tomography scan four days after admission showed an area of increased density consistent with a left occipitotemporal hematoma (Fig 2–2). The hemorrhagic infarction produced aphasia characterized by a mild degree of fluently abnormal speech with mild to moderate disturbances in comprehension and repetition, total inability to identify letters and words, and dense right hemianopia. Aphasia and agraphia cleared rapidly except for mild residual anomia and occasional paraphasias so that the patient was left with hemianopia and other features of the syndrome of alexia without agraphia. The patient was examined one year after the stroke and at 18, 24, and 30 months.

The patient was severely impaired at all levels of reading. On the Boston Diagnostic Aphasia Examination he was unable to match short words and letters to their equivalents in upper case, lower case, or cursive. The errors suggested visual confusions, such as "B" and "d," "dog" and "boy." Number reading was worse than letter reading. Handwriting was legible, but slow, with occasional distortions. No particular musical aspect of reading or playing caused difficulties, but the complexity of the task slowed the patient and so the rhythm suffered. At 20 months after the stroke, the patient wrote a seven-minute piece for chorus and orchestra in five weeks with no assistance; however, performance on musical dictation was less proficient.

This patient was similarly impaired at naming symbols in music and

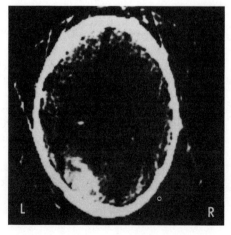

**Fig 2–2.**—Unenhanced cranial computed tomographic scan showing left occipital hematoma. (Courtesy of Judd, T., et al.: Brain 106:435–457, June 1983.)

language, made reading errors in short phrases of unfamiliar material in each system and performed at the elementary school level in both. Music symbols were more accurately identified than text and more rapidly played in their appropriate context than in isolation on a page. The differences between these music and language reading impairments were assumed to reflect distinctions in brain organization or the nature of alexia. It is difficult to explain this patient's pattern of deficits, generally characterized as a visual-verbal disconnection. However, an alternative explanation is that mild impairments in visual perception and in naming are exaggerated when combined in the tasks of reading or naming things presented visually. Neither explanation accounts for the patient's failure to show any semantic substitutions in text reading as is seen in "phonemic dyslexics."

▶ The interesting thing about this patient was that he was able to write script and read music but had great difficulty reading print. The authors point out that music recognition may be more widely distributed in the brain than reading and thus may survive when the more focally placed printed word reading is lost, especially when the patient is a skilled composer of many years experience.— R.D.C.

---

**The Human Klüver-Bucy Syndrome**
Ralph Lilly, Jeffrey L. Cummings, D. Frank Benson, and Michael Frankel (Univ. of California, Los Angeles)
Neurology (Cleve.) 33:1141–1145, September 1983                    2–7

Klüver and Bucy, in 1939, described a behavioral syndrome that followed bilateral temporal lobectomy in rhesus monkeys, which was characterized by "psychic blindness," a tendency to examine all objects orally, an irresistible impulse to touch, loss of the normal anger and fear responses, and increased sexual activity. Human Klüver-Bucy syndrome (KBS) closely resembles the primate disorder, but a more complex behavioral syndrome is seen in human beings.

Findings were reviewed in 12 patients with KBS. Five patients had Pick's disease and one had Alzheimer's disease. Four cases were related to encephalitis and two to trauma. Most if not all the features of KBS seen in monkeys after bilateral anterior temporal lobectomy were seen in these patients. Blunted affect and apathy corresponded with the placidity and loss of fear and anger observed in monkeys. Psychic blindness or visual agnosia is most often evident as an inability to distinguish among friends, relatives, and strangers. Auditory agnosia has been found in some human cases. One of the patients in this study appeared to have a tactile agnosia. Hypermetamorphosis is manifested by consistent exploration of the environment, usually manually, and the placement of objects in the mouth. Sexual overtures and comments and attempted physical contact are observed more often than actual copulation or masturbation. Nearly all patients have both aphasia and amnesia. Dementia may occur with features of KBS.

Klüver-Bucy syndrome can occur in common clinical disorders and includes all features of the original syndrome seen in lobectomized monkeys. It is invariably associated with aphasia, amnesia, or dementia. The syndrome may resolve or persist. Its partial expression suggests the presence of bilateral lesions of the medial and anterior temporal regions, as does the complete syndrome. Human KBS has little etiologic specificity.

▶ Although the Klüver-Bucy syndrome when it occurs in humans resembles the syndrome in nonhuman primates, the evolutionary advances of the human brain result in a more complex behavioral syndrome after bilateral temporal lobe damage or removal. The human syndrome manifests all of the features of that in monkeys, but, in addition, there are amnesia, aphasia, and/or dementia. Partial expression of the syndrome apparently has the same localizing significance as the complete syndrome.—R.N.D.J.

---

### Musical Hallucinations Associated With Acquired Deafness

Thomas A. Hammeke, Michael P. McQuillen, and Bernard A. Cohen (Med. College of Wisconsin)
J. Neurol. Neurosurg. Psychiatry 46:570–572, June 1983          2–8

Two patients with auditory hallucinations beginning after a long history of bilateral hearing loss were studied. The hallucinations included both unformed (tinnitus and irregular sound of varying pitch and timbre) and formed (instrumental music, singing, and voices) components, and they were repetitive. The hallucinations were affected by ambient noise levels; their content and speed were influenced by attentional and intentional factors. There was no evidence of global dementia or of epileptogenic or psychiatric disturbance.

CASE 1.—Woman, 75, a right-handed retired teacher complained of annoying musical hallucinations. The first occurred four months earlier, shortly after she discontinued antibiotic medication for a sinus infection. Computed tomographic (CT) scan showed mild diffuse atrophy; EEG revealed mixed dysrhythmic complexes throughout central and posterior regions bilaterally; brain stem auditory evoked potential (BAEP) studies showed increased interpeak latencies; somatosensory evoked potentials (SEP) showed diminished amplitude over the left cerebrum.

CASE 2.—Woman, 80, a right-handed nun, reported a three-year history of auditory hallucinations. Right ear deafness had been present for 40 years following mastoidectomy. A CT scan showed mild cerebral atrophy; EEGs taken over several years showed sharp theta waves over bilateral temporal regions, although audiovisual monitoring with the EEG showed no correlation between these waves and reported hallucinations; BAEP results and SEP studies were normal.

The features of these patients are consistent with those of other reported cases. Some investigators maintain that neural or end organ disease alone is sufficient to produce musical hallucinations or similar phenomena, postulating sensory deprivation as the mechanism. Under conditions of reduced sensory input, perception-bearing circuits are disinhibited, and perceptual traces are released that yield a reexperience of perceptions. Other investigators argue that a combination of peripheral and central dysfunction is required. These theorists point out that such hallucinations occur most frequently in elderly patients, among whom the incidence of brain pathology is increased. The neuropsychological and evoked potential studies in the present cases were suggestive of mild localized cortical dysfunction, perhaps with mild generalized atrophy. Whether the central dysfunction implied by these findings is critical, contributory, or incidental to the phenomenon is unknown.

▶ Are these musical hallucinations only one step removed from the event that probably all of us have experienced when busy of having a tune "go through our head" repetitively and irritatingly? Or are they very different? The suddenness of onset sounds like stroke superimposed on prior progressive deafness. Evidently no pathologic examination is available. Some of these hallucinations are, one presumes, actual memories of previously heard music, but the fact that their speed or content can be altered by the patient by subvocalization makes them more than memory. They were not just vocal—some were instrumental—and they were not all familiar tunes. Both patients were retired school teachers. Is this inward composition? Do you suppose Beethoven experienced this?—R.D.C.

# 3 Cerebrovascular Disease

**The Decline of Stroke**
Jack P. Whisnant (Mayo Clinic and Found.)
Stroke 15:160–168, January–February 1984                    3–1

Mortality from stroke has declined over several decades. A steady decrease since 1900 is evident in the United States (Fig 3–1). Stroke mortality in Rochester, Minn., has been consistently lower than that in the U.S. white population, particularly for the oldest persons. The average annual incidence of new cases of stroke has declined in Rochester in every five-year period since 1950. Women have shown a fairly gradual decline since 1955, whereas men have shown a sharp decline in annual incidence since 1969. The decline in men has amounted to 44% in the last 10 years of observation. A change in coding "cerebrovascular accident" as cerebral hemorrhage in 1950–1968 and as ill-defined stroke thereafter led to a considerable distortion in the mortality trend for cerebral hemorrhage (Fig 3–2). Data from Rochester show a considerable decrease in mortality from cerebral hemorrhage from 1950–1954 to 1970–1974. Mortality associated with subarachnoid hemorrhage increased in the United States from 1950 to 1970 and has declined slightly since then. These trends were not evident in the Rochester population.

The prevalence of transient ischemic attacks in the Rochester population

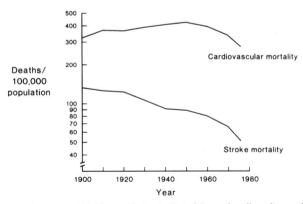

Fig 3–1.—Annual rates per 100,000 population in United States for all cardiovascular and stroke mortalities, age adjusted to 1940 U.S. population, for 1900 through 1976. (Courtesy of Whisnant, J.P.: Stroke 15:160–168, Jan.–Feb., 1984; by permission of the American Heart Association, Inc.; from Whisnant, J.P.: The role of the neurologist in the decline of stroke, Ann. Neurol. [in press]. By permission of the American Neurological Association, 14:1, 1983.)

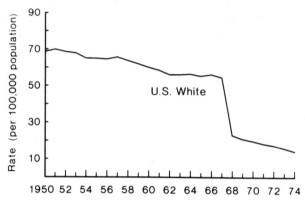

**Fig 3–2.**—Annual mortality per 100,000 U.S. white population for intracerebral hemorrhage for 1950 through 1974. (Courtesy of Whisnant, J.P.: Stroke 15:160–168, Jan.–Feb., 1984: by permission of the American Heart Association, Inc.; modified from Anderson, G.L., and Whisnant, J.P.: A comparison of trends in mortality from stroke in the United States and Rochester, Minnesota, Stroke 13:804, 1982; by permission of the American Heart Association, Inc.)

is rather low. It is unlikely that treatment of asymptomatic carotid stenosis has had any impact on the incidence of stroke. The relation of serum lipid elevations to ischemic stroke has been inconsistent. Cigarette smoking is only weakly associated with stroke. The risk of stroke is clearly increased in patients with heart disease, but only a relatively small decrease in incidence of coronary heart disease has occurred in Rochester. There is considerable variation in the incidence of ischemic stroke among diabetics, depending on other risk factors. Hypertension is clearly a powerful risk factor for stroke and is the chief factor in the declining incidence in Rochester. Treatment of hypertension may be the only significant factor in the decreases in stroke incidence and mortality. Future efforts should emphasize the control of hypertension in black populations and the effective treatment of systolic hypertension.

---

### The Continuing Decline in the Incidence of Stroke

W. Michael Garraway, Jack P. Whisnant, and Ivo Drury (Mayo Clinic and Found.)

Mayo Clin. Proc. 58:520–523, August 1983                                  3–2

It is not clear whether the recent decline in mortality from cerebrovascular disease noted in developed countries is the result of an actual reduction in the occurrence of stroke. The authors attempted to clarify the situation in the population of Rochester, Minn., where almost complete case ascertainment for stroke is possible. Review was made of 2,133 new strokes occurring during 1.5 million person-years of observation between 1945 and 1979.

The overall incidence of stroke declined steadily. Fewer than half of the number of first episodes of stroke occurred per unit of population in 1975–

1979 than in 1945–1949. Both sexes experienced a decline in stroke incidence, but in males most of the decline occurred in the last decade of the study. Persons aged 85 or more had the greatest reduction in stroke incidence. Birth cohort analysis confirmed a trend of declining incidence rates in all age groups. Rates of cerebral infarction declined consistently starting after 1950–1954. Rates of intracerebral hemorrhage fluctuated, and those of subarachnoid hemorrhage had no clear trend. Strokes of uncertain type followed a pattern similar to that of cerebral infarction.

The decline in stroke mortality was accompanied by a major reduction in the incidence of stroke. Cerebral infarction had the most marked reduction in incidence. The role of community hypertension control programs remains to be established. Substantial improvement in survival of patients with cerebral hemorrhage has recently been observed.

▶ The apparently real decline in stroke incidence is surprising. It is difficult to believe that something that now is so easy to accomplish as the control of hypertension could influence so markedly a disease that only 30 years ago was thought to be an inevitable consequence of aging. How far down the incidence rate will go and what neurologists (and neurosurgeons) will do with their spare time remains to be seen. Is the decline just a "putting off" of stroke, a shift upward of the stroke age?—R.D.C.

---

**Internal Carotid Occlusion: A Prospective Study**
R. Cote, H. J. M. Barnett (Univ. of Western Ontario), and D. W. Taylor (McMaster Univ.)
Stroke 14:898–902, November–December 1983                          3–3

---

The authors monitored 47 patients with internal carotid artery (ICA) occlusion, who had no more than a mild neurologic deficit, for an average of 34 months. All had had at least one cerebral or retinal ischemic attack in the three-month period before entry into the study. None underwent cerebrovascular bypass operations. None had other conditions possibly causing the symptoms, such as a cardiogenic source of emboli. The 39 men and 8 women had a mean age of 59 years. Twenty patients were seen with minor neurologic deficits and 27 with transient ischemic attacks only. Twenty-three patients were hypertensive, 14 had heart disease, and 7 had evidence of peripheral vascular disease. The origin of the ICA was the site of atherosclerotic occlusion in 87% of cases.

Thirteen cerebral infarctions occurred in 11 patients during follow-up, for a rate of 8% of patients per year. Seven infarctions occurred on the occluded side. The annual rate of ipsilateral stroke was 5%. The median time from entry to the study to stroke was 1.3 years. Three of the 11 strokes were severe; the other three were minor. Nine of 14 patients with initial evidence of further atherosclerotic disease on the same side as the occluded ICA had an ischemic event beyond the occlusion during follow-up. One stroke-related death occurred. About half the patients continued to have transient ischemic attacks in the region of the occluded artery. At least half the patients received antiplatelet therapy during follow-up, and four of these patients had a stroke during follow-up.

Prospective studies suggest an increased stroke rate compared with retrospective series. Whether extracranial-intracranial arterial bypass operations will improve the outlook for patients with ICA occlusion is unknown.

▶ This is a small but probably significant study of the prognosis of nonsurgically treated internal carotid artery occlusion discovered after a stroke. About half the patients continued with transient ischemic attacks, and about a quarter had a stroke during the three-year follow-up. Only half of the strokes were on the side of the occluded carotid.

In a summary article, Thompson (*Br. J. Surg.* 76:371–376, 1983) discusses his long experience with carotid endarterectomy and gives convincing evidence of both its safety and efficacy. But the situation is not simple. He is selecting his patients carefully. Is surgery better than antiplatelet agents combined with treatment of other risk factors: hypertension, hyperlipidemia, diabetes, and heart disease?

Fields, in a recent review of aspirin (*Am. J. Med.* 74:61–64, 1983), mentions an ongoing English study that will help settle the question of how much aspirin is enough and how much too much.—R.D.C.

---

**The Significance of Carotid Stenosis or Ulceration**
J. C. Grotta, R. H. Bigelow, H. Hu, L. Hankins, and W. S. Fields (Univ. of Texas at Houston)
Neurology (Cleve.) 34:437–442, April 1984                                     3–4

---

The severity of carotid stenosis or ulceration may be important in planning the management of patients with carotid-middle cerebral transient ischemic attacks (TIAs), asymptomatic carotid plaques, or asymptomatic bruits. The authors reviewed data from medically treated patients in the Aspirin in TIA study to determine whether carotid stenosis or ulceration increases the risk of ipsilateral TIA or infarction in patients with asymptomatic carotid bruits. Patients with at least one episode of monocular or hemispheric TIA in the preceding three months were randomized to receive 10 grains of aspirin or placebo twice daily and were then followed up for a mean of 15.5 months. Thirty-one patients with 35 asymptomatic carotid bruits were entered into a prospective study lasting for a mean of 28 months.

In patients with symptomatic carotid arteries, stenosis of 50% or more without ulceration was associated with an increased risk of subsequent symptoms. Ulceration was associated with an increased risk in nonstenotic vessels only. Lesion anatomy could not be related to the outcome in patients with asymptomatic arteries; the incidence of cerebral infarction was low.

Stenosis of 50% or more in symptomatic carotid arteries without ulceration is associated with an increased risk of subsequent ipsilateral cerebrovascular symptoms. The risk of subsequent infarction in patients with asymptomatic carotid arteries is low even if stenosis or ulceration is present. Factors other than angiographically identified abnormalities must influence the likelihood of subsequent cerebrovascular symptoms. Delayed events in the distribution of previously asymptomatic vessels could result from progressive changes in the artery, rather than from the initially discovered lesion itself. The anatomy of carotid lesions must be taken into account in studies of treatment in patients with TIAs.

▶ So stenosis of 50% or more increases the risk, but ulceration increases the risk only if the artery is nonstenotic. I'll have to think about that for awhile.— R.D.C.

---

**Adverse Effects on the Brain in Cardiac Operations as Assessed by Biochemical, Psychometric, and Radiologic Methods**
Torkel Åberg, Gunnar Ronquist, Hans Tydén, Siw Brunnkvist, Jan Hultman, Kjell Bergström, and Anders Lilja (Univ. of Uppsala, Sweden)
J. Thorac. Cardiovasc. Surg. 87:99–105, January 1984                    3–5

---

Some patient groups such as the elderly still have frequent CNS complications from cardiac operations, and brain dysfunction can occur in patients without clinically overt cerebral complications. The authors prospectively followed 94 patients, who underwent heart operations, by cerebrospinal fluid (CSF) analysis, psychometric testing, and brain computed tomography (CT). Coronary bypass grafting was performed in two thirds of patients and valve replacement only in one fourth. Levels of adenylate kinase (AK), lactate, and glutathione in CSF were determined 24 hours after cardiopulmonary bypass. Psychometric evaluation involved use of the synonyms, figure rotation, and figure identification tests. Fifty-three patients had both preoperative and postoperative CT studies.

A substantial increase in CSF AK activity was found in 13% of patients and a moderate increase in 46%. The enzyme is a marker of ischemic brain cell injury. The postoperative CSF AK and lactate values were not related, and no correlation with glutathione values was evident. Psychometric testing indicated a moderate postoperative decline in intellectual function. Two patients had postoperative CT evidence of cerebral infarction. Indices of brain injury did not correlate with either diagnosis or length of perfusion. Only one of five CT studies in patients with elevated CSF AK values showed cerebral infarction.

Subclinical brain injury is frequent after cardiac operations, but it is most often trivial, reversible, or both. The cause of ischemic brain cell injury in this setting is unclear, but circumstances in the operative field appear likelier to be important causative factors than microembolism. The quality of cardiopulmonary bypass and cardiac surgery may have reached a plateau.

▶ These authors confirm the suspicion that brain ischemic events during cardiac bypass surgery are relatively common although, thankfully, usually trivial.

Coronary bypass surgery may be associated more with cerebral ischemic events than is carotid surgery these days—possibly because of the necessity of the pump in the former or of the short operative time with the latter.—R.D.C.

---

**Relation of Atrial Fibrillation and High Hematocrit to Mortality in Acute Stroke**
G. D. O. Lowe, A. J. Jaap, and C. D. Forbes (Royal Infirmary, Glasgow, Scotland)
Lancet 1:784–786, Apr. 9, 1983                                    3–6

Atrial fibrillation and high levels of hemoglobin or hematocrit may be associated with an increased risk of stroke. To test the hypothesis that both atrial fibrillation and an elevated hematocrit are not only common in stroke patients but are also associated with increased mortality, the authors retrospectively analyzed the records of 320 patients with acute stroke who were hospitalized during a five-year period.

Age and coma were the only clinical factors related to mortality. None of the 57 patients who were comatose on admission survived. Mortality increased progressively with age from 36% in patients younger than 60 years to 41% in patients aged 60–69, 58% in those aged 70–79, and 66% in those aged 80 years or older ($P<.005$). Of 316 patients for whom an ECG was obtained, 78 (25%) had atrial fibrillation. The incidence of atrial fibrillation increased progressively with age from 14% in patients less than 60 years of age to 37% in those aged 80 years or older. Forty-nine (63%) of the 78 patients with atrial fibrillation died compared with 113 (48%) of the 238 without atrial fibrillation ($P<.05$). A significant increase in mortality associated with atrial fibrillation was limited to patients aged 60–69 (Fig 3–3). Of patients aged 60–79 years, 67% of those with atrial fibrillation died compared with 44% who did not have atrial fibrillation. In patients with atrial fibrillation, mortality was not significantly associated with age, although it was so in patients without atrial fibrillation. Atrial fibrillation was not significantly associated with coma, but was associated with heart murmur ($P<.0005$) and a history of heart valve disease ($P<.0005$). Both high and low hematocrit levels were associated with increased mortality, but the high mortality related to low hematocrit value was associated with a high percentage of patients over age 75 (Fig 3–4). In patients over 75 years of age, mortality was not significantly related to hematocrit level; however, there was a trend toward lowest mortality in patients with a hematocrit value of 0.40–.44. In patients younger than age 75, a greater than twofold increase in mortality was observed in those with a hematocrit value of 0.50 or more ($P<.005$). Hematocrit levels were not significantly associated with coma, blood urea levels, or creatinine levels. Other laboratory variables associated with mortality were increased mean red blood cell volume, white blood cell count, erythrocyte sedimentation rate, and globulin, urea, and creatinine levels and decreased albumin levels.

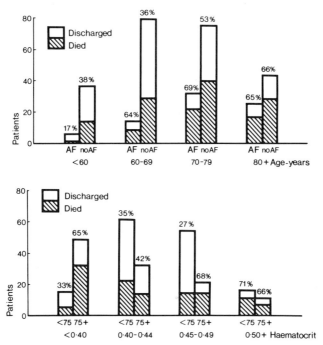

**Fig 3–3 (top).**—Mortality (%) in patients with and without atrial fibrillation in relation to age.

**Fig 3–4 (bottom).**—Mortality (%) in patients aged less than 75 and in those aged 75 or more in relation to hematocrit.

(Courtesy of Lowe, G.D.O., et al.: Lancet 1:784–786, April 1983.)

The high prevalence of and increased mortality associated with atrial fibrillation and an elevated hematocrit value in patients who sustain a stroke indicates the need for additional studies of the prevention and treatment of stroke in this group.

▶ These two medical conditions increase the likelihood of stroke. Our hematologists remain uninterested in recommending bleeding for stroke patients with high hematocrits, and adequate anticoagulation is difficult to maintain safely on an outpatient basis. Perhaps it is not too much to hope that some safer method of anticoagulation may be found in the future.

Speaking of heart disease and stroke, Francis et al. (*J. Neurol. Neurosurg. Psychiatry* 47:256–259, 1984) with the use of ambulatory monitoring have found cardiac arrhythmias in 41% of 64 patients with transient ischemic attacks. In the 21% with significant arrhythmia, treatment of the heart abnormality stopped or improved the neurologic symptoms.—R.D.C.

## Duration of Atrial Fibrillation and Imminence of Stroke: The Framingham Study

Philip A. Wolf, William B. Kannel, Daniel L. McGee, Stephen L. Meeks, Nadir E. Bharucha, and Patricia M. McNamara
Stroke 14:664–667, September–October 1983                    3–7

It was proposed that an excess of stroke occurs in patients with paroxysmal, intermittent, and recent-onset atrial fibrillation (AF) unassociated with rheumatic heart disease. The authors examined the development of stroke in relation to the duration of AF in a general population of 5,184 subjects followed prospectively for 30 years beginning in 1950. Initial ages were 30–62 years, and participants were examined every two years.

A total of 501 cases of stroke occurred, 59 in the presence of AF that was not associated with rheumatic heart disease. Strokes having an embolic source other than AF were not investigated. Atrial fibrillation contributed to the risk of stroke independently of coronary heart failure and coronary heart disease. A clustering of stroke events close to the onset of AF was apparent. In 14 patients AF was first noted during hospitalization for stroke, and 8 other strokes occurred in the first year after onset of AF. Survival after stroke in the AF group did not differ from that in all other stroke patients (17% vs. 19%). A second stroke occurred in 20% of patients without AF and in 25% of the study group, not a significant difference. Early recurrences were more frequent in the AF group, but over time the difference between the two groups narrowed.

Most strokes in persons with AF appear to be the result of cerebral embolism, although AF does reduce cerebral blood flow. Attempts to prevent strokes in patients with nonvalvular AF undoubtedly will emphasize measures that interfere with intra-atrial thrombus formation. A controlled trial of antithrombotic agents or anticoagulants to prevent stroke in patients with nonrheumatic AF is needed.

▶ The Framingham study continues to yield helpful information. Not only were strokes more frequent around the time of development of the atrial fibrillation but stroke recurrence in the first six months was twice as frequent. This finding fits well with the findings of Lowe et al. (abstract 3–6).—R.D.C.

## Why Admit Stroke Patients to Hospital?

Derick T. Wade and Richard Langton Hewer (Bristol, England)
Lancet 1:807–809, Apr. 9, 1983                    3–8

Stroke patients consume a significant proportion of health resources in England, most being related to hospital costs. Hospitalization for diagnosis should be tempered by the recognition that the need for increased diagnostic accuracy depends on the extent to which management is altered as a result. In addition, many investigations entail certain patient risks. There is no evidence to warrant the hospitalization of all stroke patients on special stroke intensive-care wards. No specific treatment method has been established as beneficial in reducing cerebral damage in stroke patients, and surgery is rarely necessary. Although referral to the hospital may be necessary to gain access to rehabilitation services, there is no suggestion that these measures must be carried out in the hospital. Certain underlying diseases may warrant hospital treatment after stroke, and hospitalization is recommended when the diagnosis is in doubt, nursing care is not available at home, active therapeutic intervention is a possibility, or the underlying cause of stroke requires investigation.

Rehabilitation in the hospital sometimes is not appropriate to the patient's needs. Many patients already are cared for at home without ever entering the hospital. Patients at home have access to their general practitioner, who is aided if necessary by hospital consultants during domiciliary visits or by outpatient referral. Rehabilitation can be carried out successfully at home, which may in fact be the best place for it. Rehabilitation at home can be closely tailored to the patient's needs and expectations, and anxiety and depression may be minimized. If limited resources are used more effectively, fewer patients will require hospitalization, and those who do require it might be discharged sooner.

▶ Certainly circumstances change one's approach. The chances are that English stroke patients receive better home physician care than American patients. Thus it is possible that most of their underlying medical problems are already recognized and treated. In the Mississippi stroke population that is not necessarily so. Of the 1,500 or so stroke patients admitted to the University of Mississippi stroke unit in the last 15 years, I can recall just one in whom there was not some underlying treatable disease. Hospital admission may be justified on that basis alone.—R.D.C.

---

**The Dichotomy of Myocardial and Cerebral Infarction**
W. Michael Garraway, Lila R. Elveback, Daniel C. Connolly, and Jack P. Whisnant (Mayo Clinic and Found.)
Lancet 2:1332–1335, Dec. 10, 1983                                    3–9

---

Declining mortality from both coronary heart disease and stroke is reported in the United States and other countries. Changes in incidence and case fatality rates for myocardial infarction (MI) and cerebral infarction (CI) were compared in the population of Rochester, Minn. A marked decline in the age-adjusted and sex-adjusted incidence of CI was observed, along with an overall decline of 14% in MI, including sudden unexpected deaths (SUD) (Fig 3–5). The reduction in adjusted incidence of CI in the same period (1950–1979) was 55%. The reduction in MI incidence resulted from the decreased incidence of SUD, especially in younger persons. The 30-day case-fatality rate after MI decreased from 50% to 35%. The proportion of CI patients hospitalized increased from 1960 on, whereas that of MI patients declined in 1975–1979 because of a reduction in the number of SUD patients admitted to the hospital or reaching the hospital alive.

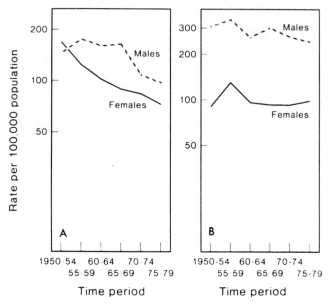

**Fig 3–5.—A**, average annual age-adjusted incidence of cerebral infarction in population of 100,000. **B**, average annual age-adjusted incidence of myocardial infarction (including sudden unexpected death) in population of 100,000. (Courtesy of Garraway, W.M., et al.: Lancet 2:1332–1335, Dec. 10, 1983.)

The decline in incidence of CI is more marked than that of MI. It can be attributed in part to the more specific effect of hypertension on the cerebral circulation than on the coronary circulation. The latter is influenced more uniformly by several risk factors. The reduction in the number of MI patients with SUD may reflect a change in the severity of MI, or a change in the mechanism of infarction. Changes in risk factor prevalence and in public perception of the diseases must be assessed in order to clarify the relative importance of changes in incidence and case-fatality rate of coronary heart disease and stroke.

► The authors of the above study further point out (*Lancet* 2:1332–1335, 1983) that cerebral infarction and myocardial infarction are not parallel, possibly because control of hypertension is less effective in preventing heart disease than stroke.—R.D.C.

---

**Reversal of Acute Experimental Cerebral Vasospasm by Calcium Antagonism With Verapamil**
Richard Leblanc, William Feindel, Lucas Yamamoto, John G. Milton, and Mony M. Frojmovic (McGill Univ., Montreal)
Can. J. Neurol. Sci. 11:42–47, February 1984                    3–10

---

Cerebral vasospasm is a major cause of mortality and morbidity in patients with aneurysmal subarachnoid bleeding. The authors evaluated

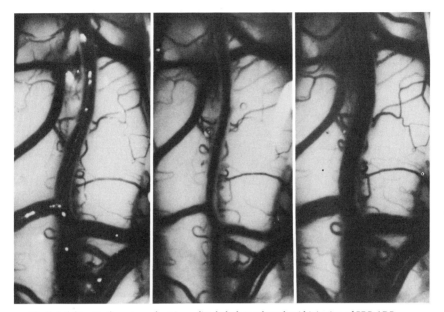

Fig 3–6 (left).—Basilar artery of cat immediately before subarachnoid injection of PRP-ADP.

Fig 3–7 (center).—Same vessel 10 minutes after subarachnoid injection of PRP-ADP, demonstrating vasoconstriction.

Fig 3–8 (right).—Same vessel five minutes after application of verapamil, showing marked vasodilatation.

(Courtesy of Leblanc, R., et al.: Can. J. Neurol. Sci. 11:42–47, February 1984.)

the calcium channel blocker verapamil in anesthetized cats in which acute vasospasm of the transclivally exposed basilar artery was produced by subarachnoid injection of platelet-rich plasma (PRP) treated with enough adenosine diphosphate (ADP) to induce platelet aggregation and secretion. Verapamil was applied topically to produce vasorelaxation, and its effects were recorded photographically for one hour.

The injection of PRP-ADP produced prompt vasoconstriction of the basilar artery (Figs 3–6 and 3–7). Topical verapamil application produced rapid, dramatic vasorelaxation of the vessels (Fig 3–8), which persisted in a decremental manner for the one-hour observation period. Reinjection of PRP-ADP produced vasoconstriction comparable to that produced initially. Reapplication of verapamil again rapidly reversed the vasoconstriction. The vasodilating effect of verapamil could not be ascribed to its pH. No significant changes in mean arterial pressure or $Pco_2$ occurred during the studies.

Topical application of a calcium antagonist consistently reversed experimental vasospasm in a transient manner in this model. It appears that a continuous supply of calcium blocker is needed as long as the vessels are exposed to spasmogen. This may limit the usefulness of systemically administered verapamil because of its hypotensive action, but calcium channel blockers, through their marked spasmolytic properties, may hold promise for use in the management of cerebral vasospasm.

▶ These observations indicate that the platelet fraction of whole blood may be involved in the genesis of acute vasospasm following subarachnoid hemorrhage and that this phenomenon can be readily reversed by calcium antagonism.—R.N.D.J.

---

**Natural History of Cerebral Complications of Coronary Artery Bypass Graft Surgery**
C. Edward Coffey, E. Wayne Massey, Kenneth B. Roberts, Steven Curtis, Robert H. Jones, and David B. Pryor (Duke Univ.)
Neurology (Cleve.) 33:1416–1421, November 1983                  3–11

---

Encephalopathy, stroke, and peripheral neuropathy have all been described after coronary bypass grafting. The authors reviewed the neurologic complications that occurred among 1,669 consecutive patients undergoing coronary bypass grafting without other procedures between 1969 and 1981. Cerebral complications occurred in 64 (3.8%) patients. A total of 75 complications occurred in these patients, who resembled those without neurologic complications in age and sex.

Fifty-seven patients had altered mental state, usually manifested as delirium one to six days after operation. Average duration of delirium was five days; it was generally benign and self-limited. Postoperative arrhythmias were more frequent in these patients than in the overall patient population. Hypoxic-metabolic encephalopathy occurred in 24 patients in relation to intraoperative or postoperative complications or both. Mortality in this group was 71%. Stroke occurred intraoperatively in nine patients and postoperatively in four. Patients with stroke more often had carotid bruits at admission than did the cohort. Five patients had seizures unrelated to past epilepsy. All responded to anticonvulsant therapy. Two patients had seizures complicating hypoxic-metabolic encephalopathy.

Cerebral complications occurred in nearly 4% of this large series of patients undergoing coronary bypass grafting. Coma from hypoxic-metabolic encephalopathy accounted for all but 1 of the 20 deaths. The surviving patients had full functional recovery. Mental alteration was the most frequent neurologic complication in this series. The cause of postoperative strokes was unclear. The management of postoperative seizures should be personalized. A better understanding of the pathophysiologic basis of these complications should help in their prevention.

▶ The true incidence and natural history of the neurologic complications of coronary bypass grafting are difficult to ascertain. These authors describe their experience with the occurrence, clinical course, and natural history of the cerebral sequelae of such surgery.—R.N.D.J.

## Manifestations of Coronary Disease Predisposing to Stroke: The Framingham Study

William B. Kannel, Philip A. Wolf, and Joel Verter (Boston Univ.)
JAMA 250:2942–2946, Dec. 2, 1983                                            3–12

The authors evaluated coronary heart disease (CHD) as a precursor of stroke in 5,184 men and women aged 30–62 who were examined during 24 years of biennial follow-up; all were free of stroke initially. Routine ECGs, chest films, and blood pressure (BP) levels were obtained; patients were assessed for CHD and cardiac failure at each examination, and the risk of stroke was ascertained.

During the 24-year period there were 344 strokes of which 60% were brain infarctions, 1,004 CHD events, and 330 instances of heart failure. Strokes occurred later in life than myocardial infarction. Overall, the five major CHD risk factors were as predictive of brain infarction as of myocardial infarction. Elevated BP and ECG evidence of left ventricular hypertrophy were the principal determinants of this predictive capacity. The dominant risk factors predisposing to stroke were hypertension, clinical signs of CHD, cardiac failure, atrial fibrillation, and ECG and radiographic evidence of a compromised coronary circulation. Persons with overt clinical manifestations of CHD had almost a threefold increased risk of stroke, and cardiac failure was associated with more than a fivefold increased risk. The risk of stroke associated with myocardial infarction was markedly higher than that for angina pectoris (Fig 3–9). Also, CHD in hypertensive persons posed a distinctly greater risk of stroke than it did in normotensive persons. However, CHD carried a substantial excess risk in those without hypertension, especially in men in whom myocardial infarction was the preponderant manifestation of CHD. The presence of CHD and coronary failure added to the risk of stroke associated with hypertension.

Strokes play a part in the larger problem of cardiovascular disease. Once coronary disease and cardiac failure occur or there is even asymptomatic

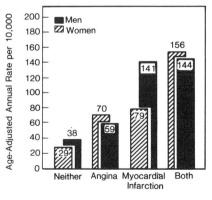

Fig 3–9.—Risk of stroke based on clinical manifestation of coronary heart disease; 24-year follow-up of individuals aged 45–84 from the Framingham Study. (Courtesy of Kannel, W.B., et al.: JAMA 250:2942–2946, Dec. 2, 1983; copyright 1983, American Medical Association.)

evidence of compromised coronary circulation, the risk of stroke is greatly increased. Control of hypertension and prevention and relief of cardiac failure, atrial fibrillation, and CHD are essential to stroke prevention.

▶ The correlation between coronary disease and cerebrovascular disease has long been apparent to most physicians. This careful and detailed study gives statistical confirmation of this correlation.—R.N.D.J.

---

**CT and Clinical Correlations in Recent Aneurysmal Subarachnoid Hemorrhage: Preliminary Report of Cooperative Aneurysm Study**
Harold P. Adams, Jr., Neal F. Kassell, James C. Torner, and A. L. Sahs (Univ. of Iowa)
Neurology (Cleve.) 33:981–988, August 1983                               3–13

---

Failure to diagnose subarachnoid hemorrhage (SAH) in less seriously ill patients is a major problem. The authors reviewed the results of computed tomography (CT) in 1,378 patients admitted to 71 different centers within

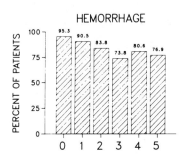

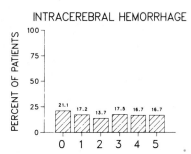

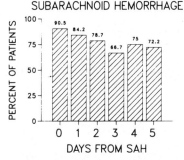

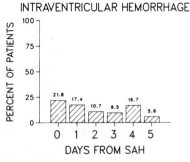

Fig 3–10.—**Upper left,** percentage of patients in whom intracranial hemorrhage was detected by CT as influenced by the interval from the occurrence of subarachnoid hemorrhage (SAH). **Lower left,** percentage of patients in whom SAH was seen on CT. **Upper right,** frequency of detection of intracerebral hemorrhage on CT. **Lower right,** percentage of patients in whom intraventricular hemorrhage was seen on CT; this incidence was significantly more common on CT performed on days 0 or 1. (Courtesy of Adams, H.P., Jr., et al.: Neurology (Cleve.) 33:981–988, August 1983.)

three days of SAH. Overall, 149 patients had neither headache nor meningeal signs when hospitalized. Evidence of subarachnoid, intracerebral, intraventricular, or subdural hemorrhage was obtained by CT in 89% of the patients.

The interval from SAH to CT examination was related to the results in patients examined within five days after the ictus (Fig 3–10). Intraventricular bleeding and SAH were more frequent in patients examined on the day of the ictus, whereas normal findings were much more prevalent in those seen two or more days after the ictus. Alert patients were more likely to have normal CT findings or only a thin local collection of SAH. Normal speech also was related to normal CT findings or only local thin deposits of subarachnoid blood, as were normal orientation and appropriate responses to commands. The lesion was detected by CT in 77% of the patients with neither headache nor nuchal rigidity and in 85% of those with either symptom. Normal CT findings or the presence of only a local thin collection correlated closely with normal motor responses. Local thick collections of blood, hydrocephalus, and intracerebral or intraventricular hemorrhage were more frequent in patients with abnormal posturing or with no motor response.

Computed tomography should be the initial diagnostic procedure in patients with symptoms suggestive of SAH. It can also detect intracranial bleeding in patients in whom SAH is not suspected clinically. The role of CT in predicting the long-term outcome in patients with SAH remains to be established.

▶ In the first few days after a subarachnoid hemorrhage, computed tomography provides highly accurate information on the site and extent of the hemorrhage. The demonstration of the presence of subarachnoid bleeding by such tomography may obviate the need for lumbar puncture and cerebrospinal fluid examination. The authors state that, if it is available, computed tomography should be the initial diagnostic study on patients with symptoms suggesting the presence of subarachnoid bleeding.—R.N.D.J.

---

### The Syndrome of Bilateral Paramedian Thalamic Infarction

Alan Guberman and Donald Stuss (Univ. of Ottawa)
Neurology (Cleve.) 33:540–546, May 1983                                    3–14

---

Acute, persistent amnesia is usually attributed to alcoholism with thiamine deficiency, head trauma, or cerebral anoxia. Bilateral paramedian thalamic infarction due to occlusion of a thalamosubthalamic perforating artery supplying both medial thalami is a less frequent cause. The authors report data on two patients in whom bilateral anterior paramedian thalamic infarction, due to occlusion of a bilaterally distributed thalamosubthalamic paramedian artery, was demonstrated on computed tomography. One patient was initially seen with transient coma, asterixis, hypersomnia, vertical gaze disturbances, profound Korsakoff amnesia, and subcortical dementia. He remained severely impaired a year later. The second patient, with a predominantly right-sided thalamic infarct, recovered well from amnesia and vertical gaze disorder.

The most consistent feature in these cases has been a Korsakoff amnesic syndrome. There is an anterograde and retrograde deficit, with impairment of both verbal and nonverbal memory. The amnesia is probably due to destruction of the dorsal median nuclei. Subcortical dementia is a frequent finding, suggesting possible importance of thalamic involvement in the mental changes of progressive supranuclear palsy and similar disorders. Transient asterixis suggests impingement of the lesion on the internal capsule. Vertical gaze abnormality may be detected only by electro-oculography. Mild aphasic disturbance similar to that found in patients with left thalamic or putaminal hemorrhage may be present.

This disorder can be considered to be a lacunar syndrome. Hypertension is often described, but embolization may sometimes be responsible. Computed tomography can confirm the diagnosis of bilateral paramedian thalamic infarction.

▶ This disorder can be called a lacunar syndrome in the distribution of the anterior paramedian thalamosubthalamic arteries. Hypertension was responsible in all the reported cases. The clinical and computed tomographic features are characteristic.—R.N.D.J.

---

## Cerebral Blood Flow and Cerebrovascular CO₂ Reactivity in Stroke-Age Normal Controls

Stephen M. Davis, Robert H. Ackerman, John A. Correia, Nathaniel M. Alpert, Jen Chang, Ferdinando Buonanno, Roger E. Kelley, Bernard Rosner, and Juan M. Taveras

Neurology (Cleve.) 33:391–399, April 1983                        3–15

---

Any effects of age alone on cerebral hemodynamics must be understood for proper interpretation of cerebral blood flow (CBF) data in patients at risk for stroke. The authors determined CBF, carbon dioxide reactivity, gray matter perfusion (Fg), and white matter perfusion (Fw) in 55 healthy persons aged 18–88 years without hemodynamically significant extracranial vascular disease. The CBF was measured by the radioxenon inhalation technique. Cerebral hemodynamics were assessed during hyperventilation in 41 persons. A representative carotid bifurcation is shown in Figure 3–11. None of the 27 participants older than 50 years of age had significant changes distal to the carotid bifurcation.

A significant linear decline in mean cerebral Fg was noted with advancing age. The age-related decline was significant for women but not for men. Cerebral Fg values were reproducible. No significant relationship was observed between mean cerebral Fw and age. Cerebrovascular carbon dioxide reactivity showed a modest, insignificant downward trend with advancing age. Cerebrovascular resistance was significantly increased in older persons.

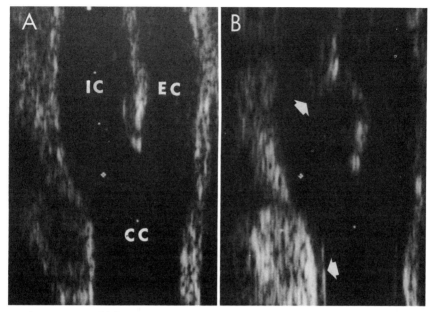

**Fig 3–11.**—Carotid bifurcation in elderly subject as seen with a high-resolution, real-time, B-mode ultrasound device. **A,** the bifurcation is normal in a midlongitudinal plane. CC, IC, and EC represent the common, internal, and external carotid arteries, respectively. White dots are cursor marks. **B,** in 55 normal stroke-age controls, the most severe disease seen was found along the posterior wall *(upper arrow)* of the carotid artery in one subject. The plaque was not as prominent anteriorly in the vessel, and the stenosis was estimated to be 50%. *Lower arrow* indicates ultrasound reflection related to normal intima. (Courtesy of Davis, S.M., et al.: Neurology (Cleve.) 33:391–399, April 1983.)

A progressive decline in gray matter CBF appears to occur in association with physiologic aging, but the mechanism is unclear. Both physiologic and pathophysiologic determinants of CBF must be considered in assessing cerebral hemodynamics in stroke-prone and ischemic stroke patients.

▶ This original and thorough study suggests that there are physiologic changes in cerebral hemodynamics associated with aging, as well as pathologic ones. The physiologic ones make older persons more stroke-prone than younger persons.—R.N.D.J.

---

**CSF Enzymes in Lacunar and Cortical Stroke**
Geoffrey A. Donnan, Peter Zapf, Austin E. Doyle, and Peter F. Bladin (Univ. of Melbourne)
Stroke 14:266–269, March–April 1983                                                      3–16

---

A distinction between lacunar and cortical infarction is important because cortical infarction is considered to be embolic in origin; however, differentiation may be difficult. The authors attempted to determine whether cerebrospinal fluid (CSF) enzyme determination can aid in de-

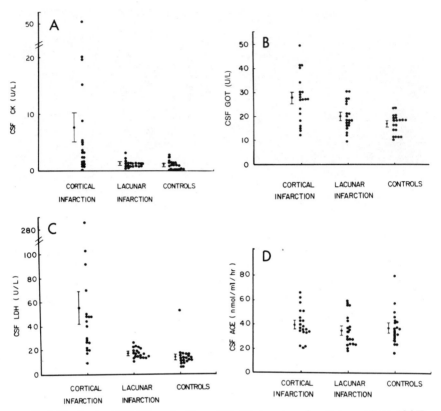

**Fig 3–12.**—Levels of CSF (**A**) creatine kinase *(CK)*, (**B**) glutamic oxaloacetic transaminase, *(GOT)*, (**C**) lactic dehydrogenase *(LDH)*, and (**D**) angiotensin converting enzyme *(ACE)* in 20 patients with cortical infarction, 20 with lacunar infarction, and in 20 controls. Mean and SEM values are shown. (Courtesy of Donnan, G.A., et al.: Stroke 14:266–269, March–April 1983.)

tecting cortical involvement and in distinguishing it from lacunar syndromes. Twenty consecutive patients with lacunar syndromes in whom the site of infarction was documented by computed tomography (CT) and 20 others with "cortical" stroke were evaluated. The latter patients had hemiplegia accompanied by cortical signs, a focal contralateral EEG abnormality, neuropsychological abnormalities, and CT confirmation of the site of infarction. The CSF values of creatine kinase (CK), glutamic oxaloacetic transaminase (GOT), lactic dehydrogenase (LDH), and angiotensin converting enzyme (ACE) were estimated.

Initial neurologic deficit scores were similar in the two patient groups. Markedly elevated levels of CSF CK were found in the patients with cortical stroke (Fig 3–12), and GOT values also were elevated. The most marked difference was in LDH levels. No elevation of ACE activity was found in either group. None of the enzyme levels was elevated in the serum, and CSF and serum levels were not correlated. Infarctions were seen to communicate with the subarachnoid CSF on CT examination in 15 patients with cortical stroke. Enzyme levels correlated both with more peripheral infarctions and with infarction size.

These findings may help explain the unpredictability of CSF enzyme elevations in stroke patients. Enzyme determinations could help distinguish cortical from lacunar stroke in some cases.

▶ A study of the cerebrospinal fluid levels of certain enzymes may be of use to distinguish between cortical and lacunar strokes and thus be of importance for management purposes, decisions about entry into stroke treatment trials, and identification and differentiation of syndrome types.—R.N.D.J.

---

**A Two-Year Longitudinal Study of Poststroke Mood Disorders: Findings During Initial Evaluation**
Robert G. Robinson, Lyn Book Starr, Kenneth L. Kubos, and Thomas R. Price
Stroke 14:736–741, September–October 1983                                   3–17

---

Depression is observed significantly more often and is more severe in patients with left hemispheric than in those with right hemispheric stroke injury. The authors attempted to identify the important factors in post-stroke mood disorders in a two-year prospective study of 103 patients seen in a one-and-a-half-year period at University of Maryland Hospital. Most were in their sixth or seventh decade. About three-fifths were men; nearly two thirds were black. Only one tenth of the patients had a family history of psychiatric disorder, but nearly one fourth had a past history of stroke. Eighty-five patients had thromboembolic infarcts, and 18 had intracerebral hemorrhage.

Signs of major depression were present in 27% of patients, and signs of dysrhythmic disorder were seen in another 20%. Nine percent were inappropriately cheerful. Among patients with lesions of the frontal or parietal-occipital lobes, those with left frontal lesions had significantly greater mean depression scores. The most severely depressed patients had the worst social functioning in the acute stroke period. Both functional physical impairment and global cognitive impairment correlated signifi-cantly with the severity of depression. The younger patients were the most severely depressed.

About one half of these unselected stroke patients had significant mood disorders. The location of the lesion probably is the most important single factor in the development of poststroke mood disorders. Patients with left frontal lesions are especially prone to depression. Age, the quality of social support, and the degree of intellectual or functional physical impairment are also factors which may either modify the neurophysiologic process or may themselves lead to depression through a different mechanism.

▶ Poststroke depressive disorders are multifactorial in their determination, de-velopment, and expression, and include both neurophysiologic-neurochemical mechanisms and psychological factors in the etiology. Patients with left frontal lobe brain injury have a greater prevalance and severity of depression than patients with lesions of other locations.—R.N.D.J.

## Nortriptyline Treatment of Poststroke Depression: Double-Blind Study

John R. Lipsey, Robert G. Robinson, Godfrey D. Pearlson, Krishna Rao, and Thomas R. Price

Lancet 1:297–300, Feb. 11, 1984                                          3–18

Many stroke patients have clinically significant depression, and patients are at high risk of depression for two years after stroke. The authors undertook a double-blind study of nortriptyline in the treatment of poststroke depression in 34 patients with thromboembolic stroke or intracerebral hemorrhage and moderate to severe depression. No severe comprehension deficit was present. Most patients were treated for six weeks. The daily dose of nortriptyline was increased from 20 to 100 mg over the study period. Fourteen of the 34 patients received nortriptyline, and 20, placebo. Eleven of the former patients completed the entire study.

The pretreatment neurologic findings were comparable in the treated and control groups, and patients who completed the study had similar degrees of cognitive impairment. Computed tomography showed similar hemispheric distributions of lesions in the two groups. Half the nortriptyline-treated patients and 60% of the placebo patients had major depression at the outset. Significantly more improvement occurred in patients given nortriptyline than in the placebo group. Responsive patients had serum nortriptyline concentrations in the therapeutic range.

Poststroke depression is a psychological reaction to the cognitive and physical impairment resulting from stroke. Nortriptyline appears to be an effective treatment for poststroke depression. Delirium has developed in treated patients. Contraindications to nortriptyline therapy include serious cardiac arrhythmias, recent myocardial infarction, heart block, urinary outlet obstruction, and narrow-angle glaucoma.

▶ The authors point out what is probably a neglected treatment area. Poststroke depression, especially as seen in a rehabilitation center, must be more common than the acute-care clinician realizes. Perhaps antidepressant drugs can be started earlier, during the subacute phase of stroke recovery.—R.D.C.

# 4 Child Neurology

**A Proposed Neuropathological Basis for Learning Disabilities in Children Born Prematurely**
Peter W. Fuller, Robert D. Guthrie, and Ellsworth C. Alvord, Jr. (Univ. of Washington)
Dev. Med. Child. Neurol. 25:214–231, April 1983                    4–1

Although the learning disabilities of children labeled "MBD" (minimal brain dysfunction) and "LD" (learning disabilities) have received considerable study, correlation with specific neuropathologic lesions has not been established. Premature infants are of particular interest because they are a high-risk group, as evidenced by the increasing numbers of survivors of neonatal intensive care units who develop MBD-LD complications. The authors studied 16 prematurely born infants ranging from 28 to 32 weeks gestation, with survival times of 13 hours to 28 days. At autopsy, 45 separate sites in each of the brains were examined for evidence of white and gray matter damage.

The histologic findings showed 10 (67%) of 15 cases for whom information was available had gray matter lesions in the hippocampus, including "old" and "recent" necrosis; 7 (47%) had extensive lipids present, and 4 (27%) had gliosis. Overall, 5 (31%) of 16 cases had necrosis, and 14 (88%) showed extensive lipid involvement in the corpus callosum. Temporal and cerebellar cortex both showed significant gray matter lesions: 5 (33%) of 15, and 6 (38%) of 16 cases, respectively. Parietal or association cortex was involved in 4 (27%) of 15 cases; the basal ganglia showed necrotic lesions in 6 (40%) of 15 cases. The brain stem was involved in 9 (56%) of 16 cases, and the thalamus-hypothalamus in 5 (33%) of 15 cases.

When the premature CNS is exposed to perinatal complications, the lesions may not be immediately symptomatic or fatal. In some cases, there should be subclinical lesions which result in little or no damage in survivors. The implications of a potential gradation in degree of neuronal loss (focal, multifocal, or diffuse in structures such as the hippocampus, corpus callosum, cerebellum, cerebral cortex, basal ganglia, and thalamus) suggest possible relationships between lesions and abnormal learning and behavior. The cerebellar lesions can result in lack of fine and gross motor control, clumsiness, and difficulty in visual-motor control. The association of necrosis, hemorrhage, and lipid-laden cells in the cerebellar deep nuclei and white matter with neonatal asphyxia and hypoxemia in the premature infants who died after seven days of age shows that such lesions may have significance in neonates who survive these complications.

The potential consequences of lesions in the corpus callosum and other commissural fibers are also intriguing. Impulses arriving from all areas of the cerebral cortex via association and commissural fibers largely terminate in the second and third layers of other cortical areas. Areas of association cortex, such as the language-association area, are of relevance for language-learning disabilities. The corpus callosum and other association fibers are among the last to complete myelination after birth. The cellular precursors of myelination (immature glial cells or oligodendroblasts) may be more at risk in the premature infant surviving with repeated hypoxic-ischemic insults. The lipid accumulation observed in young glial cells in this study may be the oligodendroblasts which are myelin precursors. The present histologic findings have shown that extensive numbers of lipid-laden cells are positively associated with the extent of various other necrotic lesions.

▶ This is a careful neuropathologic study of premature infants who died hours to days after birth. Corpus callosum involvement was common; but lesions of the hippocampus, cerebellum, cerebral cortex, basal ganglia, and thalamus were also present in many infants, and the authors suggest that these lesions could be the neuropathologic basis of minimal brain dysfunction and learning disability. It wouldn't be surprising to hear soon that nuclear magnetic resonance scanning will show such lesions in surviving premature infants and provide in vivo correlation opportunity.—R.D.C.

---

**The Long-Term Effects of Removal of Sensorimotor Cortex in Infant and Adult Rhesus Monkeys**
R. E. Passingham, V. H. Perry, and F. Wilkinson (Univ. of Oxford, England)
Brain 106:675–705, September 1983                                    4–2

---

Recovery from the effects of cortical damage is believed to be more complete if a lesion is incurred in infancy rather than adulthood. Most of Kennard's data relate to the claim that in the short term a lesion is less disruptive to infants than to adults. The authors reexamined the long-term effects of cortical sensorimotor lesions in monkeys.

Unilateral lesions were produced to maximize the chance of recovery and anatomical reorganization. Six rhesus monkeys had the sensorimotor cortex removed from one hemisphere, four of them in infancy and two at about age three years, and they were tested after at least 18 months. Six other animals had either the motor cortex or the somatosensory cortex removed in infancy or had the regions of both motor and somatosensory cortex representing the leg removed. The lesions produced in infant monkeys are shown in Figure 4–1.

Both the infant and adult monkeys recovered to a remarkable degree. They were able to walk, climb, and jump easily, but they could not grip food by using the thumb and forefinger independently of the other fingers. Adults also exhibited permanent impairment in use of the wrist and forearm. The findings fail to support the view that in monkeys the effects of lesions of the sensorimotor cortex are less severe or persistent if the damage is incurred in infancy. In the 18 months after surgery simple tests of

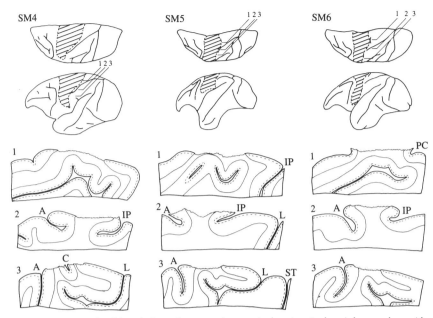

Fig 4–1.—Dorsal and lateral views of cortex and parasagittal sections in three infant monkeys with sensorimotor lesions. Lateral views show levels at which sections were taken. *A* = arcuate sulcus, *C* = central sulcus, *IP* = intraparietal sulcus, *L* = lateral sulcus, *ST* = superior temporal sulcus. (Courtesy of Passingham, R.E., et al.: Brain 106:675–705, September 1983.)

locomotion and manual skill showed no significant differences between animals that received lesions in infancy or in adulthood.

Available evidence suggests that compensation for brain damage occurs only when an animal is very immature at the time of injury. The brain of a neonatal monkey is much more mature than that of a rat or hamster. True compensation probably can only occur in monkeys if a lesion is made well before birth. There is no good evidence that the function of any area of neocortex can be subsumed by a different area of cortex. There is considerable redundancy between the functions of the association areas of the two hemispheres in adult as well as infant monkeys, but there is much less redundancy in human beings. There is no reason why changes in anatomical connections must always compensate for a loss of cortical tissue.

▶ These results do not support Kennard's conclusions made in 1942 that infant monkeys recover more completely than adults from the effects of brain lesions. Evidence from present studies suggests that compensation occurs only when the animal is very immature at the time of operation. The brain is much more mature in neonatal monkeys than in rats or hamsters. True compensation can probably only occur in monkeys if the lesion occurs well before birth, and this is probably true in human beings as well.—R.N.D.J.

**Long-Term Outcome of Children With Severe Head Trauma and Pro-longed Coma**
William J. Mahoney, Bernard J. D'Souza, J. Alex Haller, Mark C. Rogers, Melvin H. Epstein, and John M. Freeman (Johns Hopkins Univ.)
Pediatrics 71:756–762, May 1983                                      4–3

Trauma is the leading cause of death in children over 1 year of age, with head trauma being the major contributing factor. Recent advances in the management of head trauma have decreased mortality, though it has been predicted that this decline in mortality would be accompanied by a concomitant increase in morbidity in survivors. Data are reported on the long-term outcome in 46 children with significant head trauma observed between January 1976 and December 1979, who remained in coma for more than 24 hours. Two case histories illustrative of the severity of the children's problems and their outcome are presented.

Twelve (38%) of the 46 patients died. These patients were either dead on arrival (group A), or they died of causes not related to the CNS (group B), died as a result of increased cranial pressure (ICP) (group C), or died of other causes (group D). The four patients in group A were believed to be brain dead at the time of arrival; cerebral function did not return despite extensive resuscitative efforts and maintenance of vital functions for more than 24 hours. The one patient in group D appeared to have died because of hypotension. Eleven of the 12 children were declared brain dead. The mean duration of coma in the survivors was 15.5 days. Intracranial pressure was monitored in 10 of the survivors and all underwent computed tomography scanning. The patients were classified according to outcome: return to normal after trauma (class I); learning or behavioral problems (class II), further subdivided into those with similar problems prior to trauma (class IIA) and those reportedly normal before trauma (IIB); handicapping motor residua, but normal intellect (class III); and significant mental retardation, motor problems that could preclude independent functioning, or both (class IV). Of the three class IV survivors, two were less than two years of age and were the only patients in this age group who survived. Ten of 12 children younger than four years of age survived. Of the 34 survivors, 10 were in class I, 11 in class IIA, 7 in class IIB, 3 in class III, and 3 in class IV. Although children who were in a prolonged coma tended to have a poor outcome, 9 of 14 children who were in coma for more than two weeks had little or no handicapping neurologic residua.

The findings indicate that intensive medical and surgical care in patients with serious head trauma does not result in a large number of severely disabled survivors.

▶ This study shows that prolonged coma following head trauma in children has a relatively good prognosis when managed at a facility especially equipped for this problem. Other factors that influence the prognosis are skilled management at the accident site by paramedical teams, rapid transport to the facility, computed tomography scan to detect correctable lesions, and aggressive management to treat increased intracranial pressure. Similar studies on children with Reye's syndrome and near drowning demonstrate the importance of regionalized centers to manage brain injuries in children. The prognosis is usually good for those who survive.—Owen B. Evans

---

**Hypoxic-Ischemic Encephalopathy in the Newborn**
Gerald M. Fenichel (Vanderbilt Univ.)
Arch. Neurol. 40:261–266, May 1983                              4–4

---

Since asphyxia in term newborn infants is nearly always an intrauterine event, hypoxia and ischemia occur together, leading to a hypoxic-ischemic encephalopathy (HIE). The relative contributions of hypoxia, ischemia, and cerebral edema to the brain damage that occurs in infants with HIE remain to be established. Animal models are unable to duplicate exactly the human condition. Brain acidosis increases when ischemia is added to hypoxia. Although brief episodes of partial asphyxia are probably common in normal deliveries, brain damage from asphyxia is relatively uncommon. In mild encephalopathy, symptoms are maximal in the first 24 hours after birth and then decrease progressively, and consciousness is not substantially impaired except for a brief period immediately after birth. Infants with moderate encephalopathy are lethargic or obtunded for at least 12 hours after birth. Those severely affected are stuporous or comatose immediately after birth and have apnea and seizures that progress to tonic and multifocal clonic patterns in the first 24 hours. The infant's condition deteriorates 24–72 hours after birth. Survivors may be stuporous for some weeks and can be expected to have severe neurologic handicaps.

Immediate management requires attention to derangements in multiple organ systems and to systemic metabolic disorders. Infants with moderate HIE, in whom the outcome is undecided, may benefit most from treatment. It has not been documented that treatment of cerebral edema has immediate or long-term benefits in newborn infants with HIE. Even if edema is a secondary phenomenon, it can aggravate tissue necrosis by compromising the microvasculature, and attempts to relieve it are warranted. Suggested measures include fluid restriction, diuretics, hypertonic osmotic agents, and corticosteroids. Corticosteroid therapy, however, is questionable in the setting of cytotoxic edema. The author prefers phenytoin as an anticonvulsant. If necessary, diazepam, paraldehyde, or both can be added on an intermittent basis. There is no evidence that continued treatment prevents epilepsy.

► This is an important, scholarly discussion of the care of the term newborn infant who has had significant perinatal asphyxia. Because newborns at risk for neurologic handicaps resulting from perinatal asphyxia have evidences of derangements of multiple organ systems, the immediate treatment of such infants requires attention to these derangements as well as the use of anticonvulsants when indicated.—R.N.D.J.

### Relationship of Cerebral Intraventricular Hemorrhage and Early Childhood Neurologic Handicaps

Lu-Ann Papile, Ginny Munsick-Bruno, and Anne Schaefer (Univ. of New Mexico)
J. Pediatr. 103:273–277, August 1983
4–5

To determine whether cerebral intraventricular hemorrhage (CVH) is associated with early developmental or neuromotor handicaps, the authors compared the outcome in 198 surviving very-low-birth-weight infants (less than 1,501 gm) with and without CVH as determined by computed tomographic scans.

Developmental assessment was normal in 61 of the infants without CVH, suspect in 43, and abnormal in 11. Neuromotor and developmental testing of these 116 infants without CVH showed that 57 were normal, 46 had a minor handicap, and 12 had a major handicap. Seven of the latter were multihandicapped. Of the 39 infants with a grade 1 CVH (isolated germinal matrix hemorrhage), 33 were alive at one year of age; of these, 16 were not handicapped, 14 had a minor handicap, and three had a major handicap, two being multihandicapped. Nine of 18 infants with a grade 2 CVH (intraventricular hemorrhage with normal ventricular size) had no handicap, 7 had a minor handicap, and 2 had a major handicap. Evaluation of 14 infants with a grade 3 CVH (intraventricular hemorrhage with ventricular dilatation) showed that 2 were normal, 7 had a minor handicap, and 5 had a major handicap, 4 being multihandicapped. Of the 17 infants with a grade 4 CVH (intraventricular hemorrhage with parenchymal hemorrhage), 2 had no handicap, 2 had a minor handicap, 13 had a major handicap, and 10 were multihandicapped. Posthemorrhagic hydrocephalus developed in 22 infants, all with a grade 3 or grade 4 CVH. Ten of these 22 infants had a major handicap and 10 were multihandicapped. The incidence of major handicaps in these infants was similar to that in comparable infants without posthemorrhagic hydrocephalus.

The findings indicate that very-low-birth-weight infants with grades 1 and 2 CVH do not have a higher incidence of major handicaps in early childhood than comparable infants without CVH. However, there is a direct relationship between grades 3 and 4 CVH and major handicaps. Posthemorrhagic hydrocephalus does not increase the risk for major handicaps but does influence the incidence of multihandicaps.

▶ The overall incidence of major neurologic handicaps was approximately 18% in this series. This is somewhat higher than other reports. However, during the second year of the study patients were pre-selected for being at risk of developing hemorrhage. Grades 3 and 4 hemorrhage have a direct correlation with increasing neurologic handicaps. The author suggests that because the hemorrhage is usually large in these groups, brain injury resulted from compromised cerebral blood flow or compression of the periventricular white matter or, possibly, increased intracranial pressure.

The natural history of this disorder has yet to be determined. The study comes close to giving some prognosis for surviving low-birth-weight infants with intraventricular hemorrhage.—Owen B. Evans

---

**A Clinical Neuropathological Study of the Fetal Alcohol Syndrome**
K. Wisniewski, M. Dambska, J. H. Sher, and Q. Qazi
Neuropediatrics 14:197–201, November 1983                                    4–6

---

Fetal alcohol syndrome (FAS) consists of CNS dysfunction, growth deficiency, typical facial dysmorphism, and various major and minor malformations. The clinical features are better known than the pathologic abnormalities. The authors report the autopsy findings in five patients with a clinical diagnosis of FAS who died during the preceding five years. The clinical presentation was typical. The infants died at ages two days to eight months; three died in the first month after delivery. Micrencephalic brains were found in all patients. One infant had gross brain malformation, and all had microdysplasias. Single heterotopias were present in the white matter in two. In four there were glial or glioneuronal meningeal heterotopias and minimal anomalies in the organization of the cortical mantle. The gross malformations in one patient were agenesis of the corpus callosum and underdevelopment of the cerebellar vermis.

The brain is commonly affected in FAS. The spectrum of devclopmental anomalies in FAS is fairly broad, and a definite teratogenic period is difficult to identify. About one third of evaluable patients have had severe brain malformations. Microdysplasias and glioneuronal submeningeal heterotopias are among the frequent findings. Intrauterine growth retardation in FAS is usually accompanied by microcephaly. Reductions in size and weight of the brain, however, are not correlated with delayed brain maturation in these infants. The frequency of micrencephaly in FAS suggests a direct action of alcohol on the growth and development of nervous tissue. The ability of the liver to detoxify alcohol may be a factor.

▶ The developmental changes in the brains and other parts of the body that occur in infants whose mothers drank excessively during pregnancy have been termed the fetal alcohol syndrome. These authors state that not only the influence of alcohol and its metabolites but also undernutrition and the use of other drugs by the mothers should be taken into account as possible etiologic factors.—R.N.D.J.

---

**Questions Concerning Safety and Use of Cranial Ultrasonography in the Neonate**
Ira Bergman (Children's Hosp. of Pittsburgh)
J. Pediatr. 103:855–858, December 1983                                    4–7

---

Ultrasonography presently is the preferred means of assessing the size of the cerebral ventricles and the presence or absence of intraventricular hemorrhage in neonates. Ultrasound is a radiant mechanical force; few studies have attempted to determine whether it can produce subtle or delayed adverse effects. Cranial ultrasound units use real-time scanners that are pulse-echo imaging systems. Biologic effects can result from thermal and cavitational as well as from mechanical mechanisms. Marked heat build-up can occur at tissue-bone interfaces. Ultrasonic energy at very high intensities can destroy tissues, and at somewhat high intensities it can produce hemorrhagic spinal cord lesions. At clinical intensities, it has altered in vitro cell systems and disrupted the development of insect larvae. An increased number of low-birth-weight infants born to mothers having ultrasonography during pregnancy has been reported but not independently confirmed; problems leading to ultrasound study of the mother may have been responsible for low birth weight in these infants.

Risks of ultrasound-induced injury may be increased when embryonic tissues are scanned, when serial scans are made at high peak intensities, or when the intensity is inadvertently elevated. However, ultrasonography appears to be the safest, most convenient, and least expensive available means of imaging the intracranial contents of neonates, and there should be no reluctance to use it in place of CT, which involves ionizing radiation exposure. Caution is needed, however, in extending the use of ultrasound to routine examinations of all premature infants, or to serial examinations of premature infants with or without intracranial hemorrhage. Ultrasonography is indicated only when diagnostic benefit is anticipated. Exposures should be limited to those required to obtain the necessary diagnostic information. Equipment yielding high-quality images at minimal levels of intensity and duration should be used.

▶ Although ultrasonography in the neonate probably is safe, it worries some. It may take decades to prove its safety.—R.D.C.

---

**Clinical NMR Imaging of the Brain in Children: Normal and Neurologic Disease**
M. A. Johnson, J. M. Pennock, G. M. Bydder, R. E. Steiner, D. J. Thomas, R. Hayward, D. R. T. Bryant, J. A. Payne, M. I. Levene, A. Whitelaw, L. M. S. Dubowitz, and V. Dubowitz
AJR 141:1005–1018, November 1983                                    4–8

---

The authors report the nuclear magnetic resonance (NMR) image findings in 8 normal children and in 52 with a wide variety of neurologic disorders. The 28 boys and 24 girls were 13 years of age or younger. Ten had follow-up examinations. Some neonates and young infants were sedated for the study. Saturation-recovery (SR), inversion-recovery (IR), and spin-echo (SE) pulse sequences were used. Neonates also had cranial sonography, and 15 patients had computed tomography (CT).

The good gray-white matter contrast provided by IR sequences provided a means of visualizing normal myelination as well as delays or deficits in myelination. Ventricular enlargement was readily identified. Marginal edema was demonstrated with SE sequences. Abnormalities were seen in cases of congenital malformation, cerebral palsy, aminoaciduria, and meningitis. Space-occupying lesions were identified by increased relaxation times and by their mass effects. Both extrinsic and intrinsic tumors were visualized on NMR imaging.

Nuclear magnetic resonance imaging holds considerable promise for use in pediatric neuroradiology. It is the only imaging method that demonstrates myelination and permits recognition of delayed or impaired myelination. The study can provide useful data in neonates with hemorrhagic and ischemic lesions. Hydrocephalus and marginal edema are readily identified. The technique is better than CT in demonstrating posterior fossa disorders. Disadvantages include the cost of the study, the slow scanning time, and the poor demonstration of calcification. Multislice methods have reduced scanning times. A resistive magnet-based NMR device has been designed specifically for pediatric use.

▶ This study demonstrates that nuclear magnetic response has considerable potential in pediatric neuroradiologic practice, in some cases supplying information not available by CT or sonography.—R.N.D.J.

---

**Development of a Scoring System for the Milani-Comparetti and Gidoni Method of Assessing Neurologic Abnormality in Infancy**
Patricia H. Ellison, Carol A. Browning, Barbara Larson, and John Denny
Phys. Ther. 63:1414–1423, September 1983                    4–9

---

All proposed methods of neurologic assessment of infants are somewhat subjective, and interrater reliability has not been assessed as rigorously as in tests of infant development. A quantitative system could increase the usefulness of any of the methods. The authors developed a scoring system for use with the Milani-Comparetti and Gidoni method of neurologic examination of infants, and they evaluated it in assessing 999 infants confined to neonatal intensive care units for longer than 5 days. Assessments were made at ages 6 and 15–16 months, and at other intervals as scheduled by the physical therapist. Seventy-seven infants were followed to corrected gestational ages of 17–21 months.

Overall, 89 infants were considered neurologically abnormal, and 207 others had scores in the transiently abnormal range. The scoring system was useful in quantifying degrees of abnormality, distinguishing normality from abnormality, and determining different types of abnormalities. Quantification of the neurologic findings is expected to contribute to monitoring programs in neonatal intensive care units in which research is a part of follow-up. The system permits the findings for a given infant to be compared between examinations and permits findings in one group of infants to be compared with those in another. Quantitative scoring also allows more sophisticated data analyses.

▶ The scoring system herein described for the Milani-Comparetti and Gidoni method of assessing neurologic abnormality in infancy separates normal, transiently abnormal, and abnormal infants, quantitates the degree of abnormality, and distinguishes among types of abnormality.—R.N.D.J.

## Intelligence in Epilepsy: Prospective Study in Children

Blaise F. D. Bourgeois, Arthur L. Prensky, Helen S. Palkes, Barbara K. Talent, and Suzanne G. Busch (St. Louis Children's Hosp.)
Ann. Neurol. 14:438–444, October 1983                                    4–10

Many questions regarding the intelligence of epileptic patients are unanswered. The authors report the first prospective study of serial IQ changes in children with seizure disorders. Seventy-two noninstitutionalized children, aged 1½ to 16 years, underwent initial psychological study within two weeks of the diagnosis of epilepsy and then yearly for an average of four years. Over half the children began treatment before initial testing, but most children had used drugs for less than a week and none appeared to have toxic drug concentrations. Forty-five siblings were tested at the time of initial patient evaluation. The average age of patients at initial testing was 7½ years and that of siblings was 9 years.

The mean overall IQ of children with epilepsy on initial evaluation was 99.7, not significantly different from that of siblings. Scores did not change appreciably over time, although eight patients (11%) had a persistent decline in IQ of 10 points or more. Drug levels in the blood of these patients were more often in the toxic range; epilepsy was harder to control in these patients, and their seizures had begun at an earlier age. The best predictors of the ultimate IQ were age at the onset of seizures and number of drugs that became toxic to the patient. Seizure control and total number of seizures were less useful predictors.

The findings suggest that, particularly in younger children, total seizure control should not be sought at the price of repeated episodes of drug toxicity. Drug toxicity appears to be a predictive factor for a reduction in IQ during the follow-up of children with epilepsy. Neither the cause of epilepsy nor the type of seizures was correlated with a reduction in IQ scores in this study.

▶ In this prospective study two factors appeared to be associated with decline in the intelligence quotient in epileptic children: early age of onset of seizures, and a higher incidence of drug levels within the toxic range, probably because both seizures and drug toxicity have a greater impact on the developing brain. The authors suggest that, particularly in younger children, total seizure control should not be achieved at the price of repeated episodes of drug toxicity.—R.N.D.J.

## Reye's Syndrome: 20 Years On

A. P. Mowat (King's College Hosp. Med. School, London)

Br. Med. J. 286:1999–2001, June 25, 1983

The author's current thinking concerning the pathogenesis, diagnosis, and management of Reye's syndrome, an acute, rare disorder of childhood in which vomiting and coma develop three or four days after what seems at first to be a mild viral illness. The cause is unknown. There are laboratory features but usually no clinical signs of liver disease. The coma is associated with cerebral edema without cellular infiltration or demyelination. There are marked regional variations in incidence of Reye's syndrome within the United States. The prodromal illness is usually a viral respiratory tract infection, often influenza B or varicella. Profuse, persistent vomiting is associated with, or rapidly followed by, mental changes and, in some cases, delirium, seizures, and coma. Medullary coning and brain death can occur. The cerebrospinal fluid findings are generally normal. Liver biopsy shows small fat droplets in all cells without significant necrosis or inflammation. The liver returns to normal within a month. Electron microscopic examination shows loss of glycogen, lipid accumulation, and mitochondrial swelling with fragmented cristae and flocculation of the intrametrical protein.

Reye's syndrome is considered to be a self-limited derangement of hepatic mitochondria. The mitochondrial lesion presumably results from a virus-host interaction, perhaps dependent on the genetic make-up of the host and possibly modified by exogenous factors such as salicylate use. Management is nonspecific, with the goals of preventing a rise in intracranial pressure and of minimizing the metabolic abnormalities. The outcome is related to the severity of disease at admission. If only lethargy and slowed thinking are present, correction of any fluid and electrolyte deficit and maintenance of the blood sugar concentration should suffice. Unresponsive patients require intensive medical and nursing care. A cerebral perfusion pressure of at least 50 mm Hg should be maintained by using ventilatory assistance with paralysis, if necessary, and phenobarbital and morphine coma. The usefulness of dexamethasone and mannitol is unclear. Bifrontal decompressive craniotomies can be considered if other measures fail. The best results have been achieved at centers where there is increased awareness of the syndrome both in the community and by physicians.

▶ This is a succinct, practical review of the current concepts regarding Reye's syndrome and the management of patients who have it.—R.N.D.J.

---

**Paraldehyde Therapy in Childhood Status Epilepticus**
Richard G. Curless, Bernard H. Holzman, Eugene Ramsay (Univ. of Miami)
Arch. Neurol. 40:477–480, August 1983

---

Treatment of status epilepticus with phenobarbital, diazepam, or both, given intravenously, can cause respiratory arrest and hypoxic encephalopathy. The authors evaluated the use of paraldehyde as first-line treatment for status epilepticus in children. Thirteen patients aged 5 days to 17 years were studied. Seven were younger than age one year. All but one had received intravenous doses of phenobarbital, phenytoin, or both without benefit before paraldehyde was tried. Paraldehyde was given rectally to three patients, both rectally and intravenously to one, and only intravenously to the others. About half the patients received a loading dose of 0.3 gm/kg. Maintenance was usually with 0.05 gm/kg per hour of paraldehyde as a 4% solution in normal saline. The maximal total amount given was 4.5 gm/kg.

Six of the 16 treatment trials led to good seizure control and 3 to fair control. The patients who responded well received an average total dose of 0.39 gm/kg. Only one of them received an initial bolus of paraldehyde. The response was best in patients without previous neurologic dysfunction. In three patients, all given intravenous bolus therapy, respiratory arrest developed during or a few minutes after the loading dose; all recovered after being intubated. The results of treatment could not be related to the type of seizures or to the EEG abnormalities.

Rectal administration of paraldehyde may be useful for treating children with status epilepticus in whom intravenous access is not readily available. An intravenous infusion of paraldehyde can be effective with minimal complications. The risk-benefit ratio in the youngest patients has been as good as that in older patients, and the drug seems to be safe in the absence of hypotension or significant hepatic or pulmonary dysfunction. Paraldehyde has been especially useful in patients without previous neurologic disorder whose status epilepticus has been refractory to treatment.

▶ Paraldehyde has long been known to be effective in the treatment of status epilepticus, but has been used reluctantly because of its unpleasant side effects and the divergence of opinion with respect to risks, dosages, and routes of administration. These authors report good therapeutic response without complications with intravenous administration.—R.N.D.J.

---

## Childhood Migraine and Motion Sickness

Gabor Barabas, Wendy Schempp Matthews, and Michael Ferrari (Univ. Medicine Dentistry of New Jersey–Rutgers Med. School)
Pediatrics 72:188–190, August 1983                              4–13

---

As many as 55% of adults with migraine have been reported to have motion sickness, and Holguin and Fenichel reported a 23% incidence in children with migraine. The authors assessed the occurrence of motion sickness in 60 pediatric patients with seizure disorders, 60 with migraine, 42 with nonmigraine headache, and 60 with learning disability or perceptual or neurologic impairment without headache. All the groups were matched for age, with an overall mean of 11.1 years. No subject was mentally retarded or had a disorder that would preclude locomotion.

The incidence of reported motion sickness was 45% in the group with migraine and less than 8% in the three control groups. Seventy-three percent of the 37 children with motion sickness had migraine.

Motion sickness is substantially more frequent in children with migraine than among other diagnostic groups of children. It may appropriately be considered a minor diagnostic criterion for migraine. The central mechanisms involved in motion sickness are not well understood, but putative neurotransmitters seem to be involved. Migraine is known to have some relation to humoral disturbances, particularly those related to metabolism of serotonin. Theoretically both peripheral and central mechanisms may be involved in motion sickness and migraine through a common underlying neurotransmitter abnormality that is related to the relative predominance of brain stem cholinergic systems over serotoninergic ones. Hypersensitivity of the semicircular canal receptors to motion may result from intermittent vasoconstriction in the distribution of the basilar artery and ischemia in the region of its labyrinthine branches.

▶ It is suggested that a history of motion sickness may be an additional criterion in the diagnosis of childhood migraine. Hypotheses regarding common mechanisms underlying both conditions are offered.—R.N.D.J.

---

**Myasthenia Gravis in Children: Long-Term Follow-Up**
Moses Rodriguez, Manuel R. Gomez, Frank M. Howard, Jr., and William F. Taylor (Mayo Clinic, Rochester, Minn.)
Ann. Neurol. 13:504–510, May 1983                                    4–14

The natural course of myasthenia gravis in children is not adequately known, and the utility of thymectomy has not been demonstrated. The authors studied 157 patients with myasthenia gravis and analyzed the incidence of remission after treatment.

Of the 157 patients, 149 had experienced onset after one year of age (juvenile group), and 8 had persistent symptoms before one year of age (congenital group). All patients were followed up for at least 4 years; the median time was 17 years, and for thymectomy patients it was 14 years. Disease remission was defined as those instances in which anticholinesterase medication was reduced 50% and the clinical state was ameliorated.

The spontaneous remission rate for the 149 patients with juvenile myasthenia gravis was 22.4 remissions per 1,000 person-years. Figure 4–2 shows cumulative remission percentages for all patients in this group. Transsternal thymectomy was performed on 57% (85 of 149) of the juvenile-onset patients, based on severity of disease. Of this subgroup, 82% had either fulminant or moderate generalized myasthenia gravis. Remissions increased sharply to 260 per 1,000 person-years during the first postoperative year. Patients undergoing thymectomy within 12 months of onset had a significantly better remission rate (326 per 1,000 person-years) than did those who waited more than 12 months (98 per 1,000 person-years) ($P<.01$). In the early thymectomy group, 61% were in remission

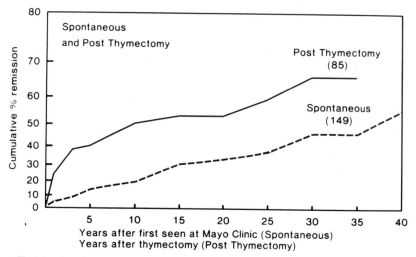

Fig 4–2.—Cumulative percentages of spontaneous and postthymectomy remissions for 149 myasthenia gravis patients less than 17 years old. (Courtesy of Rodriguez, M., et al.: Ann. Neurol. 13:504–510, May 1983.)

three years postoperatively, but only 24% of the late thymectomy patients were in remission at this time (Fig 4–3). Prednisone was given to 24% of the patients who underwent thymectomy and to 6% of the remaining persons. It was helpful in 30% of the thymectomy patients but appeared to be ineffective in the nonthymectomy subgroup.

There were eight patients with congenital myasthenia gravis; their most common signs were ptosis and external ophthalmoplegia. Involvement of bulbar musculature, generalized weakness, and respiratory problems were

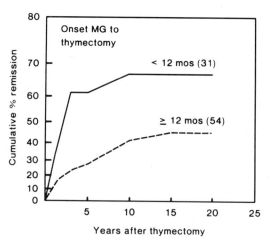

Fig 4–3.—Cumulative percentages of remission for patients who underwent thymectomy 12 months or more after onset of symptoms or less than 12 months after onset of symptoms. (Courtesy of Rodriguez, M., et al.: Ann. Neurol. 13:504–510, May 1983.)

uncommon and usually mild. One patient was treated with prednisone, and another underwent thymectomy. Neither improved, and the other patients were unchanged.

In this study, 80% of the patients with juvenile disease were estimated to be alive at age 40 years, about 90% of the expected survival for the general population. As of 1980, 42 remissions and 25 improvements occurred in the 85 thymectomy patients. In the 64 nonthymectomy patients, 22 remissions and 18 improvements occurred. The variables that influence postoperative remission are early surgery, presence of bulbar symptoms or other immune disease, absence of ocular muscle or generalized weakness, and onset of symptoms between 12 and 16 years of age. As has been noted in other studies, myasthenia gravis is often associated with other diseases, both immune and nonimmune disorders. In this report, epilepsy (four patients) and neoplasia (seven) were the most frequently associated nonimmune diseases; rheumatoid arthritis (five), juvenile-onset diabetes mellitus (three), asthma (three), and thyroid disease (three) were the most prevalent immune disorders.

▶ I have often wondered about the proper way to treat childhood myasthenia. Youssef (see abstract below) has summarized the University of Montreal experience and Rodriguez et al. the large Mayo Clinic patient group. Both found that the thymectomy clearly benefited the patients as compared with the unoperated children. It is possibly not too much to hope that eventually laboratory and clinical methods can be found to determine which youngster with myasthenia will spontaneously remit and, conversely, which one needs surgery.— R.D.C.

---

**Thymectomy for Myasthenia Gravis in Children**
Sami Youssef (Univ. of Montreal)
J. Pediatr. Surg. 18:537–541, October 1983                                    4–15

---

Myasthenia gravis is rare in childhood, and evaluation of treatment is difficult. During a 12-year period the author treated six girls and two boys less than 16 years old for myasthenia gravis. The mean age at presentation was about 12 years. There was no significant family history, and no significant associated diseases were present. None of the six children tested had AChR antibodies. All eight children were taking anticholinesterase drugs, and five received steroids as well. Two required tracheostomy before and one after operation. If possible, thymectomy was done when the disease was stable. All mediastinal thymic tissue was removed via a median sternotomy.

All of the children were alive at follow-up 1–11 years postoperatively. There was no significant postoperative morbidity. Four had acute fulminant myasthenia at the time of operation. None had nonprogressive ocular myasthenia. Thymoma was not present, but lymphoid hyperplasia was found in four specimens. Severe thymic atrophy was present in one child. All six children followed up for three or more years were in complete remission without need for medication. One child improved markedly a year after surgery, but another had a few myasthenic crises following a good initial response.

Thymectomy as soon as possible is recommended for all children except those with pure ocular myasthenia gravis. Thymectomy arrests the progress of the disease and minimizes the occurrence of benign and malignant thymomas, which in themselves are associated with a poor prognosis. Complete removal of all thymic tissue is necessary. Morbidity and mortality from thymectomy in myasthenic patients have declined markedly with improved anesthesia and respiratory care.

---

**Which Children With Febrile Seizures Need Lumbar Puncture?: A Decision Analysis Approach**
Alain Joffe, Marie McCormick, Catherine DeAngelis
Am. J. Dis. Child. 137:1153–1156, December 1983                    4–16

---

The records of 241 children, aged six months to six years, who had a first seizure with a fever were reviewed. All children who had a lumbar puncture or who were available for follow-up were included in the study. The records were reviewed for 12 preselected items in the history, physical examination, and laboratory test results. The patients were divided into those who had cerebrospinal fluid (CSF) pleocytosis and were hospitalized and those who had normal CSF findings and were sent home. The two groups were compared on the basis of the preselected items, and those showing significant differences between the two groups were calculated for the sensitivity, specificity, and positive and negative predictive value.

Thirteen children had CSF pleocytosis, and of these 11 had positive bacterial cultures. The five items that discriminated significantly between those with meningitis and those without were *(1)* visit to a physician 48 hours prior to the seizure; *(2)* seizure upon arrival at the emergency room; *(3)* a focal seizure; *(4)* suspicious findings on physical examination; and *(5)* abnormal findings on the neurologic exam. Examination abnormalities included rash or petechiae, cyanosis, hypotension, and grunting respirations. Abnormal neurologic examination findings included the presence of a stiff neck, altered muscle tone, altered consciousness, focal neurologic signs, and a bulging or tense fontanel.

An abnormal finding on the neurologic exam was the most sensitive item for detecting those children who would have an abnormal CSF. A child who had a convulsion upon arrival in the emergency room had the greatest likelihood of having cells in the CSF. No single item excluded the diagnosis of meningitis with certainty; however, when these factors were used in combination, they detected all cases of meningitis requiring in-patient therapy with a 100% sensitivity and were much more specific than the use of lumbar puncture alone in detecting patients with meningitis. If lumbar puncture had been performed in all patients in whom a single risk factor was present, it would have correctly identified all patients with meningitis, and 62% of the children would not have required the procedure.

▶ This is an interesting study that tries to determine criteria for doing lumbar punctures in children with a fever who have their first seizure. Doing a lumbar puncture on all children with this clinical picture results in a large number of unnecessary procedures. If one can assume that a careful history and physical examination have been performed and that immediate follow-up on children who did not receive a lumbar puncture is available, then the use of these criteria may spare many children from having an unnecessary procedure. In general, the absence of the five risk factors suggests that the child who appears healthy upon evaluation probably does not need a lumbar puncture.—Owen B. Evans

---

**Cerebral Perfusion Pressure in Central Nervous System Infections of Infancy and Childhood**
Kalman J. Goitein and Israel Tamir (Hadassah Univ. Hosp., Jerusalem)
J. Pediatr. 103:40–43, July 1983                                          4–17

---

Infections of the CNS may be complicated by the development of severe brain edema, which can contribute significantly to morbidity and mortality. Increased intracranial pressure can cause additional damage to the CNS by impairing cerebral blood flow, which depends on adequate cerebral perfusion pressure (CPP). When CPP is reduced as a result of elevated intracranial pressure, cerebral ischemia may develop. The authors studied CPP in 17 children, aged 45 days to 11 years; all had severe CNS infections and were in deep coma.

Eleven children (64.7%) had meningitis, five (29.4%) had encephalitis, and one had a brain abscess that developed after chronic, intractable otitis media. Maximal intracranial pressure elevations occurred during the first 36 hours after hospitalization. Eleven children survived and six died; one of the survivors died seven weeks after discharge. The mean blood pressure in survivors was $100.4 \pm 20$ mm Hg, compared with $50.0 \pm 15.8$ mm Hg in those who died ($P<.005$). In two children the shock level blood pressure was a terminal event. The mean maximal intracranial pressure in survivors was $43.3 \pm 19.6$ mm Hg, compared with $63.7 \pm 27.2$ mm Hg in nonsurvivors; this difference was not statistically significant. All children who had a minimal CPP greater than 30 mm Hg throughout the hospital course survived, whereas all with a minimal CPP of less than 30 mm Hg died. Cerebral perfusion pressure in survivors could be maintained adequately by reducing intracranial pressure. In nonsurvivors, however, noncompliance of brain tissue developed, and CPP could not be maintained at levels that would ensure adequate cerebral blood flow, thereby resulting in cerebral ischemia and death.

Continuous monitoring of arterial blood pressure and intracranial pressure is essential to the management of children with severe CNS infections, allowing early initiation of treatment when a decrease in CPP is noted. Maintenance of adequate CPP may be critical in these children.

▶ The treatment of serious infections of the CNS in children by monitoring of intracerebral pressure and providing appropriate therapy to lower it seems to be effective if the pressure responds.—R.D.C.

---

**Computed Tomographic Study of Children With Classic Autism**
Margot R. Prior, Brian Tress, Wendy L. Hoffman, and David Boldt
Arch. Neurol. 41:482–484, May 1984                                        4–18

---

Most workers view autism as a developmental disorder resulting from some organic CNS impairment. The authors performed computed tomography (CT) studies in nine autistic boys aged 9–16 years, all of whom were thought to have definite classic childhood autism. The boys had been symptomatic since infancy and were functioning at a borderline to normal intelligence level. The mean IQ was 87. No child had evidence of organic damage. All did poorly on tests designed to measure left hemispheric functions. Results of the CT studies were considered normal. There was no evidence of any asymmetry that might be related to lateralized cognitive functions.

Previous reports of abnormalities seen on CT in autistic children may have resulted from the inclusion of patients with heterogeneous disorders. Although a failure of CT to show abnormalities does not rule out the presence of structural damage at some level (e.g., in the limbic system), the present findings reinforce the view that autistic behavior can result from a variety of factors and that in patients with "pure" autism there is minimal evidence of brain abnormality of the type that is identifiable on CT scans. It is possible that biologic damage not apparent by present scanning methods is present, or that biochemical abnormalities are operative in autism.

▶ Autism continues to be elusive.—R.D.C.

# 5  Dementia and Aging

## Senile Dementia of the Alzheimer Type

Robert D. Terry and Robert Katzman (Albert Einstein College of Medicine)

Ann. Neurol. 14:497–506, November 1983                                5–1

Severe dementia was identified in about 5% of the population over age 65 in a number of community surveys, and mild to moderate dementia in about 10%. There may be 1.3 million severely demented persons in the United States today. A marked rise in incidence occurs as age 85 is approached. It is difficult to assess the role of genetic factors in the etiology of senile dementia of the Alzheimer type (SDAT). The diagnosis is ultimately a clinicopathologic one. Both primary depression and a reversible state producing cognitive deficits must be ruled out. Symmetric, usually diffuse slowing of EEG pattern is a relatively consistent physiologic correlate of progressive SDAT. Cerebral blood flow is reduced consistently, as in most disorders producing cognitive impairment. Histologic abnormalities are found in the frontal, temporal, and parietal cortex. The findings relating to aluminum in SDAT are complex. Experimental transmissibility has been claimed, suggesting an infectious cause of the disease. Some strains of scrapie agent have induced the formation of neuritic plaques resembling those of Alzheimer's disease when inoculated into the CNS of certain mouse strains.

Common psychoactive drugs are used to manage secondary behavioral problems in patients with SDAT. Treatment with tricyclic antidepressants is reasonably effective in those with intercurrent depression. Neuroleptic drug therapy is sometimes helpful in agitated, sleepless patients, but often at the cost of producing a less responsive person. Acetylcholine precursors have been tried in an attempt to overcome the cholinergic deficit, and cholinergic agonists in an attempt to prevent breakdown of acetylcholine. Gangliosides now are of interest because these drugs may produce increased sprouting and regeneration of injured nerve cells. Other speculative approaches include the use of deferoxamine to chelate aluminum and the use of interferon.

► This is a thorough and timely review of our knowledge of the senile and presenile dementias of the Alzheimer type by two recognized authorities on the subject. In spite of the prevalence of the disease, its etiology is still unknown. The role of aluminum in its etiology is disputed. Inheritance is still not understood. Viral etiology is speculative. Management of the patient is difficult. Substrate therapy has not been effective. Trophic factors, gangliosides, and aluminum chelation therapy are being investigated.—R.N.D.J.

## Alzheimer's Disease: Genetic Aspects and Associated Clinical Disorders

Albert Heyman, William E. Wilkinson, Barrie J. Hurwitz, Donald Schmechel, Alverta H. Sigmon, Tina Weinberg, Michael J. Helms, and Michael Swift

Ann. Neurol. 14:507–515, November 1983                                    5–2

Recent studies of familial factors in Alzheimer's disease have increased interest in the genetic aspects of the disorder. The authors reviewed the clinical and genetic aspects of Alzheimer's disease in 22 men and 46 women who became ill at or before age 70 years. All were seen at the Duke University Medical Center. Dementia was classified as mild in 27 patients, moderate in 28, and severe in 13. Definite brain abnormalities were seen on CT in 45 patients, and results of EEG were abnormal in 37. The probands had classic manifestations of Alzheimer's disease. Information was sought on 136 parents, 298 siblings, 558 nieces and nephews, 140 children, and 146 grandchildren of the probands.

Dementia was identified in 22 (25%) relatives of probands and was distributed among 17 families. The cumulative incidence in both the parents and siblings at age 75 was estimated to be 14%. An affected parent appeared to increase the risk of secondary dementia in siblings, but not to a significant degree. Leukemia was less frequent in first-degree and second-degree relatives than expected. Eleven persons with Down's syndrome were found in the families of six probands. Fourteen probands had a history of thyroid disease or treatment with thyroid hormone; the rate in female probands was 20%. Also, 12% of sisters of the probands had a history of thyroid disease, compared with 6% of sisters of the spouses. Occupational histories failed to indicate exposure to aluminum or other toxic agents. Parental ages at birth of the probands were not significantly different from expected. No excess of hematologic malignancies was found in relatives of the probands in this study.

▶ The results of this study indicate that early-onset Alzheimer's disease is associated with certain genetic factors including a substantial familial aggregation of dementia, an excess of cases of Down's syndrome in relatives, and a possible association with thyroid dysfunction in women.—R.N.D.J.

## CT Assessment of CSF Spaces in the Brain in Demented and Nondemented Patients Over 60 Years of Age

Knut Kohlmeyer and Abdel Raman Shamena (Central Inst. of Mental Health, Mannheim, Federal Republic of Germany)

AJNR 4:706–707, May–June 1983                                           5–3

Computed tomographic (CT) brain scans were performed in 300 patients more than age 60, half with and half without dementia, to obtain data regarding the size of the third ventricle, the lateral ventricles, and the cortical sulca in dementing diseases. The width of the third ventricle, the Huckman number, the ventricular index, and the cella media index were determined; the largest sulci in the frontal, temporal, and parietal areas were also measured, with the sum serving as an approximate sulcal index.

Nondemented patients had an increase in the width of the cortical sulci that corresponded to increasing age. Demented patients did not have this progressive increase; rather, higher values were found consistently in all age groups, although the difference between groups was statistically significant only in those aged 60–64 and 65–69 ($P<.01$ and $P<.05$, respectively). The width of the third ventricle also increased with age in both groups, but values were significantly greater only for demented patients at all ages ($P<.01$ through age 79, $P<.05$ thereafter). The Huckman number also increased progressively with age, but values were significantly greater only in the demented patients in all age groups ($P<.01$). Ventricular index values remained essentially unchanged with age in both groups, but were significantly lower in the demented patients at all ages ($P<.01$). This was also the case with the cella media index ($P<.01$). The strongest statistical relationship observed was for the lateral ventricles, which were of normal size in nondemented patients, but were markedly enlarged in the demented patients.

The findings do not support the contention that there are no correlations in older patients between CT-demonstrated enlargement of the lateral ventricles and intellectual impairment or dementia.

▶ These authors confirm what one instinctively believes. The CT scan of a demented patient is not the same as that of a normal patient of the same age. The combination of ventricular and cortical atrophy gives it its characteristic appearance.—R.D.C.

---

**Syndromes of Amyotrophic Lateral Sclerosis and Dementia: Relation to Transmissible Creutzfeldt-Jakob Disease**
Andres M. Salazar, Colin L. Masters, D. Carleton Gajdusek, and Clarence J. Gibbs, Jr.
Ann. Neurol. 14:17–26, July 1983                                        5–4

---

The clinical features of transmissible subacute spongiform encephalopathy, Creutzfeldt-Jakob disease (CJD), include a rapidly progressing neurologic syndrome of dementia, myoclonus, and pyramidal, extrapyramidal, and/or cerebellar signs with a periodic sharp-wave pattern on EEG. Brains of affected patients contain widespread spongiform changes with gliosis and neuronal loss distributed in a characteristic pattern. Until the transmissible nature of CJD was discovered, many considered its spectrum to include a syndrome of slowly progressive dementia with lower motor neuron (LMN) signs, with or without extrapyramidal signs. Known as the "amyotrophic form" of CJD, the syndrome has never been clearly defined, and its relationship to transmissible spongiform encephalopathy has remained unclear. The authors reviewed data on more than 2,000 cases of CJD and related disorders, which were described in the literature and in their own files (at the Natl. Inst. of Health, Bethesda, Md., and the Univ. of Western Australia, Perth) to clarify this ambiguity.

The clinicopathologic profiles of the 231 patients who had dementia with early LMN signs were distinctly different from those of patients with transmissible CJD: the former patients had a longer illness, and their brains lacked the typical spongiform change. Brain tissue from 33 of the patients with dementia and early LMN signs was inoculated into nonhuman primates, but only 2 specimens from atypical cases transmitted a spongiform encephalopathy; 23 were incubated from 3 to 12 years and were considered to be negative transmissions. These results show that the great majority of cases involving syndromes of dementia and early onset of LMN signs are distinct from typical cases of CJD and do not represent transmissible disease. Occasionally LMN involvement does occur in transmissible spongiform encephalopathy (CJD), but it usually appears late in the course of the disease and in the context of a more fulminant cerebral and cerebellar involvement. However, the syndromes of dementia and LMN disease may be caused by agents acting quite differently from those associated with spongiform encephalopathies.

The authors conclude that the syndromes of dementia and LMN disease are closely related to the more usual forms of sporadic and familial amyotrophic lateral sclerosis (ALS). The clinical and pathologic findings are most consistent with ALS in which the degenerative process extends to involve selectively the extrapyramidal system (substantia nigra) and the cerebral cortex (notably, the frontotemporal areas). Other diseases in which amyotrophy has been reported to coexist with dementia are Shy-Drager syndrome, striatonigral degeneration, olivopontocerebellar atrophy, progressive supranuclear palsy, and some of the spinocerebellar degenerations.

▶ This statement clarifies the relationship of chronic dementia with lower motor neuron signs to the spongiform encephalopathy of CJD. The authors feel that the ALS-dementia complex should be categorized with the more common forms of ALS.—R.D.C.

---

**Alzheimer's Disease: Focal Cortical Changes Shown by Positron Emission Tomography**
Norman L. Foster, Thomas N. Chase, Paul Fedio, Nicholas J. Patronas, Rodney A. Brooks, and Giovanni Di Chiro (Natl. Inst. of Health)
Neurology (Cleve.) 33:961–965, August 1983                    5–5

The authors performed positron emission tomography with $^{18}$F-2-fluoro-2-deoxy-D-glucose (FDG) in 13 patients with clinically diagnosed Alzheimer's disease, nine men and four women with a mean age of 59 years. All had had gradual intellectual deterioration without focal motor or sensory abnormalities. The average duration of symptoms was 3½ years. Dementia was mild to moderately severe. Three patients had predominant language deficits, four had disproportionate failure of visuoconstructive function, and six had chiefly memory loss. The EEG generally showed no localized abnormality, whereas computed tomography showed generalized cerebral atrophy. No patient was receiving medication at the time of the study.

Patients with language dysfunction had markedly reduced glucose metabolism in the left frontal, temporal, and parietal regions. Those with constructional apraxia had a hypometabolic focus in the right temporal and parietal lobes. No consistent asymmetry of hypometabolism was evident in the patients with predominant memory failure. Tests of verbal competence correlated generally with glucose utilization in the frontal and temporal lobes in the left, but not the right, hemisphere. Tests of ability to deal with two-dimensional designs and three-dimensional objects correlated with metabolism in the right parietal lobe. The degree of general dementia did not correlate closely with the mean overall rate of cortical glucose metabolism.

The findings support the view that patients with Alzheimer's disease who have specific cognitive deficits may have focal reductions in cerebral glucose metabolism, as well as a generalized reduction in metabolism. Positron emission tomographic maps of cortical metabolism in relation to performance on tests of language and visuoconstructive skills have yielded patterns generally consistent with classic localizing notions.

▶ Positron emission tomography may help to localize specific brain functions and neuronal dysfunction to a degree not previously possible.—R.N.D.J.

---

**Changes in Brain Ventricular Size With Repeated CAT Scans in Suspected Alzheimer's Disease**
Samuel D. Brinkman and John W. Largen, Jr.
Am. J. Psychiatry 141:81–83, January 1984                                      5–6

Marked variation in ventricular size with normal aging complicates the interpretation of cerebral ventricle size in computed tomography (CT) studies of demented patients. The authors performed serial CT studies in five patients (three women) with the diagnosis of probable Alzheimer's disease. Patients' ages ranged from 59 to 64 years. The diagnosis was based on psychometric evidence of significant memory and cognitive impairment, progressive dementia of insidious onset, and absence of psychiatric and other neurologic disorder and of other known causes of dementia. Multi-infarct dementia was considered to be unlikely. Published normative data were interpolated to estimate the normal rate of change in ventricular size.

Four of the five patients had increases in ventricular size that were markedly greater than the norm over periods of 15–35 months. The patient with a pattern resembling the normative graph had ventricular size markedly greater than normal at both studies.

Marked enlargement of the lateral ventricles occurred over relatively short periods in four of these five patients. Further investigation should use standardized CT scanning techniques to evaluate both demented and normal elderly subjects. A two-year interval between CT studies would seem to be adequate for distinguishing between normal aging and the morphological changes associated with atrophy.

▶ Brinkman and Largen find that a rapid change in serial CT scans that occurs with aging has significance, confirming the findings of Gado et al. (*AJNR* 4:699–701, 1983). The latter investigators also found that the degree of dementia correlates with ventricular size (*AJNR* 4:499–500, 1983) but not with CT brain parenchymal density (*Neuroradiology* 147:703–710, 1983). De Leon et al. (*AJNR* 4:553–556, 1983; ibid. 4:568–571, 1983) found by PET scanning that glucose utilization is reduced in Alzheimer's disease, especially in the region of the third ventricle and the temporal lobes.

Nice recent summaries on Alzheimer's disease and dementia are those by Henderson (*Aust. N.Z. J. Psychiatry* 17:117–127, 1983) and Kokmen (*Mayo Clin. Proc.* 59:35–42, 1984). Of interest is the recent note by Zeisel et al. (*J. Pharmacol. Exp. Ther.* 225:320–324, 1983) who found their laboratory choline and lecithin were contaminated with methylamines, substances that may form nitrosamines which are carcinogens.—R.D.C.

---

**Cerebral Vasomotor Responses During Oxygen Inhalation: Results in Normal Aging and Dementia**
Takahiro Amano, John Stirling Meyer, Takashi Okabe, Terry Shaw, and Karl F. Mortel (Baylor College of Medicine)
Arch. Neurol. 40:277–282, May 1983                                      5–7

---

Abnormal regional cerebral blood flow (rCBF) and abnormal total CBF have been reported in patients with senile dementia of the Alzheimer type (SDAT) and multi-infarct dementia (MID). The authors measured resting regional gray matter flow (Fg) and cerebral vasoconstrictor responses to 100% oxygen inhalation by the radioxenon inhalation method in 84 healthy subjects with a mean age of 55.5 years, 11 patients with SDAT, and 8 with MID. The patients with SDAT had no risk factors for stroke; those with MID had such risk factors. The patients with SDAT had a mean age of 64 years, and those with MID had a mean age of 70 years. Twenty-two of the normal subjects were matched with the demented patients for age.

Linear reductions in oxygen responses were associated with advancing age in the normal subjects. The patients with SDAT had bilateral, symmetric reductions in resting-state Fg values compared with the age-matched controls. Those with MID had no significant reduction in mean Fg values. Oxygen vasoconstrictive responses in the patients with SDAT were symmetric and similar to those in controls, whereas the patients with MID had reduced responses that were asymmetric between the hemispheres and heterogeneous within the hemispheres. Interhemispheric differences in vasoconstrictive responses were significantly greater in this group than in either the patients with SDAT or the normal subjects.

Measurements of resting-state rCBF may confirm the nature of dementia in patients with MID, but testing regional cerebral vasomotor responses during oxygen inhalation is a reliable and safe means of demonstrating asymmetric and inhomogeneous regional responses. These differ significantly from those seen in patients with SDAT and those associated with normal aging. This noninvasive test may be useful in selecting suitable patients for inclusion in therapeutic trials for various types of dementia.

▶ The testing of regional cerebral vasomotor responses during 100% oxygen inhalation is a safe, reliable, and useful means of differentiating between senile dementia of the Alzheimer's type and multiple infarct dementia, and thus of determining the therapeutic approach to the demented patient.—R.N.D.J.

---

**The Frequency of Physical Signs Usually Attributed to Meningeal Irritation in Elderly Patients**
J. A. H. Puxty, R. A. Fox, and M. A. Horan
J. Am. Geriatr. Soc. 31:590–592, October 1983                    5–8

---

Meningitis is difficult to diagnose in elderly patients because they often have nonspecific deterioration without signs of meningitis. Conversely, the presence of clinical signs may be wrongly attributed to a disease process. Nuchal rigidity may be a sign of meningitis. The authors assessed the incidence of nuchal rigidity, Kernig's sign, and Brudzinski's sign in 74 patients aged 17–83 years (mean, 51) hospitalized on an acute care medical ward and in 287 patients aged 62–92 years (mean, 79) confined to acute care or rehabilitation geriatric wards.

Nuchal rigidity was present in 35% of the patients in the geriatric wards, but in only 13% of those in the acute care medical ward (table). Also, 31% of the geriatric patients had nuchal rigidity at night, and 42% had it in the morning; all patients with nuchal rigidity at night were also affected by it in the morning. Overall, 12% of the geriatric patients and 1.5% of the medical patients had a positive Kernig's sign, and all of these also had nuchal rigidity. Brudzinski's sign was positive in 8% of the geriatric pa-

| NUCHAL RIGIDITY IN MEDICAL AND GERIATRIC PATIENTS ON ACUTE CARE WARDS | | | | |
|---|---|---|---|---|
| | Nuchal Rigidity Present | | Nuchal Rigidity Absent | |
| | Patients' Mean Age (Years) | Percentage | Patients' Mean Age (Years) | Percentage |
| Geriatric patients | 81 | 35 | 76 | 65 |
| Medical patients | 72 | 13 | 57 | 87 |

(Courtesy of Puxty, J.A.H., et al.: J. Am. Geriatr. Soc. 31:590–592, October 1983.)

tients, but in none of the medical patients; nuchal rigidity was also present in the former group. Agreement between examiners was 100% for the presence of nuchal rigidity and 89% for its absence. Patients taking psychotropic drugs, or those who had a history of akinetic-rigidity syndromes or cervical arthralgia, did not have an increased incidence of nuchal rigidity. However, nuchal rigidity was strongly associated with a history of cerebrovascular disease, the presence of confusion, an abnormal plantar response, and primitive reflexes ($P<.001$ for all).

Patients with neck stiffness but without a previous history of neurologic deficit or cognitive disorder and without primitive reflexes should be evaluated carefully for meningitis. Nuchal rigidity in patients with prior neurologic deficit, cognitive disorders, or primitive reflexes should be interpreted with caution.

▶ A nice study to solve an old problem: which patient with a stiff neck has meningitis? The authors point out that if stiff neck occurs in an elderly patient who is otherwise neurologically normal, meningitis should be seriously considered; but stiff neck in a patient with a history of neurologic disease, other neurologic findings on examination, and an absence of other signs of meningitis means only that he or she probably has increased tone in the neck muscles, and that's all.

Our knowledge of the neurology of aging has been further supplemented by Impallomeni et al. (*Lancet* 1:670–672, 1984) who found 94% of 200 consecutive patients in a geriatric department had ankle jerks elicited by striking the hammer on the examiner's hand placed against the plantar foot surface. So the ankle jerk does not disappear with aging.—R.D.C.

# 6 Epilepsy and Convulsive Disorders

**Fetal Anticonvulsant Syndrome in Rats: Dose- and Period-Response Relationships of Prenatal Diphenylhydantoin, Trimethadione, and Phenobarbital Exposure on the Structural and Functional Development of the Offspring**
Charles V. Vorhees (Children's Hosp. Research Found., Cincinnati)
J. Pharmacol. Exp. Ther. 227:274–287, November 1983            6–1

The fetal anticonvulsant syndromes thus far described are characterized by growth retardation, minor dysmorphological changes, especially of the facies, and CNS dysfunction. The author attempted to develop a murine model of these postnatal functional defects. First, the lower end of the malformation dose-response curves for diphenylhydantoin (DPH), trimethadione (TMD), and phenobarbital (PB) was established in Sprague-Dawley rats; then, postnatal behavioral teratology studies were carried out using drug doses that did not significantly increase the malformation rate.

All three drugs produced some evidence of postnatal dysfunction at the highest nonmalforming doses when administered on days 7–18 of gestation, whereas substantially lower doses produced no such effects. The use of DPH led to smaller maternal and offspring weight gains and increased offspring mortality; it also was associated with delayed auditory startle and swimming development, decreased adult rearing, and increased rotational behavior. When TMD was given, a small rise in offspring mortality resulted as well as increased adult ambulation and increased water maze errors. Administration of PB increased offspring mortality and may have influenced startle and alternation behavior. Administration of DPH at different phases of gestation showed that the most marked effects occurred during midorganogenesis, and the fewest effects occurred earlier.

Postnatal development dysfunction is produced when DPH, TMD, and PB are administered to rats in doses at or below those that produce low incidence rates of malformations. The findings support clinical observations that these drugs can produce postnatal dysfunction when administered in high doses after prenatal exposure, and they support the concept that the drugs are functional teratogens. Whether epilepsy itself also increases the risk to the embryo or fetus, or interacts with the drugs, remains to be determined.

▶ All three drugs can produce changes in neonatal rat behavior when used in utero in nonmalforming doses. These rats did not have seizures so it cannot be said as it is with humans that the effect was related to the seizure rather than to the medications. Of course the rat dosages were higher than human anticonvulsant dosages.—R.D.C.

---

**Long-Term Outcome in Children With Temporal Lobe Seizures: V. Indications and Contraindications for Neurosurgery**
Janet Lindsay, Christopher Ounsted, and Peronelle Richards (Univ. of Oxford, England)
Develop. Med. Child Neurol. 26:25–32, February 1984                    6–2

---

The authors followed 100 unselected children with temporal lobe epilepsy between 1948 and 1982. Contraindications to operation emerged before the end of school attendance in 42. Ten children were too handicapped for operation to be feasible, and 32 recovered fully without the need for operation. Remission occurred before age 13 in about three fourths of these patients. Among patients with affected relatives, those with a higher IQ were likelier to have remissions (Table 1). Twenty-nine of the other 58 patients were considered for operation, and 13 were operated on. None of the 16 who were rejected for technical reasons made an epileptic, social, or psychiatric recovery.

Four children younger than age 12 years and nine older than age 16 were operated on. Three of the younger patients had hemispherectomies. The other patients had temporal lobectomies. The most common operative findings were mesial temporal sclerosis and cortical dysplasia. All patients were relieved from habitual temporal lobe epilepsy after operation; only two have had occasional grand mal seizures (Table 2). All the adult patients were working regularly at follow-up. None has had lasting psychiatric or social difficulties. Most patients noticed a definite increase in energy and drive. Sexual indifference did not change postoperatively in the four men who were affected.

TABLE 1.—PATIENTS WITH AFFECTED KIN WHO HAD CONVULSIONS BEFORE ONSET OF FOCAL EPILEPSY: DISTINGUISHING FACTORS BETWEEN REMISSION AND NONREMISSION GROUPS

|  | Remission (N = 11) | Non-remission (N = 10) |
|---|---|---|
| Epilepsy both severe and frequent | 1 | 8 |
| Median IQ | 94 | 75 |
| Exclusion from normal school | — | 7 |
| Hyperkinetic syndrome | — | 5 |

(Courtesy of Lindsay, J., et al.: Develop. Med. Child Neurol. 26:25–32, February 1984.)

TABLE 2.—Postoperative Seizure Outcome After Temporal Lobectomy or Hemispherectomy

| Age at operation (yrs) | Pathology | Duration of follow-up (yrs) | Seizure outcome |
|---|---|---|---|
| *Lobectomy* | | | |
| 16 | Mesial temporal sclerosis | 15 | Seizure-free |
| 25 | Mesial temporal sclerosis | 9 | Up to 4 short fits/yr |
| 28 | Mesial temporal sclerosis | 8 | Seizure-free |
| 32 | Mesial temporal sclerosis | 5 | Seizure-free |
| 7 | Astrocytoma | 1 | Seizure-free 6/12; died aged 8 |
| 25 | Mixed astrocytoma/ oligodendroglioma | 10 | Seizure-free |
| 16 | Cortical dysplasia | 10 | Seizure-free |
| 20 | Cortical dysplasia | 6 | Seizure-free |
| 36 | Cortical dysplasia | 4 | Seizure-free |
| 31 | No lesion seen | 8 | Seizure-free |
| *Hemispherectomy* | | | |
| 10 | | 19 | Seizure-free |
| 10 | | 11 | Seizure-free died aged 21 |
| 11 | | 16 | Occasional nocturnal seizures |

(Courtesy of Lindsay, J., et al.: Develop. Med. Child Neurol. 26:25–32, February 1984.)

Operation need not be considered only as a last resort for the treatment of children with temporal lobe epilepsy. Children receiving drug therapy for temporal lobe epilepsy who have had no remission at the time of leaving school should be considered for neurosurgical treatment. Operation should not be delayed when deterioration occurs at an earlier age. A remarkable reversal of the social, intellectual, and character deficits associated with temporal lobe epilepsy may be observed after operation.

▶ The authors favor surgery if childhood temporal lobe seizures do not respond to drug therapy, and they feel that deterioration of behavior, particularly in school, in a child with temporal lobe epilepsy should be a warning that consideration for surgery should not be delayed much longer lest the seizures become permanently fixed.

Hermann et al. (*J. Neurol. Neurosurg. Psychiatry* 46:848–853, 1983) have studied hypergraphia in temporal lobe epilepsy and are not able to confirm the reports of excessive writing tendency in those patients. They carefully analyze the possible causes for their lack of agreement with their predecessors. One can't resist commenting that the hypergraphia may have been more on the part of the observers.—R.D.C.

## Double-Blind Study of γ-Vinyl GABA in Patients With Refractory Epilepsy

Elizabeth M. Rimmer and Alan Richens (Welsh Natl. School of Medicine, Cardiff)

Lancet 1:189–190, Jan. 28, 1984                                              6–3

A functional impairment of inhibitory transmission involving γ-aminobutyric acid (GABA) has been postulated as underlying epilepsy. The authors evaluated γ-vinyl GABA, a specific enzyme-activated irreversible inhibitor of GABA transaminase, the enzyme that metabolizes GABA, in a double-blind, placebo-controlled, crossover study in 24 patients with frequent drug-resistant seizures. The 15 females and 9 males had a mean age of 33 years. They had poorly controlled epilepsy, mainly complex partial seizures with or without secondary generalization. The mean duration of epilepsy was 21 years, and the mean seizure frequency was 5.8 per week at the time of the study. Seventeen patients were receiving more than one anticonvulsant drug. Eight patients were mentally subnormal. Either γ-vinyl GABA or placebo was given for nine weeks, the former in a dosage of 1.5 gm every 12 hours. The mean dose was 48.5 mg/kg.

Three patients were withdrawn, one because of acute confusion in the first week of γ-vinyl GABA therapy. The other patients had fewer seizures during active treatment than at baseline or during placebo administration. Fourteen patients had more than a 50% reduction in seizure frequency, and six had a greater than 75% reduction. Both complex partial and tonic-clonic seizures were reduced by active treatment. Drowsiness and mood changes were more frequent with active treatment than with placebo. Serum phenytoin concentrations were lower during treatment with γ-vinyl GABA. The clinical response could not be related to EEG changes during treatment.

It appears that γ-vinyl GABA holds promise for use in treatment of refractory epilepsy. Toxicity tests, however, have shown vacuolation of white matter in the CNS with long-term high dosage in the rat, mouse, and dog, but not in monkeys; and careful monitoring of this effect will be necessary.

▶ This looks like a step in the right direction. Evidently, GABA levels rise in animals when they are given this enzyme inhibitor. There is little doubt that some day we will have more specific drugs for the epilepsies and these authors' efforts may be pointing the way.—R.D.C.

## Long-Term Follow-Up of Absence Seizures

Susumu Sato, Fritz E. Dreifuss, J. Kiffin Penry, Deanna D. Kirby, and Yuko Palesch

Neurology (Cleve.) 33:1590–1595, December 1983                              6–4

The authors report a follow-up study of 83 patients with absence seizures documented on videotape. The 46 females and 37 males had a mean age of 10½ years at initial evaluation and a mean duration of illness of nearly four years. The mean age at follow-up was 20 years. Overall, 52% of the patients had persistent seizures at follow-up, whereas 48% were seizure free. Persistent absence seizures were present in 42% of patients at follow-up. Of the 26 who were using no antiepileptic drug at follow-up, 2 had persistent seizures. Among 35 patients in the first follow-up study, seizures recurred in 2 of 18 who had been seizure free and ceased in 5 of 17 who had reported persistent seizures.

Univariate analysis yielded four significant prognostic factors. Onset with absence seizures only was associated with a favorable outcome, as were a lack of history of generalized tonic-clonic seizures, an IQ of 90 or above, and no family history of seizures. Multivariate analysis indicated that in patients with absence seizures only, a favorable outcome was related to a lack of absence seizures with mild clonic components and an initial full-scale IQ of 90 or above. All but 3 of 16 patients with both of these factors were free of absence seizures at follow-up.

All types of seizures resolved in about 56% of the patients in this study who were seen initially with absence seizures. There was no evidence that absence seizures were transformed into complex partial seizures. The favorable prognostic factors identified by multivariate analysis for all types of seizures included normal IQ, normal neurologic findings, and a lack of hyperventilation-induced spikes and waves.

▶ The authors point out that more than 90% of patients with three or more of these significant findings from multivariate analysis stopped having absence seizures. Childhood seizures and sports are the subject of two thoughtful comments, one by a committee (*Pediatrics* 72:884–885, 1983) and one by Niall O'Donohoe (*Arch. Dis. Child.* 58:934–937, 1983); the authors of both articles are in general agreement on what a child should be allowed to do. Both agree that swimming and bathing and fishing unsupervised are dangerous, as is rope climbing and the parallel bars; but cycling, tennis, and even the contact sports are probably allowable depending on the balance of seizure control against the child's and parent's desires and fears. The trend is toward more athletic participation by the epileptic child.—R.D.C.

---

**Why Does Epilepsy Become Intractable? Prevention of Chronic Epilepsy**
E. H. Reynolds, R. D. C. Elwes, and S. D. Shorvon (King's College Hosp., London)
Lancet 2:952–954, Oct. 22, 1983                                    6–5

---

In a review of seven hospital-based and two community-based studies, and of their own 10-year prospective study of 106 consecutive previously untreated patients with epilepsy, the authors discuss the prognosis for seizure control. Although the prognosis is good in most patients, in about 25% chronic epilepsy develops. The pattern of chronicity is set early in the course of treatment. Important factors adversely affecting prognosis include the presence of partial or mixed seizure types, abnormal findings on neurologic or mental state examinations, a low IQ, a large number of seizures, and a long duration of epilepsy before referral. The influences of age at onset, presence of EEG abnormalities, and genetic and other factors are less certain. Neurologic, psychological, and social handicaps have the most profound influence on prognosis. Usually, patients who will not respond can be identified within the first two years of treatment; the longer the epilepsy remains active, the less likely is eventual remission. Most patients enter remission early in treatment. One mechanism that may underlie the evolution of chronic epilepsy was proposed by Gowers in 1881, who suggested that every seizure attack is, in part, the result of those attacks that preceded it and is the cause of those attacks that follow it. Chronic epilepsy presents a formidable challenge and may best be prevented by more effective treatment at the onset of attacks.

▶ These authors have taken up a question that bothers most neurologists: Why do seizures become established in some patients and not in others? They found through an analysis of factors that the length of time seizures occurred before proper treatment did influence the likelihood of becoming seizure free. They feel that early adequate treatment may prevent the development of chronic epilepsy. It is difficult for the physician to recommend adequate amounts of anticonvulsants to a youngster who has had only a few seizures, but that appears to be an avenue to eventual control.—R.D.C.

---

**The Treatable Epilepsies**
Antonio V. Delgado-Escueta, David M. Treiman, and Gregory O. Walsh (UCLA School of Medicine)
N. Engl. J. Med. 308:1508–1514, June 23, 1983; 1576–1584, June 30, 1983                                    6–6

---

The onset of a specific type of seizures at a specific age generally distinguishes the treatable epilepsies. Both absence and convulsive epilepsies are considered primary and generalized when the initial clinical and EEG changes suggest involvement of both cerebral hemispheres. Absence is a heterogeneous group of epilepsies. Juvenile myoclonic epilepsy should be distinguished from the difficult-to-treat infantile spasms of West syndrome and the myoclonic seizures of adolescence and adulthood that are part of the untreatable progressive heredofamilial myoclonic encephalopathies. Pure grand mal is the only type of attack in as many as 10% of all patients with epilepsy. Partial epilepsies, or focal epilepsies, are characterized by seizures in which the initial clinical and EEG changes indicate activation of a system limited to a part of one or both hemispheres. Partial seizures in children and young adults are often due to atrophic, nonprogressive structural changes resulting from birth injury or trauma and are therefore amenable to control or even cure. Rolandic epilepsy is a self-limited form of partial epilepsy of childhood.

The goal of antiepileptic drug therapy is to control seizures without producing systemic or neurologic toxicity. Valproic acid is preferred for traditional grand mal seizures, benign juvenile myoclonic epilepsy, and absence epilepsy associated with tonic-clonic seizures. Pure absence seizures are controlled with ethosuximide. Partial epilepsies are treated with carbamazepine, phenytoin, phenobarbital, or primidone. Most adults can safely use phenytoin for effective control of partial seizures, especially if diagnosed and treated early. Candidates for anterior temporal lobectomy are assessed by relating the initial warning symptoms to the nature of the psychomotor attacks as recorded on the EEG and by closed-circuit television. Surgery may be indicated if focal or regional paroxysms in one anterior temporal lobe lead to motionless staring and if there is no evidence of memory impairment (by the Wada test) in the contralateral temporal lobe. Excision of the right anterior temporal lobe is more successful than left-sided surgery, which may impair verbal memory and rote verbal memory. Lobectomy is not indicated for patients whose complex partial seizures suggest an extratemporal lobe origin.

▶ The authors point out that the prognosis in the various epilepsies depends to a large degree on the type, and they therefore go into detail to outline the clinical characteristics of each type. They recommend valproic acid as the drug of first choice for traditional grand mal, a controversial recommendation when one considers the serious liver dysfunction side effect. Coulter (*N. Engl. J. Med.* 309:1456, 1983) in a letter disagreed strongly with their recommendation for several reasons: no comparative study has been done and the cost is higher, and the drug produces side effects; however, the authors respond with more and somewhat convincing data.

Lerman, also in a letter, (ibid. 309:1455–1456, 1983) points out that in his experience, if hyperarrhythmia with infantile spasms is treated early with high ACTH doses continued over long periods, 100% recover in contrast to the feelings of Delgado-Escueta et al. regarding the often poor outlook of that syndrome.

Eldridge (an author of the study abstracted below) also responds by letter in the same issue (ibid. 309:456, 1983). For his late childhood (10 years age of onset) myoclonic recessive epilepsy, valproic acid is the drug of choice, phenytoin causing worsening.—R.D.C.

---

**"Baltic" Myoclonus Epilepsy: Hereditary Disorder of Childhood Made Worse by Phenytoin**
Roswell Eldridge, Robert Stern, Matti Iivanainen, Thelma Koerber, and B. J. Wilder
Lancet 2:838–842, Oct. 8, 1983                                                6–7

---

The authors report the clinical and genetic findings in 15 families in the United States in which one or more living members experienced the spontaneous onset of myoclonus epilepsy in youth, but did not have inclusion bodies of the Lafora type. In all, 528 individuals were identified and 126 were examined.

Of 45 individuals in sibships, 27 were affected, 15 of whom were males (Fig 6–1). None of the parents of these individuals had a history of my-

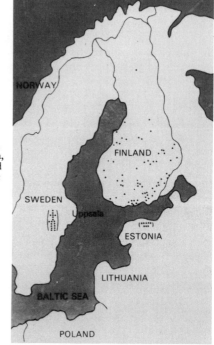

**Fig 6–1.**—Distribution of 127 patients with myoclonus epilepsy living around the Baltic Sea, including 8 from Estonia, 18 from Sweden, and 101 from Finland. (Courtesy of Eldridge, R., et al.: Lancet 2:838–842, Oct. 8, 1983.)

oclonus or generalized tonic-clonic seizures, and most were neurologically normal. One family had three relatives with myotonic dystrophy. In another, the parents were consanguinous. When verifiable, the mean age at onset was 10 years (range, 6–13 years). Myoclonus was the initial presentation in seven patients, generalized tonic-clonic seizures in four, and absence seizures in two. Electroencephalographic changes included prominent spike-and-wave discharges with generalized dysrhythmia. Abnormal activity was invariably induced by photic stimulation. Twenty-six of the 27 patients were given phenytoin at some time. In none was the drug of long-term benefit and in at least nine patients death was associated with its administration. Once treatment with valproate sodium was begun (dose, 15–25 mg/kg), eight individuals had marked improvement in neurologic and intellectual function; four of these eight came from one family. Postmortem examination revealed a marked loss of Purkinje cells in the cerebellum, but no inclusion bodies were detected.

Because the disease was limited to siblings and consanguinity of parents was confirmed in one family and thought possible in another, autosomal recessive inheritance is likely. The progression of disease in these families was more rapid than that described in earlier reports from the Baltic region (Fig 6–2). This may have been owing to a toxic effect of phenytoin, as the drug given alone or with other antiepileptic agents was associated with motor and intellectual deterioration, marked ataxia, and even death. Be-

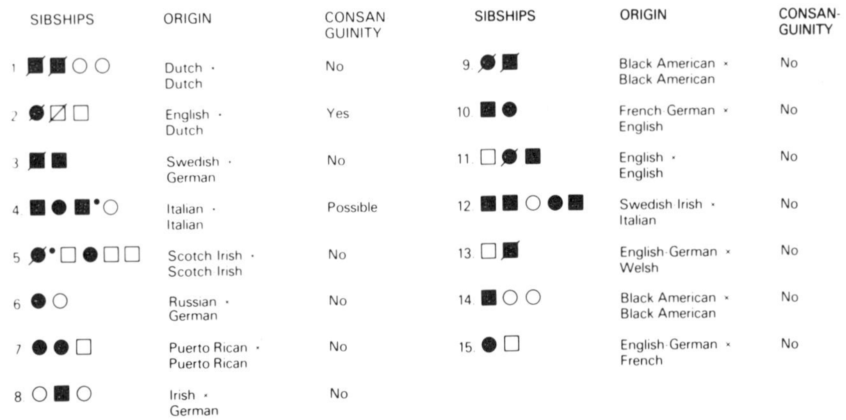

| SIBSHIPS | ORIGIN | CONSAN-GUINITY | SIBSHIPS | ORIGIN | CONSAN-GUINITY |
|---|---|---|---|---|---|
| 1. ■ ■ ○ ○ | Dutch · Dutch | No | 9. ◗ ■ | Black American × Black American | No |
| 2. ◗ ▨ □ | English · Dutch | Yes | 10. ■ ● | French German × English | No |
| 3. ■ ■ | Swedish · German | No | 11. □ ◗ ■ | English · English | No |
| 4. ■ ● ■ •○ | Italian · Italian | Possible | 12. ■ ■ ○ ● ■ | Swedish Irish · Italian | No |
| 5. ◗• □ ● □ □ | Scotch Irish · Scotch Irish | No | 13. □ ◪ | English-German × Welsh | No |
| 6. ● ○ | Russian · German | No | 14. ■ ○ ○ | Black American × Black American | No |
| 7. ● ● □ | Puerto Rican · Puerto Rican | No | 15. ● □ | English-German × French | No |
| 8. ○ ■ ○ | Irish · German | No | | | |

Fig 6–2.—Sibship pattern, geographic origins, and consanguinity in 15 families having 27 family members affected with Baltic myoclonus epilepsy living in the United States. Symbols represent the following: ▨ = male, dead; ∅ = female, dead; ● = affected female; ■ = affected male; • = aborted. Status of firstborn is shown at the left. (Courtesy of Eldridge, R., et al.: Lancet 2:838–842, Oct. 8, 1983.)

cause of the similarity in age at onset, clinical picture, and inheritance pattern in these families and those reported from the Baltic region, the term "Baltic" myoclonus epilepsy is proposed.

▶ This disorder was unknown to me until this note appeared. Reading produces belief, although I am not certain about the authors' conclusion that phenytoin injures Purkinje cells. Such cell loss in epileptics to the point of producing clinical cerebellar disorders was reported before phenytoin came on the scene. There seems little doubt that valproic acid should be the initial treatment for this type of seizure disorder. Eldridge et al. defend this thesis in a response to the review article (see abstract above) on the treatable epilepsies by Delgado-Escueta et al.—R.D.C.

---

## Relevance of a Family History of Seizures
M. Baraitser (Hosp. for Sick Children, London)
Arch. Dis. Child. 58:404–405, June 1983                                         6–8

---

Few types of epilepsy are inherited as single gene disorders; however, most types have a weak genetic component, and the presence of a family history increases the risk of an affected child. For grand mal seizures, if a parent is affected, the risk for a child is about 1 in 25 (4%). This represents a 10-fold increase from such a risk in the general population. If a parent and a sibling have had recurrent seizures, the risk is increased to 10%. In cases where normal parents have given birth to a child who had grand mal episodes, the risk for another such child is about 1 in 25 (4%).

If there is a history of petit mal, the risks are not significantly different from grand mal (4%) for siblings or offspring. Petit mal, when present in families, seldom breeds true; the increased risk is for either grand mal or petit mal. One of 33 children in the general population will have a febrile convulsion. The risk after one affected child is about 20%; if both parents and a previous child had such convulsions, the risk for another sibling increases to 33%. The most common circumstance is the family with a child having infantile spasms. Tuberous sclerosis accounts for about 10%– 20% of such patients. If this is excluded—and it is current practice to have the child examined under a Wood's lamp—the risk of epilepsy in a younger sibling is about 1.5%. There is conflicting evidence about the role of genetic vs. environmental factors in the occurrence of Lennox-Gastaut syndrome; one study has suggested a genetic risk of 7%. In benign epilepsy with rolandic spikes, the seizures are usually self-limiting; a family history is present in about 15% of all patients. If the family history shows a previously affected child, recurrence risks in subsequent offspring may be as great as 30%. In focal epilepsy, there is an increased risk to offspring of only 1%–2%; most of this risk is for generalized epilepsy rather than for focal seizures. Familial epilepsy often responds more readily to therapy than do other types.

▶ This very short article is densely written and has a lot in it. Baraitser gives the risk for a child who is a younger sibling of an epileptic child or for a child with another epileptic relative. A valuable reference for those counseling the parents of children with seizures.—R.D.C.

---

### The Sunflower Syndrome: A New Look at "Self-Induced" Photosensitive Epilepsy

Frances R. Ames (Groote Schuur Hosp. Observatory, Cape Town, South Africa) and David Saffer (Baragwanath Hosp., Johannesburg, South Africa)
J. Neurol. Sci. 59:1–11, April 1983 6–9

---

The authors report data on a mother and daughter who manifested heliotropism and arm rocking movements. The mother was sensitive to flicker, but the child was unique in initially being insensitive to flicker despite frequent heliotropic attacks. Her movements therefore cannot be interpreted as an attempt to induce epilepsy.

Girl, 13, white, had for four years manifested "hand-waving" attacks in sunlight occurring now four or five times monthly. An epileptic maternal great aunt had had generalized seizures starting at age 10 and continuing until death, during a seizure, at age 30. Her mother had identical sun-induced attacks, occasional generalized seizures, and migraine. Her older sister (aged 15) had had two generalized epileptic seizures a year ago and her EEG showed nonspecific slowing without evidence of photosensitivity. The patient had several EEGs done at ages 10–14; all except the last showed similar features. Photic stimulation with a Beckman model 5561 radiating white diffuse light with a flash intensity of 0.6 J, a duration of 10 msec, and a stimulation distance of 25 cm failed to provide conclusive evidence of photosensitivity at age 10 years (Fig 6–3) or at ages up to 14. At age 14, although no abnormalities were noted during monocular or binocular photic

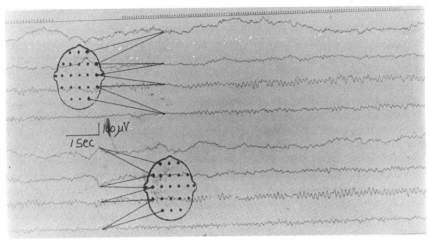

Fig 6–3.—No evidence of photosensitivity during intermittent photic stimulation in 1977 at age 10 years. (Courtesy of Ames, F.R., and Saffer, D.: J. Neurol. Sci. 59:1–11, April 1983.)

stimulation with eyes open, the response to binocular stimulation with the eyes closed was repeatedly abnormal (Fig 6–4). None of the subjective feelings noted during the heliotropic spells and no arm or any other movements occurred.

Both mother and daughter manifested two unusual episodic, stereotyped forms of abnormal behavior; one form was epileptic, of short duration, and photically induced, and the other was periodic prolonged circling not photically induced but audiogenically augmented. The attacks in both mother and daughter were unusually complex, involving arrest, heliotropism, oculoversion, torticollis or retrocollis or both, tonic posturing and repetitive movements of one arm, visual hallucinations and illusions, and absences. The profusion of symptoms and signs during attacks indicates regional discharge. One region from which such diverse effects could arise is the cingulate gyrus.

In these two patients, glaring sunlight forced the panoramic looking that involves posterior parietal area 7, which has rich reciprocal connections with the limbic lobe, including the cingulate area. Heliotropism was accompanied by arm posturing and repetitive movements that brought the abducted fingers back and forth across the eye ipsilateral to the direction of gaze. These movements may indicate seizure discharge in the cingulate circuit. There was no history of ischemic damage to the anterior cerebral artery or evidence of structural abnormalities to explain the putative cingulate involvement.

The adjective "self-induced" distorts clinical perception and encourages speculation that is premature at the present state of knowledge. This complex syndrome merits meticulous neurophysiologic and neurochemical investigation. The name "sunflower syndrome," which at least directs attention to the link between sunlight, movement, and growth in all living things, is preferred.

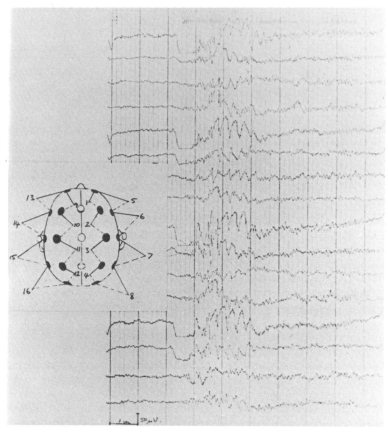

Fig 6–4.—Photoconvulsive response during intermittent photic stimulation in 1982, at age 14. (Courtesy of Ames, F.R., and Saffer, D.: J. Neurol. Sci. 59:1–11, April 1983.)

▶ These patients manifested apparent self-induced photosensitive epilepsy that was actually not self-induced. There is no question that some patients clearly induce seizures, but it is worth pointing out that not all that appear self-induced are. The patients described by the authors must be a minority.—R.D.C.

---

**Phenytoin and Folic Acid Interaction: A Preliminary Report**
Mary J. Berg, Lawrence J. Fischer, Michael P. Rivey, Boris A. Vern, Robert K. Lantz, and Dorothy D. Schottelius
Ther. Drug Monit. 5:389–394, 1983                                   6–10

Long-term phenytoin therapy sometimes reduces concentrations of folate in serum, red blood cells, and cerebrospinal fluid, necessitating folic acid supplementations. The addition of folic acid leads to a fall in plasma phenytoin concentration. The authors examined the effects of a one-mg daily dose of folic acid on the disposition of phenytoin in five male folate-deficient seizure patients treated only with phenytoin. Each had a serum folate concentration of less than 3 ng/ml and a stable seizure disorder. Free and total plasma phenytoin concentrations and urinary metabolite values were measured before and after folic acid therapy was started at a morning oral dose of 1 mg. Four patients completed 15 days of study.

Three of four evaluable patients had decreases in both total and free phenytoin concentrations after folic acid therapy. The serum folate concentration returned to normal in three patients. The extent of the fall in plasma phenytoin concentration correlated with the Michaelis-Menten parameter, $K_m$. The ratios of urinary metabolites to parent drug increased when the plasma phenytoin concentration decreased after folic acid supplementation. The percentages of phenytoin and metabolites excreted in 24-hour urine samples did not change consistently with folic acid administration.

The findings suggest a folic acid–associated increase in the oxidative metabolism of phenytoin in seizure patients given phenytoin only, with folate supplementation. Folate deficiency may limit hepatic enzyme induction, and supplementation may restore the capacity to metabolize enzyme-inducing drugs such as phenytoin. The change in total plasma phenytoin concentration appears to depend on the $K_m$ value for the given patient when folate is added in an oral daily dose of 1 mg.

▶ It is important to understand the interaction between folic acid and phenytoin, because half of the epileptic patients given the latter as an anticonvulsant will develop folate deficiency. If folic acid supplementation is used to compensate for the deficiency, the phenytoin dosage may have to be increased.— R.N.D.J.

---

**Antiepileptic Drug Therapy: Fine Tuning the Dosage Regimen**
Timothy E. Welty, Nina M. Graves, and James C. Cloyd (Univ. of Minnesota)
Postgrad. Med. 74:287–305, November 1983                                          6–11

Epilepsy affects more than two million Americans. Recent advances in antiepileptic drug therapy have led to significantly improved management; however, therapeutic drug monitoring is complicated by several factors, including individual seizure frequency patterns, the varying therapeutic ranges of the drugs used, and differences in absorption and metabolism of these drugs. Some patients benefit from minimal concentrations of antiepileptic drugs, whereas others require levels above the therapeutic range. Close monitoring is especially important at the start of treatment, during dose or drug changes, and at various disease states. Many disorders influence antiepileptic drug concentrations, and frequent measurements are necessary when a patient's homeostasis changes. Serum drug levels should be estimated whenever a change in dose or form is made, or when concomitant drug therapy is modified.

Phenytoin has a broad range of activity and is approved for use in patients with generalized tonic-clonic and partial seizures. The therapeutic range is about 10–20 mg/L, but variability may be caused in part by individual differences in free drug concentrations. The initial maintenance dose is based on body weight. Treatment for two to four weeks may be necessary to produce steady-state conditions. Dose adjustments should be made cautiously. Carbamazepine is being used on an increasing basis. The full adult maintenance dose is 7–15 mg/kg daily, but treatment is begun with a dose that is 25% of the targeted maintenance dose, increased at weekly intervals. Phenobarbital is effective against most seizure types except for absence seizures; however, it has unpredictable effects in children. Elimination of the drug is prolonged, and achievement of therapeutic serum levels may be delayed unless a loading dose is given. Adult maintenance doses are 2–4 mg/kg daily. Valproic acid is approved for the treatment of absence seizures. A loading dose is seldom necessary, and the initial recommended maintenance dose for both adults and children is 10–15 mg/kg daily. Rapid absorption and elimination of the drug make single serum level estimates difficult to interpret.

▶ Because of some unique characteristics of the commonly used antiepileptic drugs and of epilepsy itself, fine tuning of the dosage regimen on the basis of drug concentrations in serum is crucial to achieving seizure control without signs of toxicity.—R.N.D.J.

---

### Monitoring Phenytoin in Salivary and Plasma Ultrafiltrates or Pediatric Patients

Kenneth Bachmann, Robert B. Forney, Jr., and Kytja Voeller
Ther. Drug Monit. 5:325–329, September 1983                6–12

The authors determined the extent of plasma protein binding of phenytoin and the relation between salivary and plasma unbound drug levels in pediatric patients and assessed the value of using salivary measurements in monitoring treatment. Patients aged 2 to 16 years who received phenytoin, alone or with valproic acid, for seizures on an outpatient basis were included in the study. Paired samples of plasma and saliva were ultrafiltered and analyzed by a gas-liquid chromatographic procedure.

Mean phenytoin free fraction was 9.2% in 46 studies of 29 patients who received phenytoin only. Concurrent valproic acid therapy increased mean free phenytoin fraction to 13.2%, a significant elevation. Correlation between concentrations of phenytoin in salivary and plasma ultrafiltrates was excellent, with a correlation coefficient of 0.96. Mean ratio of levels of salivary to plasma ultrafiltrates in 25 patients was 1.06. Mean coefficient of intraindividual variation in free phenytoin fraction, determined three to six times in six patients taking phenytoin only, was 19.2%.

Levels of phenytoin in salivary ultrafiltrates were closely similar to those in plasma ultrafiltrates in children in this study. The substantial intraindividual variation in phenytoin free fraction and the increase in free fraction seen in patients who also received valproic acid indicate the importance of using unbound plasma levels in monitoring phenytoin. Measuring the concentration in salivary ultrafiltrates can provide a practical noninvasive means of monitoring phenytoin therapy in children. Parents can be trained to collect samples after seizure episodes. Values of unbound plasma phenytoin can be used in monitoring patients taking other anticonvulsants as well, particularly valproic acid.

▶ The close agreement between plasma and salivary ultrafiltrate phenytoin concentrations suggest that the latter should provide a practical, noninvasive means of monitoring phenytoin, especially in pediatric patients.—R.N.D.J.

---

**Painful Epileptic Seizures**
G. Bryan Young and Warren T. Blume (Univ. of Western Ontario)
Brain 106:537–554, September 1983                                6–13

The authors reviewed data on 24 cases of painful seizures that occurred among a total of 858 epileptic patients (2.8%). The patients used the term "pain" to describe a symptom that occurred first or among a series of ictal events. Patients with only postictal pain such as headache or with preictal pain that did not seem to be part of the seizure were not included in the study. Six female and 4 male patients aged 11–35 years had unilateral pain in the face, arm, leg, or trunk. One case is described below.

Girl, 14, with congenital left hemiparesis had developed seizures at age 10 which began with "burning, tingling pain" in the left forearm and progressed to "shooting pain" in the left shoulder and sometimes to macropsia and a generalized tonic-clonic seizure. Paresis was most marked in the left arm and hand, and the hand was analgesic and anesthetic distal to the wrist. Pinprick sensation was reduced in the rest of the extremity and in the left upper chest, neck, and lower face. Position sense was impaired in the left wrist. A seizure recorded on the EEG showed reduced voltage in the right central region just before the start of left arm pain, followed by quasiperiodic right central sharp waves.

At operation an area of shrunken gliotic cortex was found in the right postcentral gyrus and superior temporal area. Stimulation just above this area (Fig 6–5) produced tingling in the left forearm. Cortical epileptiform activity was present superior and posterior to the gliotic area. Resection of the atrophic area and the immediately adjacent cortex relieved the patient of seizures. The sensory deficit was slightly increased. The cortex exhibited a disorganized neuronal arrangement with dense gliosis and foci of calcification.

Six female and five male patients aged 10–46 years had pain restricted to the head. One female and two male patients aged 15–20 years had central abdominal pain. Unilateral pain consistently implicated ictal involvement of the contralateral rolandic region at the time pain was present, and in most cases pain probably was due to involvement of the primary somatosensory cortex. Cephalic pain did not localize the site of seizure origin; it probably arose through a vascular mechanism in most cases. Abdominal ictal pain reflected epileptic activity of the temporal lobe; it is unlikely to be due to a peripheral mechanism.

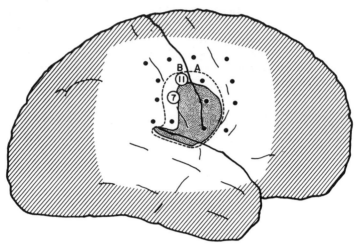

Fig 6–5.—Nonlined area was exposed at operation. Dashed line delimits excision. Stippled area is atrophic gliotic cortex. Stimulation at *A* produced flexion of forearm and hand and at *B*, left forearm tingling. Solid dots represent placement of electrocorticogram electrodes. Principal spikes were recorded at *7* and *11*. (Courtesy of Young, G.B., and Blume, W.T.: Brain 106:537–554, September 1983.)

▶ While relatively rare in occurrence, localized pain is occasionally a symptom of epileptic seizures. This study demonstrates that unilateral pain may be associated with ictal involvement of the contralateral rolandic region, probably as a result of the presence of an epileptogenic lesion in the somatosensory cortex, and that abdominal pain appears to reflect temporal lobe involvement. Cephalic pain did not, in this study, localize the site of seizure origin and probably arises by means of a vascular mechanism.—R.N.D.J.

**Phenobarbital Compared With Carbamazepine in Prevention of Recurrent Febrile Convulsions: A Double-Blind Study**
Jayne Henly Antony and Simon H. B. Hawke
Am. J. Dis. Child. 137:892–895, September 1983                          6–14

Proper treatment of febrile seizures remains controversial, but alternative drugs have been sought because of the behavioral side effects of phenobarbital and the hepatotoxicity of valproate sodium. The authors undertook a double-blind study comparing phenobarbital with carbamazepine in 72 children seen in 1977–1981 at Royal Alexandra Hospital for Children, Sydney, Australia, with recurrent febrile convulsions. All had had at least two febrile seizures, complex seizures, neurologic or developmental abnormalities, or were aged one year or younger at the onset of febrile seizures.

The initial doses of phenobarbital were 4–5 mg/kg daily and of carbamazepine, 20 mg/kg daily; both were divided into twice daily doses. The therapeutic ranges were 14–23 mg/L of phenobarbital and 5–9 mg/L of carbamazepine. Thirty-two patients received each of the drugs. Forty patients had adequate serum drug levels.

Nine of 19 (47%) evaluable patients given carbamazepine had febrile seizures. Five of the nine had recurrent seizures, and two were withdrawn from the trial and subsequently remained free of seizures on phenobarbital. Two (10%) of 21 phenobarbital-treated patients had a single febrile seizure. Covariant analysis confirmed the superiority of phenobarbital in preventing recurrent febrile seizures.

Most side effects occurred in the first six months of treatment. Five phenobarbital-treated patients and three who were given carbamazepine had unacceptable side effects. Nearly all the side effects of phenobarbital were related to overactivity. Four patients received carbamazepine after being overactive while on phenobarbital and three of them had recurrent febrile convulsions.

Carbamazepine appears to be less effective than phenobarbital in preventing recurrent febrile convulsions in children. Its effect on antidiuretic hormone may be responsible because low levels of serum sodium have been observed in some children with febrile seizures.

▶ These results confirm previous reports suggesting that carbamazepine is not as effective as phenobarbital in the prophylactic treatment of recurrent febrile convulsions in children.—R.N.D.J.

---

**Complex Partial Seizures: Clinical Characteristics and Differential Diagnosis**
William H. Theodore, Roger J. Porter, and J. Kiffen Penry (Natl. Inst. of Health, Bethesda, Md.)
Neurology (Cleve.) 33:1115–1121, September 1983    6–15

---

Most patients with complex partial seizures may be diagnosed incorrectly at referral. The authors studied 163 complex partial seizures in 40 patients who had been referred with medically intractable seizures. The 22 male and 18 female subjects had a mean age of 26 years. Seizures had begun at a mean age of 11½ years. Twenty-eight patients reported generalized tonic-clonic seizures. Five patients had a history of head injury, three had had neonatal complications, two had brain tumors, and four had infections of the CNS. One patient had an arteriovenous malformation and one had an arachnoid cyst. Ten patients exhibited intellectual impairment, but only two had localizing neurologic findings.

Mean duration of seizures was about two minutes. Distinct ictal and postictal phases usually could be distinguished; mean ictal phase lasted 54 seconds. Auras were uncommon. Automatisms were seen in nearly all instances, and 81% of seizures included automatisms of the legs and trunk. Two patients exhibited "violent" automatisms. Lapses were seen in 11 seizures in 9 patients. Only 13 patients were occasionally aware of having had a seizure. Eight patients had clusters of seizures. Seven patients had distinct postictal aphasia after 12 seizures. No specific electroclinical correlations were observed.

Complex partial seizures are short and are followed by postictal confusion. The automatisms usually are stereotyped, "primitive," and undirected. Complex partial seizures are most apt to be confused with absence seizures, but their clinical features distinguish them from other types of seizures and pseudoseizures.

▶ Complex partial seizures are short in duration, relatively uncomplicated, and often overlooked or undiagnosed. Videotape analysis provides objective criteria by which they may be identified and differentiated from other seizure types.— R.N.D.J.

---

**Clinical and EEG Estimates of Absence Seizure Frequency**
Thomas R. Browne, Fritz E. Dreifuss, J. Kiffin Penry, Roger J. Porter, and Billy G. White
Arch. Neurol. 40:469–472, August 1983                    6–16

The frequency of absence seizures is difficult to measure because of the brevity of most attacks, the minimal clinical manifestations, and the lack of reliability of parents in estimating the frequency. The authors compared various methods of estimating absence seizure frequency in 20 patients, aged 5–15 years, none of whom had previously received antiabsence medication. Seven patients were receiving phenytoin, primidone, or both, or phenobarbital for other types of coexisting seizures. Patients received placebo capsules and then 250 mg of ethosuximide three times daily in the hospital. If the frequency of seizures was not reduced by half in a week, the dosage was raised up to 1,500 mg daily. Mothers, nurses, and physicians or other trained observers estimated the frequency of attacks, and these estimates were combined with the physical and neurologic findings and the routine EEG to form a seizure index. Further, telemetered EEG studies were carried out for 12 hours in all but three patients.

Both the seizure index and the telemetered EEG estimates of seizure frequency were greater than mothers' estimates in most cases, both in the placebo period and during treatment. Trained observers found more seizures than the mothers in most cases during the placebo period, but the difference was less great during treatment. Mothers found more seizures than nurses in 16 of the 20 cases during the placebo period; there was little difference during treatment. The telemetered EEG showed the most seizures during both periods. Agreement between the telemetered EEG and other measures of seizure frequency ranged from 65% to 75%.

The telemetered EEG is the most reliable means of estimating the frequency of absence seizures. Intensive observation is the next best method. Neurologic examination and the routine EEG diagnosed absence attacks in all cases in this study and adequately determined if attacks were completely controlled by treatment in all but 2 of the 20 patients.

▶ Telemetered EEG recordings are necessary for accurate determination of absence seizure frequency and to determine drug effectiveness and adequacy of treatment.—R.N.D.J.

---

**Sexual Automatisms in Complex Partial Seizures**
Susan S. Spencer, Dennis D. Spencer, Peter D. Williamson, and Richard H. Mattson (Yale Univ.)
Neurology (Cleve.) 33:527–533, May 1983                                    6–17

---

Sexual manifestations of complex partial seizures may include automatisms, emotions, or somatosensory phenomena in the genitals. The authors report findings in four patients who experienced sexual automatisms in some or all of their seizures and who had evidence of frontal lobe abnormality. The electrode positions used are shown in relation to the important anatomical sites in Figure 6–6. The patients were among 61 seen with medically refractory complex partial seizures and were among 14 who had frontal lobe seizure foci on depth EEG study, or radiologic evidence of a structural lesion in the frontal lobe. Some patients had sexual automatisms only in some seizures, and they often were not reported by the family or the patient. Three patients had a frontal lobe seizure origin documented by depth EEG recording, and one had a calcified lesion. Frontal lobectomy revealed abnormal pathology in three patients and was followed by a reduction of 75%–100% in seizure frequency. The automatisms in these patients took the form of grasping and manipulating the genitals and pelvic thrusting.

Sexual automatisms in epilepsy are not common. Only five previous

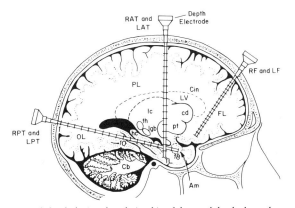

**Fig 6–6.**—Anatomical sketch depicts the relationship of the usual depth electrode array to significant cerebral structures. *RF, LF* = right and left frontal electrodes; *RAT, LAT* = right and left anterior temporal electrodes; *RPT, LPT* = right and left posterior temporal electrodes; *FL* = frontal lobe; *Cin* = cingulate gyrus; *PL* = parietal lobe; *OL* = occipital lobe; *LV* = lateral ventricle; *cd* = caudate; *pt* = putamen; *Ic* = internal capsule; *th* = thalamus; *lgb* = lateral geniculate; *hc* = hippocampus; *Am* = amygdala; and *Cb* = cerebellum. (Courtesy of Spencer, S.S., et al.: Neurology (Cleve.) 33:527–533, May 1983.)

reports of patients with clearly described sexual automatisms were found; the temporal lobe was the presumed site of origin of the seizures in all five, but the only patient studied pathologically had extension of tumor into the frontal lobe. The present patients all had a frontal lobe seizure origin. Surface EEG recordings suggested anterior temporal foci in two of the four patients. It is possible that the association area for the sexual emotion or the sexual aura is localized in the temporal lobe part of the limbic system, whereas the physical manifestation of sexuality, or automatism, is limited to the frontal lobe input into the limbic system.

▶ Sexual manifestations (automatisms, emotions, or somatosensory phenomena in the genitals) have long been thought to originate in the temporal or parietal lobes. This careful study, however, shows that in the patients under observation, sexual automatisms did not occur in patients with seizures originating in any area other than the frontal lobe.—R.N.D.J.

## A Double-Blind Study Comparing Carbamazepine With Phenytoin as Initial Seizure Therapy in Adults

R. Eugene Ramsay, B. J. Wilder, Joseph R. Berger, and Joseph Bruni
Neurology (Cleve.) 33:904–910, July 1983                    6–18

Carbamazepine compares favorably with phenytoin in double-blind, crossover studies. The authors evaluated the efficacy and safety of these agents when used as initial treatment in patients older than 17 years of age with generalized or partial epilepsy. A double-blind, two-compartment, parallel design was used, and all patients were followed up for at least six months. The initial dose of carbamazepine was 200 mg twice daily, and that of phenytoin was 100 mg twice daily. The maximal daily doses were 1,200 mg of carbamazepine and 600 mg of phenytoin. Of the 87 study patients, 37 had partial seizures only, and 27 had generalized seizures only.

Major side effects occurred in 23% of patients in each study group. A rash was the most frequent effect. One phenytoin-treated patient had severe exfoliative dermatitis. One carbamazepine-treated patient had marked cognitive impairment even though plasma levels of the drug were low. Minor side effects were common with both drugs, the most frequent being nystagmus. Five treatment failures occurred in the carbamazepine group and four in the phenytoin group. Failures were not related to seizure type. The mean blood drug levels in successfully treated patients at weeks 8–24 were 9–11 $\mu$g/ml in the phenytoin group and 4.7–6.5 $\mu$g/ml in the carbamazepine group.

Carbamazepine was as effective as phenytoin in controlling partial and generalized seizures in these patients. Overall rates of major and minor side effects were comparable with the two drugs. Carbamazepine should be considered a major anticonvulsant for use as the initial and only drug in patients with these types of seizures. A single drug can provide control in 85% of compliant patients who are adequately treated early in the course of the disorder.

▶ It is useful to know that carbamazepine and phenytoin are equally safe and effective in the single-drug therapy of generalized and focal epilepsy.—R.N.D.J.

---

**Should Alcohol Withdrawal Seizures Be Treated With Antiepileptic Drugs?**
M. E. Hillbom and M. Hjelm-Jäger (Karolinska Hosp., Stockholm)
Acta Neurol. Scand. 69:39–42, January 1984                                6–19

---

Carbamazepine, phenytoin, and valproic acid are often used (sometimes in conjunction with sedatives) in treatment and prevention of alcohol withdrawal syndrome. The authors reviewed data on 292 randomly selected patients, including 46 women, who were admitted to an alcoholism treatment facility for two weeks over a 16-month period. Age range was 23–79 years. The patients had used alcohol heavily for at least a week before admission, and all had minor symptoms of alcohol withdrawal syndrome. Two thirds of the patients received combined treatment with an anticonvulsant and a sedative-hypnotic. Typically oxazepam, pentobarbital, or clomethiazole was given for four to six days, with carbamazepine or phenytoin for at least a week. The anticonvulsant dose was gradually reduced after the sedative-hypnotic drug was discontinued.

Seizures and delirium tremens occurred during detoxification in 3% of patients. The overall frequency of seizures, including those occurring just before admission, was 10%. Seizures were more frequent in patients with previous brain injury. Several patients with seizures had taken high doses of benzodiazepines with alcohol or had used prescribed phenytoin intermittently, both with and without alcohol, or had taken toxic doses. Half the patients with delirium tremens had previously been treated for delirium. None of them had seizures during detoxification. Six of the eight patients had a history of brain injury and withdrawal seizures.

The use of psychotropic drugs, including nonsedative anticonvulsants, appears to increase acute seizure problems in patients with alcohol withdrawal symptoms. Withdrawal seizures do not warrant use of anticonvulsants out of the hospital. Intermittent alcohol abuse may be related to increasingly severe symptoms of alcohol withdrawal, including seizures. Both erratic drug-taking and drug-alcohol interactions may contribute to seizures in this setting. Patients with delirium tremens can be efficiently and safely treated with clomethiazole taken orally.

▶ These authors may have settled a question that has always concerned me. Should we or should we not recommend anticonvulsant therapy for the alcoholic who has had a seizure before coming to the hospital or who has one in the hospital? The authors feel that giving the patient anticonvulsants only adds an extra hazard, since the patient will forget the medication when he goes on a binge and thus increase the tendency to seizures when he stops drinking. Double withdrawal. So they don't do it, and I am inclined to agree with them.—R.D.C.

---

**A Prospective Evaluation and Follow-Up of Patients With Syncope**
Wishwa N. Kapoor, Michael Karpf, Sam Wieand, Jacqueline R. Peterson, and Gerald S. Levey (Univ. of Pittsburgh)
N. Engl. J. Med. 309:197–204, July 28, 1983                                              6–20

---

The authors studied 204 patients with syncope to determine how often a cause could be established together with a prognosis. Syncope was defined as sudden loss of consciousness associated with an inability to maintain postural tone that was not compatible with a seizure disorder, vertigo, dizziness, coma, shock, or other states of altered consciousness. Patients who required pharmacologic or electric cardioversion at initial presentation were excluded from the study. Mean age was 55.8 ± 19.6 years (range, 14–90 years); 119 patients were female and 85 male. Within one day of their only or last syncopal episode, 129 patients were evaluated; 50 patients were seen within two or three days of their last episode.

The most frequently associated diseases were hypertension (67 patients), history of myocardial infarction (25), history of congestive heart failure (20), history of ventricular arrhythmias (15), diabetes mellitus (23), history of stroke (17), and valvular heart disease (15). A cause of syncope was established in 107 patients. A cardiovascular cause was found in 53 patients and a noncardiovascular cause in 54. In 97 patients a specific diagnosis could not be determined (syncope of unknown origin).

Mean follow-up period was 10.6 ± 3.2 months. Of the 204 patients, 28 died and were classified on the basis of suddenness of death and type of syncope (Table 1). Patients were considered to have died suddenly if death occurred within 24 hours of onset of terminal symptoms. Cumulative overall mortality was 14% ± 2.5% at 12 months, with an overall incidence of sudden death of 8% ± 2.0%. At 12 months, mortality due to cardiovascular syncope was 30% ± 6.7%, compared with 12% ± 4.4% in

TABLE 1.—DEATHS DURING FOLLOW-UP PERIOD

| | CARDIO-VASCULAR DIAGNOSIS (N = 53) | NONCARDIO-VASCULAR DIAGNOSIS (N = 54) | SYNCOPE OF UNKNOWN CAUSE (N = 97) |
|---|---|---|---|
| | *no. of patients* | | |
| Sudden death | 11 | 2 | 3 |
| Nonsudden cardiovascular death | 2 | 0 | 0 |
| Death due to other underlying diseases | 3 | 4 | 3 |

(Courtesy of Kapoor, W.N., et al.: N. Engl. J. Med. 309:197–204, July 28, 1984; reprinted by permission of The New England Journal of Medicine.)

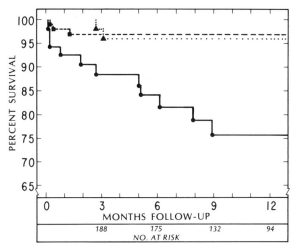

**Fig 6–7.**—Cumulative incidence of sudden death in patients with syncope due to a cardiovascular disorder *(circles)*, syncope due to a noncardiovascular disorder *(triangles)*, and syncope of unknown origin *(squares)*. (Courtesy of Kapoor, W.N., et al.: N. Engl. J. Med. 309:197–204, July 28, 1984; reprinted by permission of The New England Journal of Medicine.)

patients with a noncardiovascular cause and 6.4% ± 2.8% in patients with an unknown cause. A 24% ± 6.6% incidence of sudden death occurred in patients with a cardiovascular syncope (Fig 6–7). Among patients who died suddenly, 11 had underlying cardiovascular disease as the cause of syncope, and all 3 patients with syncope of unknown origin had chronic renal insufficiency (Table 2).

TABLE 2.—CAUSE OF SYNCOPE IN 16 PATIENTS
WHO DIED SUDDENLY

| CAUSE | NO. OF PATIENTS |
|---|---|
| Cardiovascular | |
| Ventricular tachycardia | 5 |
| Sick-sinus syndrome | 1 |
| Complete heart block | 1 |
| Myocardial infarction | 1 |
| Pulmonary embolism | 1 |
| Pulmonary hypertension | 1 |
| Aortic dissection | 1 |
| Noncardiovascular | |
| Cough syncope | 1 |
| Drug-induced syncope | 1 |
| Unknown | 3 |

(Courtesy of Kapoor, W.N., et al.: N. Engl. J. Med. 309:197–204, July 28, 1984; reprinted by permission of The New England Journal of Medicine.)

The data suggest that patients with syncope secondary to a noncardiovascular or unknown cause are not at increased risk of death unless severe underlying disease is present. The patient history and physical examination were the most useful aids in establishing a cause of syncope. Initial ECGs were frequently abnormal but seldom diagnostically helpful. Electrocardiographic monitoring also often revealed abnormalities, but in only 29 patients was it diagnostic of a cause. The EEG was abnormal in 30 patients but rarely suggested the cause of syncope. Computed tomographic head scans were similarly of little use in diagnosing cause of syncope. In agreement with previous studies, the present investigation indicates that despite detailed patient evaluation it is difficult to define the etiology of syncope. However, patients with syncope can be categorized into three diagnostic subgroups of prognostic importance.

▶ Syncope, although often "simple," is troublesome. Neurologists often, perhaps usually, are not happy with their diagnostic yield for this complaint. These authors must be fairly honest. They admitted finding the cause in just about half of their patients. They do point out the serious prognosis of syncope that has a cardiovascular basis, whereas if no cardiovascular cause is found, the prognosis is good. They also note that the EEG and the CT scan usually are not of much use, whereas the ECG and cardiac evaluation are.—R.D.C.

# 7 Extrapyramidal Disorders

**A Polymorphic DNA Marker Genetically Linked to Huntington's Disease**
James F. Gusella, Nancy W. Wexler, P. Michael Conneally, Susan L. Naylor, Mary Anne Anderson, Rudolph E. Tanzi, Paul C. Watkins, Kathleen Ottina, Margaret R. Wallace, Alan Y. Sakaguchi, Anne B. Young, Ira Shoulson, Ernesto Bonilla, and Joseph B. Martin
Nature 306:234–238, Nov. 17, 1983

7–1

Huntington's disease is a progressive neurodegenerative disorder inherited in an autosomal dominant manner. The first symptoms usually occur in the third to fifth decade of life. The gene is completely penetrant. The symptoms result from premature neuronal cell death, most marked in the basal ganglia. Most affected persons have children before the diagnosis is made. No reliable method of prenatal or presymptomatic diagnosis is available, and there is no effective treatment. Family studies showed the Huntington's disease gene to be linked with a polymorphic DNA marker that maps to human chromosome 4. The initial screen for linkage to the gene involved testing 12 DNA markers in an American family (Fig 7–1). The G8 marker is a recombinant bacteriophage from the human gene library of Maniatis et al. The G8 sequence was mapped to a human chromosome by Southern blot analysis of human-mouse somatic cell hybrids.

Chromosomal localization of the Huntington's disease gene is the first step in using recombinant DNA technology to identify the primary genetic defect. Further study is needed to determine whether the disease is genetically heterogeneous, although this seems unlikely. If heterogeneity is excluded and G8 is close enough to the Huntington's disease locus, it can be used in linkage analysis to provide prenatal and presymptomatic determination of carriers. If linkage disequilibrium exists between the two loci, the G8 marker might lead to a screening test for carriers within known

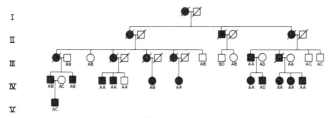

Fig 7–1.—Pedigree of American family with Huntington's disease. Circles = females; squares = males; black symbol means that an individual is affected with Huntington's disease; slashed symbol indicates an individual who died. (Courtesy of Gusella, J.F., et al.: Nature 306:234–238, Nov. 17, 1983.)

Huntington's pedigrees. Further understanding of the nature of the genetic defect may contribute to the development of effective treatment.

▶ This is an epoch-making contribution to our knowledge regarding Huntington's chorea, an important, dominantly inherited neurodegenerative disease for which there is at present no reliable method of presymptomatic or prenatal diagnosis, and no effective therapy. The chromosomal localization of the Huntington's chorea gene is the first step in using recombinant DNA technology to identify a primary genetic defect and may ultimately lead to the development of improved treatment measures. It is likely that Huntington's chorea is only the first of many hereditary autosomal diseases for which a DNA marker will provide the initial indication of the chromosomal localization of the genetic defect.—R.N.D.J.

---

**Maternal Transmission in Huntington's Disease**
Richard H. Myers, David Goldman, Edward D. Bird, Daniel S. Sax, Carl R. Merril, Miriam Schoenfeld, and Philip A. Wolf
Lancet 1:208–210, Jan. 29, 1983                                      7–2

---

Huntington's disease (HD) usually appears between the ages of 35 and 45 years, but onset of choreiform movements at ages 4 and 65 years have been reported. Late-onset HD (age 50 or later) progresses more slowly and produces less marked dementia than HD with early (20–34 years) or midlife (35–49 years) onset. Paternal transmission is more common in patients younger than age 21, and a review of data on patients with onset before age 10 showed that all inherited the gene from affected fathers. In contrast to early-onset HD, the inheritance of late-onset HD has not been described.

The effect of maternal transmission on age at onset of HD was examined in 100 unrelated pedigrees. Onset of HD was defined as the age at which involuntary movement disorder first appeared. The sample of HD patients, taken from the New England Huntington's Disease Center Without Walls, was divided into those with juvenile-adolescent onset (5–19 years), early onset, midlife onset, and late onset.

The mean age at onset in 238 cases was 41 years. The sex of the affected parent was identified for 205 of these 238 persons; 100 inherited the HD gene paternally and 105 maternally. There was a progressive increase in the proportion of maternally transmitted cases with advancing onset age in the offspring (Fig 7–2). The data indicate that HD mothers of late-onset cases also have late-onset; difficulty in identifying the affected parent in late-onset HD is usually due to death of the parent from other causes before onset of neurologic signs. High positive correlations for age of onset between all fathers and their offspring, and all mothers and their offspring, suggest that additional genes modify the expression of the HD gene. However, modifying genes of chromosomal origin do not explain the disproportionate number of early-onset cases inherited from affected fathers and late-onset cases inherited from affected mothers.

In man, extrachromosomal organelles, such as the mitochondria, are

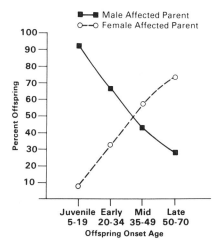

Fig 7–2.—Two hundred five patients with Huntington's disease divided into four groups according to age at onset and subdivided according to the sex of the affected parent. (Courtesy of Myers, R.H., et al.: Lancet 1:208–210, 1983.)

inherited exclusively from mothers; such maternal factors may modify the onset of HD or the expression of the gene. By this model, the juvenile- and early-onset offspring of affected fathers would be the product of the extrachromosomal factors of their unaffected mothers in combination with modifying chromosomal genes of their early-onset affected fathers. The equal distribution of 33 males and 33 females among late-onset cases in this study, as well as the finding that none of the daughters of late-onset males had late-onset HD, indicates that the modifying mechanism is not X-linked.

The hypothesis that maternally transmitted factors modify the gene for HD leads to the prediction that the correlation will be greater maternally than paternally. Although this was not statistically supported in the present study, in a larger sample of more than 500 parent-offspring pairs collected by the National Huntington Disease Roster, the maternal correlation was significantly greater. The wide range in age of onset of HD suggests that expression of the gene is modified by other factors; the authors of this study hypothesize that mitochondrial chromosomes may be involved.

▶ This supports the idea that the age of onset of Huntington's chorea is earlier if the affected parent is the father and later if the mother. The authors point to mitochondrial inheritance from the mother as the possible modifying factor. Apparently it is always beneficial—the effect of our mothers on us.—R.D.C.

---

**Huntington's Chorea Arising as a Fresh Mutation**
M. Baraitser, J. Burn, and T. A. Fazzone (Inst. of Child Health, London)
J. Med. Genet. 20:459–460, December 1983                                    7–3

---

Well-documented fresh mutations in Huntington's chorea are rarely reported. The authors encountered a well-documented case in which Huntington's chorea resulted from a new mutation.

Woman, 33, described clumsiness of her hands, a tendency to drop things easily, and frequent falling while walking. Her memory reportedly was somewhat impaired. Continuous jerky choreiform movements were noted in the hands, legs, and face, and jerky dysarthria was evident. Testing revealed impaired short-term and long-term memory and mental arithmetic ability. The patient could not maintain a grip or posture despite the absence of demonstrable weakness. Her reflexes were brisk; her gait was unsteady and poorly coordinated. The parents, aged 70 and 71, and four older siblings were healthy. Examination of the parents showed no neurologic abnormalities. The eldest of the patient's three children, a girl aged 17, had behavior problems but no neurologic abnormality.

After eight years the proband was confined to a wheelchair. The choreiform movements were worse, and memory for recent events was very poor. On computed tomographic (CT) examination, caudate atrophy was observed.

This patient fulfills all of the criteria for Huntington's chorea except for transmission of the disease. True paternity was considered highly likely in this case and was supported by examination of blood groups. The clinical features are those of classic Huntington's disease, and the diagnosis was supported by CT examination.

Findings in this patient confirm the occurrence of fresh mutations in Huntington's chorea. Published reports probably have underestimated the true incidence of new mutations in view of the difficulties inherent in confirming them.

▶ This is nearly, but not quite, an open and shut case of Huntington's chorea arising as a fresh mutation. There is a very small chance one of the parents may yet develop Huntington's chorea (a benign chorea with minimal mental symptoms in the elderly) and an even smaller chance one of the parents is not the true parent. If neither is true and if, in 10 or 15 years, the patient's 17-year-old daughter develops the disease then I too will believe in spontaneous mutations. So far I have preferred alternative explanations.—R.D.C.

### Etiology of Parkinson's Disease: A Research Strategy

André Barbeau (Clin. Res. Inst. of Montreal)
Can. J. Neurol. Sci. 11:24–28, February 1984   7–4

The author presents a "global hypothesis" for explaining the pathophysiology of Parkinson's disease and an appropriate research strategy for evaluating it. Idiopathic Parkinson's disease is seen as resulting from a generalized cellular aging process, accelerated in susceptible persons by a variety of often repetitive triggering factors that lead to a transient increase in turnover within catecholamine-producing neurons and the accumulation of free radicals. When these exceed the scavenging capacity of the cells, damage to organelles and membranes occurs and leads to the formation of Lewy bodies through an autoimmune reaction to damaged filaments and subsequent cell death. A compensatory increase in catecholamine turnover in the residual pigmented neurons of the brain stem leads to an accelerating degenerative process. The hypothesis is illustrated schematically in Figure 7–3.

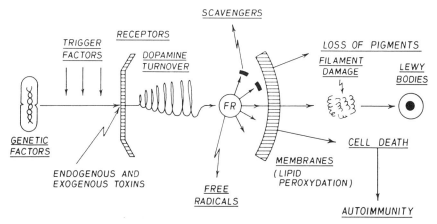

Fig 7–3.—Outline of author's "global hypothesis" on pathophysiology of Parkinson's disease. (Courtesy of Barbeau, A.: Can. J. Neurol. Sci. 11:24–28, February 1984.)

Susceptibility to parkinsonism is presumed to be genetically determined and reflected in all cells. A role for "susceptibility factors" in nonfamilial forms of the disease cannot be denied. The trigger factors are mostly those operative in all person's lives. An increase in turnover of catecholamines in central and peripheral nervous tissues is considered to be a common mechanism of action in all stressful situations. Aging is manifested by nerve cell atrophy, with a compensatory increase in connective tissues, and often the deposit of pigments. Increases in free radicals can result from purely exogenous causes as well as from nonspecific stress factors; manganese intoxication is an example. Concentrations of scavenger enzymes have been found to be reduced in the substantia nigra of parkinsonian patients. Cell loss in the substantia nigra and locus ceruleus is translated into a specific loss of the catecholamines produced in needed areas such as the striatum. The dopamine deficit is directly responsible for some parkinsonian symptoms such as akinesia.

This hypothesis can be exploited by delineating the limits of true Parkinson's disease from all phenocopies, identifying susceptible persons and the most common trigger factors, and protecting susceptible persons by increasing the functional availability of free radical trapping agents. At the same time the metabolic effects of unavoidable trigger factors can be minimized.

▶ This is a thoughtful and thorough review by a scientist who has been among the foremost investigators into the pathophysiology and neuropharmacology of the various extrapyramidal disorders, mainly Parkinson's disease and Huntington's chorea. His hypothesis should be given serious consideration by all workers in this field.—R.N.D.J.

## Cognitive Deficits in the Early Stages of Parkinson's Disease
A. J. Lees and Eileen Smith (Natl. Hosp. for Nervous Diseases, London)
Brain 106:257–270, June 1983                                                7–5

Cognitive deficits have been increasingly recognized in patients with Parkinson's disease, but it is unclear whether improved life expectancy, adverse effects of L-dopa, or simply greater clinical awareness is responsible. The authors used neuropsychological tests for frontal lobe damage to assess cognitive function in 30 mildly disabled patients seen between 1979 and 1981 with newly diagnosed idiopathic Parkinson's disease, none of whom had been treated. There were 19 men with a mean age of 59 years and 11 women with a mean age of 58. Mean duration of disease was 2.4 years. All patients had normal cranial computed tomographic studies, and none was depressed or had high ischemia scores. Most of the 30 age-matched controls were awaiting operation for disk disease or carpal tunnel syndrome.

No impairment of general intellectual function was found in the parkinsonian patients on the Wechsler Adult Intelligence Scale and New Adult Reading tests. No abnormalities were found on cognitive estimates or the Two-Choice Recognition Memory Test. The patients had significantly more difficulty than controls in shifting conceptual sets, and they produced more perseverative errors on both the modified Wisconsin Card Sorting Test and the Benton Word Fluency Test.

The subtle cognitive deficits identified in parkinsonian patients in this study might underlie the mental inflexibility and rigidity characteristic of Parkinson's disease. They could be a result of destruction of the ascending dopaminergic mesocorticolimbic pathway. The findings are similar to those described in association with frontal lobe damage, although the patients lacked clinical "frontal lobe signs." A comparable loss of dopaminergic neurons in the neighboring nigrostriatal bundle could explain the reported correlation between motor deficits and intellectual decline in patients with Parkinson's disease.

▶ A certain rigidity of thinking has been reported in Parkinson's disease before, a concept in which I for one did not believe. But here it is again and well verified. In the meantime I have gotten a little less rigid and am willing to accept it. It doesn't seem too hard to conceptualize a situation in which shifting mental activity and shifting motor activity can be equally involved.—R.D.C.

## Parkinson's Disease in 65 Pairs of Twins and in a Set of Quadruplets
Christopher D. Ward, Roger C. Duvoisin, Susan E. Ince, John D. Nutt, Roswell Eldridge, and Donald B. Calne
Neurology (Cleve.) 33:815–824, July 1983                                     7–6

The role of genetic factors in the etiology of Parkinson's disease (PD) has long been controversial. Many previous studies have relied too heavily on medical records and untrained witnesses. The authors reviewed 47 monozygotic and 18 dizygotic twin pairs, as well as the surviving members of a set of quadruplets in which the index case had a monozygotic and a dizygotic sibling. Among 43 evaluable monozygotic and 19 dizygotic twin pairs in which an index case had definite PD, only 1 monozygotic pair was definitely concordant for PD. When pairs with questionable clinical features were included, 4 of 48 monozygotic pairs and 1 of 19 dizygotic pairs were concordant.

The frequency of PD in monozygotic cotwins of index cases with PD in this series was similar to that expected in an unrelated control group matched for age and sex. The maximum concordance rate of 8% is considered an overestimate. Concordance rates can serve as a crude estimate of "heritability." The findings support the view that the chief contribution to the etiology of PD is nongenetic. No single environmental factor was identified in this study that determined the onset or course of PD. A predisposition to the disease may be acquired early in life.

▶ This detailed study by experienced clinical neurologists and neuroepidemiologists leads to the conclusion that the major factors in the etiology of Parkinson's disease are nongenetic.—R.N.D.J.

---

**Pergolide in Parkinson's Disease**
Christopher G. Goetz, Caroline M. Tanner, Russell Glantz, and Harold L. Klawans (Rush-Presbyterian-St. Luke's Med. Center, Chicago)
Arch. Neurol. 40:785–787, December 1983                    7–7

---

Pergolide mesylate is a new, synthetic, direct-acting dopaminergic agonist that is more potent than bromocriptine in rats with nigrostriatal lesions. The authors evaluated the effect of pergolide therapy in 12 men and 10 women, mean age 61, with idiopathic Parkinson's disease. The average duration of disease was 13½ years, and the average length of levodopa therapy was 9 years. All patients experienced loss of efficacy or dose-limiting side effects with previous therapy, including the on-off phenomenon in 20, dyskinesias in 19, and hallucinations in 4. Twelve patients had received bromocriptine, and four, lergotrile. Treatment began with an oral dose of 0.1 mg of pergolide daily, and the dose was increased until therapeutic effects were achieved or side effects occurred. The maximal daily dose was 6 mg.

Most parameters indicated significantly less disability after three and six months of treatment. Improvement in gait, maximal at six months, deteriorated somewhat by one year. Two patients deteriorated precipitously after six months. No new on-off phenomenon developed during pergolide therapy. The average dose at one year was 2.85 mg daily, and the daily dose of levodopa was lower in most patients. Both dyskinesia and chorea were less apparent after a year of pergolide therapy. Sleep abnormalities progressed in several patients. Hallucinations improved in all instances, but two patients experienced mild hallucinations during pergolide therapy. Several patients had temporary akathisia early in the course of treatment, and some had orthostatic hypotension transiently. No persistent rise in the levels of transaminases was observed.

Most of these parkinsonian patients have done well with pergolide therapy, experiencing reduced drug-related side effects after a year. Pergolide may be a more selective dopaminergic agonist than previous medications. No significant incidence of cardiac disease was associated with its use in this series.

▶ Pergolide seems to be an improvement over Sinemet in this study with the added advantage that hallucinations improved. It is my understanding that it may take two more years for pergolide to be accepted for general use in the United States. I hope it is not longer.

An excellent short review of the current treatment of Parkinson's disease is a recent *Lancet* editorial (1:829–830, 1984). A comprehensive analysis of most aspects of the disease appears in the *Canadian Journal of Neurological Sciences* (11:[Suppl.], 1984) and includes more than one opinion on subjects such as whether dopamine agonists should be given early or late. (Early may be best.)

Freed (*Biol. Psychiatry* 18:1205–1267, 1983) gives us an in-depth summary of the situation with regard to brain transplant (which is being used experimentally as therapy for Parkinsonism) and concludes that "a useful clinical application, although probably years away is by no means an unreasonable goal."—R.D.C.

---

**Comparison of Pergolide and Bromocriptine Therapy in Parkinsonism**
P. A. LeWitt, D. C. Ward, T. A. Larsen, M. I. Raphaelson, R. P. Newman, N. Foster, J. M. Dambrosia, and D. B. Calne (Nat'l. Inst. of Neurological and Communicative Disorders and Stroke)
Neurology (Cleve.) 33:1009–1014, August 1983                    7–8

---

The authors compared the efficacy and toxicity of pergolide and bromocriptine in 27 outpatients with Parkinson's disease, 19 men and 8 women with a mean age of 59 years. Mean duration of symptoms was 11 years. Nine patients had uncomplicated or mild disease that responded well to levodopa, and 15 had advanced parkinsonism or problems with levodopa therapy. Two patients had not received levodopa, and another was not on medication at the time of the study.

Pergolide mesylate was provided in 0.1- and 0.5-mg capsules and bromocriptine mesylate in 1- and 2.5-mg capsules in a double-blind crossover design. There were no upper dose limits. Twenty-four patients completed the study on both drugs.

All patients but two had improved control of parkinsonism on ergot therapy, and the two drugs provided comparable control in both the mildly affected and the more severely disabled patients. Optimal doses of both drugs varied substantially among patients. Eleven patients elected to continue with pergolide at the end of the study; seven favored bromocriptine. The pergolide-treated patients have shown continued benefit for as long as 13 months. Adverse effects were comparable with the two treatments. Only one patient had increased levels of liver enzymes, which were associated with the development of unilateral pleural fibrosis. The disorder improved after drug therapy was discontinued.

Pergolide and bromocriptine exhibited comparable therapeutic and adverse effects in these patients with Parkinson's disease. Both clinical benefit and toxicity vary from one patient to another, making careful individual adjustment of medication necessary. Routine surveillance is required to detect asymptomatic, potentially serious toxicity.

▶ It has been found that certain other dopaminergic ergoline derivatives are as effective as bromocriptine in the treatment of Parkinson's disease, even though their neurochemical action differs from that of the one originally used. In this study there was little difference in the efficacy of pergolide as compared with bromocriptine. Another drug of this group, lisuride, is equally efficacious therapeutically, but appears to have a somewhat greater hepatotoxicity.—R.N.D.J.

**Bromocriptine in Long-Term Management of Advanced Parkinson's Disease**
J. David Grimes and Mohamed N. Hassan (Univ. of Ottawa)
Can. J. Neurol. Sci. 10:86–90, May 1983                    7–9

The duration and long-term quality of treatment effects from bromocriptine in advanced Parkinson's disease are unclear. The authors followed 37 patients with advanced disease, who initially responded to bromocriptine therapy, for 12–50 months (mean, 28). The patients, with an average age of 67 years, had had classic Parkinson's disease for a mean of nine years. All were levodopa responders who had been treated with the drug for a mean of five years. Eight patients were receiving anticholinergics as well, 12 received amantadine, and four received both. Twenty-eight patients had end-of-dose deterioration, and nine had disabling bradykinesia. All but seven patients had levodopa-induced dyskinesias. Bromocriptine usually was begun in a dose of 2.5 mg and increased in 2.5-mg increments at intervals of five to seven days. Sinemet therapy was often reduced as the dosage of bromocriptine was increased.

Patients received bromocriptine for a mean of 28 months. The peak drug effect was apparent by three months and was maintained for a mean of 22 months. At peak effect the clinical response was variable, but 8 patients had marked and 18 had moderate improvement. Eight patients have had sustained improvement at peak effect without changes in therapy for an average of 29 months. Eight others did not maintain their peak clinical responses. Twenty-one patients maintained the peak effect for an average of 14 months before loss of response was detected. A late increase in end-of-dose deterioration was arrested by increasing the frequency of dosing in six patients. Sinemet-induced dyskinesias were reduced in 26 of 30 patients and became slightly worse in 2. Twenty-nine patients have continued to use bromocriptine. Anticholinergics were stopped in five, with no worsening of parkinsonism. Bromocriptine was stopped in four patients because of severe confusion with hallucinations. Three patients developed mild cold-sensitive digital vasospasm that was not dose limiting. Gastrointestinal problems were minimal.

Addition of bromocriptine is an effective measure in some patients with advanced Parkinson's disease. Results are best in younger patients without dementia who have end-of-dose deterioration and levodopa-induced dyskinesias. If initial improvement is lost, further benefit can usually be obtained by carefully adjusting the dosage and timing of both bromocriptine and levodopa.

▶ With cautious introduction and intermittent dosage adjustment, bromocriptine can be of long-term benefit to patients with advanced Parkinson's disease. The majority of patients have a gradual late fall-off in effect which can frequently be reversed with dosage adjustment.—R.N.D.J.

---

**New Form of Familial Parkinson-Dementia Syndrome: Clinical and Pathologic Findings**
Marina Mata, Katerina Dorovini-Zis, Mary Wilson, and Anne B. Young (Univ. of Michigan)
Neurology (Cleve.) 33:1439–1443, November 1983          7–10

---

The authors describe a family in which three siblings had a syndrome of parkinsonian features, mental deterioration, pyramidal signs, and abnormal eye movements starting in the third decade. The index patient noticed paucity of movement and impaired manual dexterity in his mid-20s and then developed rigidity, a postural tremor with flapping movements of the arms, and slurred speech. He became increasingly rigid and bradykinetic, and dementia was evident by age 30, with unintelligible speech and worse rigidity and cogwheeling. Computed tomography (CT) showed diffuse cortical and deep cerebral atrophy with ventricular enlargement. A younger brother developed similar clinical features from age 24 years and was found on CT to have diffuse cortical atrophy and mild ventricular enlargement. Intelligence was at the low end of the average range.

Neuropathologic study of the older sister, who had developed rigidity and slowness of movement and severe dementia before dying at age 31, revealed changes resembling those of progressive supranuclear palsy or the Parkinson-dementia complex of Guam. Severe, bilaterally symmetric degeneration of the substantia nigra with marked reactive gliosis was seen (Fig 7–4). Astrocytic gliosis was prominent in the periaqueductal gray matter. The globus pallidus showed some neurofibrillary degeneration and mild neuronal depletion but no gliosis. The hippocampus was severely involved. Neurofibrillary tangles were only occasionally seen in cortical neurons other than in the temporal lobe.

This disorder does not fit any previously described syndrome causing

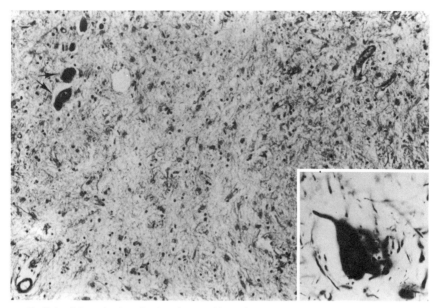

Fig 7–4.—Substantia nigra showing gliosis and loss of neurons. A few pigmented neurons remain. Phosphotungstic acid–hematoxylin; original magnification, ×132. Inset shows neurofibrillary tangle. Cajal's pyrimidine silver nitrate; original magnification, ×825. (Courtesy of Mata, M., et al.: Neurology [Cleve.] 33:1439–1443, November 1983.)

progressive extrapyramidal and pyramidal findings with dementia in the third decade. It could be a new entity in the spectrum of extrapyramidal degenerative disorders of early life. Inheritance appears to be of the autosomal dominant type with low penetrance and expression, although autosomal recessive inheritance cannot be excluded.

▶ The authors suggest that this is a new entity in the spectrum of extrapyramidal diseases of early life, probably inherited as an autosomal dominant.—R.N.D.J.

**Delayed Neurologic Sequelae in Carbon Monoxide Intoxication**
Il Saing Choi (Yonsei Univ., Seoul, Korea)
Arch. Neurol. 40:433–435, July 1983                              7–11

The author reviewed the records of 2,360 victims of acute carbon monoxide intoxication who were examined between 1976 and 1981. Delayed neurologic sequelae developed in 65 subjects, representing 2.75% of the entire group and 12% of those admitted to the hospital. The 40 women and 25 men had a mean age of 56 years; none was younger than age 30 years. The mean lucid interval before symptoms began was 22 days. Neurologic abnormalities were likelier with a longer duration of unconsciousness at the time of acute intoxication, but they sometimes occurred even when the mental state was clear during the event. The most common disorders were mental deterioration, urinary or fecal incontinence, or both, and gait disturbance. Seven of 17 computed tomographic studies showed areas of decreased density. Six of the 36 patients followed did not improve, and 3 others died of infection. Recovery took place after an average of three to six months. Five of the 27 patients who recovered had mild memory disorders, and 1 had parkinsonism. One patient developed a glioblastoma of the corpus callosum two years later. Treatment with corticosteroids, aspirin, and cerebral vasodilators was ineffective in preventing or alleviating the neurologic sequelae.

The cause of delayed neurologic abnormalities in patients with carbon monoxide intoxication is unclear. A direct myelinotoxic effect is unlikely, and delayed demyelination has not been observed after experimentally induced cerebral edema. Apart from mental deterioration, incontinence, and gait disturbance, there may be signs of damage to frontal lobes and basal ganglia. Cerebellar signs are rare. The signs and symptoms characteristically fluctuate during the clinical course. The prognosis is relatively good. The only predisposing factors identified are age and severity of anoxia during the acute episode.

▶ Delayed neurologic sequelae after carbon monoxide intoxication are common and have characteristic features. The prognosis is relatively good.— R.N.D.J.

---

**High-Dosage Anticholinergic Therapy in Dystonia**
Stanley Fahn (Columbia Univ.)
Neurology (Cleve.) 33:1255–1261, October 1983                    7–12

---

The author studied the effects of anticholinergic drugs on dystonia in an open-label study of 23 children and 52 adults with torsion dystonia of various causes and distribution patterns of involuntary movements. Dosages were gradually increased until a beneficial effect was observed or intolerable adverse effects developed. Initially, trihexyphenidyl was administered; later, the adults were given ethopropazine.

The children and adults responded differently to high-dose anticholinergic therapy. Fourteen (61%) of the 23 children had a sustained and moderate to dramatic response to trihexyphenidyl (average daily dose, 41 mg). Six of eight Ashkenazic children improved, and one of two autosomal dominant children had a dramatic response, achieving a normal appearance. Definite improvement occurred in 8 of 11 children with generalized dystonia and in 5 of 10 children with segmental dystonia, but not in either of the 2 with unilateral dystonia. The median duration of improvement was five years, and the longest was 13 years.

Twenty (38%) of the 52 adults experienced sustained and moderate to marked improvement. Only one adult improved dramatically, in contrast to this response in four children. Except for dystonia secondary to stroke or infection, improvement occurred in all etiologic categories. Definite improvement occurred in both adults with autosomal dominant dystonia, but in only 8 of 18 Ashkenazim and 9 of 28 adults with idiopathic dystonia. Overall, 46% of the adults with generalized dystonia, 42% with segmental dystonia, 43% with Meige syndrome, and 38% with torticollis responded. In adults the average daily dosage was 24 mg of trihexyphenidyl and 350 mg of ethopropazine. Fewer than 50% of the adults received treatment for two years or more, the longest duration being seven years. Most adults treated for less than one year stopped taking medication because of adverse effects. Of the 26 adults who continued treatment with some benefit, 12 were taking trihexyphenidyl and 14 were taking ethopropazine. Except for weight loss in one child and first-day worsening in two, no child discontinued medication because of adverse effects.

Although treatment with anticholinergic drugs was not effective in all patients, it was beneficial enough to warrant continuation in the initial phase of treatment of dystonia.

▶ Fahn points out that one must push the dose of antichollingergic drugs to get a response, and then not all patients will respond. He first used trihexyphenidyl and later added ethopropazine.—R.D.C.

---

**Dystonia Musculorum Deformans Improved by Bromocriptine**
J. C. Gautier and A. Awada (Hôpital de la Salpétrière, Paris)
Rev. Neurol. (Paris) 139:449–450, June–July, 1983          7–13

---

The authors evaluated bromocriptine in a woman 25 years of age who had had severe dystonia musculorum deformans since age 14 years. No similar cases were reported in the family. Torsion spasm and a cogwheel phenomenon in both upper extremities were observed. The abnormalities resolved on treatment with bromocriptine in a dose of 22.5 mg daily and reappeared when the dose was progressively reduced. The patient was leading a normal life at university after a year of treatment with 12.5 mg of bromocriptine daily.

▶ There may be many varieties of and causes for dystonia musculorum deformans. This contribution discusses a possible treatment that should be tried in the cases of patients with this progressive and heretofore untreatable condition.—R.N.D.J.

---

**Three Years of Continuous Oral Zinc Therapy in Four Patients With Wilson's Disease**
T. U. Hoogenraad and C. J. A. Van den Hamer
Acta Neurol. Scand. 67:356–364, June 1983          7–14

---

Left untreated, Wilson's disease invariably has an unfavorable outcome. Treatment with penicillamine increases cupriuresis, resulting in a negative copper balance and, usually, clinical improvement. However, lifelong treatment is necessary to prevent renewed accumulation of copper; also, D-penicillamine is a potentially toxic drug. Because excessive dietary zinc decreases copper absorption from the gastrointestinal tract, the authors evaluated the effectiveness of oral zinc therapy (100–400 mg three times daily) in four patients with Wilson's disease. Oral zinc sulfate was the only medication the patients received to influence their copper balance over a three-year period. The effect of therapy was monitored by physical examinations, oral $^{64}$Cu loading tests, and determination of plasma copper, zinc, and ceruloplasmin concentrations, as well as by measurement of urinary copper excretion.

All four patients responded favorably to oral zinc therapy. In three patients, the aim of therapy was to stabilize their clinical condition, as all three were effectively decoppered prior to the trial. All three showed a slight additional improvement. The fourth patient, who had biochemical and clinical signs of abnormal copper storage, had a dramatic response to oral zinc therapy; the most serious symptoms remaining at the end of three years were dysarthria and stammering. All four patients tolerated the medication well, and there were no toxic side effects.

The results suggest that oral zinc sulfate therapy may be an important alternative treatment in patients with Wilson's disease. However, the dosage required to suppress copper absorption varies from patient to patient, thus frequent determination of plasma zinc, copper, and ceruloplasmin concentrations is necessary.

▶ This is a new approach to the treatment of Wilson's disease with the use of oral zinc before meals to decrease copper absorption from the gastrointestinal tract. It sounds promising, although whether anyone will do a comparative study of this treatment vs. other treatments is questionable. At least it appears to be a good alternative method of treatment if penicillamine is not tolerated.— R.D.C.

---

## Fluphenazine and Multifocal Tic Disorders

Christopher G. Goetz, Caroline M. Tanner, and Harold L. Klawans (Rush-Presbyterian-St. Luke's Med. Center, Chicago)
Arch. Neurol. 41:271–272, March 1984        7–15

---

Haloperidol is the standard treatment for Tourette's syndrome and chronic motor tic disorders of childhood, but significant side effects may impair its usefulness. The authors undertook a five-year, open-label study of fluphenazine in 21 patients with multifocal tic disorders who were intolerant of haloperidol. The 16 males and 5 females had an average age of 22 years. Symptoms had developed at an average age of 6½ years. Eighteen patients had tics and involuntary vocalizations, and three had compulsive stereotypic behaviors without vocalizations. Haloperidol had been used for an average of about 2½ years, with an average efficacy at tolerated dosage of only 35%. Sedation, dysphoria or depression, and decreased concentration were the most common effects. Fluphenazine was begun in a dosage of 0.5 mg daily and increased to an average of 7 mg daily after withdrawal of haloperidol.

The average group tic frequency decreased by 21% with fluphenazine therapy. Control was better than with haloperidol in 11 patients. In two patients the frequency of tics increased, and haloperidol therapy was resumed. Ten of the 11 patients who had better control of tics by fluphenazine continued to show improvement after a mean follow-up of 2.3 years. All but five patients reported fewer side effects when taking fluphenazine, whereas three felt that they were worse than with haloperidol. No new side effects were described. An improved therapeutic index was evident in 11 patients. Three patients with increased side effects stopped using fluphenazine.

Fluphenazine is an alternative drug for use by patients with multiple tics who do not tolerate haloperidol. Frequently, side effects are reduced without loss of tic control. Multiple treatment trials are warranted in patients with tic disorders who are intolerant of any single agent. A long-term, double-blind, prospective trial of fluphenazine would be useful.

▶ Fluphenazine can be an effective treatment for multiple tics in patients with dose-limiting side effects related to haloperidol.—R.N.D.J.

---

**Pure Psychic Akinesia With Bilateral Lesions of Basal Ganglia**
Dominique Laplane, Michel Baulac, Daniel Widlöcher, and Bruno Dubois (Hôpital de la Salpétrière, Paris)
J. Neurol. Neurosurg. Psychiatry 47:377–385, April 1984          7–16

---

The authors report data on three patients who exhibited dramatic psychic akinesia after recovering from toxic encephalopathy; none had more than a mild motor disorder. The akinesia was reversible on stimulating the patient. Two patients also had stereotyped behaviors resembling compulsions. All had CT evidence of bilateral basal ganglia lesions.

Man, 41, experienced convulsive coma for 24 hours after being stung on the arm by a wasp; he then exhibited intensive choreic movements—alleviated by treatment with thioproperazine—and gait impairment. The abnormalities decreased in the next several months, but mild dementia developed and persisted over the next 12 years. All activities were much reduced, and the patient spent many days doing nothing but did not seem bored. He described a "blank mind." Dreaming continued to occur, although the patient's fantasy life was impoverished. On stimulation by external events or another person, he could perform rather complex tasks correctly, e.g., playing bridge. Intellectual function was within the normal range. Stereotyped activities (e.g., mental counting and accompanying gestures) began two years after the episode of encephalopathy. Very mild choreic movements were noted, but there was a permanent facial rictus with tic-like facial and jaw movements. On computed tomography (CT), low-density areas were identified in the internal part of the lentiform nucleus bilaterally (Fig 7–5). Dramatic improvement occurred when clomipramine therapy was instituted. The patient was able to initiate talking and other activities, but the stereotyped behavior continued.

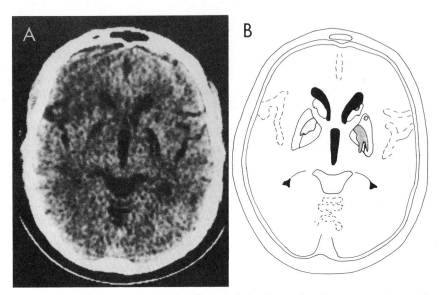

Fig 7–5.—**A,** CT scan 42 mm above the orbitomeatal plane showing low-density areas in the internal part of the lentiform nucleus bilaterally. **B,** schematic representation of same view. (Courtesy of Laplane, D., et al.: J. Neurol. Neurosurg. Psychiatry 47:377–385, April 1984.)

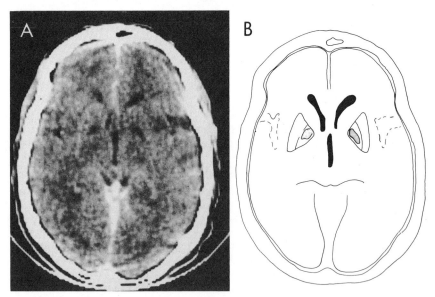

Fig 7–6.—**A,** CT scan 40 mm above the orbitomeatal plane showing two low-density areas almost symmetrically placed in the internal part of the lentiform nucleus. **B,** schematic representation of same view. (Courtesy of Laplane, D., et al.: J. Neurol. Neurosurg. Psychiatry 47:377–385, April 1984.)

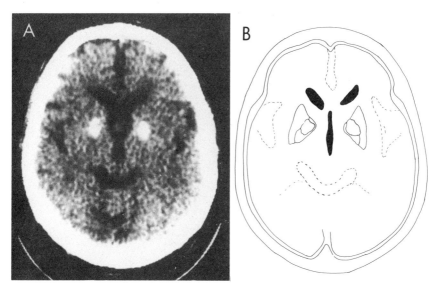

Fig 7–7.—**A,** CT scan 45 mm above the orbitomeatal plane showing two bilateral abnormal areas with spontaneous high density corresponding to calcified lesions in the internal part of the lentiform nucleus. **B,** schematic representation of same view. (Courtesy of Laplane, D., et al.: J. Neuro. Neurosurg. Psychiatry 47:377–385, April 1984.)

The patient died after massive aspiration of food; autopsy was not performed.

Spontaneous psychic akinesia was the chief disorder in all three patients. Both mental and behavioral activities were markedly reduced, but the akinesia was dramatically reversible by stimulation. The stereotyped behavior seen in two patients consisted mainly of counting, sometimes paced by finger movements. The CT abnormalities were in the deep forebrain at the level of the basal ganglia (Figs 7–6 and 7–7). The mental symptoms may be caused by encroachment of the lesions on the anterior limb of the internal capsule, involvement of the ventral extension of the pallidum within the substantia innominata, interruption of ascending fiber bundles, or involvement of cholinergic cells in the basal nucleus of Meynert.

▶ So here is an additional example of the psychic side of basal ganglia dysfunction—psychic akinesia.—R.D.C.

# 8 Headache and Head Pain

**Is Migraine Food Allergy? A Double-Blind Controlled Trial of Oligoantigenic Diet Treatment**
J. Egger, J. Wilson, C. M. Carter, M. W. Turner, and J. F. Soothill (Hospital for Sick Children, London)
Lancet 2:865–868, Oct. 15, 1983                                8–1

The authors evaluated the effect of an oligoantigenic diet in 88 children with severe and frequent migraine.

Of the 88 children who completed the oligoantigenic diet, 78 recovered completely, 4 had considerable improvement, and 6 did not improve. All but 8 of the 82 who improved relapsed upon reintroduction of one or more of the implicated foods. In addition to headache, other associated symptoms that improved included abdominal pain, behavior disorder, aches in limbs, seizures, rhinitis, asthma, and eczema. Reintroduction of excluded foods in 40 children showed that 55 substances provoked symptoms. Most children reacted to cow's milk, and all but one of these also reacted to cheese. However, 13 children who reacted to cheese showed no reaction to cow's milk. The median time until symptom recurrence was two days (range, less than one hour to more than seven days). Symptoms usually disappeared within 2–3 days (range, less than 1 to 21 days). Nondietary provocation of migraine before treatment was reported by 38 of the successfully treated children. Forty-five (52%) had positive skin prick test results with one or more of five antigens routinely used to identify atopic individuals; 63 children (72%) had positive reactions to one or more of 28 antigens. However, only three patients would have recovered if they had avoided only those foods to which they had a positive skin prick test reaction. High serum IgE levels were detected in 28% of 64 children, but IgE antibodies were not helpful in identifying causative foods. Except for two children who resumed a full diet and drug treatment, all continued to follow their oligoantigenic diets without symptoms or evidence of adverse effects.

Most children with severe, frequent bouts of migraine recovered when an appropriate diet was instituted. A wide range of foods was involved, thus an allergic process rather than a metabolic idiosyncracy would appear to be responsible for the occurrence of symptoms.

▶ Having been a childhood migraineur, I am able to buy this. In this study the most common foods producing headache were cow's milk, egg, chocolate, orange, and wheat, with peanuts and grapes down the list, both of which have given me terrible headaches. Their oligoantigenic diet for each meal consisted of one meat (lamb or chicken), one carbohydrate (rice or potato), one fruit (banana or apple), and one vegetable (brassica); and a vitamin supplement was given once a day. The diet was continued for three or four weeks. It is interesting that benzoic acid was in sixth place on their list of common precipitants. This is used as a preservative in commercial soda pop (squash). The authors point out that the skin tests are not reliable indicators of migraine-producing foods in children.

Glover et al. (*Headache* 23:53–58, 1983), Peatfield et al. (*J. Neurol. Neurosurg. Psychiatry* 46:827–831, 1983) and Merrett et al. (*J. Neurol. Neurosurg. Psychiatry* 46:738–742, 1983) are busy attempting to identify the dietary factors responsible for migraine, and they point to a possible deficiency of phenolsulfotransferase P enzyme as the critical defect.—R.D.C.

---

**Migraine as an Etiology of Stroke in Young Adults**
Leo J. Spaccavento and Glen D. Solomon (USAF Med. Center, Wright-Patterson AFB, Ohio)
Headache 24:19–22, January 1984                                  8–2

Stroke in young adults is rare in western populations. Risk factors for atherosclerosis have been absent in recent large series of young stroke patients. The authors reviewed the records of 15 patients, aged 20–40 years, seen between 1975 and 1980 with the diagnosis of stroke due to ischemic cerebrovascular disease. Extensive studies including computed tomography, cerebral angiography, or both were carried out. The eight women and seven men had an average age of 28 years when stroke occurred. Four patients (27%) had a documented past history of classic migraine, and three of them had migraine attacks at the time of stroke. The fourth patient had a history of migraine with basilar artery symptoms and had a lateral medullary syndrome. The migraine patients had an average age of 24 at the time of stroke. Three other patients had valvular heart disease, and one each had sickle cell anemia and postinfectious dural sinus thrombosis. No cause was apparent for six cases.

PREVALENCE RATES OF KNOWN OR POSSIBLE RISK FACTORS FROM SERIES THAT INCLUDED MIGRAINE AS A RISK FACTOR

| | Migraine | Ethanol/Drugs | Oral Contraceptives | Hypertension | Heart Disease |
|---|---|---|---|---|---|
| Hindfelt and Nilsson (n = 64) | 7 (11%) | 4 (6%) | 8 (12.5%) | 12 (19%) | 4 (6%) |
| Hilbom and Kaste (n = 76) | 21 (28%) | 29 (38%) | 20 (26%) | 11 (14%) | 8 (11%) |
| Spaccavento and Solomon (n = 15) | 4 (27%) | 0 | 0 | 0 | 3 (20%) |
| Total (n = 155) | 32 (21%) | 33 (21%) | 28 (18%) | 23 (15%) | 15 (10%) |

(Courtesy of Spaccavento, L.J., and Solomon, G.D.: Headache 24:19–22, January 1984.)

No evidence of premature atherosclerotic disease was found in this series of 15 young stroke patients. Migraine was the only identifiable risk factor in about one fourth. The prevalence rates of migraine as a possible risk factor for stroke in this and other series are shown in the table. Three of the authors' four patients had their strokes during usual migraine attacks. Most migraine attacks are preceded by cerebrovascular vasoconstriction occurring during the prodrome. Decreased regional cerebral blood flow has been demonstrated. Arterial vasospasm alone can produce cerebral ischemia, and other risk factors in migraine patients can produce thrombo-occlusion and cerebral ischemia. A careful history should be obtained from all young stroke patients to detect migraine.

▶ I invite you to read this article if you feel as I did that migraine does not produce strokes in young adults. The case histories are convincing. Three of four patients had had sensory or ocular symptoms with previous migraines, symptoms that may mark the subgroup of migraineurs at increased risk for stroke. Perhaps this group would most benefit from the calcium channel blockers (see abstract 8–4).

Speaking of migraine, Blau (*Lancet* 1:444–445, 1984) has proposed a new and simpler definition of migraine: "Episodic headaches lasting 2 to 72 h[ours] with total freedom between attacks. The headaches must be associated with visual or gastrointestinal disturbances, or both. The visual symptoms occur as an aura before, and/or photophobia during, the headache phase. If there are no visual but only alimentary disturbances, then vomiting must feature in some attacks." It is a restrictive definition and should slim down the numbers in therapeutic trials.—R.D.C.

---

### Changes in Regional Cerebral Blood Flow During Course of Classic Migraine Attacks

Martin Lauritzen, Tom Skyhøj Olsen, Niels A. Lassen, and Olaf B. Paulson (Bispebjerg Hosp., Copenhagen)
Ann. Neurol. 13:633–641, June 1983                   8–3

The authors used the $^{133}$Xe intraarterial injection method to study regional cerebral blood flow (rCBF) after carotid arteriography in 13 patients with classic migraine. Radionuclide washout was recorded by 254 collimated detectors covering the lateral aspect of one hemisphere.

A characteristic migraine attack developed in 9 of the 13 patients after carotid arteriography. A series of rCBF studies carried out 5–10 minutes apart showed a wave of reduced blood flow originating in the posterior part of the brain and progressing anteriorly through the parietal and temporal lobes in eight of the nine patients. Relative to mean hemispheric blood flow, the mean decrease in blood flow in these regions was 24%. Oligemia was also observed in the frontal lobe in seven patients and appeared to be independent of the posterior oligemia because it did not cross the central or lateral sulcus. The calculated rate of progression of the spreading oligemia was 2.2 mm/minute, and rCBF in the oligemic areas ranged from 34 ml/100 gm$^{-1}$/minute$^{-1}$ to 67 ml/100 gm$^{-1}$/minute$^{-1}$. The appearance of focal symptoms did not coincide with the spread of oligemia in a corresponding primary sensorimotor area. Typically, the spread of oligemia began before the patient experienced any focal symptoms, reaching the primary sensorimotor area after symptoms attributable to that area began. In addition, the oligemia persisted in this area after the focal symptoms disappeared. Also, the oligemia spread to other regions without causing new focal symptoms.

The observed time course and intensity of the reduction in rCBF in these patients with induced migraine suggest that spreading oligemia is not the cause of focal symptoms in classic migraine. The rate at which oligemia spread, and its dependence on major macrostructural and microstructural changes, may indicate a relationship with Leao's spreading depression. If so, the spread of oligemia may be an epiphenomenon accompanying spreading depression, and focal migraine symptoms may be the result of prolonged inhibition of cortical neurons after spreading depression.

▶ This is an interesting and instructive study. The authors precipitated migraine by an angiogram and then watched by blood flow techniques the spread of oligemia, which began before the patient had any symptoms. One supposes that they are correct in assuming that migraine precipitated by angiography is the same as spontaneous migraine. They bring up again the question as to whether the vascular changes are secondary to Leao's spreading depression.

A recent note on the treatment of migraine in the emergency room may be of use: the author found that 96 of 100 patients were completely relieved in an hour by the injection of intramuscular chlorpromazine (1 mg/kg of body weight to a maximum of 100 mg) (Iverson, K.V.: *Ann. Emerg. Med.* 12:756–758, 1983).—R.D.C.

---

### The Pharmacology of Calcium Channel Antagonists: Novel Class of Antimigraine Agents?
Stephen J. Peroutka (Johns Hopkins Hosp.)
Headache 23:278–283, November 1983                                   8–4

---

Calcium channel antagonists, which are vasodilators, prevent the influx of extracellular calcium into vascular smooth muscle. Their unique pharmacologic properties provide a theoretical basis for their use in the treatment of both common and classic migraine. The author reviewed the pharmacologic effects of these drugs.

The calcium channel antagonists block the final common pathway of vascular smooth muscle contraction by preventing the entrance of calcium through the membrane channels, regardless of whether the channel is voltage sensitive or receptor operated. Thus, these drugs bypass the agonist receptor sites, blocking all vasoconstriction that is dependent on extracellular calcium. In addition, the vascular effects of the calcium channel antagonists are preferential for intracerebral vs. peripheral arteries. Theoretically, the degree of selectivity of these agents should allow increased cerebral blood flow without producing systemic hypotension. Flunarizine and cinnarizine, two specific calcium antagonists, and cyproheptadine and amitriptyline, two nonspecific antagonists, appear to be effective in the treatment of migraine. This suggests that the latter two drugs, which are traditional antimigraine agents, may produce their clinical effects through blockade of calcium channels. Additional studies will determine whether calcium channel antagonists are of therapeutic value in the treatment of migraine and other types of vascular headache. Because the calcium channel antagonists bypass the sites of action of the various endogenous vasoactive substances implicated in the pathogenesis of migraine, they may be useful in direct evaluation of the vascular theory of migraine.

▶ The calcium channel antagonists are a recently developed class of vasodilators that prevent the influx of calcium into vascular smooth muscle. This novel class of vasodilators provides a powerful tool for critical evaluation of the vascular theory of migraine.—R.N.D.J.

## Therapeutic Impact of Temporal Artery Biopsy

S. Hall, S. Persellin, J. T. Lie, P. C. O'Brien, L. T. Kurland, and G. G. Hunder (Mayo Clinic and Found.)
Lancet 2:1217–1220, Nov. 26, 1983                                                    8–5

Proper management is uncertain when the patient's clinical picture suggests giant cell arteritis but temporal artery biopsy findings are negative. The authors followed up 134 patients who underwent temporal artery biopsy between 1965 and 1980. Initial biopsy results were positive for giant cell arteritis in 46 patients and negative in 88. The findings in these two groups are compared in the table. Age and sex distributions in the groups were comparable. Generous biopsy samples were obtained in this series. The overall clinical features were remarkably similar in the two groups, except for the more frequent finding of jaw pain or claudication

FINDINGS IN 134 PATIENTS WITH TEMPORAL ARTERY
BIOPSY

|  | Biopsy positive (n = 46) | Biopsy negative (n = 88) |
|---|---|---|
| Median age (range) in years | 74 (55–92) | 69 (47–90) |
| % female | 57 | 72 |
| Number with unilateral/bilateral biopsy | 31/15 | 39/49† |
| Median (range) length of tissue examined in cm | 4·0 (0·8–9·5) | 5·0 (0·5–17.5) |
| Median ESR (range) in mm/h* | 95 (50–126) | 83 (5–126) |
| Median haemoglobin (range) in g/l | 116 (87–141) | 120 (71–162) |

*Westergren.
†P<.001; chi-square test.
(Courtesy of Hall, S., et al.: Lancet 2:1217–1220, Nov. 26, 1983.)

in those with positive results, as well as the more frequent detection of clinical abnormality over the temporal artery in this group.

Those with negative biopsy results were followed up for a median of 70 months. Polymyalgia rheumatica was the final diagnosis in 31 patients in whom no other symptoms or signs developed during follow-up. Nine patients had infectious disorders, and other connective tissue disease developed in eight. Giant cell arteritis eventually was diagnosed in eight patients.

Only 9% of patients in this series with initially negative findings on temporal artery biopsy subsequently required long-term steroid therapy for giant cell arteritis. Biopsy correctly predicted the need for steroid therapy for this diagnosis in 94% of the patients. The high predictive value of a negative biopsy result may be due in part to the fact that a large sample was obtained and also that bilateral biopsies were done when the first results proved negative. Temporal artery biopsy should be done in all patients suspected of having giant cell arteritis before long-term, high-dose corticosteroid therapy is undertaken.

▶ This is a helpful article from the Mayo Clinic. In the authors' large series of cases of temporal arteritis they found artery biopsy correctly predicted the subsequent need for corticosteroid therapy in 94% of their patients. They performed repeat biopsies when suspicion remained after a negative biopsy and performed bilateral biopsies in some cases, but the chief reason for their outstandingly successful prediction was the length of artery taken; the mean length was 5.4 cm!—R.D.C.

# 9 Infections of the Nervous System

**Measles Encephalomyelitis: Clinical and Immunologic Studies**
Richard T. Johnson, Diane E. Griffin, Robert L. Hirsch, Jerry S. Wolinsky,
Susi Roedenbeck, Imelda Lindo de Soriano, and Abraham Vaisberg
N. Engl. J. Med. 310:137–141, Jan. 19, 1984                      9–1

An acute perivenular inflammatory and demyelinating disorder is the most common neurologic complication of measles. Acute measles encephalomyelitis is distinct from both subacute inclusion body encephalitis in immunodeficient patients and subacute sclerosing panencephalitis. The authors reviewed the findings in 19 patients seen with measles encephalomyelitis during summer epidemics of measles in Lima, Peru, between 1980 and 1983. The 10 males and 9 females had a median age of five years. All patients had typical measles, and most developed signs of encephalomyelitis one to eight days after the rash, when defervescence had occurred.

Ten patients had sudden obtundation or confusion, and six had generalized seizures. Only three had antecedent headache and nuchal rigidity. Fever usually recurred or increased abruptly within 12 hours of the onset of neurologic signs. Nine patients in all had seizures. Motor deficits were frequent but of variable severity. Only one patient had cerebellar ataxia as the only focal neurologic abnormality. Only three cerebrospinal fluid protein values exceeded 100 mg/dl. Thirteen of 18 patients had lymphocytic pleocytosis, but only four counts were greater than 100 cells/cu mm. Only 1 of 12 samples had an elevated IgG index. Proliferative lymphocyte responses to human myelin basic protein were significantly more frequent than in patients without encephalomyelitis or those with other neurologic disorders. All patients were able to return home, but only 1 of the 10 reexamined was free from sequelae. The final status showed little relation to the severity of initial illness.

Measles encephalomyelitis may not depend on viral replication within the CNS, since intrathecal synthesis of antimeasles antibody is lacking. Abnormal lymphoproliferative responses to myelin basic protein are also observed after varicella or rubella and in patients with encephalomyelitis after rabies vaccination, suggesting a common immune-mediated pathogenesis for a perivenular demyelinating disorder. The profound immune suppression resulting from measles virus infection may explain why measles is the most common cause of postinfectious demyelinating disease.

▶ Studies on patients with postinfectious encephalomyelitis complicating measles virus infections support the hypothesis that this demyelinating disease has a pathogenesis similar to that of experimental allergic encephalomyelitis. Although the frequency of natural measles infections in the United States has been markedly reduced by the use of a live virus vaccine, measles infections are still widespread in the rest of the world, and measles encephalomyelitis remains a serious and frequent cause of childhood disability and death.—R.N.D.J.

## Subacute Sclerosing Panencephalitis: An Immune Complex Disease?

Ana Sotrel, Seymour Rosen, Michael Ronthal, and David B. Ross
Neurology (Cleve.) 33:885–890, July 1983                                          9–2

Subacute sclerosing panencephalitis (SSPE) is a progressive, slowly evolving viral disease characterized by myoclonic jerks, typical changes seen on EEG, and high measles virus antibody titers in the serum and cerebrospinal fluid (CSF). The authors report evidence of deposition of antigen-antibody complexes in cerebral vessels of a patient with SSPE.

Woman, 19, experienced left-sided incoordination and underwent personality changes six months previously in early gestation. A generalized seizure occurred in the last month of pregnancy, and phenytoin therapy was begun after delivery of a healthy infant. The patient was disoriented in time and had a childlike affect with inappropriate giggling and tearfulness. Left homonymous hemianopia was noted, as well as myoclonic jerks of the left extremities. Bilateral ankle clonus occurred, with extensor plantar responses. On CT a nonenhancing area of low density was seen in the right parietal lobe, and EEG showed diffuse paroxymal, pseudoperiodic, triphasic discharges. The CSF gamma globulin level was 41% of the total protein. The measles antibody titer in CSF was elevated at 1:16, and the titer in serum was 1:256. The patient deteriorated over the next months and was discharged to a chronic care institution.

Measles virus was not isolated from a right parietal lobe brain biopsy specimen. Extensive necrosis was present, with plasma cells, lymphocytes, microglia, hypertrophic astrocytes, and lipid-laden macrophages in the white matter. Electron microscopy showed intramembranous electron-dense deposits consisting of tubular and annular profiles in the walls of about two thirds of the capillaries. Similar clusters of tubular profiles were seen in some myelinated axons. No viral particles were observed. Immunofluorescence study with measles antiserum showed granular deposits along the vessel walls and prominent intervascular punctate areas. Staining was not obtained with preimmune serum.

Measles virus antigen-antibody complexes were demonstrated in cerebral vessels in this patient with confirmed SSPE. She may be the first in whom vascular immune complex deposits in the CNS were demonstrated ultrastructurally and by immunofluorescence. Immune complexes trapped in the cerebral vasculature could be important in the pathogenesis of CNS manifestations of systemic immune complex diseases and persistent viral infections of the brain.

▶ This apparently is the first demonstration of immune complexes in the blood vessels of the central nervous system.—R.N.D.J.

### Treatment of Neurosyphilis With Chloramphenicol: A Case Report

Barbara Romanowski, Elout Starreveld, and Andrew J. Jarema (Social Hygiene Services, Edmonton, Alberta, Canada)

Br. J. Vener. Dis. 59:225–227, August 1983                    9–3

Penicillin is the accepted treatment for syphilis, but treatment failures have occurred in neurosyphilis treated with procaine and benzathine penicillin. In penicillin-allergic patients, tetracycline or erythromycin fail to pass the blood-brain barrier. The authors report data on a case of general paresis that was successfully treated with chloramphenicol, which does achieve adequate levels in the cerebrospinal fluid (CSF).

Man, 49, was seen after two months of dizziness, loss of balance, and pain in his right knee. He reported feeling anxious and nervous. There was no reported extramarital sexual contact in the past 10 years, and no genital ulceration had been noted at any time. Serologic testing had been negative 26 years earlier. The patient was allergic to penicillin. He was nervous and suspicious when examined and had tremulous speech. Palmomental reflexes were positive bilaterally, and there was a fine tremor of the outstretched hands. Syphilis serology was positive and lymphocytic pleocytosis was found in the CSF. Bacterial and viral cultures were negative. Results of serologic testing of the wife's serum were negative. Computed tomography (CT) of the brain showed a small area of decreased density in the posterior aspect of the left basal ganglia. Chloramphenicol, 1 gm every six hours for two weeks, was given intravenously. Clinical and CSF abnormalities were less marked at the end of treatment, but the patient presented three months later with leg weakness, impaired judgment and recent memory, hypokinesia, and slight rigidity of all extremities. Results of a repeat CT study were normal. An EEG showed mild dysrhythmia. The patient was mentally and physically stable a year after treatment, but was unable to return to work.

This patient clearly had symptoms and signs of general paresis. Although the neurologic abnormalities were not resolved, the treatment was considered successful. Intravenous chloramphenicol may be more appropriate than tetracycline for use in penicillin-allergic patients with neurosyphilis.

▶ Intravenous administration of chloramphenicol achieves adequate concentrations in the CSF and therefore may be a more appropriate agent than tetracycline and erythromycin for the treatment of patients with neurosyphilis who are allergic to penicillin.—R.N.D.J.

---

### Chronic Partial Denervation Is More Widespread Than Is Suspected Clinically in Paralytic Poliomyelitis: Electrophysiological Study

A. Cruz Martinez, M. C. Pérez Conde, and M. T. Ferrer (Ciudad Sanitaria "La Paz," Madrid)

Eur. Neurol. 22:314–321, September–October 1983                    9–4

The cause of late, slowly progressive weakening of previously affected muscles in patients who sustained an acute attack of poliomyelitis at a young age is unclear. The authors analyzed the clinical and electromyographic (EMG) findings in 34 selected patients who had paralytic poliomyelitis during infancy. Motor unit fiber density per uptake area of a special electrode was also determined in the extensor digitorum communis (EDC) muscle in 24 patients.

Patients ranged in age from 10 to 64 (mean, 37.5) and were studied 9–62 years (mean, 36.1 years) after the poliomyelitis attack. The most common physical signs were muscle wasting and reduction of muscular strength. These signs were observed in a lower limb in 21 patients (61.6%), unilaterally in an upper and a lower limb in 5 (14.7%), in both lower limbs in 5 (14.7%), in all 4 limbs in 2 (6%), and in an upper limb in 1 (3%). Seventeen patients (50%) reported slow progression of muscle weakness; deterioration occurred in the affected muscles in 6 patients (35.4%), only in apparently unaffected muscles in 8 (47%), and in affected and unaffected muscles in 3 (17.6%). The other 17 patients did not report deterioration of function, although the mean number of years elapsed since the attack was significantly less in this group ($P<.01$). Fibrillation potentials were detected in seven patients, all of whom reported deterioration of function. An increment in the mean duration of motor unit potentials and a loss of motor units were observed in 87.5% of the patients. Increases in polyphasia as great as 20% (mean, 9.1%) were found in 37% of the muscles. A slight reduction in motor conduction velocity on the peroneal nerve was seen in only 7% of the patients. Automatic EMG analysis revealed a great increase in mean amplitude in weak muscles, as well as in hypertrophic and other muscles that had normal strength. Motor unit fiber density was increased in the EDC muscle in 20 (83%) of 24 patients, even though the EDC was clinically normal in 21 of them. The increases in mean EMG amplitude and in motor unit fiber density were significantly greater in the weaker muscles (both $P<.01$).

The results confirm that partial denervation followed by collateral reinnervation in poliomyelitis is more widespread than is clinically suspected and affects apparently preserved muscles. The late functional deterioration reported by some patients always occurs in muscles that were damaged previously and are partially depleted of motor units. Widespread neurogenic involvement of muscles can be significant in the late functional deterioration of patients who have had paralytic poliomyelitis.

▶ This may relate to the continuing mystery of the relationship of poliomyelitis to amyotrophic lateral sclerosis. Some who have had poliomyelitis years before continue to notice muscle jumps here and there. Does this study give us the reason? It appears also that some deterioration of the affected muscles with aging can be expected. But these do not make amyotrophic lateral sclerosis.— R.D.C.

---

**Herpes Zoster Ophthalmicus and Delayed Ipsilateral Cerebral Infarction**
Dennis N. Bourdette, Neil L. Rosenberg, and Frank M. Yatsu

Neurology (Cleve.) 33:1428–1432, November 1983                    9–5

Twenty-six cases of herpes zoster ophthalmicus (HZO) and delayed ipsilateral cerebral infarction have been previously reported. The authors describe five new patients with acute cerebral infarction that occurred five weeks to six months after HZO. All had infarcts of the cerebral hemisphere ipsilateral to the HZO, and one also had a cerebellar infarct. The sex distribution in all 31 reported cases was nearly equal. Average age was 55 years. Average interval from onset of HZO to stroke was eight weeks. Several stroke syndromes occurred, most of sudden onset. Several patients had transient ischemic attacks before or after the stroke. The most consistent angiographic finding was segmental narrowing or occlusion of the proximal middle cerebral artery or a major branch ipsilateral to the HZO. The proximal anterior communicating artery, posterior cerebral artery, or distal carotid artery was occasionally affected. Autopsies showed necrotizing arteritis of multiple small vessels.

Zoster arteritis can evolve as a result of HZO and lead to a range of stroke syndromes. The risk appears to be low, but the association is not rare. The pathogenesis of HZO angiitis is unclear, but it might be a result of viral invasion of vessels. The virus could reach intracranial vessels by traveling along the ophthalmic nerve branches that supply intracranial arteries and the meninges. A definite diagnosis of zoster arteritis is impossible short of biopsying intracranial vessels, but the clinical diagnosis can be confirmed by arteriography. The usefulness of corticosteroids, anticoagulants, or antiplatelet drugs in the management of patients with presumed zoster arteritis is unknown. Any regimen should recognize that most patients have limited duration of risk of stroke and a low risk of death due to stroke.

▶ Zoster arteritis can develop as a consequence of herpes zoster ophthalmicus and result in a variety of stroke syndromes. The development of delayed ipsilateral cerebral infarction after herpes zoster ophthalmicus is not rare.— R.N.D.J.

---

**Intracranial Complications of Acute and Chronic Infectious Ear Disease: A Problem Still With Us**
David Gower and W. Frederick McGuirt (Bowman Gray School of Medicine)
Laryngoscope 93:1028–1033, August 1983                                    9–6

---

There are only infrequent reports of CNS complications of infectious ear disease. Because of the lack of familiarity with these potential complications and the masking of developing CNS complications by antibiotic therapy, early recognition of these problems is less likely than it was in the past. The authors report the findings in 100 children with CNS complications of middle ear disease identified among 334,884 hospital admissions from 1962 through 1981.

In all, 76 children, 63 with acute and 13 with chronic ear disease, had meningitic complications; 24 children, 17 with acute and 7 with chronic ear disease, had nonmeningitic complications (Table 1). Fifty-six of the

TABLE 1.—Correlation of Type of Central Nervous
System Complication With Type of Infectious
Ear Disease

| CNS Complication | No. of Patients | Ear Disease Acute | Ear Disease Chronic |
|---|---|---|---|
| Meningitic | 76 | 63 | 13 |
| Nonmeningitic | 24 | 17 | 7 |
|    Brain abscess | 6 | | |
|    Subdural effusion | 5 | | |
|    Lateral sinus thrombosis | 5 | | |
|    Otitic hydrocephalus | 5 | | |
|    Subdural empyema | 3 | | |
| | 100 | 80 | 20 |

(Courtesy of Gower, D., and McGuirt, W.F.: Laryngoscope 93:1028–1033, August 1983.)

TABLE 2.—Meningitis Secondary
to Ear Disease

| Age | Ear Disease Acute | Chronic |
|---|---|---|
| 0-1 | 39 | — |
| 1-10 | 17 | 3 |
| 10-20 | 2 | 4 |
| 20-30 | — | — |
| 30-40 | 1 | 2 |
| 40-50 | — | 1 |
| 50-60 | 1 | 1 |
| 60+ | 3 | 2 |
| | 63 | 13 |

(Courtesy of Gower, D., and McGuirt, W.F.: Laryngoscope 93:1028–1033, August 1983.)

76 children with meningitis were less than 10 years of age (Table 2); most were treated with antibiotics only. *Hemophilus influenzae* type B and *H. influenzae* nontyped were the most common organisms cultured from the cerebrospinal fluid (CSF). Death occurred in 5 (7.9%) of the 63 children with meningitis secondary to acute otitis media and in 4 (30.7%) of the 13 with meningitis due to chronic ear disease. Of the 24 children with nonmeningitic complications, 3 had subdermal empyema, 5 had subdermal effusion, 6 had brain abscess, 5 had lateral sinus thrombosis, and 5 had otitic hydrocephalus. One child with brain abscess died.

These findings demonstrate that CNS complications of otitis media still occur and that the traditional paths of infectious spread have not changed. The resulting mortality remains high. Meningitis secondary to ear disease should be considered carefully in children who have fever and are lethargic and irritable.

▶ It's clear that in spite of the antibiotics we have not conquered middle ear disease and to ignore it may still be fatal.—R.D.C.

---

**Toxoplasma Encephalitis in Haitian Adults With Acquired Immunodeficiency Syndrome: Clinical-Pathologic-CT Correlation**
M. Judith Donovan Post, Joseph C. Chan, George T. Hensley, Thomas A. Hoffman, Lee B. Moskowitz, and Susan Lippmann (Univ. of Miami)
AJR 140:861–868, May 1983                                                  9–7

---

*Toxoplasma* encephalitis typically occurs in adults with immunologic impairment. Although usually progressive and fatal, it can be treated successfully with sulfadiazine and pyrimethamine when detected early. However, diagnosis may be difficult. To define the usefulness and specificity of computed tomography (CT) in the diagnosis of this disease, the authors retrospectively analyzed the clinical and laboratory findings and CT abnormalities in eight Haitian adults with *Toxoplasma* encephalitis.

*Toxoplasma gondii* infection was identified at autopsy in five patients and on brain biopsy in three; the final diagnosis was established using the immunoperoxidase method and electron microscopy. All eight patients, six of whom had been in the United States for 24 months or less, had severe idiopathic immunodeficiency syndrome. All had peripheral lymphocytopenia, and six were being treated with antituberculosis medication when the neurologic symptoms developed. All eight were febrile and had an altered mental status; three had seizures, four had focal neurologic deficits, and four had headache. The CT scans obtained before treatment showed a multiplicity of intraparenchymal lesions in seven patients that were bilateral in six and affected the cerebral hemispheres in all seven. Edema and a mass effect were noted around the lesions. The basal ganglia were affected in seven patients, and the corticomedullary junction in the cerebral hemispheres was also commonly involved. Focal enhancement of the lesions after administration of contrast medium was seen in six patients, and hypodense areas in two. Patterns of focal uptake included ring or nodular enhancement. The ring-enhancing lesions were hypodense centrally and usually had thin, smooth margins. The enhancing nodules were smooth, sharply defined, and best demonstrated on coronal views. Serial scans demonstrated progression of the abnormalities and the appearance of new lesions (Figs 9–1, 9–2, and 9–3).

Neither type of contrast uptake nor density measurement was useful in differentiating toxoplasmosis from other intracranial infections. However, despite this lack of specificity, CT confirmed the presence of multiple intracranial lesions and determined the magnitude of mass effects, size of the ventricles, and extent of edema. It was also particularly useful in localizing lesions for biopsy, with optimal visualization obtained on axial and coronal scans 5-mm thick with double-dose contrast medium injection. For these reasons, CT is recommended in patients with a clinical presentation similar to that described.

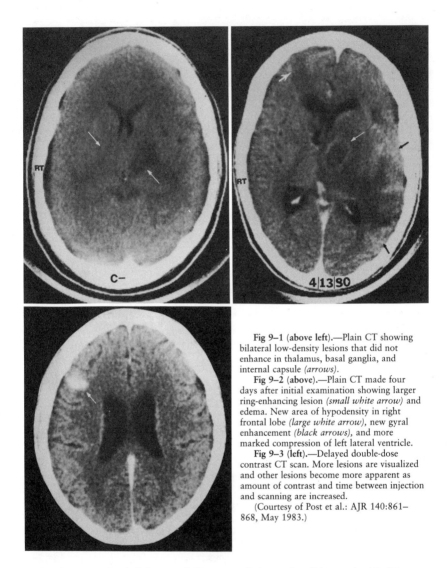

**Fig 9–1 (above left).**—Plain CT showing bilateral low-density lesions that did not enhance in thalamus, basal ganglia, and internal capsule *(arrows)*.

**Fig 9–2 (above).**—Plain CT made four days after initial examination showing larger ring-enhancing lesion *(small white arrow)* and edema. New area of hypodensity in right frontal lobe *(large white arrow)*, new gyral enhancement *(black arrows)*, and more marked compression of left lateral ventricle.

**Fig 9–3 (left).**—Delayed double-dose contrast CT scan. More lesions are visualized and other lesions become more apparent as amount of contrast and time between injection and scanning are increased.

(Courtesy of Post et al.: AJR 140:861–868, May 1983.)

▶ Immunologically deficient patients not only have *Candida* meningitis (abstract 9–9) but *Toxoplasma* encephalitis. This disease, difficult to diagnose with certainty, should be considered when the characteristic CT scan picture is seen in an appropriate patient. The same situation has been reported from France (Guilbeau, J.C.: *J. Radiol.* 64:347–351, 1983).—R.D.C.

---

**Cerebral Cysticercosis Treated Biphasically With Dexamethasone and Praziquantel**

Lawrence D. deGhetaldi, Robert M. Norman, and Arthur W. Douville, Jr.
Ann. Intern. Med. 99:179–181, August 1983

9–8

The diagnosis of cerebral cysticercosis, an infection of the CNS caused by the larval stage of the pork tapeworm, *Taenia solium*, has increased in the United States, probably because of the widespread availability of CT and the increased influx of immigrants from endemic areas. Treatment is limited for the most part to relieving manifestations of the infection. The authors describe the successful treatment of cerebral cysticercosis with high-dose corticosteroids followed by a course of praziquantel, an anti-parasitic agent.

Mexican woman, 29, had generalized major motor seizures not preceded by head trauma or drug use; she had no family history of neurologic disorder. She had traveled to Mexico 11 and 3 years previously. Mild right facial paresis and weakness of dorsiflexion of the right foot were present. Results of routine serum tests were normal, as was the blood count. Cerebrospinal fluid (CSF) examination showed an opening pressure of 320 mm CSF, four leukocytes/cu mm with 100% polymorphonuclear neutrophils, a protein level of 27 mg/dl, and a glucose level of 68 mg/dl. Results of bacteriologic cultures were negative. Multiple low-density cystic lesions and numerous intracranial calcifications were seen by CT in both cerebral hemispheres. Twelve isolated cysts were identified, with one 3-cm cyst seen in the left parasagittal area, which probably explained the right leg weakness. Plain films of the thighs showed multiple soft tissue calcifications. Serum and CSF complement fixation and serum indirect hemagglutination titers for cysticercosis were not diagnostic. Phenytoin and phenobarbital therapy resolved the seizure activity and improved right leg strength. The patient was rehospitalized 10 months later with intermittent headaches and weakness and focal seizure activity in the right leg. Phenytoin and phenobarbital levels were within the therapeutic range. A contrast-enhanced CT scan showed marked enlargement of the left parasagittal cyst, which was surrounded by significant edema. Treatment with oral dexamethasone (4 mg four times daily) produced dramatic resolution of the right leg weakness, disappearance of the right Babinski's sign, and decreased frequency of focal seizure activity. At discharge she was advised to take dexamethasone, phenytoin, and phenobarbital.

The patient was readmitted two months later to start praziquantel therapy. Prior to treatment, CT showed resolution of the pericystic cerebral edema, but there was no change in the size or number of cysts. Praziquantel therapy was begun at 50 mg/kg/day in three divided doses for 14 days; dexamethasone and anticonvulsant medications were continued. On the third day of treatment the patient had a diffuse headache, a low-grade temperature, and signs of mild meningismus. Lumbar puncture revealed an opening pressure of 310 mm CSF; CSF contained 61 leukocytes/cu mm with 80% neutrophils and 20% lymphocytes; total protein concentration was 40 mg/dl; and glucose level was 51 mg/dl. Radioimmunoassay of the CSF for anticysticerci IgG was 2+ reactive, consistent with active infection. The headache, meningismus, and fever resolved without additional treatment, and the 14-day course of praziquantel was completed uneventfully. The patient was discharged taking anticonvulsant therapy and a tapering course of steroids. One month after the course of praziquantel, she no longer had right leg weakness or focal seizures. A CT scan at this time showed a reduction in size of all intracerebral cysts. Six weeks after treatment, examination of the CSF showed an opening pressure of 260 mm CSF; four leukocytes/cu mm (60% lymphocytes, 28% neutrophils, and 12% eosinophils), and normal glucose and protein levels. At four months, a CT scan showed complete disappearance of all intracerebral cysts. The patient tolerated complete weaning of steroids; she regained full motor function of the right lower limb, with no return of generalized or focal seizure activity.

Although it is unlikely that this regimen affects end-stage or calcified lesions, it may serve as an alternative to surgery in patients with overwhelming infection or in whom the position of a cyst rules out surgery. Steroid therapy before or during treatment with praziquantel is advocated. Scanning with CT is essential in the diagnosis and follow-up of patients treated with praziquantel.

▶ The medical treatment of cerebral cysticercosis with these agents is new. They appear to be a real hope for patients with a difficult therapeutic problem.—R.D.C.

---

### Candidal Infection in the Central Nervous System

Stuart A. Lipton, William F. Hickey, James H. Morris, and Joseph Loscalzo
Am. J. Med. 76:101–108, January 1984                                    9–9

---

Candidiasis has become the most prevalent cerebral mycosis found at autopsy. The authors reviewed 13 autopsy cases of CNS candidiasis, among 28 cases of systemic candidiasis, and another case in a patient with systemic candidiasis who was treated and is alive. The eight females and six males were aged 16–87 years. Various clinical and pathologic patterns of cerebral involvement were observed. Central nervous system candidiasis was suspected during life in only six patients and was documented in only three. The most common initial sites of recognized infection were the urine, airways, and blood, followed by the skin. All patients had risk factors for opportunistic infection, most frequently antimicrobial therapy for acute bacterial infection and immunosuppressive therapy for chronic disorders or renal transplantation. *Candida* organisms were recovered from the CSF in only three cases.

Scattered intraparenchymal microabscesses were observed at seven autopsies. Two patients had gross abscesses. Three had noncaseating granulomas, and four had glial nodules. Vascular involvement by *Candida* was seen in three patients, two of whom had true vasculitis with thrombosis and luminal proliferation of *Candida*. Only two patients had meningeal infection. One patient had candidal fungous balls in the temporal lobe in association with disseminated cerebral aspergillosis.

A more aggressive diagnostic approach to cerebral candidiasis is warranted, particularly in immunocompromised patients and drug addicts. Tissue biopsy and serologic testing are indicated, besides standard fungous studies of body fluids, whenever candidiasis is a possibility. There is no convincing evidence that intrathecal amphotericin B therapy is superior to intravenous treatment. A large candidal abscess may have to be surgically evacuated. A mycotic aneurysm may also necessitate operation.

▶ In renal transplant patients and those who are immunologically suppressed for other reasons, *Candida* has come to the front. This is a serious problem in renal transplantation centers.

An interesting sidelight on immunity and disease is the finding by Hoffman et al. (*J. Gerontol.* 38:414–419, 1983) that among Guamanians the immune system changes markedly with age, suggesting a relationship to the high prevalence of the amyotrophic lateral sclerosis–dementia–parkinsonism complex on Guam.—R.D.C.

---

**Disinfection Studies With Two Strains of Mouse-Passaged Scrapie Agent: Guidelines for Creutzfeldt-Jakob and Related Agents**
R. H. Kimberlin, C. A. Walker, G. C. Millson, D. M. Taylor, P. A. Robertson, A. H. Tomlinson, and A. G. Dickinson
J. Neurol. Sci. 59:355–369, June 1983                                    9–10

---

Scrapie agent and the related etiologic agent of Creutzfeldt-Jakob disease (CJD) both possess physicochemical stability, which makes disinfection difficult. The need for better techniques has been emphasized by reports of iatrogenic transmission of CJD by the use of implanted electrodes that were inadequately sterilized between patients. It is hoped that the various methods studied for disinfecting scrapie agent will be applicable to agents of CJD.

Experiments involved two strains of intracerebrally passaged scrapie agent: 22A, chosen for its resistance to heating, in VM mice ($Sinc^{p7}$); and 139A, commonly used in scrapie research, in CW mice ($Sinc^{s7}$). Autoclaving, hypochlorite, phenolic disinfectant, permanganate, sodium dodecyl sulfate (SDS), and Tego (dodecyl-di(aminoethyl)-glycine) were the treatments investigated. Agent sources were brains taken from the mice at the clinical stage of scrapie, when infectivity titers are highest.

Scrapie strain 139A was relatively sensitive to autoclaving, with heating to 126 C for longer than 30 minutes producing the maximal detectable loss of 6.9 log units; no infectivity was found after heating to 136 C for 4–32 minutes. Similar treatment of 22A scrapie reduced the titer by only 1.4 log units, and significant infectivity remained after heating at 126 C for two hours; the maximal detectable loss of 5.6 log units was obtained by heating at 136 C for four minutes or longer. Treatment of 139A with Hycolin (0.6% chlorinated phenols) for 30 minutes had virtually no effect on titer; incubation for 16 hours was no more effective than for 1 hour. The decrease of 22A titer was even less after incubation for 1–16 hours.

An inactivation factor of $10^4$ should be the minimum achieved for disinfection purposes. By this criterion, 0.2% permanganate and 4% Hycolin were found to be unsuitable for scrapie or CJD disinfection; 10% Lysol was as ineffective as Hycolin. The noncorrosive agent SDS was found to be ineffective in the treatment of whole brain homogenates at ambient temperature, even after long exposure times. Hypochlorite was the best chemical reagent for disinfection of scrapie. Exposure for four hours or longer to hypochlorite having at least 1,000 ppm chlorine produced an inactivation factor of $10^4$–$10^5$; 0.5 hours of exposure to hypochlorite with 10,000 ppm available chlorine yielded similar results. The present findings suggest that the previously recommended procedure of autoclaving at 121 C for one hour is inadequate to disinfect high titers of scrapie; a temperature of 136 C is needed.

Until recently, there were no laboratory animal models of CJD that were reproducible or economical for infectivity titrations. However, CJD has recently been transmitted to rodents, and it would be useful to check the present results with hypochlorite and autoclaving in this CJD system. Still, it is the mouse model of scrapie that will continue to be used for such work because of the availability of agent strains and the relative safety.

▶ For those who are worried about their operating rooms after biopsy for CJD (and who is not?) this may give help. The authors found hypochlorite kills the mouse scrapie agent better than autoclaving or any other method. Hospital infection committees should read this article with interest.—R.D.C.

---

**Neurologic Abnormalities of Lyme Disease: Successful Treatment With High-Dose Intravenous Penicillin**
Allen C. Steere, Andrew R. Pachner, and Stephen E. Malawista (Yale Univ.)
Ann. Intern. Med. 99:767–772, December 1983                    9–11

Lyme disease is characterized by erythema chronicum migrans developing at the site of a tick bite, followed in some cases by neurologic or cardiac abnormalities. Many patients become arthritic weeks to years later as a result of the bite. The authors used high doses of penicillin administered intravenously to treat patients in whom neurologic abnormalities developed despite previous oral antibiotic therapy. The use of penicillin is based on the finding that the disease is caused by a spirochete, which was also recovered from the cerebrospinal fluid of a patient with neurologic involvement. Twelve patients with meningitis caused by Lyme disease who were referred for neurologic problems received 3.3 million units of sodium penicillin G intravenously every four hours for 10 days.

Headache and stiff neck developed within a mean of five weeks after onset of the initial illness. Four patients also had cranial neuritis, most often facial palsy; two had motor or sensory radiculoneuropathy, and four had both cranial and peripheral radiculoneuropathies. All 12 patients had abnormal spinal fluid findings. Three patients had more intense pain and low-grade fever in the early phase of treatment. Neurologic pain usually resolved during treatment, and motor deficits began to improve. No patient relapsed after treatment was stopped. Fifteen previous patients who were treated with prednisone in daily doses of 40–60 mg required treatment for a mean of 30 weeks. Meningitis symptoms resolved more rapidly in the penicillin-treated patients, and fewer of them became arthritic.

High doses of penicillin given intravenously are effective in patients with neurologic abnormalities caused by Lyme disease. The finding of recurrent meningitis symptoms is a helpful clue to Lyme disease, and serologic testing often is helpful. Oral tetracycline therapy might be considered in patients allergic to penicillin, as in tertiary syphilis. The addition of steroid therapy does not appear to hasten the resolution of neurologic abnormalities.

▶ The suspicion continues that Bannwarth's syndrome in Europe and Lyme disease in this country are similar. Both are tick borne and both are suspected to be caused by a spirochete—a *Borrelia* (*Dtsch. Med. Wochenschr.* 108:577–580, 1983) in Bannwarth's syndrome and the *Ixodes dammini* spirochete in Lyme disease. Their clinical pictures also are similar (*Nervenarzt* 54:640–646, 1983). Now Steere and co-workers find Lyme disease responds to high-dose intravenous penicillin. It would not be surprising to read next year that Bannwarth's syndrome also responds to the same antibiotic.—R.D.C.

# 10 Intoxications Affecting the Nervous System

**Adult Inorganic Lead Intoxication: Presentation of 31 New Cases and Review of Recent Advances in the Literature**
Mark R. Cullen, James M. Robins, and Brenda Eskenazi (Yale Univ.)
Medicine 62:221–247, July 1983                                    10–1

The authors reviewed findings in 31 adults who were exposed to metallic lead or inorganic lead compounds; all had measurable impairment of at least one organ system known to be associated with lead exposure, with no other apparent cause found after appropriate examination. Thirty of the patients were males, and the mean age was about 40 years. Thirty patients were exposed to lead occupationally, and one while stripping paint from his house. The mean duration of exposure was about nine years. All patients but one were aware of their exposure to lead at the time of presentation.

Nine patients had no complaints when first seen, and no predominant complaints were noted in the group overall. The most common findings were abdominal pain, fatigue, and headache. Organ involvement is related to type of presentation in the table. All of the patients with hemolysis had moderately severe anemia, whereas the hypoproliferative anemias were consistently very mild. All patients with hemolysis had an acute onset of symptoms and abdominal pain. Basophilic stippling was infrequent. Abnormal glomerular function was rare. None of the 18 patients who had formal neuropsychological testing had completely normal findings, with visuomotor coordination and rapid motor control being most often impaired. Four patients were depressed at presentation, and three others had a history of depression. All of the patients were removed from lead exposure, and 10 with high burdens and major dysfunction were chelated with intravenous calcium ethylenediamine tetraacetic acid without complications. The effects of treatment were generally favorable in the 18 patients followed up. The rapidity of symptomatic and functional responses tended to parallel the duration of lead exposure.

Measurement of the blood lead level remains the best single means of determining whether a clinical syndrome is related to lead exposure. Both acute and chronic forms of clinical lead intoxication occur in adults, as well as a "late" syndrome of gout, chronic renal failure, and encephalopathy. Both acute and chronic intoxication have been treated successfully

Comparison of Prevalence of Involved Organs in Patients With Acute Versus Those With Insidious or Asymptomatic Presentations

| Organ system dysfunction | Acute presenters (N = 6) | Insidious/asymptomatic presenters (N = 25) | Significance* |
|---|---|---|---|
| Hematologic | 5 (83%) | 4 (16%) | p <.01 |
| Gastrointestinal | 6 (100%) | 10 (40%) | p <.01 |
| Renal | 2 (33%) | 10 (40%) | NS |
| Rheumatologic | 1 (17%) | 6 (24%) | NS |
| Endocrine/reproductive | 3 (50%) | 13 (52%) | NS |
| Neurologic/psychiatric | 4 (67%) | 17 (68%) | NS |

*Using chi-square analysis.
(Courtesy of Cullen, M.R., et al.: Medicine 62:221–247, July 1983.)

by removing patients from exposure and by chelation, but only the hematologic and gastrointestinal tract effects have been reversed completely.

▶ My ignorance of the clinical syndrome of lead poisoning in adults was badly exposed by this article. A variety of mental, neurologic, and psychological symptoms result from chronic lead poisoning in adults, but only eight of the 31 had evidence of peripheral nerve involvement. The reader would be well advised to obtain and mark this excellent summary reference for future reading.—R.D.C.

### Alcoholism: Images, Impairments, Interventions

Paul S. Hill (Texas A & M Univ.)
Postgrad. Med. 74:87–99, November 1983                    10–2

Alcoholism, though treatable, is unfortunately often unrecognized by physicians, partly because of cultural stereotypes and partly because of denial by those affected. Most alcoholics are married and employed, and they most commonly consume beer. Alcoholism should be considered a primary disorder rather than a symptom of underlying personality or mental disorder. Vigilance and a functional, adaptive attitude on the part of the physician are necessary to diagnose alcoholism. The diagnosis is based on the pattern of alcohol use, impaired social or occupational functioning, and evidence of tolerance or withdrawal. Pathologic drinking patterns include the daily use of alcohol as a prerequisite for adequate functioning, going on binges, experiencing blackouts, and making repeated attempts to reduce excessive drinking. The physician should avoid asking questions that elicit defensive responses and guarded replies. It may be helpful to talk to the spouse or another family member who is close to the patient. Alcoholism tends to run in families. Blood alcohol determinations are an underused test, and determination of serum gammaglutamyl transpeptidase activity may also be useful diagnostically.

The first step in intervention is to persuade the patient to accept the diagnosis. Confrontation by family members or employers may be necessary. Any treatment program should include adequate medical supervision, patient education, and psychotherapy focusing on direct problem-solving in everyday life and on coping with feelings. Traditional insight-oriented dynamic therapy has been generally ineffective in the management of alcoholism and may even be harmful. Participation in Alcoholics Anonymous is usually considered the single most important factor in helping alcoholics to remain sober, but any effective program must involve family members. Disulfiram treatment can be an effective deterrent to the impulsive consumption of alcohol if the patient's physical status permits its use. Close follow-up is an essential part of the management of alcoholism. Alcoholics who are recovering should not use sedatives or hypnotics, and use of narcotic drugs increases the risk of relapse.

▶ This is a concise, well-delineated summary of the syndrome of alcoholism, with specific emphasis on the role of the primary care physician in diagnosis, intervention, treatment, and follow-up care. Because the alcoholic is characteristically defensive and denies the diagnosis, the physician must be persistent and honest when confronting the patient. Effective treatment is available through programs comprising patient and family education, psychotherapy, medical supervision, involvement in Alcoholics Anonymous, and follow-up care; and avoidance of psychoactive and sedative drugs is also important.— R.N.D.J.

### Cerebellar Degeneration Caused by High-Dose Cytosine Arabinoside: Clinicopathologic Study

Marc D. Winkelman and John D. Hines (Case Western Reserve Univ.)
Ann. Neurol. 14:520–527, November 1983                                    10–3

High-dose cytosine arabinoside (Ara-C) therapy can induce remissions in patients with acute nonlymphocytic leukemia and malignant lymphoma whose disease is refractory to conventional therapy, but cerebellar degeneration may occur as a complication of treatment. The authors reviewed data on 15 men and 10 women, mean age 42, who received high-dose Ara-C therapy between 1979 and 1982. Of these, 23 had hematologic malignancy refractory to conventional treatment, 1 had newly diagnosed leukemia, and 1 had refractory orbital osteosarcoma. The drug was given intravenously in a dose of 3 gm/sq m of body surface area every 12 hours for six days. Ten patients also received 4'-(9-acridinylamino)-methanesulfon-m-anisidine, two received doxorubicin, and three were given daunorubicin.

Four of the 25 patients sustained irreversible cerebellar ataxia during high-dose Ara-C therapy. A fifth patient was ataxic but could not be fully

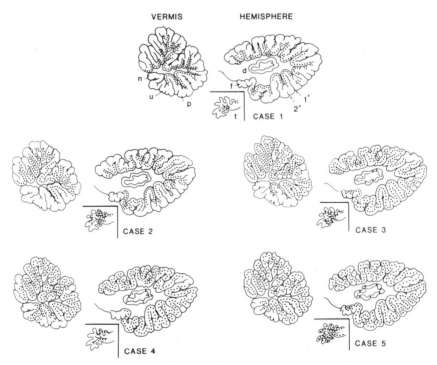

Fig 10–1.—Drawings show sites of Purkinje cell loss in five patients with cerebellar degeneration caused by treatment with high doses of cytosine arabinoside. Dots indicate areas of cortex depleted of Purkinje cells and show involvement of deep nuclei (*d*). Inset represents the cerebellar tonsil (*t*). 1° = primary cortical sulcus; 2° = secondary cortical sulcus; n = nodulus; u = uvula; p = pyramis; f = flocculus. (Courtesy of Winkleman, M.D., and Hines, J.D.: Ann. Neurol. 14:520–527, November 1983.)

evaluated neurologically. The first signs were noted after five to seven days of treatment; ataxia peaked in severity in the next two to three days and then remained stable for two to six days before improvement began. No patient recovered completely, and four remained unable to walk, feed themselves, or speak intelligibly. Other patients experienced reversible cerebellar abnormalities with mild symptoms, e.g., nystagmus or cogwheel ocular pursuit movements. The chief cortical abnormality in irreversible ataxia was a loss of Purkinje cells, the patterns of which are shown in Figure 10–1. None of the patients with reversible ataxia was examined at autopsy. Those with and those without irreversible ataxia did not differ significantly in age, duration of malignant disease before treatment, type of treatment, or survival after treatment.

High-dose Ara-C therapy carries a risk of irreversible cerebellar degeneration. The complication occurred in 17% of the present patients with refractory hematologic malignancies. The use of high-dose therapy should be reevaluated and all treated patients followed prospectively by a neurologist. If severe or progressive ataxia develops, treatment should be withdrawn.

▶ Patients with either leukemia or lymphoma who are resistant to conventional chemotherapy sometimes respond to high-dose cystine arabinoside therapy. These investigators, however, found that arabinoside given in such doses may cause cerebellar degeneration with characteristic clinical and pathologic features. Further studies are necessary to see if it is possible to prognosticate, before instituting such therapy, which patients are at risk for such complications.—R.N.D.J.

---

**Intoxication From Accidental Marijuana Ingestion**
Diane Weinberg, Arthur Lande, Nancy Hilton, and David L. Kerns (Children's Hosp. Med. Center of Northern California, Oakland)
Pediatrics 71:848–850, May 1983                                              10–4

---

Adverse effects have been described in adults absorbing marijuana via inhalation or by the oral and intravenous routes. The authors report data on three children who accidentally ingested marijuana by eating cookies that contained it. A girl, aged three years, was seen to have an ataxic gait and a voracious appetite and exhibited a labile affect with euphoric smiling alternating with fear and crying. She became increasingly stuporous, but recovered uneventfully within six hours, as did the other two children, a brother aged four years and a girl aged two. The boy was ataxic and had similar but less marked signs. The younger girl was the least affected child, with only a mild hand tremor and slight ataxia.

Marijuana is less completely absorbed when ingested than when inhaled, and the onset of effects is slower. Nausea, vomiting, and dizziness may occur, and there may be an increased appetite for sweets. Dose-related tachycardia is seen, and there may be transient bradycardia after severe overdose. Patients may be somnolent or euphoric, and there may be mood changes and decreased attention span. Severe intoxication can result in decreased motor coordination, ataxia, slurred speech, and muscular jerking. Management is supportive. The environment may have to be adjusted if the patient is agitated. The manifestations of acute marijuana intoxication in young children are similar to those in older patients.

In an addendum, the authors report that another child, a girl aged two, was seen more recently with tachycardia, inappropriate crying, and a fine tremor after she ingested $\Delta^9$-tetrahydrocannabinol. She recovered within five hours.

▶ As the use of marijuana increases, physicians, especially pediatricians, should be alert to the possibility of accidental oral ingestion by young children. This article describes the adverse effects experienced by young children following such ingestion.—R.N.D.J.

---

**Sensory Neuropathy From Pyridoxine Abuse: A New Megavitamin Syndrome**
Herbert Schaumburg, Jerry Kaplan, Anthony Windebank, Nicholas Vick, Stephen Rasmus, David Pleasure, and Mark J. Brown
N. Engl. J. Med. 309:445–448, August 25, 1983          10–5

---

Pyridoxine is now being used in body-building regimens and as a remedy for premenstrual syndrome. High doses have been used to treat schizophrenics and autistic children, and also for childhood hyperkinesia. The authors investigated seven adults with ataxia and severe sensory dysfunction that followed consumption of large amounts of pyridoxine.

Woman, 27, had increased difficulty walking about two years after she began taking 500 mg of pyridoxine daily for premenstrual edema. Intake was increased to 5 gm daily a year before presentation. Lhermitte's sign developed, and the patient had become progressively unsteady on walking and had noticed difficulty in handling small objects. She could walk only with a cane and had a broad-based, stamping gait. Pseudoathetosis of the outstretched arms was marked. All limb reflexes were absent. Muscle strength was normal, but all sensory modalities were markedly impaired in all extremities, and there was mild change in touch-pressure and pinprick sensations on the cheeks and lips. No sensory nerve action potentials were elicited, and results of somatosensory evoked-response tests were negative. Motor nerve conduction and the electromyogram were normal. Gait and sensation began improving two months after withdrawal of pyridoxine. At seven months the patient could walk steadily unaided and had returned to work. Reflexes remained absent, and marked impairment of vibratory sensation persisted in the feet. Other sensory modalities were improved. Evoked-response studies showed improvement in central conduction.

The clinical findings were similar in all seven cases. The maximum daily consumption of pyridoxine ranged from 2 to 6 gm. In no case had pyridoxine benefited edema or underlying psychiatric disorder. All patients improved substantially after pyridoxine withdrawal, and two patients followed for two to three years have recovered almost completely.

Pyridoxine megavitaminosis appears to be the sole cause of this disorder. The pathogenesis of pyridoxine neurotoxicity is unclear, but vulnerability of the neurons of the dorsal root ganglia to circulating toxins has been proposed. Safe concentrations of pyridoxine use must be established, and megavitamin therapy for behavioral disorders should be discouraged unless its value can be clearly demonstrated in controlled studies.

▶ Long-term megavitamin ingestion is practiced with significant frequency and is generally considered to be both safe and effective. Overuse of any substance is to be avoided, and it is important for both the laity and the medical profession to know that overuse of the so-called essential vitamins may be associated with serious unknown manifestations.—R.N.D.J.

---

**Intracerebral Hemorrhage and Oral Amphetamine**
Hugh Harrington, H. Allen Heller, David Dawson, Louis Caplan, and Calvin Rumbaugh
Arch. Neurol. 40:503–507, August 1983                                                                 10–6

---

Intracerebral hemorrhage has been associated with intravenously administered amphetamine and related compounds. The authors report findings in four patients who sustained intracerebral hemorrhage after the oral or nasal use of such drugs.

Man, 60, was hospitalized after 36 hours of confusion and clumsiness of the left hand. He was taking diethylproprion HCL for obesity; four or five tablets were taken on the day that symptoms began. The patient was disoriented and unable to calculate or draw a clock. Examination showed left homonymous hemianopia, slight weakness of the left arm, and a left extensor plantar response.

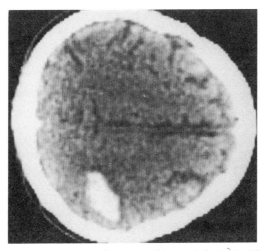

Fig 10–2.—High-convexity CT section shows area of increased density in right posterior parietal region consistent with hemorrhage. (Courtesy of Harrington, H., et al.: Arch. Neurol. 40:503–507, August 1983; copyright 1983, American Medical Association.)

Sensation was impaired in the left extremities. The blood pressure was 198/100 mm Hg. Cranial computed tomography (CT) showed an area of increased density 2 × 3 cm in size in the right posterior parietal region (Fig 10–2) that did not enhance with contrast. The patient improved rapidly but sustained a focal seizure involving the left arm two weeks later after taking two diethylproprion tablets during the previous week. Constructional apraxia, clumsiness, and astereognosis of the left hand were noted. The blood pressure was normal, and CT showed no new bleeding. Angiography disclosed occlusion of several small vessels in the posterior circulation and irregular vessels in the right middle cerebral territory. An early-draining vein was noted near the site of bleeding. Anticonvulsants were given. At discharge the patient had a slight sensorimotor deficit remaining in the left hand but was well otherwise.

Two of the four patients had abnormal-appearing cerebral vessels seen on angiography. Seven similar patients were described previously. Only half of the patients had used drugs illicitly. Drug doses were sometimes low. Most patients remained conscious, but they often were disoriented or confused. Four patients became unresponsive and later died, resulting in a mortality of 36%. The hemorrhages usually occurred in the cerebral white matter, and they may have been related to a drug-induced rise in blood pressure or to damage to cerebral vessels. Physicians who prescribe amphetamines and related drugs, or who treat drug abusers, should be aware of the possibility of intracerebral hemorrhage, especially in young men with symptoms or signs suggestive of the presence of such hemorrhage.

▶ It is important to know that intracerebral hemorrhage may follow oral or nasal use of amphetamines and related compounds, even on the first occasion of their use and even when used for nonrecreational purposes.—R.N.D.J.

# 11 Multiple Sclerosis

**Multiple Sclerosis: The Present Position**
W. I. McDonald (Inst. of Neurology, London)
Acta Neurol. Scand. 68:65–76, August 1983

Multiple sclerosis was one of the earliest diseases to be described in a modern manner, but more than a century later, its cause remains unknown and there is little that will alter its course. Both environmental and genetic factors have been implicated. The risk of disease in persons of northern European and Jewish stock depends on where they live, and clusters of cases have occurred in a restricted area in a circumscribed period. Infection may be acquired in childhood, and a virus is often implicated because of knowledge of neurotropic viruses that produce the cardinal features of multiple sclerosis such as demyelination and relapses and remissions. The rarity of multiple sclerosis in some ethnic groups suggests that a genetic factor may be involved in its etiology. Evidence implicating the HLA-D/DR region is the strongest. There are suggestions that immune mechanisms may be involved in the pathogenesis of multiple sclerosis, but precisely how these mechanisms operate remains to be determined, and it has yet to be shown definitively that the observed immune changes are primary and causally related to the development of lesions.

It is unlikely that measures aimed at eliminating viruses will be helpful at present. Nevertheless, interferon therapy has been tried. It seems more reasonable to attempt to modify the pathogenesis of the disease by immune stimulation or immunosuppression. The value of immunosuppression has not been conclusively established. Immune stimulation with transfer factor is not of established value. There is evidence favoring some beneficial effect of azathioprine on the course of multiple sclerosis, but the author uses it only in patients with clinically definite disease who have fairly frequent relapses or whose condition is deteriorating steadily, and who have persistent neurologic deficit. It is possible that monitoring of T-lymphocyte levels will be useful in selection of patients for treatment. Serial nuclear magnetic resonance (NMR) scanning may offer a better way of identifying patients who are continuing to develop new lesions and for whom risky treatment would be justified.

▶ This is a thoughtful, detailed review of the present status of our knowledge in regard to multiple sclerosis. As far as etiology is concerned, environmental factors are important, and the evidence seems to point to an infectious factor. However, there is also a genetic contribution, which is probably multifactorial and related to immune regulation. We are unlikely to be able to modify the disease by tackling the environmental agent but may be able to do so by manipulating the pathogenesis, although an effective way of doing so is yet to be defined.—R.N.D.J.

## The Predictive Value of Cerebrospinal Fluid Electrophoresis in "Possible" Multiple Sclerosis

Dwight Moulin, Donald W. Paty, and George C. Ebers

Brain 106:809–816, December 1983

11–2

The authors undertook a prospective study of 250 patients with "possible" multiple sclerosis to determine the predictive value of cerebrospinal fluid (CSF) oligoclonal banding for the subsequent development of clinically definite multiple sclerosis (CDMS). A total of 183 patients had objective evidence of white matter disease and clinically unifocal involvement, usually of the optic nerve, brain stem, or spinal cord. Oligoclonal IgG banding (OB) was found in 83 of these patients during a mean follow-up of 34 months.

The patients with and those without OB were similar in age at onset and in major sites of anatomical involvement. The mean duration of disease was longer in those with OB. During follow-up, CDMS developed in 24% of those with and in 9% of those without OB (table), a significant difference. Substantial numbers of patients in both groups had evidence of dissemination on electrophysiologic testing, but those with OB had significantly more electrophysiologic abnormalities.

A possible relationship between OB and the number of lesions or degree of dissemination of multiple sclerosis was evident in this study. The high frequency of banding early in the course of disease may reflect the fact that most lesions are clinically silent and that many lesions may be present at the time of clinical onset. Repeated CSF electrophoresis may prove useful in confirming the diagnosis. In addition, patients with monosymptomatic demyelination who have OB appear to be at a greater risk for the development of clinically disseminated disease than OB-negative patients are. Whether all patients with OB will ultimately have clinical multiple sclerosis remains to be determined.

COMPARISON BETWEEN OLIGOCLONAL BANDING-POSITIVE (OB +) AND OLIGOCLONAL BANDING-NEGATIVE (OB −) PATIENTS IN THE DEVELOPMENT OF DISSEMINATED DISEASE (BASED ON CLINICAL AND LABORATORY FINDINGS)

|  | Percentage developing clinically definite MS | Percentage developing laboratory probable MS |
|---|---|---|
| OB + | 20/83  (24 %) | 39/62 (63 %) |
| OB − | 9/100 ( 9 %) | 36/79 (46 %) |
|  | $P < 0.01$ | $P < 0.05$ |

(Courtesy of Moulin, D., et al.: Brain 106:809–816, December 1983.)

▶ This may be the beginning of more complex correlation of spinal fluid findings with the clinical picture in multiple sclerosis (MS). It is not too much to hope that eventually we will have a computer program that can receive patient examination data, including CT or NMR scan and spinal fluid, and get out a prediction and perhaps even a recommendation for treatment.

Whitaker (*Ital. J. Neurol. Sci.* 2:153–157, 1983) reviewed myelin basic protein and multiple sclerosis recently, and Hughes (*J. Neurol.* 230:73–80, 1983) did the same for immunologic treatment of MS. Both are balanced comments on the state of the art. Ilyas and Davison (J. Neurol. Sci. 59:85–95, 1983) find that peripheral blood lymphocytes from MS patients demonstrate a hypersensitivity to brain gangliosides that may be more disease specific than the hypersensitivity to myelin basic protein. Another step nearer a non-CSF diagnostic test?—R.D.C.

---

**Multiple Sclerosis After Age 50**
John Noseworthy, Donald Paty, Thomas Wonnacott, Thomas Feasby, and George Ebers (Univ. of Western Ontario)
Neurology (Cleve.) 33:1537–1544, December 1983                    11–3

---

The authors found that multiple sclerosis (MS) developing after age 50 is not rare and is commonly misdiagnosed. Findings in 79 patients with MS that developed after age 50 were compared with those in 527 patients

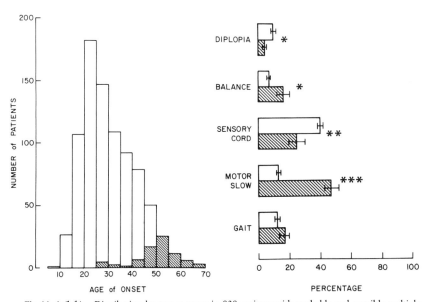

**Fig 11–1 (left).**—Distribution by age at onset in 838 patients with probable and possible multiple sclerosis. All those seen for the first time after age 50 (79 patients) are represented by the shaded bars.

**Fig 11–2 (right).**—Bar graphs indicate the initial symptoms of multiple sclerosis in patients with early-onset and late-onset (shaded areas) disease. *$P<.05$; **$P<.01$; ***$P<.001$.

(Courtesy of Noseworthy, J., et al.: Neurology 33:1537–1544, December 1983.)

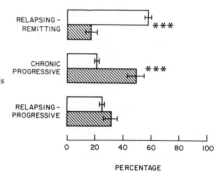

**Fig 11–3.**—Clinical course of multiple sclerosis in 527 patients with early-onset (before age 50) disease and in 79 patients with late-onset (after age 50, shaded areas) disease. \*\*\*P<.001. (Courtesy of Noseworthy, J., et al.: Neurology 33:1537–1544, December 1983.)

in whom the disease developed at an earlier age (Fig 11–1). Most patients with late-onset MS received initial diagnoses from neurologists of a neurologic disorder other than MS. However, 53 of the 79 patients with late onset of disease had clinically definite or probable MS. Sex distribution and mean duration of disease at the most recent evaluation were similar in the late-onset and control groups.

The chief symptoms at the onset are depicted in Figure 11–2. Older patients more often had slow deterioration of motor function, whereas in younger ones sensory symptoms and signs of cord dysfunction were the first indications of MS. Late-onset MS often was progressive from the outset, but relapsing-remitting disease predominated in the controls (Fig 11–3). Late-onset MS progressed more rapidly than did early-onset MS. Relapsing-remitting disease has the most favorable prognosis regardless of age at onset. Electrophoretic findings in cerebrospinal fluid (CSF) were comparable in the two groups, as were evoked response abnormalities.

Multiple sclerosis developing after age 50 is more frequent than previously thought and is relatively difficult to diagnose, even for neurologists. It should be considered in older persons who have neurologic dysfunction. Both CSF electrophoresis and evoked potentials recording are of diagnostic aid. It is possible that older patients have had active disease for a considerably longer time than duration of their symptoms would indicate. The progressive course typical in older patients with MS may reflect age-related changes in immune function.

▶ Permission is given to make the diagnosis of MS in older persons. One wonders if there has been a forgotten episode of neurologic dysfunction many years before, possibly even in childhood. The suggestion that the progressive type of MS may relate to aging rather than to duration of disease is interesting.

Blaivas and Barbalias (*J. Urol.* 131:91–94, 1984) in a careful analysis of the urologic function of men with MS comment on the problem of detrusor–external sphincter dyssynergia—they feel it may herald, or at least mark the patient as having, more serious involvement. And Hawkes et al. (*Br. Med. J.* 287:793–795, 1983) reviewed their data on the effect of dorsal column stimulation on bladder control. They conclude, "at present stimulation of the dorsal column does not have a place in the routine management of multiple sclerosis."—R.D.C.

**Prolonged Follow-Up of Abnormal Visual Evoked Potentials in Multiple Sclerosis: Evidence for Delayed Recovery**
W. B. Matthews and Marian Small (Radcliffe Infirmary, Oxford, England)
J. Neurol. Neurosurg. Psychiatry 46:639–642, July 1983                    11–4

The authors report a case in which the latency of the P100 component of the pattern-evoked visual response (VEP) was shown in serial recordings to be prolonged after onset of optic neuritis, but normal after another 3.5 years.

Woman, 27, developed right optic neuritis. Her VEP was initially recorded one month after onset, acuity being R:6/9 and L:6/5. The left (normal) eye showed P100 at 100.5 ms and 16 μV; the right eye at 166.8 ms and 6.3 μV. By January 1978, right eye amplitude was reduced, latency being 156.4 ms (3.0 μV); left eye response remained normal. In June 1981, the right eye showed a normal response, 103 ms and 11.1 μV with a small peak at 143.9 ms; the left eye (previously normal) showed a late P100 at 155 ms and 6.6μV. The test was repeated seven years later with similar results.

Persistent prolongation of the VEP latency after recovery from retrobulbar neuritis has frequently been reported and is the basis for using the method to diagnose multiple sclerosis (MS). The less common finding of a subsequent return of P100 latency to normal as found in the above patient prompted the authors to reexamine a group of 21 patients who had shown either a bilateral or unilateral VEP abnormality on initial examination. At the initial VEP, all patients had definite, probable, or possible MS; at follow-up, some had been reclassified, but all had MS. Recordings were made from 42 eyes; average follow-up time was 6.7 years. Upon initial VEP, 15 patients had a bilateral abnormality. Six patients had a unilateral abnormality; the latency remained constant in the normal eye of five of these patients, and in the remaining patient latency increased from 99 to 128 ms in the normal eye. Among the abnormal eyes (26), the mean latency remained unchanged (initial, 134.4 ± 17.8 ms; follow-up, 133.9 ± 24.8 ms). Overall, latency ranged from 99.7 to 157.6 ms in the follow-up group, with 10 eyes showing an improvement in latency from initial testing.

Although in most patients examined at follow-up the P100 latency and amplitude either remained constant or improved (in a few instances to normal), no patient had the same long-term improvement associated with normal visual acuity that occurred in the patient described above. Such improvement appears to be a rare phenomenon, raising questions regarding the underlying pathophysiology. It has generally been accepted that the persistent prolongation of the VEP is the result of persistent demyelination, although the restoration of function is difficult to explain. There is little evidence of remyelination in MS, and the persistent abnormalities in evoked potentials are not unexpected. The present results suggest that a slow healing process may occur. In patients with progressive disease this may not be detectable; however, patients in whom abnormal VEPs were recorded soon after the introduction of this technique should be reexamined.

▶ This paper is good news. It may indicate that improvement can take place in

MS as long as three to six years after a worsening. This has significance, since we are entering the era of adequate MS treatment. Another interesting study is that by Ebers et al. (*Neurology (Cleve.)* 34:341–346, 1984) showing with enhanced computed tomography that at least half the patients with exacerbated disease had more than one lesion, which confirms the common clinical situation of many symptoms appearing more or less simultaneously.—R.D.C.

---

**Unsuspected Multiple Sclerosis**
Joseph J. Gilbert and Mark Sadler
Arch. Neurol. 40:533–536, September 1983                              11–5

---

Some patients with clinically diagnosed multiple sclerosis (MS) survive for a prolonged time without severe disability, and autopsies may show plaques in sites not correlating with clinical observations. The authors report findings in five patients in whom demyelinating plaques typical of MS were found at autopsy although neurologic disease was not suspected before death. The cases were among 2,450 autopsies performed in hospitals in London, Ont., on patients aged 16 and older in 1974–1981. The lesions were typical of inactive old plaques of MS with demyelination and some relative axonal preservation, mild to moderate fibrous gliosis, and perivenular lymphocytic infiltration. Most lesions were periventricular in lo-

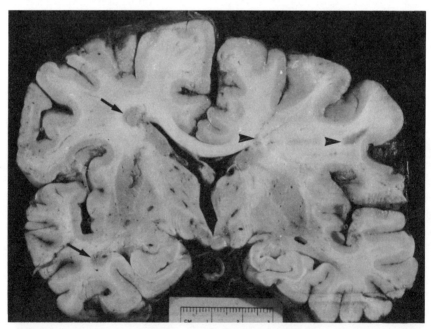

**Fig 11–4.**—Coronal section of brain at level of mammillary bodies shows periventricular multiple sclerosis plaques *(arrows)* and white matter plaques *(arrowheads)*. The cortical changes and shifts resulted from traumatic lesions. (Courtesy of Gilbert, J.J., and Sadler, M.: Arch. Neurol. 40:533–536, September 1983; copyright 1983, American Medical Association.)

cation (Fig 11–4). They were relatively small except in one patient. Two patients had thalamic lesions and two had brain stem lesions. A single lesion was found in the one spinal cord examined.

Multiple sclerosis found unexpectedly at autopsy has been infrequently reported. Previous minor, transient episodes of neurologic dysfunction may not be recalled by affected patients, or may be considered unimportant by the clinician. Subtle neurologic abnormalities may be overlooked or dismissed as insignificant when the primary complaints arise from outside the CNS. If axons are preserved in a plaque, complete conduction block may not occur. Small plaques developing in nonstrategic areas of the CNS may not produce overt symptoms or signs. Most of the lesions are in the hemispheres and are relatively small. Major lesions in the brain stem and cerebellum were not present in this series of patients.

▶ Most experienced neurologists are aware that a few minimally sized lesions typical for MS plaques are sometimes found in the brains of patients who have died of unrelated diseases but who were known to have had one or two transient minor episodes of undiagnosed neurologic disease. This report indicates that unanticipated lesions with the histopathologic features of MS may also be found in the brains of persons in whom no neurologic disease had been suspected during life. This knowledge alters the generally accepted perception that MS is always a progressive, ultimately crippling disease.—R.N.D.J.

---

**Persistent Neurological Deficit Precipitated by Hot Bath Test in Multiple Sclerosis**
Joseph R. Berger (Univ. of Miami) and William A. Sheremata (McGill Univ.)
JAMA 249:1751–1753, Apr. 1, 1983                                    11–6

Use of the hot bath test to diagnose multiple sclerosis (MS) has been advocated by investigators who state that permanent sequelae will not occur. The authors describe four patients with an initial diagnosis of "possible MS" who had substantial, prolonged neurologic debilitation after testing.

Woman, 25, whose mother had "definite MS," had fallen repeatedly during a period of several days and had suddenly lost vision after a quarrel. There was no light perception, but there was an apparent response on optokinetic testing. There was motor impersistence in all extremities, with a mildly ataxic gait. Muscle stretch reflexes were brisk, but the plantar responses were equivocal. Vision returned in several hours. A psychiatrist concluded that the patient was hysterical. Neuroophthalmologic evaluation yielded normal findings. In a hot bath test in which the oral temperature was kept at 38.6 C for five minutes, vision decreased and did not improve on cooling, and the patient was blind next day. A blurred right optic disk margin and nerve head elevation were seen, with a small hemorrhage. The papillitis resolved in the week that followed, and vision improved over three weeks, but the patient continued to fall. Gait difficulty was present a year later, and eight years after recovery, left eye pain, loss of vision, and severe ataxia developed, and examination showed moderate paraparesis, bilateral Babinski's reflexes, and marked loss of proprioception in the lower limbs. Minimal improvement occurred over the next months, after which the patient was lost to follow-up.

Two of the four patients had visual impairment in conjunction with hot bath testing. Another patient developed hemiplegia after each of two heat tests. New symptoms have also developed in patients exposed to climatic heat. Existing neurologic signs have worsened with increasing body temperature in many patients with other neurologic disorders. Long-lasting deficits may be produced in patients with MS. Explanations of the impairment associated with hyperthermia include "stress," edema in demyelinated areas, and the release of humoral substances.

Caution is indicated in using the hot bath test, especially in patients with acute neurologic deficits and during early convalescence. Clinical judgment is the key to diagnosis of MS, and various laboratory measures and computed tomography may be helpful.

▶ Most of the more conservative neurologists have been extremely reluctant to advise or even permit the use of the so-called hot bath test in patients with "possible multiple sclerosis." They have seriously questioned Poser's statement that the procedure is completely harmless and have adhered to the old adage "primum non nocere." This article confirms their apprehensions. In addition, with the refinement of laboratory procedures, the introduction of evoked potential studies, and, finally, the development of computed tomography and nuclear magnetic resonance, the hot bath test can be discarded, as it should have been many years ago.—R.N.D.J.

# 12 Myasthenia Gravis

**Prognosis of Ocular Myasthenia**
Christopher T. Bever, Jr., Abdias V. Aquino, Audrey S. Penn, Robert E. Lovelace, and Lewis P. Rowland (Columbia Univ.)
Ann. Neurol. 14:516–519, November 1983                                    12–1

Although patients with pure ocular myasthenia gravis are generally not considered candidates for thymectomy, a few do later experience generalized myasthenia. The authors reviewed the course of 108 patients who were seen between 1957 and 1967 with a diagnosis of myasthenia gravis and who had only ocular symptoms at the outset. All were followed up for at least six months without surgical treatment. Of all patients seen in this period with myasthenia gravis, 53% had solely ocular involvement initially.

The risk of generalization declined with an increasing duration of solely ocular symptoms. The median time to generalization in 53 patients was less than one year, and in only 9 patients did generalized myasthenia develop after two years. All but 3 of 20 respiratory crises or deaths occurred among the 44 patients in whom generalized myasthenia developed within two years of onset. The chance of remission decreased slowly with increasing duration of solely ocular disease. Eighteen patients had at least one month of remission, and the duration of remissions averaged 4.8 years. Older age at the onset was associated with a poorer outcome. Fourteen of the 20 respiratory crises and deaths from myasthenia occurred among the 46 patients having onset of disease after age 50 years. Five of 20 patients who had systemic curare tests had oropharyngeal or limb muscle weakness on testing; ocular symptoms remained in all 5 during an average follow-up of 15 years. Of the patients whose ocular symptoms remained, five experienced generalized symptoms during follow-up, and three had respiratory crisis.

Neither systemic curare testing nor the response to repetitive nerve stimulation can predict the outcome in patients seen initially with purely ocular myasthenia gravis. The risk of generalization appears to decline with increasing duration of solely ocular symptoms; the risk of respiratory crisis or death from myasthenia also may decrease.

▶ Only a minor percentage of patients with myasthenia gravis limited to the extraocular muscles eventually develop generalized myasthenia, but it would be helpful if one could differentiate early in the course of their disease between those who have and those who do not have a favorable prognosis. This study of the prognosis of purely ocular muscle myasthenia shows that the longer the duration of the ocular myasthenia the less likely the patient is of developing generalized disease, and the earlier the onset of the ocular myasthenia, the less the chance of its becoming generalized. Neither systemic curare tests nor responses to repetitive nerve stimulation have prognostic value.—R.N.D.J.

---

**Long-Term Corticosteroid Treatment of Myasthenia Gravis: Report of 116 Patients**
Robert M. Pascuzzi, H. Branch Coslett, and T. R. Johns (Univ. of Virginia)
Ann. Neurol. 15:291–298, March 1984                                    12–2

The authors reviewed the results of long-term corticosteroid therapy in 116 patients with disabling myasthenia gravis (MG) and no major contraindications. Steroids were used in all patients except for those with chiefly ocular myasthenia and in some with mild, nonprogressive ocular and limb weakness. The 41 males and 75 females had a mean age at treatment of 45 years. Sixteen patients had a thymoma. Follow-up ranged from 8 months to 17 years. Prednisone was begun in a dose of 60–80 mg daily until sustained improvement occurred, after which alternate-day therapy was instituted. The dose was reduced in 10-mg increments at two-month intervals as long as improvement was maintained.

Disease in 28% of the patients remitted, and another 53% improved markedly. Many patients had an initial exacerbation, and 10 required intubation or ventilatory assistance. Sustained improvement began about three weeks after the start of treatment, and the mean time to peak improvement was about nine months. Maximum improvement was maintained for a mean of nearly four years. Some patients required only a low maintenance dose of prednisone. About 20% of the patients later had significant exacerbations. Overall, 68% experienced side effects, the most common being a cushingoid habitus and weight gain. All but 1 of 11 patients who had a thymoma at the time of prednisone therapy improved markedly or had a remission. Age was the best predictor of a good response to steroid therapy. Eight of 51 patients having thymectomy and 5 of 42 unoperated-on patients could discontinue taking all medication. Two of the six patients who failed to respond to prednisone treatment may have had familial or congenital MG.

High-dose prednisone therapy can rapidly induce marked improvement or remission in many patients with MG. Management is simplified by a reduction in requirements for cholinesterase inhibitors. Patients can resume normal activities quickly, and morbidity from thymectomy is much reduced.

▶ This is good confirmation of the usefulness of corticosteroids in the treatment of myasthenia. It's not of course the perfect treatment we are all hoping for, but it certainly is adequate for holding actions and for a few patients is all that is necessary.—R.D.C.

---

**Thymectomy for Myasthenia Gravis**
Donald G. Mulder, Christian Herrmann, Jr., John Keesey, and Hannibal Ed-

wards (UCLA Med. Center, Los Angeles)
Am. J. Surg. 146:61–66, July 1983                                                12–3

Between 1954 and 1981, 781 patients with myasthenia gravis were seen by the authors; thymectomy was performed in 249 patients. Operative age ranged from 2 to 78 years (mean, 35 years); 40 patients were 20 years of age or younger, 49 patients were 50 years of age or older; mean age of female patients was 31, mean age of male patients was 42 years. Preoperatively, 9 patients had mild generalized symptoms, including ocular involvement (class I); 136 patients had moderately severe generalized disease, including bulbar involvement (class II); 84 patients had acute, generalized, and bulbar impairment (class III); and 20 patients had chronic, marked, generalized, and bulbar involvement (class IV). Mean length of time between onset of symptoms and thymectomy was 3.5 years. Median sternotomy is the incision of preference and was used in all patients.

Information was available for 205 of 249 patients, with a mean follow-up time of 7.5 years. In the remaining 44 patients, the follow-up period ranged from 2 months to 10 years (mean, 4 years). The remission rate was 51% (126 of 249 patients), being somewhat higher for female (56%) than for male (36%) patients (table). Two patients died at operation; the other 13 deaths were late, and most were due to pulmonary complications. The presence of a thymoma (51 patients) was unfavorable, particularly if it was invasive. Among these patients, the remission rate was 37% (19 of 51 patients), and 68% benefited from operation. Prognosis was more favorable in those without thymoma; of the 198 patients, 107 (54%) had remission and 91% benefited from thymectomy. Female patients had the highest favorable response (94%). Administration of prednisone on alternate days was effective in enhancing the effect of thymectomy in those patients with little or no improvement.

There was no correlation between the histologic appearance of the thymus (excluding thymoma) and surgical result; patients with a normal gland had a 51% remission rate, and those with thymic hyperplasia had a 52% remission rate. Approximately 67% of patients with more mild disease (class I or II) underwent remission, compared with 33% in class III and 25% in class IV. Time from onset of symptoms to thymectomy among

RESULTS AFTER THYMECTOMY FOR MYASTHENIA GRAVIS

| Postoperative Status | Male Patients | Female Patients | Total |
|---|---|---|---|
| Remission | 24 (36%) | 102 (56%) | 126 (51%) |
| Improvement | 26 (39%) | 64 (35%) | 90 (36%) |
| No change | 7 | 10 | 17 |
| Worse | 1 | 0 | 1 |
| Dead | 8* | 7* | 15 |
| Total | 66 | 183 | 249 |

*Includes two operative deaths.
(Courtesy of Mulder, D.G., et al.: Am. J. Surg. 146:61–66, July 1983.)

females who underwent remission was 2.7 ± 2.1 years, and among male patients it was 4.4 ± 2.2 years. Therefore, a shorter interval between onset of symptoms and thymectomy was found to be favorable. Of 78 patients followed up for more than 10 years, 37 were in remission and 37 were in class I (total 95%). Of the 26 patients followed up for 10–24 years, 20 had at least a 15-year period of observation; 14 of the 20 were still in remission after 15 years, and 6 patients were in class I (100% improvement). The authors conclude that most patients with myasthenia gravis will improve after thymectomy and that benefits will persist over an extended period of time in a high percentage of patients.

▶ In the child neurology section (chapter 4), comments are made on thymectomy in children. This report adds to the growing evidence that thymectomy is useful.

For those with an interest, the autobiography of Geoffrey Keynes (*The Gates of Memory,* New York, Oxford University Press, 1983) makes good reading. His persistence in thymectomy in spite of early bad results might not be possible in this age of research committees. The book also is otherwise delightful.—R.D.C.

---

### Exacerbation of Myasthenia Gravis After Removal of Thymoma Having Membrane Phenotype of Suppressor T Cells

Yasuo Kuroda, Ken-ichiro Oda, Ryuji Neshige, and Hiroshi Shibasaki (Saga Med. School, Japan)
Ann. Neurol. 15:400–402, April 1984                    12–4

---

The thymus appears to have an important role in the genesis of myasthenia gravis. The authors describe a patient with myasthenia associated with a thymoma having a suppressor T-cell membrane phenotype. Thymectomy led to both exacerbation of the disease and a marked increase in the serum titer of acetylcholine receptor (AChR) antibody, as well as a fall in circulating suppressor T cells.

Man, 27, experienced fatigability and muscle weakness a month previously. He had moderate blepharoptosis and moderate weakness of the facial and bulbar muscles and of the shoulder girdle and arm muscles. A constant lymphocytosis was present. The antinuclear antibody test results were positive, but a lupus erythematosus test yielded negative results. The serum AChR antibody level was elevated at 11.7 pmol/ml. Repetitive muscle stimulation led to decremental responses. An anterior mediastinal mass 6 × 6 cm in size was seen on computed tomography. An edrophonium test gave positive results. Muscle strength improved a little with pyridostigmine therapy. A thymoma associated with thymic hyperplasia was removed. Nearly all lymphocytes in the tumor reacted with mature T cells and with suppressor/cytoxic T cells (OKT8). A substantial number of OKT8 cells were present in the serum before thymectomy.

The patient became progressively weaker after thymectomy; diplopia and difficulty in walking developed despite continued pyridostigmine bromide therapy. Marked weakness of the facial and bulbar muscles was noted, with evidence of dysphagia. The pelvic girdle muscles also were weak. Respirations were labored. A marked increase in the AChR antibody titer occurred. Ambenonium chloride therapy was not helpful, but improvement occurred when high-dose prednisolone therapy was begun; the AChR antibody titer declined. A marked fall in peripheral blood OKT8 cells occurred after thymectomy. Prednisolone therapy led to a fall in all T-cell populations.

These findings illustrate the complex and variable etiopathogenic relationship between myasthenia gravis and the thymus. A large-scale study is needed to determine whether there is a special association between the membrane phenotype of thymoma in myasthenia gravis and the effect of thymectomy.

▶ There is a memory that before we knew about T cells this happened—but to a lesser degree—after removal of a hyperplastic thymus for myasthenia. The patient later spontaneously improved.—R.D.C.

# 13 Neuro-Ophthalmology

---

**Amaurosis Fugax: The Results of Arteriography in 59 Patients**
Harold P. Adams, Jr., Steven F. Putman, James J. Corbett, Brian P. Sires, and H. Stanley Thompson (Univ. of Iowa)
Stroke 14:742–744, Sept.–Oct., 1983                                        13–1

---

Amaurosis fugax is a recognized warning symptom of impending cerebral or retinal infarction and is considered to be a reliable sign of carotid artery disease. The authors reviewed the cerebral arteriographic findings in 59 patients with transient monocular blindness, representing about 86% of all patients seen with amaurosis fugax in a seven-year period. The 34 men and 25 women were mostly older than age 55 years. One patient had involvement of both eyes. All had had recent symptoms. Eleven patients also had had episodes considered to represent hemispheric transient ischemic attacks (TIAs), and eight had evidence of vertebrobasilar TIAs. Five patients had had strokes, two with residual neurologic abnormalities.

Fifteen patients had stenosis of the origin of the internal carotid artery. Eight others had prominent plaques without significant stenosis or ulcerations. Two patients had external carotid stenosis, and one had isolated ophthalmic artery stenosis. Ten patients had complete occlusion of the internal or common carotid artery. Nineteen patients had normal angiographic findings; five had other identifiable causes of visual symptoms, and seven others had atherosclerotic disease in the contralateral carotid artery, innominate artery, or a vertebral artery. The arteriographic findings could not be related to the clinical features, nor were noninvasive studies a reliable indicator. Ten of the 11 patients with symptoms of hemispheric TIAs, and all 5 with previous strokes had abnormal arteriograms.

Arteriography is the single most reliable means of diagnosis in patients with amaurosis fugax, and all patients should be assumed to have carotid artery disease, although other causes of embolism should be ruled out. A complete evaluation for cardiac, hematologic, and other vascular disorders is warranted.

► Patients with amaurosis fugax are a heterogeneous group, and their visual symptoms should not be considered a specific indication for the presence of stenosis of the internal carotid artery.—R.N.D.J.

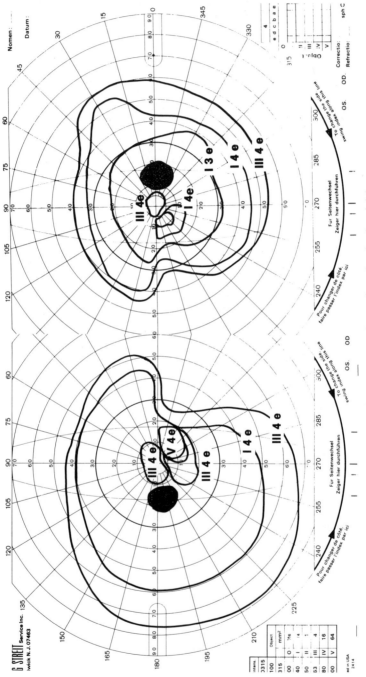

Fig 13–1.—Visual field examination showing binasal wedge-shaped defects. (Courtesy of Ford, C.S., et al.: South. Med. J. 76:1060–1062, August 1983.)

**Drusen-Associated Visual Field Defects and Hemorrhages**
C. Stephen Ford, José Biller, and Richard G. Weaver (Bowman Gray School of Medicine)
South. Med. J. 76:1060–1062, August 1983                    13–2

Visual field defects associated with drusen are less rare than was previously thought.

Woman, 30, with amblyopia ex anopsia due to esotropia and high hyperopia in the left eye, was referred two months after a severe bitemporal headache with nausea and vomiting, followed by a persistent monocular deficit in the inferior nasal quadrant of the left eye. A bitemporal headache several weeks later was followed by clouding in the inferior temporal quadrant of the right eye. Confrontation testing showed bilateral inferior field cuts, chiefly in the nasal quadrants (Fig 13–1). Funduscopy showed bilateral optic nerve drusen (Fig 13–2) and a small hemorrhage overlying the right optic disk. A cranial computed tomographic study was normal.

The visual field defects found in patients with optic drusen are usually asymptomatic and observed only on careful testing. Progression occurs in about half the patients with drusen-related field defects. Enlargement of the blind spot is the most common change, followed by nerve fiber bundle defects and concentric constriction of the field. Central vision is rarely affected. Retinal and disk hemorrhage is a rare complication, but it is sometimes responsible for symptoms of drusen. There may be splinter hemorrhages overlying the disk, vitreous hemorrhages, or subretinal hemorrhages.

The unusual disk vasculature associated with drusen is probably responsible for the retinal hemorrhages, and it may be the primary patho-

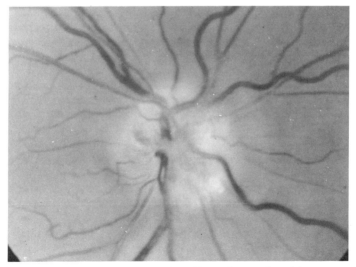

Fig 13–2.—Right fundus showing hyaline bodies and hemorrhage overlying disk. (Courtesy of Ford, C.S., et al.: South Med. J. 76:1060–1062, August 1983.)

genetic defect in drusen. Altered axoplasmic transport and abnormal axonal calcium metabolism have also been implicated in the pathogenesis of drusen.

▶ It is important for physicians to be aware of the fact that visual field defects and retinal hemorrhages can occur as complications of optic nerve drusen.—R.N.D.J.

# 14 Neuropathies

**The Natural History of Acute Painful Neuropathy in Diabetes Mellitus**
A. G. Archer, P. J. Watkins, P. K. Thomas, A. K. Sharma, and J. Payan
J. Neurol. Neurosurg. Psychiatry 46:491–499, June 1983                    14–1

Nine diabetics presented with intolerable persistent pain in the feet and legs. All were male, aged 32–61 years, except for an adolescent aged 13 years. Five were insulin dependent, and the remainder received insulin for treatment of the neuropathy. Assessment was made at time of onset of symptoms and an average of five years later (four–six years in seven patients, and 9–12 months in two patients). The characteristic symptom complex involved weight loss and persistent pain distally in the lower limbs. Tingling paresthesia was reported by some patients. Contact discomfort was present in all cases and was associated with intense hypersensitivity of the skin.

Weight loss was severe, averaging 14.2 kg (range, 9.5–27 kg), amounting to a mean loss of 19.4% (range, 12%–35%). In every instance pain began after a decrease in weight. The major symptoms coincided with the point of maximal loss; all patients became depressed and anorexic during the most severe symptoms. One patient became so cachectic that he was considered elsewhere to have disseminated malignancy. Despite the considerable weight loss, there were no abnormalities of motor function.

Improved control of diabetes with insulin was associated with weight gain and a subsequent diminution in the severity of symptoms. No medication consistently relieved symptoms, although relief of insomnia was one of the most important facets of treatment. Relief of cutaneous discomfort was achieved with loose clothing and the use of a cradle to elevate bedclothes; foot pains were reduced by discarding shoes.

Impotence was present in all the adult patients and, with one exception, has persisted. However, all of the other major symptoms ceased to be distressing within 6 months after onset in 7 patients and after 10 months in 2 patients. Thereafter, symptoms decreased with clear end points in 6 patients; by the second assessment, none had suffered a relapse.

Sural nerve biopsies of three patients in the acute stage of neuropathy showed degeneration of myelinated nerve fibers of all diameters and also of unmyelinated axons; there was a mild degree of demyelination. There was a striking lack of correlation of these neuropathies with other complications of diabetes. Six patients had no evidence of retinopathy at first assessment, and only one of three patients with retinopathy also had evidence of nephropathy. This suggests that acute painful neuropathy is not due to microvascular disease. This is in agreement with the current view that symmetrical peripheral neuropathy is secondary to metabolic disturbance, although it may at times result from multifocal proximal lesions.

It is concluded that acute painful diabetic neuropathy is a distinct syndrome, which occurs in insulin-dependent or non-insulin-dependent patients, regardless of duration of disease, and is unrelated to other diabetic pathologies. It is also distinct from other types of painful diabetic sensory polyneuropathy.

▶ The neuropathy of diabetes can be discouraging and depressing to both the patient and the physician. Of great importance is the fact that the severe manifestations subsided in all cases within 10 months and did not recur in a six-year follow-up. Although only 51% went into what is called a complete remission, another 36% improved, making a total benefited percentage of 87%.

Agardh et al. (*Acta Med. Scand.* 213:283–287, 1983) report consistent improvement in nerve conduction velocities in patients with diabetic neuropathy when they were shifted from oral hypoglycemic agents to insulin.—R.D.C.

---

**Treatment of Severely Painful Diabetic Neuropathy With an Aldose Reductase Inhibitor: Relief of Pain and Improved Somatic and Autonomic Nerve Function**
Jonathan Jaspan, Ricardo Maselli, Kevin Herold, Cynthia Bartkus (Univ. of Chicago)
Lancet 2:758–762, October 1, 1983                                              14–2

Disabling pain is one of the serious sequelae of diabetic neuropathy. The sorbitol pathway has been implicated, and its role has been confirmed by animal studies in which specific aldose reductase inhibitors have been used. The authors evaluated Sorbinil, an aldose reductase inhibitor, in 11 patients with severe pain from diabetic neuropathy that had failed to respond to many drugs. All were insulin-dependent patients who had been incapacitated by severe, chiefly lower limb, pains. All patients had distal, predominantly sensory polyneuropathy, and two had signs of severe autonomic neuropathy also. Sorbinil was given in a single daily dose of 250 mg. Eight patients also received a placebo in single-blind fashion.

Individual pain scores are shown in Figure 14–1. Eight patients had moderate to marked relief from symptoms, generally starting after three to four days of treatment, and two others had equivocal responses. All four patients with diabetic amyotrophy had striking improvement in pain and some improvement in proximal leg muscle strength. Sensation appeared to be improved in three of these patients. Pain worsened in seven of eight responders when Sorbinil was stopped, generally after some delay. Autonomic nerve function improved significantly in six of the seven patients tested. Nerve conduction velocities improved in four of seven patients, in association with clinical improvement. No drug toxicity was observed, although another patient had a rash and was withdrawn from the study.

A potent aldose reductase inhibitor considerably relieved severe neuropathic pains in many diabetics in this study. Nerve conduction velocities improved, as did autonomic nerve function in many patients. Aldose re-

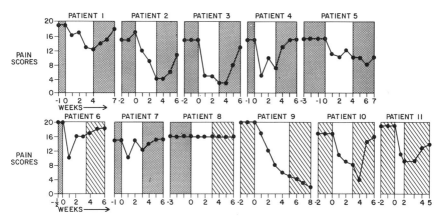

Fig 14–1.—Individual pain scores of 11 diabetic patients. Stippled areas represent placebo periods, open areas indicate Sorbinil therapy, and hatched areas denote periods when patients received nothing. (Courtesy of Jaspan, J., et al.: Lancet 2:758–762, Oct. 1, 1983.)

ductase inhibitors may be valuable in the treatment of symptomatic somatic and autonomic neuropathies complicating diabetes.

▶ Diabetic neuropathy can be extremely painful and resistant to all therapeutic endeavors. These investigators report the use of an aldose reductase inhibitor with resulting relief of pain and improvement in somatic and autonomic nerve function as well. This may be the first advance in the treatment of this severe complication of diabetes. It certainly merits further investigation.—R.N.D.J.

---

**The Treatment of Experimental Allergic Neuritis by Plasma Exchange**
M. L. P. Gross, R. I. Craggs, R. H. M. King, and P. K. Thomas (Royal Free Hosp. School of Medicine, London)
J. Neurol. Sci. 61:149–160, October 1983                                    14–3

Experimental allergic neuritis (EAN), a demyelinating disease of the peripheral nervous system inducible in laboratory animals by inoculation of peripheral nerve antigens in Freund's complete adjuvant, is similar to Guillain-Barré syndrome or acute inflammatory polyneuropathy in man. Reportedly, patients with the latter disease, as well as those with its relapsing and chronic progressive forms, improve after plasma exchange. The authors assessed the effect of plasma exchange in 16 rabbits with EAN randomly assigned to control or treatment groups when the disease reached clinical grade 2 or worse.

Four of the eight control animals had severe progressive disease, and two died; four others had acute disease of two to three weeks' duration. Seven days after plasma exchange, five of the eight treated animals experienced improvement in mean clinical grade (MCG) from 2.5 ± 1.1 to 1.4 ± 0.5 ($P<.05$). Fourteen days after the exchange, seven of the eight treated animals had improved to an MCG of 0.75 ± 0.7 ($P<.005$). The eighth animal showed neither improvement nor deterioration at days 7 and 14. The treated animals were more alert, lively, ceased to lose weight, and had less neurologic impairment. Of the four surviving control animals, one recovered but relapsed on day 84, one experienced slow progressive disease, and the other two remained well until perfused. Two treated animals were perfused at day 33 for histologic comparison with controls, another two remained well for more than 130 days, and the remaining four relapsed at 28, 29, 35, and 51 days after plasma exchange, respectively, although the relapsing illness was mild or moderate. Histologically, the relapsing animals had neural lesions consistent with the clinical findings. The two animals that did not relapse showed well-established remyelinating lesions caused by the original disease. In treated animals only a small proportion of demyelinated fibers was observed at any time.

Plasma exchange produces a significant benefit in EAN. However, the mechanism for this improvement has not been established, and further study of the effects produced by plasma exchange is necessary.

▶ Such an animal study showing that plasma exchange produces improvement in experimental allergic neuritis is useful in the debate on the sometimes similar improvement with the Guillain-Barré syndrome. This was a controlled study, and I think it will stand the test of time.—R.D.C.

---

**Mechanism of Pseudotumor in Guillain-Barré Syndrome**
Allan H. Ropper (Massachusetts Gen. Hosp.) and Anthony Marmarou (Med. College of Virginia)
Arch. Neurol. 41:259–261, March 1984                                      14–4

---

It has been proposed that in pseudotumor associated with Guillain-Barré syndrome (GBS), increased amounts of cerebrospinal fluid (CSF) protein lead to an absorption block or increase the oncotic pressure enough to raise the CSF volume. The authors report a case showing that, as in idiopathic pseudotumor, resistance to CSF outflow (Ro) is increased in GBS with pseudotumor, but that the effect cannot explain the observed elevation of CSF pressure.

Man, 27, developed joint pain and muscle aching after an upper respiratory infection, followed in two weeks by weakness on stair climbing and pain in the proximal limb muscles. A CSF protein concentration of 727 mg/dl was documented. Muscle power was reduced in the upper and lower extremities at admission five weeks after onset of symptoms. Sensory tests were normal. The tendon reflexes were hypoactive or absent. Weakness progressed slowly despite four plasma exchanges. Ocular pain and mild frontal headache developed, and papilledema was observed, with a CSF pressure of 45 mm Hg. The CSF protein concentration at this time was 605 mg/dl; cells were absent. A computed tomographic study and radionuclide cisternogram were essentially normal. The CSF pressure fell gradually during a month of prednisone therapy, and the papilledema resolved.

Studies of CSF dynamics showed initially elevated CSF pressure and Ro, with return toward normal over three weeks. The CSF production rate

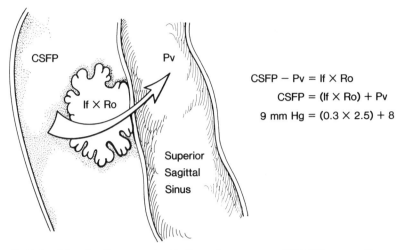

$$CSFP - Pv = If \times Ro$$
$$CSFP = (If \times Ro) + Pv$$
$$9 \text{ mm Hg} = (0.3 \times 2.5) + 8$$

**Fig 14–2.**—Subarachnoid space, arachnoid villus, and venous system. *CSFP,* CSF pressure; *Pv,* venous pressure; *If,* CSF production rate; and *Ro,* resistance to CSF outflow. Numbers indicate approximate normal values in millimeters of mercury. (Courtesy of Ropper, A.H., and Marmarou, A.: Arch. Neurol. 41:259–261, March 1984; copyright 1984, American Medical Association.)

was normal or slightly elevated. The pressure-volume index was initially elevated but later was close to normal. The highest value for Ro was less than five times the normal value at 10.8 mm Hg/ml per minute.

The mechanism of elevated CSF pressure in patients with GBS appears to be similar to that in patients with idiopathic pseudotumor. A threefold to fivefold rise in Ro, however, does not adequately explain the rise in CSF pressure and papilledema (Fig 14–2). Pseudotumor apparently is due chiefly to an increase in effective venous pressure at sites of CSF absorption, passively reflected as increased CSF pressure. The vascular explanation may also indicate why extremely high intracranial pressures are tolerated by patients with pseudotumor but not by those with cerebral masses or hydrocephalus, in whom the pressure impinges on the vasculature, eventually impeding cerebral blood flow. The role of CSF protein in pseudotumor associated with GBS, poliomyelitis, and spinal tumors is uncertain.

▶ These investigators suggest that pseudotumor cerebri results mainly from an increase in effective venous pressure at sites of cerebrospinal fluid absorption; it is passively reflected as raised cerebrospinal fluid pressure. The role of the cerebrospinal fluid protein in pseudotumor associated with the Guillain-Barré syndrome remains unexplained.—R.N.D.J.

**Proposed Mechanism of Ataxia in Fisher's Syndrome**
Allan H. Ropper and Bhagwan Shahani (Massachusetts Gen. Hosp.)
Arch. Neurol. 40:537–538, September 1983                    14–5

Many reports have appeared of Fisher's variant of Guillain-Barré syndrome with ophthalmoplegia, areflexia, and ataxia. The ataxia has suggested the possibility of lesions of the CNS. The authors report data on a patient with Fisher's syndrome in whom a disparity was found between proprioceptive information from the muscle spindles and kinesthetic information from joints and other proprioceptors.

Man, 43, with indolent rheumatoid spondylitis, awoke with horizontal diplopia several days after a viral syndrome and began staggering while walking. Acroparesthesias developed, and incoordination of the arms was noted. Bilateral sixth nerve palsies, absent pupillary light reactions, and mild ptosis were present on the third day of illness. Slight facial and lower extremity weakness, but normal sensation, were noted on examination. The patient was areflexic and had a wide-based, unstable gait. Complete internal and external ophthalmoplegia was present the following day, along with decreased vibratory sense in the great toes, a more ataxic gait, and severely ataxic finger-to-nose motion. Pinprick sensation was mildly impaired in the toes. Joint movements were perceived better distally than proximally, and perception was worse on the left, the side of greater ataxia.

Accelerometry showed a tremor that resembled cerebellar ataxia more than a "neuropathic" tremor on reaching out the upper extremity. The proprioceptive silent period (SP) in the right biceps was of normal duration, but the SP of the abductor digiti minimi was absent. In wrist extensors the proprioceptive SP was present, but less clearly than in the biceps. Minimal motor slowing was noted, with absent ulnar, median, and sural sensory nerve action potentials. There was no evidence of denervation.

This patient had typical features of Fisher's syndrome. Sense of joint position was reduced proximally and was normal distally, but muscle proprioceptive function appeared to be normal. Ataxia due to abnormal peripheral nerve function can be attributed to a disparity between proprioceptive and kinesthetic inputs, making it unnecessary to postulate cerebellar ataxia in this syndrome. Both joint capsule and muscle spindle receptors use large-diameter myelinated fibers, but peripheral nerve abnormalities may not be related solely to the diameter of the axons.

▶ These authors express the belief that their neurophysiologic studies give information sufficient to explain the ataxia and that a CNS lesion does not have to be present to explain the "cerebellar" ataxia that is an essential part of the clinical picture in Fisher's syndrome. This is at best a moot point. There is increasing evidence in the medical literature that Fisher's syndrome, long considered to be a variant of the Guillain-Barré syndrome, is in fact a brain stem encephalitis, a self-limited disease that remits spontaneously in most cases and carries a relatively benign prognosis (Al-Din et al.: *Brain* 105:481–495, 1982). The current authors give no information about the clinical course and outcome of this patient. More information will be necessary before central lesions can be ruled out as an explanation of the ataxia and internal and external ophthalmoplegia in this case.—R.N.D.J.

---

**Supranuclear Eye Movement Disorders in Fisher's Syndrome of Ophthalmoplegia, Ataxia, and Areflexia: Report of a Case and Literature Review**

Otmar Meienberg and Ernst Ryffel (Univ. of Berne, Switzerland)
Arch. Neurol. 40:402–405, July 1983

14–6

The authors report findings in a patient who had a series of ocular signs consistent with supranuclear lesions, some of which have rarely or never been described in association with Fisher's syndrome.

Man, 59, had impaired equilibrium and noted awkward hand movements two weeks after the start of an upper respiratory tract infection; diplopia developed four days after onset of symptoms. Examination three days later showed severe ataxia of the trunk and lower limbs, and moderate ataxia and dysmetria of the upper extremities with generalized areflexia. Slight ptosis and complete palsy of upward gaze were present. No convergence was possible, but minimal conjugate downward gaze was preserved. Restricted abduction was more marked on the right (Fig 14–3). There was no evidence of Bell's phenomenon. The pupils were slightly dilated and unreactive to light but showed a minimal near response. Dysarthric speech was noted. Computed tomography findings were negative, but sural nerve studies showed slight slowing of conduction velocity and an abnormal polyphasic potential; the CSF protein level was elevated at 144 mg/dl. Infrared oculography showed nystagmus with a larger amplitude in the abducting eye. All saccades were slower than normal. The ataxia resolved completely within seven months, but areflexia persisted. Convergence spasm was much less marked seven months after onset of symptoms. The vertical vestibulo-ocular reflexes remained abnormal. Downward gaze was the first component to improve. Bell's phenomenon was apparent during recovery.

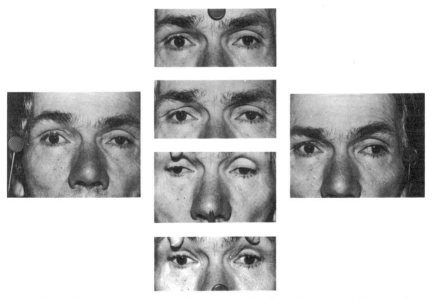

Fig 14–3.—Most marked eye movement disorder occurred on day 7. **Center, top to bottom,** complete upward-gaze palsy; only slight ptosis on straight-ahead gaze; no convergence possible; minimal conjugate downward gaze preserved. **Left,** no adduction on right and left gaze; **right,** restriction of abduction, greater on right. (Courtesy of Meienberg, O., and Ryffel, E.: Arch. Neurol. 40:402–405, July 1983; copyright 1983, American Medical Association.)

Eye movement disorders consistent with a supranuclear lesion have been described in many patients with Fisher's syndrome. The most common findings have been mild ptosis despite severe ophthalmoplegia, preservation of Bell's phenomenon despite paralysis of voluntary upward gaze, horizontal dissociated nystagmus, and conjugate palsies of vertical gaze. Convergence spasm has been reported only once, and rebound nystagmus and vertical vestibulo-ocular reflex disorder have not been noted previously in these patients. Also reported previously are EEG abnormalities consistent with a brain stem lesion. Most patients with Fisher's syndrome exhibit signs of both peripheral and central eye movement disorders.

▶ These authors conclude that "most patients with Fisher's syndrome exhibit a combination of peripheral and central eye movement disorder signs," and apparently accept the belief that the syndrome is not entirely peripheral in origin. In an accompanying editorial A. H. Ropper states, "Neurologists must resist the tendency to attribute all unusual clinical signs to the CNS without considering the incomplete understanding of peripheral nervous system pathophysiology" (*Arch. Neurol.* 40:397–398, 1983). On the other hand, Al-Din et al. have recently expressed the belief that cases with this symptom complex should be considered cases of brain stem encephalitis, a distint clinical entity with a benign prognosis (*Brain* 105:481–495, 1982).—R.N.D.J.

# 15 Neurologic Complications of Systemic Disease

**Neurological Complications of Acquired Immune Deficiency Syndrome: Analysis of 50 Patients**
William D. Snider, David M. Simpson, Surl Nielsen, Jonathan W. M. Gold, Craig E. Metroka, and Jerome B. Posner
Ann. Neurol. 14:403–418, October 1983                    15–1

Neurologic complications of acquired immune deficiency syndrome (AIDS) are seen in a significant proportion of cases. The authors reviewed data on 50 patients with AIDS and neurologic complications, who were evaluated at Memorial Sloan-Kettering Cancer Center and New York Hospital from January 1980 through January 1983. All were male homosexuals, intravenous drug abusers, or recently arrived Haitian refugees. All

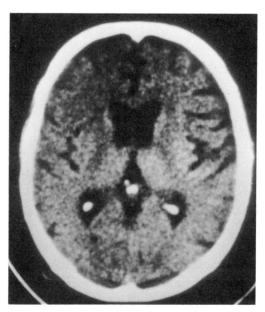

Fig 15–1.—Unenhanced computed tomography scan demonstrating generalized cerebral atrophy and periventricular white matter lucencies in patient with clinical picture of "subacute encephalitis." (Courtesy of Snider, W.D., et al.: Ann. Neurol. 14:403–418, October 1983.)

were aged 25–56 years. A specific neuropathologic diagnosis was made at autopsy in 16 cases.

The most common form of CNS infection, seen in 18 cases, was subacute encephalitis (Fig 15–1). All autopsy studies showed moderate cerebral atrophy, and most showed changes of diffuse viral infection in the gray and white matter of the cerebrum, cerebellum, brain stem, and spinal cord. Five patients had *Toxoplasma gondii* infection, three had possible *Mycobacterium avium* intracellular infection, two had progressive multifocal leukoencephalopathy, two had cryptococcal meningitis, and one had *Candida albicans* infection of the brain. Neoplasms included four meningeal lymphomas, three primary lymphomas of brain, one epidural lymphoma, and one epidural plasma-cytoma. Six patients had vascular complications, including three with cerebral hemorrhage, and eight had changes of peripheral neuropathy which usually was characterized by painful dysesthesias. Three patients had a focal mass lesion of unknown etiology. Four had aseptic meningitis and one had polymyositis. Retinopathy occurred in 10 patients, most often the cotton-wool spots previously described in AIDS.

The chief neurologic problem in these patients with AIDS was a progressive dementing encephalitis apparently caused by cytomegalovirus. Patients with AIDS also are highly susceptible to certain malignancies such as lymphoma. Patients with a history of opportunistic infectious disease, especially *Pneumocystis carinii* infection, are at the highest risk of neurologic complications. *T. gondii* infection can be treated with sulfadiazine and pyrimethamine. Nutritional factors and chemotherapy may contribute to the peripheral neuropathy seen in some patients with AIDS.

▶ This is the first detailed, documented account of the effects of acquired immune deficiency syndrome on the central and peripheral nervous systems. Fifty patients with manifestations of the syndrome had such complications. Central nervous system involvement included infection, tumors of the lymphoma variety, vascular complications, and undiagnosed central nervous system problems. Peripheral neuropathy occurred in eight patients.—R.N.D.J.

---

**Neuropsychiatric Syndromes After Gastric Partition**
Michael Sassaris, Rao Meka, G. Miletello, C. Nance, and Fred M. Hunter (Louisiana State Univ.)
Am. J. Gastroenterol. 78:321–323, June 1983                    15–2

---

The authors encountered four patients with a neuropsychiatric syndrome secondary to vitamin B complex deficiency; all were seen within 2½ to 9 months after gastric partition for morbid obesity. All four patients, none of whom had vitamin supplementation, reported protracted vomiting and weight loss of 52–100 lb. All had a peripheral neuropathy, and two also had confusion and loss of memory for recent events.

Woman, 40, weighing 304 lb, underwent gastric partition surgery but was seen six weeks later because of a two-week history of nausea and vomiting. She had lost 52 lb since the surgery. Nausea and vomiting recurred and persisted; an upper gastrointestinal tract x-ray series showed narrowing of the partition site with obstruction. Vomiting continued after revision of the partition, and endoscopy showed a patent partition site 10–11 mm in diameter. The patient became confused and lethargic, but was able to respond to commands. Nystagmus was present in all directions of gaze. Muscle tone was reduced in the legs, and tendon reflexes were absent; deep tendon reflexes were decreased in the upper extremities. Poor sensory responses were noted. The patient was significantly improved two days after institution of thiamine and trace metal supplementation. Her mental status improved gradually, and motor function improved with physical therapy. The patient weighed 190 lb nine months postoperatively. She tolerated meals well and was able to ambulate with a walker, but occasional loss of memory for recent events persisted. She was taking one multivitamin capsule a day.

Similar neuropsychiatric abnormalities may occur after jejunoileal bypass surgery for obesity, in alcoholics, and in patients with a variety of gastrointestinal tract disorders associated with persistent vomiting. The present patients did not have full-blown Wernicke's syndrome or Korsakoff's syndrome. Thiamine supplementation is important in the management of postgastric partition patients. Patients who lose weight rapidly should be monitored closely for signs of early neuropathy and should receive preventive supplementation. Vitamin B complex replacement was helpful in the present patients, but three of the four were left with residual limb weakness or memory loss.

▶ Gastric partition is a stapling of the stomach to form a tube to the duodenum so that only small amounts of food can be accommodated at one time. An occasional postoperative stenosis leads to vomiting, which with reduced food intake over a period of time results in thiamin and other B vitamin deficiencies. I believe some of Korsakoff's patients were persistent vomiters.—R.D.C.

---

### Localized Brain Stem Ischemic Damage and Ondine's Curse After Near-Drowning

M. Flint Beal, Edward P. Richardson, Jr., Robert Brandstetter, E. Tessa Hedley-Whyte, and Fred H. Hochberg
Neurology (Cleve.) 33:717–721, June 1983                                    15–3

---

Poor neurologic outcome is a serious result of near-drowning necessitating cardiopulmonary resuscitation. The authors report findings in a patient with limited brain stem dysfunction after a near-drowning incident.

Male, 19 years, lost consciousness when hit in the right temple by a rock while swimming; he was rescued after 90 seconds and subjected to cardiopulmonary resuscitation. He was apneic, comatose, and areflexic when hospitalized. The brain computed tomographic and ECG findings were normal. Consciousness returned within 24 hours, but mechanical ventilation remained necessary. Examination showed diffuse hyporeflexia, nystagmus in all fields of gaze, no palatal motion, and weak tongue protrusion. Sensations of pain and temperature were impaired only in the face. Aspiration pneumonitis developed, and subtotal gastrectomy was

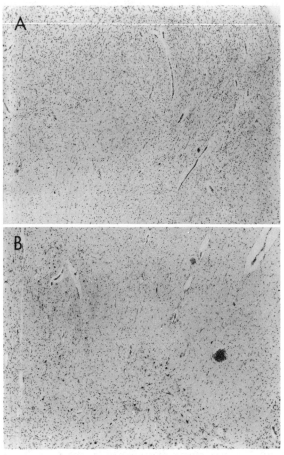

**Fig 15–2.—A,** posterior quadrant of medulla oblongata at level of posterior column nuclei. Neuronal loss is so severe that these nuclei cannot be discerned. Cresyl violet; original magnification, ×37. **B,** posterior column nuclei at same level as at left from an age-matched normal control. The nucleus of the fasciculus gracilis *(left)* and the fasciculus cuneatus *(right)* are seen clearly. Cresyl violet, original magnification, ×37. (Courtesy of Beal, M.F., et al.: Neurology [Cleve.] 33:717–721, June 1983.)

done for upper gastrointestinal tract bleeding after three weeks. Pain perception was impaired in all trigeminal divisions. Marked dysmetria of all extremities was noted. The epiglottis was flaccid and the vocal cords paralyzed in partial adduction. Some return of laryngeal motion was noted a month later. Chronic alveolar hypoventilation was present despite tracheostomy. Aspiration continued after cricopharyngeal myotomy. After four months there was horizontal nystagmus and no gag reflex was present; memory was normal, and the visual fields were full. Full power was present, but all extremities remained spastic and dysmetric. No cortical deficit was apparent. Apneic spells occurred during sleep. The patient was discharged after six months, but was found dead in bed two months later.

Autopsy showed chronic aspiration pneumonitis and acute patchy bronchopneumonia. Marked neuronal depletion was noted bilaterally in the lower brain stem (Fig 15–2). The nucleus gracilis, nucleus cuneatus, nucleus of the tractus solitarius, nucleus ambiguus, and nucleus retroambiguus were most markedly affected. Secondary degeneration of the internal arcuate fibers and the medial lemnisci was observed, and lipid-filled macrophages were present. Extensive gliosis was noted throughout the reticular formation of the medulla. The vestibular nuclei showed neuronal loss and gliosis bilaterally.

Diverse morphological abnormalities have been associated with hypoxic-ischemic damage to the brain. The forebrain and cerebellum are most vulnerable in adults, whereas in young infants the brain stem may be preferentially affected. The findings in the present case support previous concepts of the anatomical localization of the respiratory centers. Failure of automatic respiration has also been described in disorders such as encephalitis, Shy-Drager syndrome, Leigh's disease, brain stem infarction, and multiple sclerosis; and in some instances, the lesions were topographically similar to those in the present patient.

▶ The neuropathologic findings support the previous concepts of the anatomical location of the human respiratory centers. The destruction of these by anoxic-ischemic damage caused failure of automatic respiration.—R.N.D.J.

---

**Cancer Incidence in an Area of Radioactive Fallout Downwind From the Nevada Test Site**
Carl J. Johnson
JAMA 251:230–236, Jan. 13, 1984                                              15–4

---

Exposures in southwestern Utah to radioactive fallout from atmospheric nuclear tests in Nevada between 1951 and 1962 were followed by smaller exposures between 1962 and 1979 because of venting of underground nuclear detonations. The incidence of cancer in a 1951 cohort of 4,125 Mormon families in southwestern Utah living near the test site was compared with that occurring in all Utah Mormons between 1967 and 1975. Although 288 cancer patients were identified, only 179 were expected. Leukemia was most prominent between 1958 and 1966, being 3.6 times more frequent than expected; the excess of leukemia persisted into the period 1972–1980. An excess of thyroid cancer appeared early, and a notable excess occurred later. Excess breast cancers occurred in the later period, and gastrointestinal tract cancers also were more frequent than expected, as were melanoma, bone cancer, and brain tumors. A subgroup of patients with a history of acute effects from fallout had an increased incidence of cancers of several types, including leukemia. The ratio of cancers of more radiosensitive organs to all other cancers in the high-fallout area was 24% higher between 1958 and 1966 than that for all Utah Mormons, and 53.5% higher in the period 1972–1980.

The temporal trend of excess cancer appears to be consistent with the experience of Japanese survivors of the atomic bomb detonations. The largest increment of cancer in Utah probably is yet to come. An excess of radiation-induced cancers throughout the state can be expected, because an excess of childhood leukemia has already been reported for all of Utah. A survey of chromosomal aberration rates in persons who experience fallout symptoms may be useful. Study of the reproductive effects of fallout exposure also is needed.

► Inclusion of this article in a volume on neurology is difficult to justify except for its importance; however, the incidence of brain tumors was increased in the fallout area. The study seems to be valid although Land et al. (*Science* 223:139–144, 1984) feel that a previous study (Lyon et al.: N. Engl. J. Med. 300:394–402, 1979) was not valid for the reported increase of childhood leukemia in the same area. One guesses that at the time those tests were carried out we did not have information on the long-term effect of fallout from the Japanese experience.—R.D.C.

---

**Neurologic Manifestations of Essential Thrombocythemia**
Joseph Jabaily, Harry J. Iland, John Laszlo, E. Wayne Massey, Guy B. Faguet, Jean Brière, Stephen A. Landaw, and Anthony V. Pisciotta
Ann. Intern. Med. 99:513–518, October 1983                                  15–5

---

Essential thrombocythemia is a primary clonal myeloproliferative disorder characterized by persistent thrombocytosis of unknown cause. The authors recognized essential thrombocythemia in a patient during investigation of a transient ischemic attack. A review was made of the neurologic findings in 33 patients with definite essential thrombocythemia enrolled in the Polycythemia Vera Study group, a prospective follow-up investigation. The patients were randomized to treatment with radiophosphorus or melphalan, with the goal of maintaining the platelet count below 600,000/μl, and were followed for at least six months.

Twenty-one patients had neurologic symptoms at some time. They did not differ from the other patients with respect to demographic or clinical factors, but were followed for a longer time. The most common symptoms were headache and paresthesias, followed by evidence of posterior and anterior cerebral circulatory ischemia, visual disturbances, and in two

| Frequency of Neurologic Complaints Associated With Essential Thrombocythemia | |
|---|---|
| Manifestation | Patients ($n = 33$) |
| Headache | 13 |
| Paresthesiae | 10 |
| Posterior cerebral circulatory ischemia | 9 |
| Anterior cerebral circulatory ischemia | 6 |
| Visual disturbances | 6 |
| Epileptic seizures | 2 |

(Courtesy of Jabaily, J., et al.: Ann. Intern. Med. 99:513–518, October 1983.)

instances, seizures (table). Of 29 neurologic episodes, 17 occurred before initial myelosuppressive therapy was started, and 6 during periods of hematologic relapse. The occurrence of neurologic relapse could not be related to treatment, although it was more frequent in patients given radiophosphorus than in those given melphalan.

Neurologic manifestations are common in patients with definite thrombocythemia. The platelet count should be determined in those with neurologic complaints. The fact that most neurologic manifestations occurred at presentation or during hematologic relapse emphasizes the importance of keeping the platelet count below 600,000/μl.

▶ This is a relatively rare disorder which responds beautifully to treatment and in which there seems little doubt that the increase in platelets leads to stroke. The platelet count is worth looking at twice. And speaking of platelets, there is a clue (Stewart et al. *Lancet* 2:479–481, 1983) that analysis of plasma β-thromboglobulin (of platelet origin) levels may detect which patients with transient ischemia are at greater risk for stroke.—R.D.C.

# 16 Miscellaneous Conditions Affecting the Nervous System

**Neuropathology in Seven Cases of Locked-In Syndrome**
Michel Reznik (Univ. of Liège, Belgium)
J. Neurol. Sci. 60:67–78, July 1983                    16–1

The term "locked-in syndrome" refers to a clinical state in which patients are quadriplegic and mute but are awake and able to communicate by eye movements. Such a state differs from coma and akinetic mutism with which it has been confused. Whereas akinetic mutism is due to lesions in various brain areas, locked-in syndrome has always been attributed to brain stem dysfunction, the extent of which has not been clearly defined. The neuropathology of seven patients with locked-in syndrome was compared with that of three patients with akinetic mutism; all of the disorders occurred after brain stem vascular disease (nine infarctions and one hematoma).

With conventional techniques after formalin fixation, the extent of lesions in the brain stem was analyzed in these 10 cases and compared with other observations of brain stem vascular disease lacking similar clinical evolution. Other reports of locked-in syndrome have noted that symptoms have been provoked by diverse diseases of the brain stem, including pontine myelinolysis, multiple sclerosis, tumor invading the pons, head trauma, and pontine abscess. Case 4 in this study was due to a recent hemorrhage of the fourth ventricle that infiltrated and destroyed the tegmentum of the pons. The majority of locked-in syndrome cases, however, have been induced by a softening of the brain stem, as corroborated by the present report.

The extent of brain stem lesions causing locked-in syndrome varies; however, on the basis of this study and others, it is clear that most patients who have this syndrome after ischemic damage have a ventral pontine infarction with variable extension to adjacent areas. Most frequently, there is bilateral necrosis of the basis pontis involving the rostral and middle segments. Tissue destruction may be restricted to the ventral pons (cases 3 and 7), or may include variable destruction of the tegmentum (cases 1, 2, and 5). Ischemic lesions centered on one or both cerebral peduncles have also been observed (case 6) (Fig 16–1). In the seven cases of locked-in syndrome, the reticular nuclei were affected in all but one. There were few changes in the locus ceruleus, which is thought to be a major agent in cerebral cortex stimulation. However, in the three cases of akinetic mutism, the locus ceruleus was completely destroyed in one case, and its

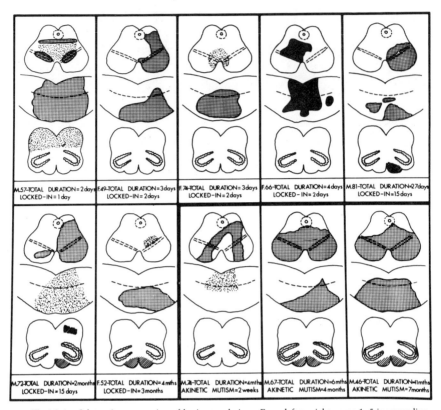

**Fig 16–1.**—Schematic presentation of brain stem lesions. From left to right, cases 1–5 in upper line and cases 6–10 in lower line. *Crosshatched* areas indicate softening or necrosis; *dotted* areas, edema or slight demyelination; *diagonal* lines, secondary demyelination; and *black* areas, recent hematoma. (Courtesy of Reznik M.: J. Neurol. Sci. 60:67–78, July 1983.)

projections to the brain were probably destroyed in another. It is concluded that although most of the clinical signs can be explained by pathologic findings at autopsy, it is not yet possible to specify the brain stem lesions responsible for the locked-in syndrome.

The prognosis of patients with locked-in syndrome is uncertain; some survive for long periods and others die within a few hours after onset. Cases 9 and 10 showed the longest survival times despite exhibiting the largest areas of brain stem destruction (in addition to basal ganglia lesions).

▶ This is a careful neuropathologic study of the locked-in syndrome. The authors point out that the preservation of an intact medulla oblongata and of most of the midbrain, particularly the periaqueductal area, seems to be necessary. The lesion in some cases seems to extend up into the lower midbrain.

A frightening report comes across the desk describing this syndrome in a young man who had chiropractic neck manipulation (*Ann. Emerg. Med.* 12:648–650, 1983). And the subject of chiropractic brings up backache. Waddell and Hamblen, orthopedists of Glasgow (*Practitioner* 227:1167–1175, 1983) have a clear no-nonsense comment on their experience with backache. In a series of 900 patients, 100 of whom had spinal pathology, they found that no patient who was between the ages of 20 and 55 and who had no previous medical˙disease, systemic symptoms, thoracic pain, limitation of lumbar flexion, raised erythrocyte sedimentation rate, or abnormal spine x-rays turned out to have spine pathology. Quite a statement.—R.D.C.

---

**Recombinant DNA and Neurologic Disease: The Coming of a New Age**
Roger N. Rosenberg (Univ. of Texas at Dallas)
Neurology (Cleve.) 33:622–625, May 1983                                    16–2

---

The author discusses the potential of using complementary DNA (cDNA) hybridization patterns in evaluating patients with genetic and metabolic disorders involving the nervous system. Using cDNA, which has constituent bases complementary to the template messenger RNA (mRNA), it is possible to make a series of recombinant DNA plasmid clones matching the total number of mRNAs transcribed in a given tissue. Species of mRNA isolated from brain tissue obtained at autopsy are intact and stable and can be used for protein translation with high fidelity. A library of cloned cDNA complementary to cerebral cortical mRNAs has been made, and construction of a library from cerebellar cortical mRNAs is in progress. Soon, clones for most important neuronal and glial proteins will be available. The nucleotide sequence of the genes can then be determined and chromosome assignment made by somatic cell hybridization or by direct in situ hybridization of the probe to the chromosome. The number of gene copies per cell will be measurable, and mRNA levels in specific brain areas can be quantitated using labeled recombinant cDNA probes.

These methods were used to identify patients with α-thalassemia and sickle cell disease, and they may well prove useful in identifying mutations in genetic neurologic disorders, as well as in antenatal diagnosis. Recombinant DNA methods can be expected to be most useful in elucidating the biochemical defects in dominantly inherited disorders, e.g., Huntington's disease, myotonic muscular dystrophy, neurofibromatosis, and the spinocerebellar degenerations. The associated DNA polymorphisms are essentially inherited bystanders, but they are effective markers of genetic disorders if close enough to the genes of interest. It should be possible through prenatal identification of heterozygotes to prevent or eliminate lethal disorders in one generation of an affected family. Gene therapy also is a possibility in the near future. The reinduction of fetal genes to compensate for a mutant defective adult gene may have particular relevance to late-onset degenerative diseases.

▶ This article reviews recent advances in molecular biology. The author postulates that neurologists will soon become familiar with and grow to rely on DNA hybridization patterns in evaluating patients with genetic and metabolic disorders and, in the near future it is hoped, will be able to apply specific gene therapy to their patients.—R.N.D.J.

---

### Hemifacial Spasm: Results of Microvascular Relocation
David Fairholm, Jiunn-Ming Wu, and Kan-Nan Liu
Can. J. Neurol. Sci. 10:187–191, August 1983                    16–3

---

The authors have treated hemifacial spasm by posterior fossa craniotomy and vascular relocation on the grounds that microvascular compression of the seventh nerve in the cerebellopontine angle is responsible for the disorder. Eleven men and nine women with a mean age of 47 years were operated on. All presented with typical disabling unilateral contractions of the face. Computed tomography (CT) and angiography ruled out structural mass lesions. Previous treatments had included partial facial nerve section, thermodenervation, and pharmacotherapy with carbamazepine and steroids. All patients had progressive spasms. Presently the diagnosis is confirmed by contrast enhanced CT only.

Unilateral craniectomy was performed via a suboccipital retromastoid approach. The compressing arterial loop (Fig 16–2), which usually arises from the anterior inferior cerebellar artery or the vertebral artery, was relocated away from the root entry zone and held by a notched Teflon sponge.

Sixteen patients had immediate relief of hemifacial spasm. The patient with glossopharyngeal neuralgia had relief of both pain and spasms. One patient improved three weeks after operation. Two patients had reexploration; in one the sponge had slipped and in the other a previously unidentified vessel was relocated. Both patients recovered completely. Another patient refused reexploration. Four patients had decreased hearing after operation; this condition has persisted in one of them. Two patients had mild transient facial weakness after operation. No patient has had recurrent spasms on follow-up for 18 months or longer. Aberrant vascular loops often compress the root entry zone of the facial nerve in patients with hemifacial spasm, and relocation leads to relief of the spasm.

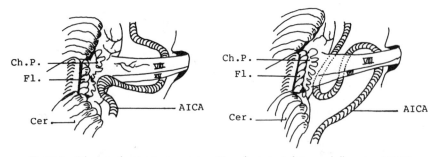

**Fig 16–2.**—Schematic drawing to represent position of anterior inferior cerebellar artery *(AICA)* on seventh nerve. *VII* = seventh nerve; *VIII* = eighth nerve; *CH P* = choroid plexus; *Fl* = flocculus; *cer* = cerebellum. (Courtesy of Fairholm, D., et al.: Can. J. Neurol. Sci. 10:187–191, August 1983.)

▶ These results give further support to the theory that hemifacial spasm is caused in many instances by vascular compression of the seventh nerve at the root entry zone. Surgical relocation of the offending vessel often gives permanent relief. This procedure is possible with little risk with modern anesthesia and microsurgical techniques.—R.N.D.J.

---

**Hand Difficulties Among Musicians**
Fred H. Hochberg, Robert D. Leffert, Matthew D. Heller, and Lisle Merriman (Massachusetts Gen. Hosp.)
JAMA 249:1869–1872, Apr. 8, 1983                                    16–4

---

The authors reviewed experience with 49 musicians who were seen for neurologic, rheumatic, or musculoskeletal difficulties and with 51 others evaluated through correspondence. A majority of the subjects were pianists. Median age was 37.5 years. The musicians had begun playing at an average age of eight years, and they practiced five to six hours a day on average.

The initial symptoms often included pain, weakness, tightening, cramping, and loss of control of the hand. The pianists most frequently reported loss of control while playing, loss of speed, loss of facility in rapid passages, and decreased endurance. The right upper limb was affected in most instances. Symptoms most often affected the fourth and fifth fingers. About half the patients examined had weakness or decreased bulk or tone in the muscles. Many exhibited abnormal positioning with curling or drooping of digits. Tendon contracture was seen in one fifth of patients. Inflammation of tendons or synovium accounted for 42% of the cases examined; tendinitis was the most common diagnosis, but nerve disorders accounted for almost the same proportion of cases. Nerve entrapment was evident in 15% of patients. Many patients had tried nonsteroid anti-inflammatory drugs, and many were involved in physiotherapy. Several had had surgical exploration. Most patients were managed by physiotherapy and anti-inflammatory agents, and the majority of those with inflammatory tendon symptoms have improved. Needle electrode-assisted biofeedback is being evaluated in patients with motor control difficulties.

Tendinitis of the finger extensors is a common problem in musicians. Neurologic disorders account for about a third of clinical difficulties in musicians. A large majority of affected musicians have a good prognosis with conservative measures, but recurrences are frequent. New treatment methods are needed for patients who have nerve entrapment and motor control problems.

▶ This article reaches no conclusions other than that there is need for further research to determine both cause and means of prevention of such complications. The authors apparently consider that the cause is always "organic"— inflammatory, neuromuscular, and some nerve entrapment syndromes. They consider only musicians in this article, but similar disorders occur in others too: "writer's cramp," "typist's cramp," and the "occupational neuroses" of Gowers, Osler, and Wilson. What are the authors results with biofeedback, behavioral modification therapy, and conditioning? This is certainly an area that needs further study, since these symptoms, which often occur in early life, may necessitate change of career and definite alteration of one's goals for the future.—R.N.D.J.

---

## Comparison of Thyrotropin-Releasing Hormone (TRH), Naloxone, and Dexamethasone Treatments in Experimental Spinal Injury

Alan I. Faden, Thomas P. Jacobs, Michael T. Smith, and John W. Holaday
Neurology (Cleve.) 33:673–678, June 1983                                    16–5

---

There is evidence implicating endogenous opiates in the pathophysiology of spinal cord injury. Opiate antagonists such as naloxone have improved functional neurologic recovery in animal studies, but they may enhance posttraumatic pain. Thyrotropin-releasing hormone (TRH) may act in vivo as a partial physiologic opiate antagonist that spares analgesic systems. The authors compared naloxone and TRH in cats in which the cord was injured by the Allen method at the C7 level. Treatment was begun an hour after injury; both agents were given in a bolus of 2 mg/kg, followed by 2 mg/kg per hour for four hours. Controls received 0.5 mg of dexamethasone per kg followed by 0.5 mg/kg per hour or physiologic saline.

Cats given naloxone or TRH showed a rapid rise in mean arterial pressure compared with controls, and pressures were better maintained in these groups. Functional neurologic scores were highest in the TRH group a week after injury, and the differences were maximal at six weeks, when TRH-treated animals had significantly higher scores than both naloxone- and corticosteroid-treated cats. Scores were higher in naloxone-treated cats than in saline controls, but the differences from corticosteroid-treated cats were not significant. The typical TRH-treated cat had normal motor function, whereas the typical naloxone-treated cat had nearly normal forelimb function and mild spasticity in the hindlimbs. The typical corticosteroid-treated or saline-treated cat had marked spasticity or ataxia, or both, in all limbs. Survival was significantly better in the TRH- and naloxone-treated groups. No significant histologic differences were found in the various treatment groups, and the histologic and neurologic scores were not significantly correlated.

Thyrotropin-releasing hormone was beneficial to cats with spinal cord injury in this study, in comparison with both naloxone and dexamethasone. Thyrotropin releasing hormone appears to be potentially ideal for use in treatment of human beings with cord injury because of its lack of effect on analgesic systems and its high therapeutic index.

▶ These authors had previously shown that both naloxone and TRH improved neurologic functional recovery after experimental spinal injury. These further studies confirm the value of both in such injury, but show that TRH is the more effective. Corticosteroids, on the other hand, did not prove to be of benefit in the present study.—R.N.D.J.

### The Discovery, Proof and Reproof of Neurosecrection (Speidel, 1917; Scharrer and Scharrer, 1934)

Harvey B. Sarnat (Univ. of Calgary)
Can. J. Neurol. Sci. 10:208–212, August 1983                    16–6

The CNS was not considered an organ of internal secretion until Scharrer and Scharrer demonstrated neuroendocrine function in the brains of both vertebrates and invertebrates in the mid-1930s. Speidel had described neurosecretory cells and correctly interpreted their function in 1917. He studied the spinal cord of the skate and later that of other species of fish. The Scharrers proposed that the cytoplasmic granules present in neurons of the paraventricular and supraoptic hypothalamic nuclei of fish are secretory hormones transported by axons to the pituitary. Subsequent studies in many vertebrate species supported this conclusion. However, some workers continued to reject the concept of neurosecretory cells as late as 1940.

Neurosecretion has been shown to be a widespread function of neuroepithelial cells, present in all animals having a nervous system. All classes of vertebrates have neurosecretory activity within the CNS. The early ancestor of all vertebrates probably was a marine nemertine worm, and

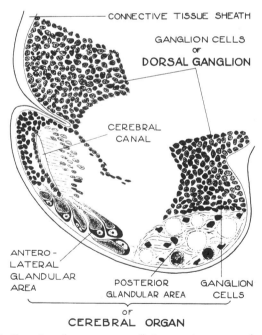

Fig 16–3.—This illustration of neurosecretory cells in nemertine worm predated development of hypothesis that these obscure animals are little-evolved descendants of ancestral prevertebrates. "Drawing of horizontal section through cerebral organ and part of dorsal ganglion of Cerebratulus lacteus. There is uninterrupted transition of nerve cells from cerebral organ into dorsal ganglion. Bouin, nitrocellulose, 20u, van Gieson; × 300." (From Scharrer, B.: J. Comp. Neurol. 74:109–130, 1941. Courtesy of Sarnat, H.B.: Can. J. Neurol. Sci. 10:208–212, August 1983.)

surviving species of this phylum have a "brain" that is essentially a secretory organ (Fig 16–3). Scharrer discovered neurosecretion in nemertines years before it was recognized that certain structures of these worms are potentially homologous with a dorsal notochord, a primordial thyroid, and other vertebrate organs. As long ago as 1900 Metcalf described a "gland arising by the transformation of nerve cells" in tunicates, simple protochordate animals with many organs that resemble those of embryonic vertebrates more than those of invertebrates.

▶ Comparative neuroanatomy and evolutionary theory have made many contributions to an understanding of the human nervous system. This interesting historical article outlines the development of our knowledge of neurosecretion.—R.N.D.J.

---

### Dominant Spinocerebellar Ataxia: Genetic Counseling
J. F. Jackson, R. D. Currier (Univ. of Mississippi), and N. E. Morton (Univ. of Hawaii)
J. Neurogenetics 1:87–90, September 1983                    16–7

---

The dominantly inherited spinocerebellar ataxias (SCAs) probably are a heterogeneous group of disorders within which at least one subtype of olivopontocerebellar atrophy (OPCA 1) is due to a single gene at a locus near HLA on human chromosome 6. Linkage of OPCA 1 with the major histocompatibility locus on chromosome 6 has been demonstrated in some kindreds but not in others.

The disease presents gradually, usually at age 20–40 years, with imbalance, clumsiness, staggering, ataxic speech, pathologic reflexes, and sensory loss of the posterior column. Progressive ataxia and severe dysar-

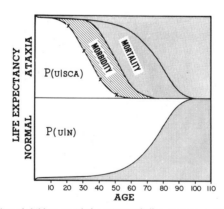

**Fig 16–4.**—Probability of children at risk for spinocerebellar ataxia to receive gene for ataxia (*upper half of diagram*) and to remain unaffected at indicated ages $P(u/SCA)$. Morbidity is indicated by *diagonal lines* and mortality by *shaded* area. Lower half of diagram shows life table general mortality for at-risk children who remain unaffected $P(u)/N$, having received normal gene rather than ataxia gene. (Courtesy of Jackson, J.F., et al.: J. Neurogenetics 1:87–90, September 1983.)

thria precede death, at age 50–60 years, due to inanition and respiratory infection.

Data on age at onset were collected from pedigrees of dominant SCA. Probability of children at risk of receiving the gene for ataxia and that of remaining unaffected at varying ages are shown in Figure 16–4. Data on age at onset can be combined with information from informative matings by using histocompatibility determination to indicate linkage status. Prior probability of affection status when the SCA gene is in coupling with HLA type in the at-risk person is 0.85 when the father is affected as a result of recombination occurring at a 15% frequency. Probability is 0.7 when the mother is affected. When the data indicate repulsion, with the HLA haplotype received from the parental chromosome with the normal rather than the SCA gene, the risk is 0.15 for children of affected fathers and 0.3 for children of affected mothers. The likelihood of disease developing when the HLA haplotype received is in repulsion with the SCA gene declines considerably during the reproductive age period, and postponing childbearing may be a strong consideration for such persons.

▶ Dominantly inherited spinocerebellar ataxia poses a problem in genetic counseling because of the late onset of symptoms and signs of the disorder. These authors cite helpful advice that can be given to members of families at risk for this disorder.—R.N.D.J.

---

**The Natural History of Back Pain**
M. O. Roland
Practitioner 227:1119–1122, July 1983                                    16–8

---

Back pain affects nearly all persons at some time in their lives. It represents a frequent problem for physicians, who have little effective treatment to offer. In contrast with practices in the United States, physicians in Britain make roentgenograms of only 5% of the patients who complain of back pain. One in every 200 patients on average eventually undergoes laminectomy. Men are seen only slightly more often than women, but they are twice as likely to have a diagnosis of disk prolapse and twice as likely to have a laminectomy. The peak age at consultation is 45–64 years. "Mechanical" causes are almost always present, and most patients have "nonspecific mechanical back pain." Ongoing research into the basic anatomy and pathophysiology of the spine should improve diagnosis of the various causes of back pain.

Pain of shorter duration is more likely to resolve fairly rapidly; only about 10% of patients continue to have pain for more than four weeks. Only 7% of patients are off work for more than a month. There is good reason to be encouraging to patients with backache. Limited straight-leg raising worsens the outlook. A thorough examination is not likely to yield more prognostic information, but it helps to reassure the patient. There is more than a threefold chance of the patient complaining of further back pain in the following year.

Treatment does not influence the eventual outcome in most patients seen in general practice with nonspecific back pain. Analgesic treatment does not alter the natural course of the disorder, and anti-inflammatory agents and muscle relaxants usually are not of much value. Bed rest shortens the time to functional recovery. Isometric exercises to strengthen the pelvic and abdominal muscles are probably as helpful as conventional exercises and may be less likely to make the patient worse.

▶ The author is an English general practitioner, not an orthopedist or a neuro-surgeon. He sees the patient with back pain first. It's good to know the great majority will recover if left alone—it may not seem so to the specialist who sees the patients with difficult, complicated, and chronic low back pain.—R.D.C.

---

**Recent Advances in Understanding Brain Capillary Function**
Gary W. Goldstein and A. Lorris Betz (Univ. of Michigan)
Ann. Neurol. 14:389–395, October 1983                                        16–9

---

Methods are now available for isolating and studying microvessels from the brain and for growing the endothelial cells in tissue culture. A model

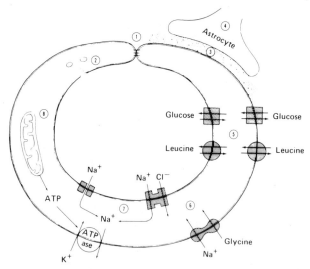

Fig 16–5.—Model of brain capillary. Tight junctions *(1)* that join endothelial cells in brain capillaries are continuous and complex, and they limit diffusion of large and small solutes. Few pinocytotic vesicles *(2)* are found in cytoplasm; this potential route for transendothelial transport is inoperative in normal brain capillaries. Basement membrane *(3)* provides structural support for capillary and may influence endothelial cell function. Foot processes of astrocytes *(4)* encircle capillary but do not create permeability barrier. Transport carriers *(5)* for glucose and essential amino acids facilitate movement of these solutes into brain. Active transport systems *(6)* appear to cause efflux of certain small amino acids from brain to blood. Sodium ion pores and sodium chloride carriers on luminal surface of endothelial cell and $Na^+$-$K^+$-ATPase on antiluminal surface *(7)* account for movement of ions across brain capillary. Mitochondria *(8)* produce ATPase needed for energy-dependent transport processes. Not shown are receptor sites for agents that may regulate permeability of this barrier. (Courtesy of Goldstein, G.W., and Betz, A.L.: Ann. Neurol. 14:389–395, October 1983.)

of the brain capillary is shown in Figure 16–5. In contrast with capillaries in other organs, the membrane fusion at junctional contacts between the endothelial cells is continuous, separating the luminal contents from the interstitial fluid of the brain. The structure of the intercellular fusion is complex. Changes in the integrity of the tight junctions might underlie enhanced permeability of the blood-brain barrier after various insults and manipulations. Transendothelial vesicular transport, or pinocytosis, is a potential route for the movement of plasma into brain tissue. The basement membrane may be able to bind selected compounds based on electric change, but whether this binding influences barrier function is uncertain.

Some polar molecules such as D-glucose and the essential large neutral L-amino acids rapidly cross the capillary wall. It seems likely that glucose carriers are present on both the luminal and the antiluminal surfaces of the endothelial cells. Transport carriers for large neutral amino acids are also present. Since the same carrier facilitates the movement of several amino acids into brain, a potential for competition exists. The antiluminal location of $Na^+$-$K^+$-ATPase in brain capillary endothelial cells is similar to the cellular polarity of many fluid-transporting epithelial cells. Transport carriers for small neutral amino acids may exhibit a similar polar distribution between the luminal and the antiluminal surfaces of the capillary wall.

The use of cultured brain capillary endothelial cells may enhance understanding of carrier-mediated transport processes. Cultured endothelial cells may also be useful for studying factors that activate capillary proliferation in brain lesions.

▶ The endothelial cells in brain capillaries form a blood-brain barrier which limits and controls the movements of solvents between blood and brain. They also contain specialized transport systems that facilitate the transfer of some solutes and actively pump other solutes from brain to blood. Methods have been developed to isolate microvessels from brain to grow brain capillary endothelial cells in tissue culture. This review summarizes knowledge of brain capillary function.—R.N.D.J.

---

**Brain Microvessel Endothelial Cells in Tissue Culture: A Model for Study of Blood-Brain Barrier Permeability**
Phillip D. Bowman, Steven R. Ennis, Kyle E. Rarey, A. Lorris Betz, and Gary W. Goldstein (Univ. of Michigan)
Ann. Neurol. 14:396–402, October 1983                                    16–10

---

Defects in brain microvessel function occur in a wide range of neurologic disorders, and the resultant breakdown of the blood-brain barrier can lead to edema and produce further brain injury from increased intracranial pressure or inadequate tissue perfusion. The authors developed a method of isolating microvessels from bovine brain and releasing and growing the endothelial cells in tissue culuture to evaluate formation and disruption of the barrier. The cultured cells contain factor VIII/Willebrand antigen, the most specific marker for endothelial cells. Frequent tight junctional complexes and few pinocytotic vesicles are observed, as in cells in vivo. The barrier was altered by removing extracellular calcium or by treatment with high concentrations of arabinose.

Exposure of monolayers of endothelial cells to calcium-free solution or treatment with 1.6M arabinose led to distinctive morphological changes in the intercellular contacts, with return of a normal structure in control medium in both instances. Exposure to calcium-free medium was followed by retraction of cells from one another and loss of the ability to form continuous sheets. The rate of movement of $^{14}$C-sucrose across the monolayer was increased by 120%. Arabinose treatment was followed by removal of water from the cells and the appearance of craters in or near the junctional complexes. Transcellular flux was increased by 40%.

The integrity of the brain microvessel endothelial cell barrier can be assessed by morphological and tracer methods. The system should prove to be useful for investigating blood-brain barrier function and its reactions to injury.

▶ This article describes a method of isolating microvessels from brain and of growing brain capillary endothelial cells in tissue culture. Following return of these cells to control medium, a normal structure was reestablished, and it was possible to assess the effect of these treatments on transcellular permeability—R.N.D.J.

---

### Central Serotonergic Nerves Project to the Pial Vessels of the Brain

Lars Edvinsson, Amanda Degueurce, Danielle Duverger, Eric T. MacKenzie, and Bernard Scatton
Nature 306:55–57, Nov. 3, 1983
16–11

Serotonin has been strongly implicated in the etiology of several cerebrovascular diseases, including stroke, migraine, and vasospasm. Studies have suggested that an indoleaminergic system of perivascular nerves exists in the large cerebral arteries of the lamprey. It also has been observed that cerebral arteries (e.g., the vertebrobasilar system of the rabbit) and microvessels in various species may take up serotonin and 5-hydroxytryptophan. However, neither the large cerebral arteries nor the microvessels directly control, or alter, cerebral blood flow. Rather, as in other vascular beds, the arterioles and small arteries are the major elements of resistance. The authors used immunocytochemical and neurochemical techniques to investigate the presence of central serotonergic innervation of pial arteries and arterioles in the rat.

With the use of indirect immunofluorescence techniques and highly specific, well-characterized antibodies to serotonin, immunocytochemistry studies revealed perivascular, serotonin-containing fibers in the pial blood vessels (Fig 16–6). The organization of the nerve plexuses was similar to that of other vasomotor nerves previously observed in the pial vessels (nerve fibers containing norepinephrine, acetylcholinesterase, vasoactive intestinal polypeptide, and substance P). The serotonin-immunoreactive

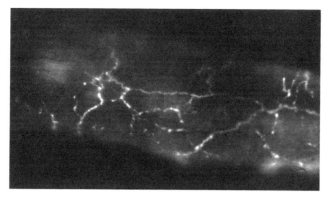

Fig 16–6.—Perivascular serotonin-containing nerve fibers in walls of pial arteries; original magnification, × 176. (Courtesy of Edvinsson, L., et al.: Nature 306:55–57, Nov. 3, 1983.)

fibers in the major cerebral arteries formed plexuses with fibers running in all directions, whereas the smaller pial arteries had only a few or a single nerve fiber.

Biochemical studies detected substantial concentrations of serotonin and its metabolite 5-hydroxyindoleacetic acid in the pial vessels when compared with cortical tissue. Experiments with the neutrotoxin 5,7-dihyroxy-tryptamine fully supported the presence of serotonergic innervation of pial vessels. Additional studies showed that serotonergic innervation of pial vessels did not originate from the small, intensely fluorescent cells of the superior cervical ganglion, and also excluded the possibility that the noradrenergic terminals in cerebral vessels take up and store serotonin. Rather, most of the serotonergic innervation of the pial vessels originated from the median and dorsal raphe, with both nuclei contributing equally. However, the two ascending serotonergic pathways may project to two demarcated cortical regions. The intracranial mast cells also contained serotonin. However, as selective raphe lesions decreased serotonin concentrations in pial vessels, the possibility that serotonin was located in perivascular mast cells is almost certainly ruled out.

The results demonstrate serotonergic innervation of the pial circulation that has a largely central midbrain origin. These serotonergic nerves may be involved in the physiologic regulation of the cerebral circulation and, in addition, may play a role in the etiology of serotonin-related cerebrovascular disorders.

▶ Whether or not the discovery of centrally originating serotonergic nerves on the pial vessels will help us to understand migraine and possibly even stroke remains to be seen. What could the function of a nerve impulse mediated by serotonin be?—R.D.C.

# NEUROSURGERY

———

OSCAR SUGAR, M.D.

# Introduction

This YEAR BOOK is the last for which I shall be an editor. Its publication in 1985 marks 30 years since I first began, as assistant for Dr. Percival Bailey, to help with the editorial work. I had been abstracting articles for some years before then, and Dr. Bailey was kind enough to have my name put on the cover and flyleaf of the 1953–1954 series, published in 1954, in anticipation of putting me to work with actual editing in the following year.

The 1954–1955 YEAR BOOK was published in 1955. The Neurology section, edited by Dr. Roland Mackay, comprised 207 pages; the Psychiatry section, under Dr. S. Bernard Wortis, 203. Dr. Bailey and I had 179 pages, with an introduction by Dr. Bailey quoting an order, dating from 1950, forbidding lobotomy operations in the Soviet Union, as well as a quotation from an address by Pope Pius XII in 1952, in which the Pontiff declared that a person did not have the right to agree to a procedure which diminished or abolished "his human personality." Nevertheless, such operations were being done, and Dr. Wortis selected for the Psychiatry section of that YEAR BOOK 11 articles on frontal lobe operations done for psychiatric reasons, and seven more articles were abstracted in the Neurosurgery section. Most of these dealt with schizophrenic disorders, but the only article abstracted in the 1984 YEAR BOOK dealt with obsessive compulsive states; none were selected for 1985. In spite of the President's Commission (see the 1980 YEAR BOOK, p. 432), psychosurgery is frowned upon by many physicians, especially psychiatrists; and since the referral for psychosurgical operations perforce comes from psychiatry, the number of operations has become minuscule, even though there is ample evidence that cingulotomy, at least, does not affect intelligence or personality.

Hemispherectomy and cortical excisions for intractable epilepsy, especially of what was then called the psychomotor variety, were reported in 1955, and they appear again in 1985; hemispherectomy for inoperable tumor was occasionally performed in the mid-1950s, but not now; commissurotomy for intractable seizures is occasionally done now, but not then. Treatment of seizures by stereotactic means was then coming into vogue, and a variety of new instrument models was described. Dr. Bailey's interest in brain anatomy and stereotaxis culminated in the *Atlas* (Schaltenbrand, G., Bailey, P. [eds.]: *Einführung in die Stereotaktischen Operationen mit einem Atlas des Menschlichen Gehirns*. Stuttgart, Thieme, 1959) to which he was a major contributor, along with Professor Georges Schaltenbrand and other collaborators. Stereotaxy has now become so commonplace that little description of the apparatus is to be found in the current articles on its use in implantation of radioactive materials and its use in combination with computerized scanning and with lasers.

Surgical treatment of movement disorders was hotly debated 30 years ago; Cooper wrote of deliberate occlusion of the anterior choroidal artery to create a lesion in the basal ganglia, while Guiot and Fénelon described different open operations to attack the same regions. Spiegel and Wycis described the first use of stereotaxy to localize targets for electrocoagulation for abolition of tremor. Such procedures are rarely done now, thanks to the development of L-dopa and its allies, but there are still neurosurgeons (Gillingham, for instance) who find them useful when medication has failed.

In the field of diagnosis, the current YEAR BOOK is heavily endowed with unthought of procedures such as computerized scanning, nuclear magnetic scanning, and B-ultrasound. A-mode ultrasound was occasionally being used in 1955 for diagnosis of midline shift and, rarely, for transdural diagnosis; the modern use of B-ultrasound at operation in various parts of the body was unavailable. Ultrasonic therapy for frontal lobe operations for pain was described, but soon fell into disuse. Angiography was still in its developmental stages, concerned with attempted differential diagnosis of tumors by angiographic patterns, with a new apparatus for serial picture taking, and with vertebral angiography, both by catheter insertion into arteries of the arm and by percutaneous injections in the neck. Complications were sufficiently frequent and disturbing that four articles described them in the 1955 YEAR BOOK, commenting on the need for newer contrast materials—which have now appeared and are taken for granted, especially when used in small amounts via femoral catheterization, not yet developed 30 years ago. Ventriculography, with air or with iodinated materials is apparently so well known now—and so readily replaced with scanning devices—that no specific articles on this diagnostic aid are included now.

Controlled hypotension for neurosurgical procedures was just being introduced, along with hibernation for head injury. The former is now an accepted technique; the latter has been revived and is much in dispute chiefly in the form that uses barbiturates to mitigate the effects of severe brain swelling after injury. Hypothermia as a part of hibernation has largely been given up, except for rare occasions for very difficult vascular procedures.

Intracranial hemorrhages were of interest when they were of traumatic origin, but a few articles appeared on hemorrhages in the brains of newborn infants, chiefly having to do with postmortem material; now the emphasis is on causation and treatment in preterm and newborn infants with intraventricular and intracerebral hemorrhage; these are matters of concern thanks to the development of special intensive care units and superspecialization of pediatricians. The section on trauma was anything but prominent 30 years ago, perhaps in part because of the infrequent admission of such patients to the University of Illinois Hospital. The circumstances are now quite different, with articles on the proper indications for radiography. (It would have been unthinkable in 1955 to omit radiographs of the skull of a patient who had been in an accident.) Similarly, the occasional nonoperative "treatment" of patients with extracerebral hematomas would have been considered malpractice then, if anyone had written about it.

The importance to neurosurgeons of infections of the nervous system has been magnified by the widespread use of a spectrum of antibiotics, especially after shunting of ventricular or spinal fluid; this was not common practice in 1955, when Matson wrote of the use of Torkildsen's ventriculocisternostomy (a procedure too often neglected by current neurosurgeons) and of the procedure he invented, which involved shunting fluid by catheter surrounded at one end by cerebrospinal fluid and by a ureter at the other (after nephrectomy). Valved shunts were not yet invented; they are commonplace now.

The arguments about the best way of treating cerebral abscesses (drainage vs. excision, for instance) continue; now, however, there is also the possibility of giving cortisone products to reduce edema and following the course of the abscess with computed scanning while giving antibiotics.

About half of the relatively few articles in 1955 concerned with brain tumors dealt with detection by roentgenographic means, chiefly with radioactive isotopes. Isotopic localization is now used only when there is doubtful result from using other imaging techniques. Boron neutron capture therapy is no longer used (except possibly in Japan in a research project). Histologic and gross anatomical study of brain tumors was included in 1955, as anticipated by Dr. Bailey's long association with histiogenesis of brain tumors. His opposition to Kernohan's classification of tumors, as well as that of Globus and Cares, is included in the older YEAR BOOK. Only a few articles dealt with operation—and none with chemotherapy. Most had to do with radiotherapy from external sources, including the betatron, and Dr. Bailey's interest in pathology was reflected in his choice of articles on the effects of roentgen therapy on the brain and spinal cord. External radiation with stereotactic apparatus now being used in a few centers in the world was not yet invented, and internal sources for radiation (brachytherapy) were not yet developed, as they are now. The early diagnosis and successful total extirpation of acoustic tumors was so rarely effected that there were no articles on this subject in the 1955 book, as there are now—including some articles on the use of lasers in attacking these and other brain tumors.

There was, in 1955, one article on surgical treatment of arteriovenous malformations and two on aneurysms. Embolization, now used in vascular lesions and tumors, had yet to be developed. A single article on thrombosis of the carotid artery contrasts with the current extensive survey of endarterectomy, dissolution of clots with streptokinase, and extracranial-intracranial shunts. Placement of omentum, muscle, or isolated temporal arteries on the brain to increase circulation to ischemic areas, a procedure that is now available, reflects the development of microneurosurgery and widespread use of the operating microscope.

Disorders of the spine and its canal were put together in a single chapter, including myelographic diagnosis, trauma (chiefly the nonsurgical treatment of the aftereffects of paraplegia), epidural abscess, metastases, and epidural granuloma. These contrast with the extensive newer studies on scanning the spine and its contents, spinal cord operations for pain, and nonionic water-soluble contrast media for diagnosis (instead of iodized oils with *their* complications).

The pathology and treatment of trigeminal neuralgia was much discussed in 1955, with subtemporal decompressions of the trigeminal apparatus described in three articles—one by Taarnhøj, another by Stender, and a third by Love and Svien—but without obvious rationale. The concept of vascular compression now so commonly held had not been developed, and current decompressive operations are done from the posterior fossa approach with apparently improved results. Current percutaneous treatments of trigeminal and glossopharyngeal neuralgia were yet to be developed (except for alcohol injections of branches of the trigeminal nerve).

Herniated lumbar disk was the subject of a few articles, one of which dealt with complications of operations, such as damage to major abdominal vessels (fortunately not a prominent problem in current neurosurgery). Fusions were being done, chiefly from behind, but there was at least one article on interbody lumbar fusions. Thomas's demonstration of the effect of papain on rabbit cartilage was published in 1956, almost 10 years before Smith published case reports on its use in herniated disks. In 1985, the YEAR BOOK notes the widespread use of chymopapain and some of the arguments about its dangers. The single article on chronic myelopathy from cervical arthrosis contrasts with the various anterior and posterior approaches now being used with and without fusion for cervical root and spinal cord disability.

The changing background of neurosurgical practice and training probably accounts for the lack of articles on the sympathetic nervous system now; in 1955 there was interest in the anatomy of the autonomic nervous system, sympathectomy for causalgia (still useful, but relatively uncommonly carried out by neurosurgeons) and also sympathectomy for hypertension (no longer done by anyone, apparently, owing to the development of medical treatment). Neurosurgeons are rarely involved now in the surgical treatment of Ménière's syndrome, which was to be found in the 1955 YEAR BOOK (but is now apparently the exclusive prerogative of the otologists).

The first hint of the use of cortisone and its derivatives was the use of ACTH for operations around the sella turcica; prednisolone and dexamethasone are accepted now as commonly used measures to reduce edema around tumors; the role of these materials after trauma is as yet unsettled. Miscellaneous articles in the current YEAR BOOK include minutiae of operations on brachial plexus and peripheral nerve, rhizotomy for spasticity, and direct electrical recording from cranial nerves at operation.

The 1984 YEAR BOOK contained 241 pages of a larger format than ever before in this series; the 1985 YEAR BOOK contains 281 pages. I am indebted to the management of Year Book Medical Publishers for permitting the gradual expansion of the volume to try to keep pace with the enormous increase in articles of interest to neurosurgeons. I particularly wish to thank Mrs. Caroline Scoulas, the managing editor, and her colleagues and predecessors for numerous courtesies and excellent cooperation.

And to Dr. Robert Crowell, my successor, go my hopes that he will bear the burden of the editorial chair with the expertise, patience, and goodwill that he has shown in the past.

Hail and farewell.

OSCAR SUGAR, M.D.

# Brief Interesting Notes

▶ Abstracts from the 34th annual meeting of the German Neurosurgical Society held in Mannheim in 1983 are to be found in *Acta Neurochirurgica (Wien)* (68:123–168, 1983). Chief subdivisions for the symposia include metastatic tumors of the central nervous system and neurosurgery of geriatric patients. The latter was subdivided into topics dealing with tumors, intraorbital masses, disk operations, aneurysms, spontaneous hemorrhages, and hematomas (chronic subdural). In the section of "free topics" may be found articles on such topics as computer-assisted myelography for cervical root compression syndromes, extracranial and intracranial bypasses, cervical spondylosis, intradiskal injection of nucleolysin (collagenase), spasmodic torticollis, evoked potentials, cerebral metabolism.

▶ I know no way of summarizing adequately the article by Matsushima et al. on microsurgical anatomy of the veins of the posterior fossa (*J. Neurosurg.* 59:63–105, 1983). The numerous illustrations are essential for the understanding of the complex anatomy described in the text. The anatomical information regarding veins includes their relationships with the nerves, particularly those at the foramina of the base of the skull, which are themselves poorly visualized through the small openings permitted by standard microsurgical techniques. I can only reiterate what has been said before about the other articles in this series: Study them!

▶ Rapid correction of hyponatremia can be dangerous and is considered by R. Laureno (*Ann. Neurol.* 13:232–242, 1983) to be the major cause of central pontine myelinolysis. He has produced the syndrome and pathological findings in animals by making them hyponatremic with vasopressin and water infusions and then giving 3% sodium chloride intravenously. The evidence appears very precise. However, hyponatremia is also a dangerous disorder, which is not always properly reversed by water restriction alone. Perhaps there is a compromise that might be of value, i.e., to give intravenous 1.5% saline solution and to give the entire dose in a period of several hours. Certainly one should avoid the pernicious practice of giving patients with head injury or other neurological-neurosurgical disorders 5% dextrose in water or ½ normal saline solution as a maintenance intravenous infusion unless there is evidence of salt-retaining disorder.

▶ Unilateral papilledema may occur in benign intracranial hypertension, according to Sher et al. (*JAMA* 250: 2346–2347, 1983). In one instance, declining vision was reversed by optic nerve "sheathotomy" through a left medial orbitotomy incision.

▶ Pulsatile tinnitus may be due to an enlargement of the jugular vein at the jugular bulb. Buckwalter et al. (*Laryngoscope* 93:1534–1539, 1983) describe this rare syndrome, which is best diagnosed by retrograde jugular venography and is responsive to ligation of the internal jugular vein. It is a disorder of the right side.

▶ Perfluorooctyl bromide (PFOB) has been used to study radiographic diagnosis of tumors in animals. Patronas et al. (*J. Neurosurg.* 650–653, 1983) report excellent visualization of experimental brain tumors in rats after intravenous injection of this material (an 8-carbon-chain material in which all hydrogens attached to carbon are replaced by fluorine (except for 1 bromine substitution).

Larger animals and computed tomographic scanning (permitting the use of smaller amounts of material) may precede similar work in humans.

▶ Positron emission tomography (PET) provides a quantitative measure of local tissue radioactivity and hence an in vivo autoradiogram. Herscovitch et al. (*J. Nucl. Med.* 24:782–789, 1983) have analyzed the computer simulation of regional blood flow by using a blood radiotracer and have concluded that it would have value for measurement of regional flow with PET in man. In a subsequent article (*J. Nucl. Med.* 24:790–798, 1983) Raichle et al. describe flow measurements using intravenously administered water $^{15}O$ and positron emission techniques in anesthetized adult baboons. They compared the results with blood flow measurements made with a standard tracer technique using residual detection of similarly labeled water injected into the internal carotid artery. Over a blood flow range of 10–63 ml/min/100 gm, the two techniques were remarkably similar. For flows exceeding 65 ml/min/100 gm, cerebral blood flow was progressively underestimated owing to the known limitation of brain permeability to water. Theoretical extrapolations based on the differences between baboon and human brains in permeability to water indicate that the PET flow estimates will appreciably underestimate so-called true blood flows from direct arterial injection only when the flow exceeds about 55 ml/min/100 gm. Problems with sampling of arterial blood in humans are estimated to be less than 1 in 1,000. One single normal human adult was studied with this technique without complication and with results showing various regional flows of from about 30 to about 60 ml/min/100 gm (while the flow in the superior sinus was as high as 65 ml/min/100 gm).

▶ Imaging signals from nuclear magnetic resonance scans can be used to measure quantitatively blood flow in the internal jugular vein, according to Singer and Crooks (*Science* 221:654–656, Aug. 12, 1983). The "slice" of head is determined by the scanner (e.g., 7 mm), and the size (area) of the vessel studied can be measured, to produce a volume of blood seen in the scan. The selected volume is magnetically depolarized with a radiofrequency pulse. After a specified time, a second radiofrequency pulse is provided which tips all the fresh blood protons entering the selected plane during the time specified by 90 degrees. The tipped protons are then imaged by a spin-echo technique to provide picture elements (pixels) providing a voltage directly proportional to the volume of blood that flows into the volume scrutinized. By selecting different times of entry of blood, various pixel voltages can be read out through a computer program integrating the signals in the vessel area related to time and producing a rate of blood flow (milliliters per second) determined by the measured time to refill the vessel after the nuclear magnetic resonance pulse. Calculations for blood flow in the internal jugular veins of one of the authors (Crooks) at the level of a transverse section through nose and ear gave flow rates of 0.344 and 0.501 ml/sec for left and right veins respectively. The authors believe it is possible to visualize any vessel and to measure its blood flow quantitatively and thereby monitor effectiveness of treatments involving the vascular system.

▶ In 11 patients studied with computed tomography by Ahmadi et al. (*Am. J. Neuroradiol.* 4:131–136, 1983), direct internal carotid-cavernous fistulas were present. In three others, exclusive dural cavernous sinus malformations were found. Specific details of filling of superior ophthalmic veins (or of occlusion indicating thrombosis!) could be described, as well as enlargement of extraocular muscles, swelling of eyelids, edema of the conjunctiva, etc. It is true that in most instances, clinical manifestations alone may lead to the diagnosis of fistula. At times, when only part of the symptom complex is manifested (e.g., proptosis without bruit), diagnosis may be obscure, and a baseline computed tomographic scan may give a clue as to the diagnosis before the definitive diagnostic arteriography is done.

▶ Following the widespread acceptance of digital venous angiography, the same technique has been applied to cerebral arteriography by the digital subtraction technique. Its advantages, according to Kelly et al. (*J. Neurosurg.* 58:851–856, 1983) include reduced procedural time and decreased burden of contrast material, which is safer for the patient. There can be an appreciable savings in film and processing costs, particularly valuable in low-volume thoracic aortograms in patients who need spinal angiography. With virtually immediate feedback, the radiographer can advance a catheter selectively from one vessel to another, administering hand-injected doses of contrast material. The authors suggest the possibility that arterial injection digital subtraction angiography may replace conventional serial angiography as a definitive diagnostic procedure.

▶ Vertex isotope sinogram after injection intravenously of a bolus of 20 mCi of technetium 99m can show very detailed anatomy (and obstruction) when the technical modifications (utilizing computer enhancement) suggested by Kapp et al. (*Surg. Neurol.* 19:450–452, 1983) are followed. Such lesions should be considered routinely in the differential diagnosis of intracranial hypertension of obscure etiology.

▶ What appears to be the first recorded instance of computerized tomography in a patient with fat embolism is described by Sakamoto et al. (*Neuroradiology* 24:283–285, 1983). Computed tomographic scans done within the first few days after the patient, age 18 years, was injured in a motorcycle accident showed no abnormalities. About a week later, multiple low-density areas appeared in the frontal white matter. They disappeared within the following two weeks while subdural effusions appeared in the frontoparietal areas, only to gradually diminish as neurologic recovery progressed.

▶ Apparently the first report of computed tomography of the head after a lightning strike to the head is that of Mann et al. (*AJNR* 4:976–977, 1983). There was subarachnoid hemorrhage as well as bleeding into the left basal ganglia with extension into the left ventricular system with shift of midline to the right. There was a persistent leak from the left ear. At autopsy after death on the 13th day there were two basal skull fractures, subarachnoid hemorrhage, and basal ganglion and intraventricular hemorrhage.

▶ Naloxone may have a role to play in the treatment of head injury according to experimental work in cats carried out by Hayes et al. (*J. Neurosurg.* 58:720–728, 1983). The benefits may be chiefly from counteracting hypotension, but the drug also appears to be useful in antagonizing respiratory depression associated with spinal shock and electroconvulsive shock.

▶ In western Europe and North America, hydatid-cyst disease is rare. The 11 cases reported from Turkey by Pamir et al. (*Surg. Neurol.* 21:53–57, 1984) represent 3.8% of all diagnosed and surgically treated cases of spinal compression in the 10-year period involved. Almost half of the patients were under age 30. On 10 cases, the cysts were epidural; the other had intradural but extramedullary cysts. All those with epidural cysts also had bone involvement. Block of contrast material was found in the thoracic area in seven cases; in the lumbar L 1–3 area in the other four. Systemic infection with *Echinococcus* has recently been successfully treated with mebendazole; it was used in two cases after operation, with no symptoms. Whether it will prove to be valuable overall remains to be seen. The basic treatment remains laminectomy with removal of the cysts, followed by washing with hypertonic saline solution. The benefits of the latter are uncertain.

The widespread use of air travel and the increasing frequency of intercontinental flights, make the dissemination of information in articles like this one by Pamir et al. imperative. Hydatid cysts are one cause of spinal cord compression; they are very rare in the United States and Western countries in general. Whether more advanced scanning techniques will accelerate diagnosis is unclear; certainly if the vertebrae are involved anterior to the cord, as with tuberculosis and cancer, approach by anterior vertebral resection and cord decompression may be a preferred route, but computerized scanning might well show the exact locus of a cyst and hence direct the approach more accurately than when tomography and myelography are used.

▶ A review of 19 cases of "pituitary abscess" reported in the literature since 1970 has been carried out by Bjerre et al. (*Acta Neurochir.* 68:187–193, 1983). The frequent association of negative cultures from these "abscesses" with previous sterile meningitis and endocrine disturbances and concurrent rhinorrhea is probably due to the presence of a normal reaction to infarction of a pituitary adenoma. The authors contend that the pituitary abscess is not a bacterial infection, as is commonly assumed. The purulent material in nine patients was sterile; bacteria were cultured in eight and fungi in two. Pleocytosis in the cerebrospinal fluid is ascribed to irritation from necrotic material spilled into the subarachnoid space. Bacterial growth in "pituitary abscess" is ascribed to perioperative contamination or bacterial invasion into the sella through a defect in the sellar floor.

▶ In a review of 23 patients with thoracic disk protrusions operated on between 1973 and 1982, Maiman et al. (*Neurosurg.* 14:178–182, 1984) emphasize the advantages of the lateral extracavitary approach in providing access without routinely entering the pleural cavity. Anesthesia dolorosa after section of the thoracic (intercostal) nerve root was relieved in one patient when the ganglion was removed. Air myelography or computed tomography was used for diagnosis. Spinal angiography was always done to be able to avoid a radiculomedullary artery. The rib removed in this approach is subsequently used for insertion as grafts in the openings made in the vertebral bodies. Russell Patterson, in discussion, considers this to be a good approach, but he is not persuaded that it has significant advantages for disk removal alone (not considering malignant tumors) over the approach through the pedicle (which does not require a postoperative body case or spine fusion). He emphasizes that for cancer, the grafts used should extend from one intact vertebral body above to one below.

▶ In a group of 268 consecutive adult patients with malignant glioma, Ruff and Posner (*Ann. Neurol.* 13:334–336, 1983) found 36% who developed clinical signs of systemic venous thrombosis (within 96 weeks after surgery; confirmed by radiocontrast venography). The patients all had elastic bandage wrappings of the legs during craniotomy. In a subsequent group of 117 patients with similar tumors, there was added intermittent pneumatic compression to both calves during craniotomy and for 8–12 hours postoperatively using inflatable knee-length boots inflated by air-driven pumps. The incidence of venous thrombosis was very significantly decreased in the second group in the first six postoperative weeks (3.42% vs. 25%); in subsequent postoperative periods there was no difference in incidence of venous thrombosis. Anticoagulant therapy with heparin-warfarin sequence was well tolerated by the patients who did develop thrombosis, with reduction in fatal pulmonary embolism without increasing the risk of intracranial hemorrhage. The authors believe that patients with malignant tumors should be considered for prophylactic antithrombotic therapy prior to craniotomy. It seems to me that the incidence of venous thrombosis is unusually high (an earlier study of 334 patients is reported to have shown an incidence of phlebitis of 27.5%).

▶ An unusual case of multicentric glioma is reported by Nonaka et al. (*Neurol. Med. Chir.* [*Tokyo*] 23:751–754, 1983). After neuroradiological investigation indicated two tumors (one on the medial side of the right frontal lobe and one in the opercular region of the left frontal lobe in this woman, age 54), operation was done by two separate craniotomies. The right medial frontal tumor was a glioblastoma, and the left one, an oligodendroglioma. Computed tomographic scan and operative findings indicated complete independence of these two masses, and angiography had shown how different the vascularizations were.

▶ A hypothalamic hamartoma consisting of normal glial tissue produced a mass in the suprasellar area in a boy, age 10 months, who had precocious puberty. The endocrine changes were reversed after partial intracapsular resection at 18 months. Based on this case and literature review, Alvarez et al. (*J. Neurosurg.* 58:583–585, 1983) advise early surgical treatment in cases of precocious puberty.

▶ The mechanism of formation of edema around brain tumors is still unclear; the frequency and amount of edema around meningiomas is much debated. When the edema is judged on the basis of changes in computed tomographic scans, according to Gilbert et al. (*Neurosurg.* 12:599–605, 1983), there is no relationship between occurrence or degree of edema and location, type, vascularity, mitoses, necroses, calcification or cortical invasion by meningioma. The larger the meningioma, however, the more the edema, and the edema is a potent factor in occurrence of clinical signs and symptoms. The possibility is again raised that a humoral agent from the tumor induces vasogenic edema in the adjacent brain.

▶ Two new cases of meningioma of Meckel's cave have been reported by Butti et al. (*Surg. Neurol.* 20:305–309, 1983). Total removal was possible in each case, and no other treatment was needed for relief of pain in the face, which was the initial complaint in each patient. The subtemporal intradural approach was used in each. Perhaps those critics who object to the inclusion of the technique of subtemporal trigeminal rhizotomy in neurosurgical treatises should temper their criticism.

▶ According to Imai et al., there have been reported five cases of intracranial meningioma presenting as a neck mass along nerves or lymph nodes. They report the first case in which the neck mass was a distended internal jugular vein filled with meningioma. It proved to have intracranial origin in the right posterior parasagittal and parieto-occipital areas, with involvement of the superior sagittal and right lateral sinuses, sigmoid sinus, and jugular bulb, and it extended down into the cervical jugular vein. Histologically, the tumor was of the transitional type without obvious evidence of malignancy. Computed tomographic scans, angiograms, and retrograde cervical venograms were useful in delimiting the extent of the tumor, which was removed in two operations staged six months apart. The ultimate outcome in this woman, age 37, is not apparent in the text (*Neurol. Med. Chir.* [*Tokyo*] 23:233–238, 1983).

▶ Reports from Israel call attention to the occurrence of intracranial meningiomas in individuals who were exposed to low-dose ionizing radiation during childhood for treatment of tinea capitis. Comparison of such meningiomas with those occurring in nonirradiated patients has been made by Soffer et al. (*J. Neurosurg.* 59:1048–1053, 1983). Those receiving childhood radiation are much more apt to have meningiomas at the calvarium than at the skull base, and to have high recurrence rates, as well as multiple tumors. Irradiated persons are also more likely to have head and neck tumors, psychiatric disorders, permanent electroencephalographic disorders, and visual evoked response abnormalities.

▶ The transseptal transsphenoidal approach that is used for pituitary tumors is also useful in attacking tumors of the clivus, according to Laws (*Otolaryngol. Head Neck Surg.* 92:100–101, 1984). He summarizes the experience with 13 patients at the Mayo Clinic with this form of surgery over a period from 1974 to 1982. This route gives good decompression when the tumor is midline. No form of surgery, he says, is apt to give cure with any approach to the larger, invasive extensive tumors.

▶ In three young women, Turpin et al. (*Sem. Hop. Paris* 59:2369–2372, 1983) found chronic hydrocephalus due to aqueductal stenosis as the only obvious abnormality to explain amenorrhea at ages 17–18 years. Skull films showed enlargement or flattening of the sella turcica and digital impressions. Computed tomograms showed dilatation of lateral and third ventricles. Endocrine assays showed normal prolactin and gonadotrophic hormones, although levels of estrogens were decreased. Ventriculoatrial shunt was followed by appearance of menstrual periods in two patients; the third has not yet been operated on because of the presence of a papilloma of the lateral ventricle which might cause bleeding.

▶ A review by Parkinson and Stephensen of the association of white blood cell count (in the blood) and outcome of subarachnoid hemorrhage in 171 patients (*Surg. Neurol.* 21:132–134, 1984) shows a striking correlation when the peripheral white cell count is over 20,000 on admission, regardless of the clinical grading scheme. At levels below 20,000 there was no correlation between count and grade and outcome (22% death rate). At levels above 20,000 there is a 90% death rate, no class A or B outcomes, and no admission clinical grades of 1 or 2. Why this should be so is not discussed.

▶ An unusual article by Henderson et al. (*J. Neurol. Neurosurg. Psychiatry*

46:437–439, 1983) relates the travels in London and Scotland over the previous year of a young man feigning subarachnoid hemorrhage. Folger et al. (*Neurology* [*NY*] 31:638–639, 1981) entitled their article "Neurologic Munchausen syndrome." And in the *JAMA,* a letter to the editor (250:1976–1977, 1983) points out the vagaries in spelling of the eponym and gives their origin. There *was* a Baron Hieronymous Karl Friedrich, Freiherr von Münchhausen, who apparently told tall tales at times, but when his countryman Rudolph Eric Raspe fled to England and composed fantastic stories, he published them in English, and used the name Baron Munchausen, without the umlaut and without the second "h," i.e., *Münchhausen* became *Munchausen.* The editor of the letters section of the *JAMA* promises henceforth to use the anglicized version in deference to history and the memory of the German baron.

▶ Posttraumatic facial nerve paralysis is not always permanent, and treatments are not agreed upon. Three patients with immediate, complete posttraumatic paralysis are presented by Brodsky et al. (*Laryngoscope* 93:1560–1565, 1983). In each case, electroneurography and electromyography showed complete nerve degeneration and muscle denervation. Despite these results, late surgical decompression was done (2.5, 3, and 14 months after injury). All had good return of facial function within six months of surgery. The authors hence suggest that although it is commonly ageed that early exploration after traumatic facial nerve palsy is worthwhile, late exploration at *any* time—I am not sure they really mean that—is worthwhile. In none of these three cases was the nerve totally disrupted; spicules of bone impinged on the nerve, and dislocated ossicles impinged on the area of the facial canal.

▶ Four instances of suprascapular nerve entrapment are described by Sarno (*Surg. Neurol.* 20:493–497, 1983) in three women. The entrapment neuropathy was similar to a radiculopathy of the fifth cervical nerve with pain in the shoulder, neck, and head and radiation of pain down along the arm. Myelography was done in only one patient and was within normal limits (in spite of atrophy of the hypothenar muscles on one side, which remains unexplained by the author). In the other cases, clinical findings, electromyography, and diagnostic block of the suprascapular nerve were used for confirmation of the diagnosis of entrapment. There are no reports indicating that the paraspinal cervical muscles or the deltoid muscles were studied by electromyography. (I trust they were.) And I do not understand the note in table 1, patient 3, which says, "Right median nerve at wrist is closed, as in [is?] right ulnar nerve at elbow." The author also writes. "It is a rare entity . . . ."

▶ Some experiments by Botney and Fields (*Ann. Neurol.* 13:160–164, 1983) indicate a mechanism for the benefits of using amitriptyline for treatment of chronic pain syndromes. An intraperitoneal dose of morphine in lightly anesthetized rats did not in itself change the latency of the tail flick reflex. When amitryptyline was given intrathecally, the analgesic effect of the morphine was enhanced, and it became effective. Systemic injection of the antidepressant did not have this same potentiating effect. They suggest that the relevant anatomical site of action of the amitryptyline is the spinal terminals of descending monoaminergic neurons which form a link in the intrinsic opioid-mediated analgesia system.

OSCAR SUGAR

# 17 Anatomy and Physiology

**Variations in the Pattern of Muscle Innervation by the L5 and S1 Nerve Roots**
Adam Young, John Getty, Andrew Jackson, Ernest Kirwan, Michael Sullivan, and Christopher Wynn Parry
Spine 8:616–624, September 1983                    17–1

The L5 or S1 nerve roots are involved, either singly or in combination, in 90% of patients with nerve root compression secondary to disk protrusion or degenerative changes in the lumbar spine. Reliable knowledge of the anatomical pattern of innervation of muscles by these roots is an essential prerequisite for clinical and electromyography (EMG) diagnosis.

The authors report surgical findings in 56 females and 44 males, mean age 43.2 years, seen at the Royal National Orthopaedic Hospital, London. The patients were operated on for L5 or S1 root entrapment, and the findings were compared with the diagnosis predicted by EMG. Direct electrical stimulation of these roots was carried out on 50 patients at surgery, and the muscle innervation pattern in the leg was determined. Bony anomalies were studied in 12 patients to determine their nature and the validity of clinical and EMG diagnosis in such cases.

Using the pattern of segmental innervation adapted from Marinacci, preoperative EMG predicted the level of root pathology correctly in 84 patients. There was little difference in reliability according to involvement of the L5 or the S1 root, or both. Of 28 patients with L5 involvement alone, 24 (85.7%) received the correct diagnosis. When only S1 was involved, the diagnosis in 11 of 14 (78.5%) was correct, as it was in 44 (83%) of 53 when both roots were involved. When clinical and contrast radiologic diagnostic methods were compared with EMG in localizing affected nerve roots, there was no significant difference if only one root was involved. However, when both roots were affected EMG was significantly the best method. Of the five patients lacking obvious root pathology at surgery, all had normal EMG results preoperatively. There were no false-positive results, but an incorrect EMG diagnosis was made in 16 patients. However, detection of root pathology at surgery depends on the surgeon's subjective assessment.

The perioperative electrical studies confirmed the essential reliability of the innervation pattern proposed by Marinacci, and also showed that most muscles have a dual innervation, with one nerve root being dominant. However, in eight patients (16%) a marked departure from the normal pattern was found. Of the 12 patients with congenital defects of bony segmentation, 7 (58%) had unusual innervation patterns; preoperative

EMG results were erroneous in 6 of these patients, indicating that diagnostic errors were more common in this group. In four patients with sacralized L5 or 4 mobile lumbar vertebrae, unusually dominant L5 nerve roots with marked overlap of innervation were noted. Whenever anomalous bony segmentation is encountered, the likelihood of variable nerve root innervation should be appreciated. In such cases, both nerve roots in question should be explored at surgery.

▶ Nikolai Bogduk of the University of Queensland, St. Lucia, Australia, has been writing about the anatomy of the lumbar spine for some years now. His most recent essay, on the innervation of the lumbar spine, appears in *Spine* (8:286–293, 1983). The lumbar disks are innervated posteriorly by the sinuvertebral nerves (more formally known as the rami meningei), and branches of the rami communicantes and ventral root rami send twigs to the lateral portions of the disk. The sinuvertebral nerves innervate the posterior longitudinal ligament and the anterior ligament receives branches from the gray rami. Medial branches of the lumbar dorsal rami supply many of the near-the-midline muscles, the interspinous ligament, and the lumbar zygapophyseal joints. Only the ventral (anterior) part of the dural sac is innervated by the sinuvertebral nerves, which thus basically are ventrally distributed. Each zygapophyseal joint receives nerves from (at least) two consecutive segmental nerves. Encapsulated, unencapsulated, and free nerve endings typical of other synovial joints are to be found in the capsules of the lumbar facet joints (zygapophyseal joints). The lateral branches of the first three lumbar dorsal rami are the ones that become cutaneous; presumably this accounts for the frequent depiction of cutaneous zones on the lower back as lacking representation from the fourth and fifth lumbar nerves.

Putting together information from Young et al. and from Bogduk emphasizes the importance of detail. An electromyographer who ignores the paravertebral muscles takes away the possibility of distinction between a root and a plexus lesion; the diagnostician who ignores the sinuvertebral nerves misses the phenomenon of pain in the leg being mimicked by disturbance of the facet joints, which have the same root innervations as the sciatic nerve.—O.S.

---

**Anatomy and Significance of Fixation of the Lumbosacral Nerve Roots in Sciatica**
David L. Spencer, George S. Irwin, and J. A. A. Miller (Univ. of Illinois, Chicago)
Spine 8:672–679, September 1983                                    17–2

---

Although the concept of fixation of the extrathecal intraspinal lumbosacral nerve roots in sciatica seems clinically valid, fixation has not been confirmed anatomically. The authors examined the anatomy of 54 pairs of lumbosacral nerve roots in nine fresh adult cadavers, 21–64 years of age, with no evidence of spinal trauma or other spinal pathology. Dural ligaments were identified fixing the dura and nerve roots at their exit from the main dural sac to the posterior longitudinal ligament and vertebral-body periosteum proximal to the intervertebral disk. The dural attachments were especially well developed at the L5-S1 level. Distal fixation was noted at the intervertebral foramen where the epineural sheath of the spinal nerve was attached. The arrangement was seen to be such that the spinal nerve was strongly connected to the surrounding structures forming the intervertebral foramen.

Mechanical analysis of the anatomical findings suggests that pressure can be applied to the extrathecal nerve root by a disk protrusion without compression of the nerve root against the posterior elements. When a contact force is present on the nerve root, traction forces are exerted on the attachments of the dural ligaments and the pedicular periosteum and connective tissue at the foraminal exit of the spinal nerve. Anatomical variation in fixation may help explain why there is no direct correlation between sciatic symptoms and the apparent size of a disk protrusion and why some protrusions are asymptomatic. The dural ligaments may contribute to sciatica both by tethering of the nerve root over a disk protrusion, leading to a pressure-induced neuropathy, and by the application of traction forces to the posterior longitudinal ligament and vertebral periosteum, producing the somatic component of the sciatic pain syndrome.

▶ The mysteries of the causation of sciatica have been stubbornly resistant to investigation. Spencer and his associates invoke small dural ligaments to fix the nerve roots against protrusions so as to produce pressure-induced neuropathy but also to apply traction forces to the posterior longitudinal ligament and vertebral periosteum and thereby produce somatic pain. Other structures whose distortion appears to induce similar pain in the back and leg include the ligaments around the facet joints, and, according to another article in the same issue of *Spine* confusing pain may also arise from intra- and extradural adhesions.

Incidentally, I protest the use of the phrase "specimens were harvested" (as used in the article by Spencer et al.) to describe the removal of parts of cadaver spines. At least in conventional usage, "to harvest" means to obtain that which has ripened as a crop. I realize that there is an extended usage that condones a meaning of that which is gained or won by effort, for certainly removing parts of cadaver spines requires effort. But why not just use the simple English of "specimens were taken" (or "removed"). De gustibus . . . .

▶ Anomalies of the lumbosacral nerve roots are receiving more and more attention, since they may be responsible for a lack of sciatica in patients with herniated disks, or a lack of documented neurologic deficits. Among the 16 cases presented by Neidre and Macnab (*Spine* 8:294–299, 1983) are three types: conjoined roots, arising in a common dural sheath (type I); two nerve roots that make their exit through one foramen (type II); adjacent nerve roots that are connected by an anastomotic root or branch (type III). The recognition of the type I anomaly is particularly important to avoid root or dural damage in trying to displace a root during diskectomy. Nerve root anomalies should be suspected in all cases of "failed disk surgery."—O.S.

## Microsurgical Anatomy of Spinal Subarachnoid Space

Haring J. W. Nauta, Eugen Dolan, and M. Gazi Yasargil
Surg. Neurol. 19:431–437, May 1983                                    17–3

Much dissection in operations for intradural tumor or vascular malformation of the spinal cord takes place in the subarachnoid space, making an understanding of the anatomy of the spinal arachnoid membranes and associated structures important. The authors performed microdissections of the subarachnoid space in 13 specimens of adult spinal cords with no antemortem evidence of spinal pathology and compared the findings with those made at operation. Ten specimens were removed by an anterior approach and three by a posterior approach.

A distinct longitudinal midline dorsal septum that was variably fenestrated was present in nearly all specimens, typically extending from the midcervical region to the upper lumbar level (Fig 17–1). A series of dorsolateral septa was present on each side, each element being oriented along the oblique course of the dorsal rootlets clustered at each segmental level. These septa extended from the dorsal root entry zone to envelop the dorsal

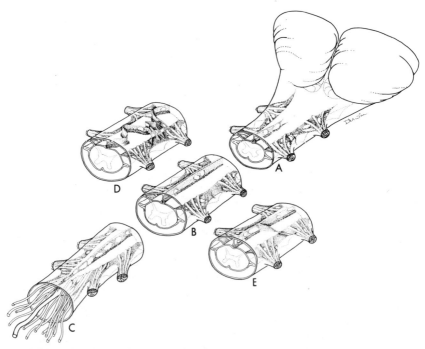

Fig 17–1.—A, B, and C show the midline dorsal septum and the dorsolateral septa, emphasizing their rostrocaudal continuity; two variations are shown. In D, the midline dorsal septum is carried in a tortuous course like that of the midline dorsal vein. As the septum and vein are swept laterally, bridging partitions may interconnect the midline dorsal septum with the dorsolateral septa. In E, a transverse arachnoid septum appears as a variant interconnecting the midline dorsal septum with the dorsal lateral septa of one side, creating a posterior cul-de-sac. (Courtesy of Nauta, H.J.W., et al.: Surg. Neurol. 19:431–437, May 1983; reprinted by permission of the publisher; copyright 1983, Elsevier Science Publishing Co., Inc.)

rootlets and attach to the outer arachnoid membrane dorsolaterally. No arachnoid condensations or septations were seen along the ventral surface of the cord. The pia mater appeared to condense laterally to form the dentate ligament, which was attached to the outer arachnoid and through this to the overlying dura about halfway between the root exits. Variations were seen even between different segmental levels of the same specimen.

Knowledge of the arachnoid septations can promote the smoother opening and subsequent reclosure of the arachnoid and can help guide the dissection of some spinal arteriovenous malformations and benign tumors. If an arachnoid cul-de-sac is present after removal of a tumor, an arachnoid cyst might be avoided by breaking down the arachnoid septations.

---

**Jugular Foramen: Anatomical and Computed Tomographic Study**
David L. Daniels, Ian L. Williams, and Victor M. Haughton (Med. College of Wisconsin, Milwaukee)
AJNR 4:1227–1232, Nov.–Dec. 1983                    17–4

---

The authors determined the computed tomographic (CT) appearances of the jugular foramen in a dry skull and in patients imaged at several planes from −15 degrees to +30 degrees to the canthomeatal line. Four patients with symptoms of a jugular foramen lesion were imaged at a plane +30 degrees to the canthomeatal line, which is perpendicular to the intraforaminal course of cranial nerves IX through XI. Sections 5 mm and 1.5 mm thick were obtained at 5 mm below the internal auditory canal

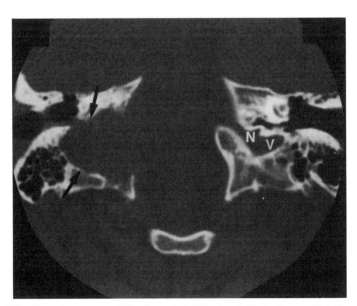

Fig 17–2.—Normal pars nervosa *(N)* and vascularis *(V)* and eroded juglar foramen *(right)* in a patient with large glomus jugulare tumor *(arrows)*; CT section is +30 degrees to the canthomeatal line. (Courtesy of Daniels, D.L., et al.: AJNR 4:1227–1232, November-December 1983.)

to locate the foramen. Iodinated contrast material was injected intravenously.

The pars nervosa and pars vascularis were visualized on CT images made at planes parallel to and positive to the canthomeatal line (Fig 17–2). Cranial nerves IX, X, and XI were demonstrated in contrast-enhanced scans made at +30 degrees to the canthomeatal line. The osseous margins of the jugular foramen were best demonstrated in planes parallel and positive to the canthomeatal line. Structures within the jugular foramen can be identified precisely enough to excude an intracanalicular mass. A gantry angle parallel or positive to the canthomeatal line should be used to evaluate the osseous anatomy of the foramen and to exclude osteolytic changes.

---

**Effect of Cranioplasty on Cerebrospinal Fluid Hydrodynamics in Patients With the Syndrome of the Trephined**

H. Fodstad, J. A. Love, J. Ekstedt, H. Fridén, and B. Liliequist (Univ. of Umeå, Sweden)

Acta Neurochir. (Wien) 70:21–30, 1984                    17–5

The so-called syndrome of the trephined (ST), or postconcussive syndrome, consists of headache, vertigo and tinnitus, fatigue, lack of concentration, memory disorder, and mental depression in postcraniectomy patients. Dyspraxia, limb paresis, and seizures also may occur. The symptoms may be aggravated by changes in body position or performance of the Valsalva maneuver. The authors undertook hydrodynamic cerebrospinal fluid (CSF) studies by the CSF infusion technique before and after cranioplasty in 23 men and 17 women, mean age 47 years, with cranial bone defects. The most common diagnoses leading to operation were trauma and meningioma. Six patients had an intracerebral abscess postoperatively. The mean interval from craniectomy to cranioplasty was 15 months. Repair was by a modified Woringer technique using mesh-reinforced methylmethacrylate.

Fourteen patients had symptoms of ST that were worsened during performance of the Valsalva maneuver or by changes in body position; their symptoms were relieved by repair of the cranial bone defect. Symptoms in 8 other patients with "partial" ST were more or less relieved by cranioplasty and were unaffected by positional changes or by performing the Valsalva maneuver. Twelve patients had neurologic defects related to the primary disorder, whereas 6 had no ST or neurologic deficit. The presence of ST was not dependent on the size of the cranial defect. Resting pressures of the CSF, which were in patients with ST or a deficit, were significantly higher after cranioplasty. Sagittal sinus pressure increased significantly in the patients with ST, as did pulse variations at resting pressure. Conductance and the pressure difference across outflow paths were unaltered by cranioplasty in all patient groups.

True ST occurs chiefly in patients having a flaccid cranial bone defect in the region of the dural sinuses. Removal of part or all of the sagittal sinus may make the adjacent cortical regions susceptible to the effects of extradural pressure on local cerebral blood flow. Postcraniectomy symptoms are relieved by cranioplasty in these patients as the CSF hydrodynamics are normalized.

▶ "Postconcussive syndrome" as a synonym for the syndrome that follows trephination or craniectomy seems inappropriate; concussion is used conventionally to imply that there has been sufficient motion of the brain to "shake it up"; I trust that trephination alone does not do this to the brain.

There are some instances in which the bony defect is large (as after removal of a large flap after infection) and hemiplegia results after removal of the bone. Reconstitution of the rigid contours may be followed by disappearance of the weakness.—O.S.

---

**Pulmonary Extravascular Fluid Accumulation Following Intracranial Injury**
Robert C. Mackersie, Janet M. Christensen, Lawrence H. Pitts, and Frank R. Lewis (Univ. of California, San Francisco)
J. Trauma 23:968–975, November 1983                        17–6

---

An association between pulmonary edema and acute intracranial injury has been documented both experimentally and clinically. The authors made serial measurements of extravascular lung water (EVLW) by the double-indicator thermal green dye technique in patients with severe intracranial injury who were comatose, had no other major septum disorder, and required mechanical ventilation and hemodynamic monitoring. All 18 patients studied had Glasgow Coma Scale scores below 8. Thirteen patients had sustained head trauma, and five had spontaneous intracranial bleeding. Fifteen patients were initially studied within 24 hours of the presumed time of injury. The mean duration of study was 3½ days.

Half the patients had elevations of EVLW more than 2 SD above the control mean at some time and were considered to have pulmonary edema. Values remained elevated in these cases for the duration of the study. No significant differences in intracranial pressure, pulmonary microvascular pressure, or pulmonary vascular resistance were noted. The mean EVLW peaked 48 hours after injury in the patients with pulmonary edema, and mean intracranial pressure peaked at the same time. A small but significant correlation was found between these parameters for both groups of patients. With one exception, postmortem gravimetric data correlated with the clinically measured EVLW. Three of four patients in the edema group had gross and microscopic evidence of pulmonary edema at autopsy, but none of three in the other group had microscopic evidence of pulmonary edema at autopsy.

Neurogenic pulmonary edema occurred in half of these patients with severe head trauma or spontaneous subarachnoid bleeding. Its clinical course is prolonged. Increased pulmonary microvascular permeability appears to be important in the pathogenesis of this disorder. Intracranial pressure may have a small effect on edema formation, but probably is not its major determinant. Blood gas exchange abnormalities can occur after intracranial injury in the absence of increased EVLW. The mechanism of production of the pulmonary edema remains unclear.

▶ There remains a considerable gap in our knowledge of the way in which disturbances within the head cause such changes in the lungs and in the conduction system of the heart, which produce electrocardiographic changes capable of simulating coronary artery disease and myocardial infarction such as may occur after subarachnoid hemorrhage.—O.S.

# 18 Diagnosis

▶ ↓ One can anticipate continuing concern on the part of the regulators of medical care as to the propriety of performing roentgenograms of the skull in the emergency care of patients with head injury. Advertisements appear (e.g., *Surg. Neurol.* 20:352) asking for information about significant problems arising in patients with apparently minor head injuries, as part of the examination by the Bureau of Radiological Health of the Food and Drug Administration of the cost-effectiveness of x-ray examinations of the skull in the management of head injuries.

A retrospective review of records of 207 patients with known traumatic intracranial masses has been carried out by Cooper and Ho (Neurosurgery 13:136–140, 1983). Skull fractures were found in 37% of these patients. Only one patient had been completely intact neurologically, had a skull fracture, was sent out, and later returned because of neurologic deterioration (from epidural hematoma, which was successfully removed). In commenting, J. T. Hoff (who is on the Skull Panel of the FDA investigation mentioned above) points to the difference in radiologists' and neurosurgeons' approaches to the problem and promises that the outcome of the Skull Panel study will be ready in six months.

It is of some interest that the authors (and the comment makers, including H. A. Freed) do not refer to the salient factor that really has an impact on clinical practice: malpractice.

Skull roentgenograms were an unimportant factor in the management of patients with head injury and did not eliminate the need for complete and serial neurologic evaluation, according to North and Pollack (*South. Med. J.* 76: 468–470, 1983). Films of 106 consecutive patients admitted to the emergency department of a Kansas City hospital were analyzed with regard to the need for hospital admission, length of stay, and choice of therapy. Traffic accidents accounted for injuries in 42 patients, household accidents in 39, assault in 9, and sports in 5. Only 2 had multiple abnormal neurologic findings in addition to abnormal skull films; 2 others had abnormal films and only a single abnormal neurologic finding, and in the fifth patient with fracture, no neurologic abnormality was detected. Thirty patients were discharged from the emergency department without eventful clinical courses. Of 76 hospitalized patients, prolonged hospitalizations were related to extracranial problems. One patient was observed for 24 hours, was diagnosed to have a concussion, and was readmitted 32 days later because of deficits which led to removal of a subdural hematoma. His films did not show any skull abnormalities. The authors are of the opinion that a skull series should be done only when medically indicated; they claim medical literature overwhelmingly shows that withholding radiologic investigation did not incite litigation (but they do not give a specific reference for this statement). They also state that a radiologically proved skull fracture was not considered sufficient reason for hospitalization in the absence of positive neurologic findings. I find this a foolhardy opinion in view of the rapidity of formation of epidural hematomas, especially in children, from bleeding of a meningeal vessel torn by a temporal fracture.

A hospital management trainee, P. Elsen (*Acta Neurochir.* 68:315–318, 1983) has analysed costs of diagnosis of brain tumor before and after installation of a computed axial tomography apparatus at l'Institut Jules Bordet in Brussels. There was a decrease in the cost amounting to 25% after the computed tomography (CT) scanner was installed as compared with the years 1974–1975. Days of hospitalization (1980–1981) were fewer, and there was less frequent utilization of expensive procedures such as air studies, isotope studies, and angiography; furthermore, the risk to the patient from CT as compared with the other techniques is less.

Unfortunately, the mood of the legislatures of the United States is such that I anticipate a great problem with getting nuclear magnetic resonance scanners, and the older problems with computed tomography scanners (v.s.) are already being repeated. Speakers on the subject of escalating medical costs are asking, not whether new devices are worthwhile, but whether we can afford them. Malpractice *is* a potent reason to ask for more diagnostic aids; unfortunately, there is a certain inertia about bundling up a sick patient to send him or her to another center for a more sophisticated test, and doctors are being sued for not doing this. For a given hospital, not having a nuclear resonance scanner means a fall in the number of patients, less income, and more economic problems. There are now several reports indicating that it is not enough to have a scanner; the hospital should also have an in-house surgical (and neurosurgical) team always available to handle emergencies. Otherwise, these reports suggest, ambulances should not take patients to the nearest hospital with a CT scanner but to the nearest one that also has a ready-and-waiting surgical team.—O.S.

---

**Interpretation of Nuclear Magnetic Resonance Tomograms of the Brain**
Gwan Go, Piet van Dijk, André L. Luiten, Addie A. Brouwer-van Herwijnen, Ijsbrand C. L. van der Leeuw, Richard L. Kamman, Louk M. Vencken, Jan Wilmink, and Herman J. C. Berendsen
J. Neurosurg. 59:574–584, October 1983                    18–1

---

The authors performed nuclear magnetic resonance (NMR) tomography in cats in which brain edema was induced by creating freezing lesions in the cerebral cortex (Fig 18–1). Nuclear magnetic resonance tomograms also were made in patients with such disorders as epidermoid and arachnoid cyst, glioblastoma, chordoma, and arteriovenous malformation. Longer $T_1$ values seemed to correlate well with tissue with higher water content. Fatty tissue appeared quite dark on $T_1$ maps, and it appeared very white on inversion recovery images. Bone of the cranial vault showed up as a dark circle with areas of a lighter inner layer representing the marrow. Saturation recovery images exhibit poor contrast between gray matter and white matter. A low signal characterizes structures containing cerebrospinal fluid on these images. Artifacts can result from disturbances of the magnetic field by ferromagnetic dental implants or foreign bodies.

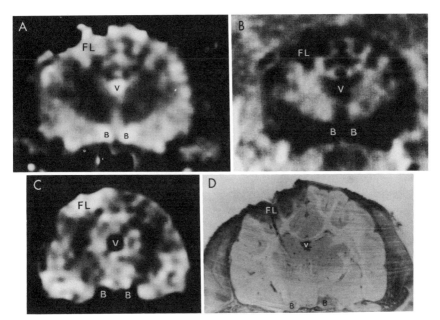

Fig 18–1.—Parts **A**, **B**, and **C** show frontal nuclear magnetic resonance tomograms of a freezing lesion *(FL)* in a cat: **a**, $T_1$ map indicating $T_1$ differences, such as the long $T_1$ of the freezing lesion and of the cerebrospinal fluid in third ventricle *(v)* and basal cisterns *(B)*; **B**, inversion recovery image; **C**, saturation recovery image. Part **D** shows section through brain corresponding to the tomogram, showing the Evan's blue–stained freezing lesion. (Courtesy of Go, G.K., et al.: J. Neurosurg. 59:574–584, October 1983.)

The appearances of NMR tomograms are determined by parameters of imaging, comprising the sequence of radiofrequency pulses. The sequence determines which of the relaxation properties are predominantly expressed in the image and the NMR characteristics of the tissues imaged, including proton density and relaxation times. Fluid flows also seem to influence the images. Inversion recovery images with enhanced $T_1$ influence provide a good differentiation between gray matter and white matter, and saturation recovery images may distinguish between structures such as cysts that exhibit protracted $T_1$ relaxation times.

▶ When an atlas of NMR pictures is available, I think it will be easier to understand the value of the various imaging sequences that are available. Huk et al. (*J. Comput. Assist. Tomog.* 7:468–475, 1983) describe a Siemens system producing slice thicknesses of 11 mm and pixel size of 2.2 × 2.2 mm. In the SE 1 mode (spin echo; saturation recovery), pathologic tissues (which have a long $T_1$ or $T_2$ relaxation time) are displayed as darker-than-normal brain areas. Pictures show the effect more clearly with low-grade astrocytoma than with meningioma. Because of the short relaxation time of protons in lipids, a lipoma is displayed as an intensely white area. In this SE mode, differentiation between white matter and gray matter is poor, because the components of the signals due to the longitudinal relaxation time $T_1$ and the transverse relaxation time $T_2$ cancel one another. With the SE 3 mode (long repetition time), spins recover more completely, and gray and white matter are clearly differentiated, with the white matter appearing darker than the gray. Cerebral edema, astrocytoma, meningioma, lipoma, and metastases are easily demarcated as white densities, and so are changes of multiple sclerosis and Wilson's disease. Differentiation of tumor from edema is not so easily seen with this mode—although the two are easily distinguished with the SE 4 mode—and ventricles and other standard anatomical areas are harder to see.

In the inversion recovery mode, strong dependence on $T_1$ gives a striking difference between white and gray matter. Tumors now may be dark to black, and surrounding edema may have decreased signal intensity. Tumors not readily seen in SE 1 mode may be easily distinguished in the inversion recovery mode. Demyelinated areas are dark in this mode. Cerebrospinal fluid cavities are dark; lipomas and resolving hematomas appear as bright, well-defined regions. The authors believe a consensus is gradually being reached on the advantages and disadvantages of the various techniques for study of differing pathologic conditions.

A special article by Karstaedt et al. (*Surg. Neurol.* 19:206–214, 1983) from the Department of Radiology at Bowman Gray deals with the physics of NMR in a way that helps in understanding this new diagnostic apparatus. The clinical applications are also briefly illustrated. This background information makes for more understanding by neurosurgeons and gives a basis for informed exchange of ideas with radiologists. As is always the case, communication between these two groups of specialists enhances the ability of the radiologist to help solve the problems of the neurosurgeon.—O.S.

---

**Nuclear Magnetic Resonance Imaging of Posterior Fossa: 50 Cases**
G. M. Bydder, R. E. Steiner, D. J. Thomas, J. Marshall, D. J. Gilderdale, and I. R. Young
Clin. Radiol. 34:173–188, March 1983                                        18–2

Nuclear magnetic resonance (NMR) scan findings were reviewed in 50 patients with a clinical diagnosis of posterior fossa disease who also underwent x-ray computed tomographic (CT) examination. Two normal persons also were studied. The most common clinical diagnoses were brain stem infarction, multiple sclerosis, brain stem tumors, and vascular occlusion or obstruction. A variety of NMR pulse sequences reflecting proton density, $T_1$, $T_2$, and blood flow were used. Imaging was performed in the transverse coronal and sagittal planes. Computed tomography was carried out with contrast enhancement by intravenously administered sodium and meglumine iothalamate as clinically indicated. Repeated free induction decay (RFID) sequences were used to demonstrate blood flow effects, but showed little gray-white matter contrast. The inversion-recovery scans showed high levels of gray-white matter contrast and were used for the basic anatomical detail. Spin echo images highlighted pathologic change against the comparatively featureless appearance of the surrounding brain.

Frequently, NMR provided diagnostic information not available from the CT scans. Lesions not seen on CT were recognized in patients with infarction and multiple sclerosis. In other cases, there was more precise definition of mass effects, edema, and anatomical relationships. Extrinsic and intrinsic tumors were readily distinguished, as were brain stem and cerebellar tumors. Malignant tumors generally were associated with more edema than were benign tumors. Arnold-Chiari malformations were demonstrated on sagittal scans. In patients with known vessel occlusion or obstruction, a corresponding reduction in blood flow was recognized in RFID scans. In an irradiated patient, more extensive changes were seen in the surrounding brain on NMR imaging than on CT scanning. However, CT was more useful than NMR imaging in demonstrating calcification and bony erosion. In some instances, CT showed the margin between a tumor and surrounding edema or brain tissue better than NMR did.

Imaging with NMR is a versatile, noninvasive means of demonstrating a wide range of disorders within the posterior fossa. The multiple sequences available and the sensitivity of NMR imaging to pathologic change are important advantages, as is the lack of known hazard. The chief limitation at present is the slow speed of the study, but multislice options may shorten imaging times in the near future.

▶ Nuclear magnetic resonance was able to detect 11 of 12 lesions in the series presented by McGinnis et al. (*J. Comput. Assist. Tomogr.* 7:575–584, 1983). Ten patients were known from CT studies to have lesions of the posterior fossa; two had histories and examinations compatible with such a diagnosis, but the CT scans were normal. Inversion recovery, saturation recovery, and spin echo pulse sequences were used, and compared with corresponding CT sections. The absence of bone artifacts makes NMR advantageous over CT for study of the posterior fossa. Inversion recovery images were able to depict all six intrinsic mass lesions, but only three of six extrinsic masses. Spin echo images demonstrated four of five extrinsic lesions, including two missed by inversion recovery. Saturation recovery images demonstrated lesions in only two of six patients. Nuclear magnetic resonance has an advantage over CT in being completely noninvasive. With the current NMR techniques, no clear differentiation between tumor and peritumoral edema was possible.

In three patients, diagnosis of adult Arnold-Chiari malformation was made as indicated by clinical symptomatology angiograms and CT scans. Ventricular shunts and decompressions were used for treatment. Lack of sustained improvement led to reexaminations, which disclosed intrinsic brain stem tumors. All three died within two years of onset of symptoms. Phillips et al. (*Neurosurgery* 13:345–350, 1983) point out the difficulty in differentiating between adult onset of symptoms in Arnold-Chiari malformation and those of posterior fossa and brain stem neoplasms. The possibility of concurrent disorders was not discussed. I would take issue (on the basis of the published photographs) with the authors' assertion that there is a lack of direct evidence of expanding cerebellar or brain stem mass in the posterior fossae of cases 1 and 3; both lateral angiograms appear to show the basilar artery pressed up against the clivus which, taken together with the herniated vessels on the tonsils, would have warranted suspicion of a posterior fossa mass. However, it has been true in a number of patients and in a number of radiographic studies that tumors are present but cannot be demonstrated until they reach some finite size. I concur with discussor Levy: wait for NMR to be used for difficult cases!—O.S.

---

## Nuclear Magnetic Resonance Imaging of the Spine
Michael T. Modic, Meredith A. Weinstein, William Pavlicek, Daniel L. Starnes, Paul M. Duchesneau, Francis Boumphrey, and Russel J. Hardy, Jr. (The Cleveland Clinic)
Radiology 148:757–762, September 1983                     18–3

---

The authors compared standard diagnostic examinations including high-resolution computed tomography (CT), myelography, and plain radiography. Potential spinal axis disease was evaluated in 40 patients, aged 14–72, by nuclear magnetic resonance (NMR) using a 0.35-Tesla superconducting magnet in 30 and a 0.15-Tesla resistive magnet in 10. Saturation recovery pulse sequence techniques were used in all patients. Those with possible trauma, tumor, developmental abnormality, or disk disease also had at least one inversion recovery image taken through the sagittal plane of the spinal cord. Spin echo images of two patients with tumors were also obtained. Abnormalities were grouped into extradural, intradural, extramedullary, and intramedullary lesions.

When evaluated by standard techniques and by NMR, 15 patients were considered normal. In the cervical region, the fourth ventricle, cervical medullary junction, and cerebellar tonsils and their relationship to the foramen magnum were delineated. The level of the foramen magnum was demarcated by a high signal intensity representing fat, both within the marrow in the clivus and occipital bone and in the soft tissue just superior to the dens. Extradural lesions were observed in 17 patients; 11 had degenerative bony changes or a herniated disk diagnosed by myelography, CT, or both. On saturation recovery images, incursions or displacement of the cervical cord agreed with findings on the contrast myelogram. However, extradural defects seen with the latter were more pronounced. The invading elements (herniated disk, hypertrophied soft tissue, or bone) could not be visualized with NMR except in one patient with a hypertrophic spur. In two patients with metastatic extradural blocks of the subarachnoid space, NMR was as diagnostic as contrast myelography. In two traumatic dissections of the spinal cord, the fractured vertebral bodies, neural arch, and their encroachment on the neural canal and cord were accurately seen with NMR. Intradural-extramedullary lesions were found in four patients, including one metastatic malignancy, two Arnold-Chiari malformations, and a lipomeningocele with a tethered cord in the lumbar region. The lipoma had a very high intensity signal, and the extent of the neural arch defect and the continuity of the lipoma with subcutaneous fat were outlined. Tethering of the cord at L3 was better demonstrated by NMR than by conventional studies (Fig 18–2).

Overall, NMR provided accurate anatomical delineation and superior tissue characterization compared with results on CT or plain radiography. Further, NMR was excellent in evaluation of the foramen magnum region

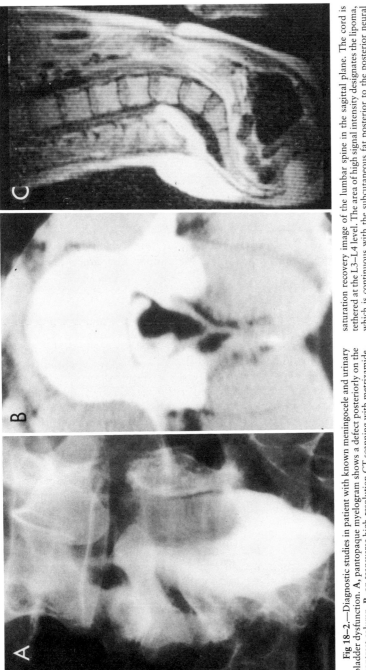

**Fig 18–2.**—Diagnostic studies in patient with known meningocele and urinary bladder dysfunction. **A,** pantopaque myelogram shows a defect posteriorly on the contrast column. **B,** on transverse high-resolution CT scanning with metrizamide, an area of decreased attenuation is seen to impinge on the subarachnoid space posteriorly; also, a defect is noted in the neural arch. **C,** lateral two-dimensional saturation recovery image of the lumbar spine in the sagittal plane. The cord is tethered at the L3–L4 level. The area of high signal intensity designates the lipoma, which is continuous with the subcutaneous fat posterior to the posterior neural arch defect. (Courtesy of Modic, M.T., et al.: Radiology 148:757–762, September 1983.)

and is the preferred means of diagnosing syringomyelia (two patients in this series) and Arnold-Chiari malformation. Although NMR was accurate in diagnosing spinal cord trauma and spinal canal block, disk abnormalities were not visualized. Also, cortical bone provides no NMR signal but is well visualized on CT and plain radiographs. In evaluation of the neural foramina, nerve roots, and intervertebral disk spaces—all requiring thin sections and high spatial resolution—CT remains more accurate than NMR.

▶ For the moment, CT remains the imaging method of choice for evaluating suspected lumbar disk rupture, according to a study of 14 patients by Chafetz et al. (*Am. J. Roentgenol.* 141:1153–1156, 1983). Of 16 ruptured disks seen by CT, 12 could also be recognized on NMR, but with less ease. It is likely that with increasing sophistication of equipment and of its use, disk hernias will be more readily diagnosed by NMR in the future.—O.S.

---

**Complications in Cerebral Angiography: A Comparison Between the Non-Ionic Contrast Medium Iohexol and Meglumine Metrizoate (Isopaque Cerebral)**
I. O. Skalpe and Inge Marie Anke (Tromsoe Univ. Hosp., Norway)
Neuroradiology 25:157–160, June 1983                                    18–4

Serious complications still occur occasionally after cerebral angiography. The authors compared the occurrence of complications with the new non-ionic contrast medium iohexol and the ionic medium meglumine metrizoate in a double-blind trial of 100 patients referred for cerebral angiography. The femoral route was used in 99 cases. The iodine content of metrizoate was 280 mg/ml and that of iohexol was 300 mg/ml. Injected volumes were 50 ml in the aorta, 10 ml in the common carotid artery, 8 ml in the internal carotid artery, and 7 ml in the vertebral artery. The types of angiographic findings were about the same in the two groups of patients.

Iohexol clearly was better tolerated than metrizoate with respect to both pain and unpleasantness during injections. Two patients had transitory paresis after iohexol injection. One of them had marked stenosis of the right internal carotid artery, but the other had normal angiographic findings. Another patient with attacks of ataxia and dysarthria had an attack that lasted several days shortly after angiography with iohexol.

There was no significant difference in the occurrence of serious side effects with iohexol and meglumine metrizoate. The complications occurring in the iohexol group in this study seemed more likely to be due to thromboembolism than to contrast medium toxicity. Nonionic contrast mediums may be less toxic to the diseased brain than ionic agents. Much less discomfort is experienced by patients given nonionic agents via external carotid injections. In addition, this new nonionic compound is stable in solution, whereas nonionic, more expensive metrizamide must be put into solution just before use.

▶ General anesthesia should be avoided during procedures involving the use of contrast agents for vascular visualization, according to Junck and Marshall (*Ann. Neurol.* 13:469–484, 1983). The level of consciousness is too valuable an indicator to permit its being obscured by anesthesia. Any sign or symptom of neurologic dysfunction dictates that the catheter be withdrawn into the aorta—and usually the procedure should be terminated. Good systemic support is the essential aspect of treatment of neurologic complications. Premedication with prednisone (50 mg every six hours for three doses) and diphenhydramine (50 mg intramuscularly, one hour before the procedure) is advocated when contrast use is essential even though there is a history of an idiosyncratic reaction. In addition to a discussion of the chemistry, osmolar effects, and other aspects of intravenous contrast materials, the authors also present comparisons of iophendylate and metrizamide as intrathecal agents, but do not include the newer nonionized triiodobenzoic acid derivatives.

In spite of the effectiveness of intravenously administered diazepam in control of status epilepticus, most neurologists do not consider this medication given by mouth to be of much value in the routine treatment of epilepsy. However, given intravenously, it appears to be helpful in preventing seizures following administration of meglumine diatrizoate for contrast enhancement in computerized tomography studies of the brain. Diazepam (5 mg) was given slowly intravenously followed immediately by the contrast material. In the series of 284 patients with known or suspected brain metastases that was studied by Paganu et al. (*AJR* 140:787–792, 1983), 188 were found to have metastases. Seizures after contrast material injection occurred in 3 of 96 patients given prophylactic diazepam and in 14 of 92 patients with metastases but no prophylactic diazepam.

Although there is a section of the paper headed "Presence, Site, Activity, and Number of Brain Metastases," I could not find any discussion of the possibility that patients with metastases in the central region were (or were not) more apt to have seizures or that the randomization was in sufficient numbers to eliminate locus of metastasis as a factor in the results. From the standpoint of genesis of focal seizures, "clearly, it is a preexisting seizure focus in patients with brain metastases that allows the intravenous administration of contrast media to induce a seizure. Furthermore, this focus is peculiar to the metastatic lesion as patients with either other focal brain lesions, such as infarctions, or epileptic foci, such as in idiopathic epilepsy, have a much lower risk of intravenous contrast media–associated seizures."

I should like to protest the use of the word *seize* as an intransitive verb as in this article; viz., "Despite persistent accumulation of contrast media [sic], the patient did not seize." There is little reason, I believe, to abandon the verb *convulse*—which has no essential meaning other than to shake violently—for seize, which means to clutch, take hold of, in a transitive manner, as in "to seize an idea." But then I also do not appreciate the use of nouns as verbs in scientific literature (e.g., "we lesioned the cat's brain" for "we made a lesion in the cat's brain").—O.S.

### Digital Subtraction Angiography With Intravenous Injection: Assessment of 1,000 Carotid Bifurcations

Gary W. Wood, Robert R. Lukin, Thomas A. Tomsick, and A. Alan Chambers (Univ. of Cincinnati)

AJR 140:855–859, May 1983                                18–5

The authors examined the usefulness of digital subtraction angiography (DSA) for evaluating the carotid bifurcation for vascular occlusive disease. The first 500 patients referred for carotid DSA in a 19-month period were included in the study. Sixty-two patients also had standard carotid arteriography near the time of the digital examination. Patients typically were aged 50–80 years. Digital subtraction angiography was done for asymptomatic carotid bruit, ischemic symptoms, nonspecific symptoms, postoperative follow-up, and contraindications to direct arteriography. Studies were done using diatrizoate meglumine or diatrizoate sodium, to a total volume of 35–50 ml of contrast material, injected usually into the basilic or cephalic vein. Three angiographic sequences in various oblique projections typically were obtained.

Diagnostic-quality results were obtained in imaging 97% of common, 93% of internal, and 90% of external carotid segments at the bifurcation. Estimation of the degree of stenosis was in agreement with the standard arteriographic findings in 97 of 98 common carotid segments, in 94 of 95 internal carotid segments, and in 79 of 91 external carotid segments. The sensitivity of DSA was 93%, its specificity was 94%, and its accuracy was 94%. Two thousand digital angiograms now have been done with no related deaths. As many as 10% of patients with known angina have had anginal attacks in close relation to contrast injection. Urticaria and nausea and vomiting occurred about as often in patients having intravenous urography.

Digital subtraction angiography appears to be accurate in identifying patients with significant carotid occlusive disease. Internal carotid stenosis at the bifurcation was accurately assessed in over 90% of individual artery evaluations in this study. Intracranial arterial segments often were satisfactorily imaged, but not consistently so.

▶ On the basis of experience with DSA in 78 patients with suspected extracranial carotid arterial disease, who also had conventional angiography, Russell et al. (*Surgery* 94:604–611, 1983) believe that DSA is a good method for evaluating bifurcation disease, but it has limitations. They maintain that its accuracy is little better than that reported by newer noninvasive and spectral analysis methods. It is more expensive and too invasive to replace noninvasive imaging. The accuracy is not sufficient to obviate use of conventional angiography, especially when a negative or nondiagnostic subtraction study is obtained. In discussion, Pairolero from the Mayo Clinic asserted that the role of DSA should be limited and should be based on the clinical picture. Transient ischemic attacks and amaurosis fugax should be investigated with conventional angiography, since digital subtraction technique fails to visualize the plaque from which the emboli come in about two thirds of the cases. J. P. Elliott of Detroit believes the future of DSA may lie in the intraarterial approach.

An assessment of DSA in 1,000 carotid bifurcations has been made by Wood et al. (*AJNR* 4:125–129, 1983). They used a criterion of 60% or greater reduction in diameter of the internal carotid artery to indicate a positive examination; with this, they found sensitivity, specificity, and accuracy of digital subtraction venous angiography to be 94% as compared with standard angiography. They excluded angiographic features other than carotid bifurcation stenosis for the purposes of this study since satisfactory imaging of carotid ulceration and intracranial arterial disease was inconsistent.

Based on correlations between DSA, selective carotid arteriography, and surgical findings. Earnest et al. (*Mayo Clin. Proc.* 58:735–746, 1983) consider intravenous DSA to accurately depict atherosclerotic lesions in the cervical carotid arteries. It is not adequate for the detection of intracranial vascular disease. About a fifth of patients referred for the venous subtraction technique have unsatisfactory examinations because of motion artifact or insufficient levels of contrast material. Modifications can increase the yield from digital subtraction venous angiography, but at the cost of increased radiation exposure, transient renal complications, congestive heart failure, infarction, or extravasation of contrast material. In this study, detection of lesions having an important impact on patient management (5%) is almost nine times greater than the incidence of permanent neurologic complications from conventional selective angiography in patients with suspected cerebrovascular disease. The authors use intravenous angiography as a screening examination primarily for asymptomatic patients in whom cerebrovascular disease is suspected, including those with carotid bruits and negative studies (indirect tests), or as a postoperative evaluation of patients who have undergone endarterectomy.

The question of peripheral vs. central injection of contrast material for intravenous digital subtraction angiography has been analyzed by Modic et al. (*Radiology* 147:711–715, 1983). The former was by a catheter whose tip lay 8 inches cephalad to the puncture site in the antecubital fossa; the central injection was by a catheter placed under fluoroscopy in the superior vena cava. When intracranial views were desired, 50 ml of contrast material was used; for carotid bifurcation studies, 40 ml. Either location of the catheter gave views of the carotid bifurcations that were good. The central injection did give better detail of small intracranial vessels.

Weinstein et al. (*Radiology* 147:717–724, 1983) analyzed intraarterial subtraction angiograms in comparison with conventional arterial angiography. The digital subtraction study can reduce greatly the amount of film, is safer, but does not have quite the spatial resolution of conventional angiography. In 70 cases studied, the digital subtraction arterial study was satisfactory for diagnosis; its chief disadvantage is the smaller field size. However, it seems likely that conventional angiography will be replaced, in most instances, by the digital subtraction version.

On the other hand, Neufang et al. (*ROFO* 139:160–166, 1983), while agreeing that for certain problems, digital subtraction arteriography can replace conventional arteriography, believe that the small field size and good spatial resolution still render conventional angiography as the basic form of investigation for some conditions, especially for detecting small carotid ulcerations and detail in cerebral vessels.

Resolution in angiograms done by intravenous subtraction angiography is admittedly inferior to that of conventional arteriography. Nevertheless, DeFilipp et al. (*Radiology* 148:129–136, 1983) point out that the venous subtraction technique does provide images of diagnostic usefulness, sufficient in many cases to allow clinical and therapeutic decisions to be made. Since the subtraction angiograms thus produced are less risky and less costly than conventional arterial catheterization, the authors consider the former to be justifiable in selected intracranial disease entities. Among these may be intracranial tumors, vasospasm after subarachnoid hemorrhage, lesions of the sella, dural sinus occlusion, and posttherapeutic embolization. Direct arteriography must be used where detailed vascular analysis is needed (except for studies of the dural sinuses which are well outlined).

The duplex scanner used by Eikelboom et al. (*Surgery* 94:821–825, 1983) provided a real-time B-mode image of the carotid arteries along with a pulsed Doppler recorder; a digital fast Fourier spectrum analyzer was used. Digital video subtraction angiography was carried out and was compared with conventional angiography with regard to accuracy in quantifying internal carotid artery disease. The most striking failure of the duplex scanner was the inability properly to classify normal vessels and those with minor lesions, for the scanner overestimated the degree of disease in these cases. Some improvement is anticipated from replacing the medium-focus scan head with a short-focus transducer. Digital subtraction angiography seemed to recognize normal carotid arteries with acceptable accuracy (12 of 14 cases) but is limited in classifying arteries with minor lesions. Stenoses and occlusions were always correctly distinguished, but some high-grade stenoses were missed. Currently, the authors believe it to be proper to perform carotid endarterectomy without conventional angiography only when there is complete agreement between digital subtraction angiography and duplex scanning.

Detailed studies of noninvasive methods of evaluating the condition of the carotid arteries continue. Spence et al. (*Can. J. Surg.* 26:556–558, 1983) found no abnormalities in 3 of 22 patients with severe stenosis of more than 80% and obtained normal findings in 1 of 9 patients with total occlusion. Combination of B-mode ultrasonography with spectral analysis of the Doppler signal should reduce error. Such studies should not be used to replace angiography but to help select patients for angiography for whom that study might otherwise be contraindicated because of advanced age or cardiac disease. It seems to me that our efforts should rather be in the direction of development and use of less toxic agents for angiography, which really is the definitive study before considering operation.—O.S.

---

**Gas-CT Cisternography for Detection of Small Acoustic Nerve Tumors**
Livia G. Solti-Bohman, David L. Magaram, William W. M. Lo, Christina T. Wade, Richard M. Witten, Franklin H. Shimizu, E. Michael McMonigle, and A. K. Raja Rao
Radiology 150:403–407, February 1984                                    18–6

---

The gas–computed tomography (CT) cisternogram effectively demonstrates intracanalicular acoustic tumors and avoids reactions to contrast material, but questions persist regarding false-positive findings. Findings were reviewed in 200 outpatients referred for gas-CT cisternography because of unilateral hearing loss or tinnitus and either positive results on brain stem electric response audiometry or abnormal findings on petrous bone radiographs. The average age was 48 years. Fourteen patients had bilateral studies. An additional 112 examinations were done in the following year. Patients were scanned in the decubitus position after lumbar intrathecal injection of 4–5 ml of filtered oxygen, using a GE 8800 CT/T scanner. Some early patients had 1–2 ml of Pantopaque instilled for subsequent pluridirectional tomography.

Abnormal findings were obtained in 6.5% of studies. Eleven of the 13 patients who were followed up after surgery had acoustic tumors, and 1 each had a meningioma and granulomatous inflammation of the eighth nerve. The results of four studies (1.9%) were interpreted as equivocal. Findings on subsequent Pantopaque studies were negative in 2 of these 4 patients. One study showed insufficient gas in the cerebellopontine angle cistern, which may have caused the abnormality. Either the seventh or eighth cranial nerve or both nerves were identified in 87% of examinations in which high-contrast retrospective analysis was performed. A small tumor can be missed if a relatively large canal is only partially examined (Fig 18–3). Extra caution is required if the filling defect does not show a convex surface, if the amount of gas is marginal, or if the canal is small. No patient experienced headache during the procedure, but most developed headache afterwards.

Interpretation of the gas-CT cisternogram is nearly always straightforward. Rather than viewing a given cisternogram as positive or negative, each apparent nonfilling of the internal auditory canal should be assessed carefully. Nonfilling of a small canal may not be abnormal, and either the contralateral canal should be assessed or a Pantopaque study carried out.

▶ I find it difficult to believe that it is important to use oxygen passed through

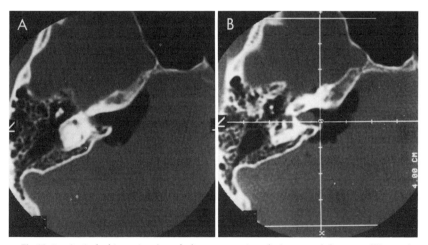

Fig 18–3.—**A,** single thin section through the upper portion of a large canal shows gas filling to the fundus without evidence of tumor. **B,** a few millimeters below the view in **A,** a bulging mass typical of a tumor is seen. (Courtesy of Solti-Bohman, L.G., et al.: Radiology 150:403–407, February 1984.)

a micropore filter instead of ordinary room air, since only 4–5 ml of gas is needed for such a study. It certainly adds to the expense.

Gas cisternography of the cerebellopontine angle may be more readily interpreted in light of the anatomicoradiologic study carried out by Braun et al. (*Neuroradiology* 26:3–7, 1984). They explored the posterior fossa with CT after injecting the arteries and veins of the cerebellopontine angle with opaque materials (such as gelatinous barium sulfate) in cadavers. Particularly notable is the constant relation of the superior petrosal vein to the trigeminal nerve, as seen in angiograms or in CT scans.

The earliest symptoms of acoustic neurinoma found by Harner and Laws (*Mayo Clin. Proc.* 58:721–728, 1983) were unilateral hearing loss, tinnitus, and disequilibrium. Facial numbness, facial weakness, and headaches were more prominent as the disorder progressed. Aside from hearing loss, the more prominent physical findings included decreased corneal reflex, nystagmus, and facial hypoesthesia. Acoustic reflex tests and the brain stem evoked response were the most useful additional tests in those with some residual hearing. The most accurate roentgenographic test was computed tomography with dye enhancement with or without the use of air contrast. The aim of diagnosis is to identify acoustic neurinomas sufficiently early that surgical removal would be safe and leave minimal deficit. As more small tumors have been studied, the value of caloric testing has been declining; but the manner of testing as outlined in this paper is probably inferior to that used by other neuro-otologists who claim a higher value of vestibular testing.—O.S.

---

**Intraoperative Neurosurgical Ultrasound in Localization and Characterization of Intracranial Masses**
Jonathan M. Rubin and George J. Dohrmann (Univ. of Chicago)
Radiology 148:519–524, August 1983                                           18–7

---

The authors reviewed the findings on intraoperative real-time ultrasonography in 70 patients who had 72 intracranial mass lesions that were thought to be tumors preoperatively or that proved to be tumors at biopsy or resection. There were 55 supratentorial and 17 infratentorial lesions in the series. All were assessed preoperatively by computed tomography (CT) or angiography. Most studies were done using a device with a specially adapted in-line scan head containing transducer elements of 3, 5, and 7.5 MHz. Nineteen operations were done on patients with cystic masses. In two patients the surface of the brain was studied by immersion of the scan head in a water path created by flooding the operative field.

All but two lesions were located by intraoperative ultrasonography. A superficial meningioma was obscured by the near-field artifact of the scan head in one patient, and a small parietal mass was missed in a patient who previously had subarachnoid bleeding. At least nine lesions were initially thought to be tumors but were not; these included inflammatory masses, hemorrhages, and arteriovenous malformations. In several patients with cystic tumor, ultrasonography confirmed the presence of fluid in the face of equivocal CT findings, or provided additional information on the

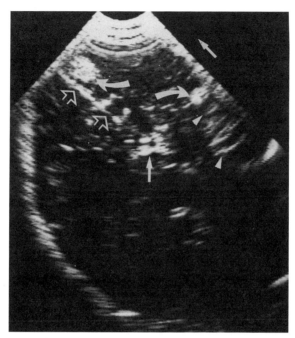

**Fig 18–4.**—Coronal ultrasound section obtained at surgery shows two small lesions *(curved arrows)*. Both were removed under ultrasonic guidance. The superior mass was an old, sclerotic arteriovenous malformation, and the inferior mass was a hemangioma. The falx *(hollow arrows)* is seen at an angle because the scan head was positioned on the dura mater covering the right hemisphere. The choroid plexus is seen passing through the foramina of Monro into the third ventricle *(arrows)*, and the right middle cerebral artery *(arrowheads)* can be seen running up to the hemangioma. The curved, echogenic white line at left is the left side of the skull. (Courtesy of Rubin, J.M., and Dohrmann, G.J.: Radiology 148:519–524, August 1983.)

fluid collection. The findings in a patient in whom two small lesions were identified are shown in Figure 18–4. The study was helpful in determining the extent of lesions before opening the dura. Biopsies were performed in 13 lesions under ultrasonic guidance. Three lesions less than 1 cm in size were removed successfully under ultrasonic guidance.

Intraoperative real-time ultrasonography is a safe, reliable means of localizing and characterizing a wide variety of intracranial masses. The technique is a dynamic, extremely flexible one and allows the neurosurgeon to assess the brain in much greater detail than is possible with most methods. The technique may be used to guide biopsies and to aid the removal of small lesions.

▶ In the same issue of *Radiology* (148:525–527, 1983) Shkolnik et al. describe experiences with four supratentorial, three infratentorial, and one intraventricular tumor. Only the latter (a choroid plexus papilloma) did not demonstrate both solid and cystic components on intraoperative real-time ultrasonic sector scanning. One parietal lobe ependymoma was subcortical and was not apparent without the ultrasound. In one cerebellar astrocytoma, gross tumor removal was found to be incomplete by ultrasonic imaging, which led to additional excision of gross tumor tissue. The authors' remark that CT fails to display the mass in the orientation presented at operation should be amended by the words "ordinary CT imaging," for certainly coronal (and even other planes) of tomography would be useful and are possible.

Accurate placement of a burr hole 16 mm in diameter permits the use of ultrasonography for postoperative as well as intraoperative scanning. Enzmann et al. (*Neuroradiology* 26:57–59, 1984) used a Diasonics DS30 neonatal unit with a 5- or 7.5-MHz probe to direct intraoperative biopsy of a "hematologic malignancy" (lymphoma). Radiation therapy was given, and postoperative follow-up was possible via the same burr hole. Accurate placement of the burr hole is obviously important, as is skill in interpreting echoencephalograms.

Ultrasound has also been used for diagnosis in patients with removal of part of the cranium (by prior neurosurgery). Gooding and Edwards (*Radiology* 148:561–562, 1983) used a 3.5- or 5-MHz transducer overlying a cranial defect in 15 male patients to determine the status of the ventricles. Acoustical gel was used as coupling agent without need to shave the head. The lateral ventricles were well visualized, but in three patients, the third ventricle could also be seen—and in one, the fourth ventricle. Midline shift, porencephalic or arachnoid cyst corresponded well with CT scans. In two other patients, both with frontal lesions, ultrasound was not effective in demonstrating the ventricles.

Scans obtained by Merritt et al. (*Radiology* 148:513–517, 1983) demonstrated tumors, abscesses, arteriovenous malformations, and hematomas in the brains of 15 patients. An attempt to visualize a cyst through a 15-mm burr hole in another patient was unsuccessful. Scans were obtained in 37 infants and children using the anterior fontanelle in the course of placement of ventricular shunts. The scanning procedure allowed proper placement of the ventricular end of the shunt system and resulted in fewer short- and long-term complications. Optimal placement of the tip of the shunt anterior to the foramen of Monro was readily achieved. The number of revisions of shunts has appreciably decreased since ultrasonic monitoring was introduced.

Roux and co-workers (*Neurochirurgie* 29:31–35, 1983) have successfully used ultrasonography, first through surgical defects and then in eight intraoperative cases. Abscesses and hematomas were located, and biopsy was performed through a 3-cm craniotomy or through a bone flap. Such biopsy of deep lesions should, in these authors' opinion, be done only if classic stereotactic procedure is not considered necessary and if the mass is larger than 1.5 cm in diameter and not too deeply situated.

At times, cortical incision is made to allow access to a subcortical tumor, which may have been located originally by ultrasonic technique. Sometimes, the tumor is not readily found. Voorhies et al. (*J. Neurosurg.* 60:438–439, 1984) suggest the use of a small cottonoid marker at the end of the incision. Repetition of the ultrasonic search will then show the relation between the cottonoid and the tumor and allow the latter to be more readily found.—O.S.

▶ ↓ Previously, Dohrmann and others have described the use of ultrasound at operation on the spinal canal and the use of a trough of saline solution in which to immerse the transducer. In the following abstract, the authors describe the utility of ultrasonic examination when the disturbing bone echoes have been removed by a previous operation.—O.S.

---

**Spinal Cord Imaging Using Real-Time High-Resolution Ultrasound**
Ira F. Braun, B. Nagesh Raghavendra, and Irvin I. Kricheff
Radiology 147:459–465, May 1983                                    18–8

---

It often is difficult to assess patients who present postoperatively with new or recurrent symptoms of cord involvement, even using myelography and computed tomography. Ultrasonography was evaluated for use in spinal cord imaging where laminectomy or a congenital neural arch defect has provided an acoustic window to the contents of the spinal canal. High-resolution real-time sector-scanner systems operating at 5 and 7.5 MHz have been used. Scans were obtained with patients in the prone, decubitus, and upright positions. Sagittal and transverse images were obtained routinely. The time-gain compensation was individualized to obtain optimal visualization of the intraspinal contents.

The spinal canal and its contents were imaged adequately in all 10 patients examined. A well-defined echogenic interface marked the boundary of the cord in both normal and pathologic cases. Pulsatile motion of the cord and small vascular structures on the anterior and posterior cord surfaces were seen routinely. A dilated central canal or linear cyst was visualized, as was cyst formation within a tumor (Fig 18–5). Solid cord tumors appeared hypoechoic, isoechoic, or slightly hyperechoic. Spinal cord atrophy was observed in two cases. Three patients had a pseudomeningocele, with the cerebrospinal fluid collection appearing as a homogeneous acoustic window.

Real-time imaging of the spinal cord in selected patients permits the rapid location of an area of interest and the comparison of normal and abnormal structures from image to image. No definite correlation has been made between sonographic appearances and histologic findings. Ultrasonography can help detect cystic regions within cord tumors, which sometimes define the rostral and caudal extent of tumors. Use of higher frequency transducers may lead to greater accuracy in visualizing smaller cystic structures associated with cord neoplasms. Neonatal syringohydromyelia and meningocele can be evaluated with this approach. Ultrasonography may be useful in guiding the percutaneous puncture of intraspinal cysts.

---

**Intraoperative Spinal Sonography: Adjunct to Metrizamide CT in Assessment and Surgical Decompression of Posttraumatic Spinal Cord Cysts**
Robert M. Quencer, Berta M. M. Morse, Barth A. Green, Frank J. Eismont, and Patricia Brost (Univ. of Miami)
AJR 142:593–601, March 1984                                    18–9

---

Real-time sonography was used to examine the spinal contents in 10

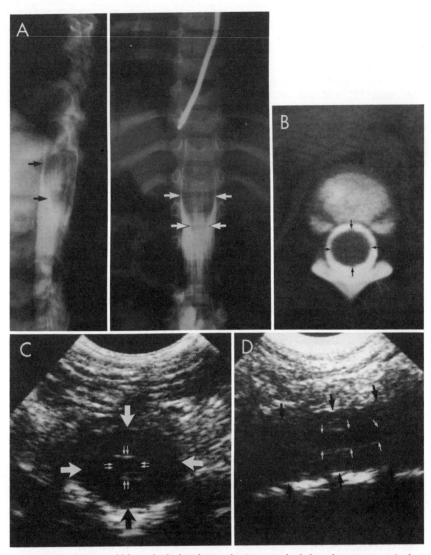

**Fig 18–5.**—Five-year-old boy who had undergone laminectomy for holocord astrocytoma. **A,** thoracolumbar myelography (lateral projection on *left,* anteroposterior projection on *right*), performed with use of aqueous contrast material, shows cord expansion in low thoracic-conus region *(arrows).* **B,** axial computed tomogram, obtained after myelography with aqueous contrast material through low thoracic cord, shows expanded cord *(arrows)* that almost fills entire spinal canal. No intramedullary cyst is noted. **C,** transverse ultrasound image of lower thoracic cord shows cord filling limits of canal *(black arrows),* unlike computed tomographic image obtained in same region (**B**). Well-defined central, echo-free area *(small arrows)* may represent intramedullary cyst. **D,** longitudinal ultrasound image of region shown in C also shows cord appearing to fill entire canal *(large arrows).* Central intramedullary cystic area *(white arrows)* centered in longitudinal plane is visualized. As predicted, intramedullary intratumoral cyst was encountered during surgery. (Courtesy of Braun, I.F., et al.: Radiology 147:459–465, May 1983.)

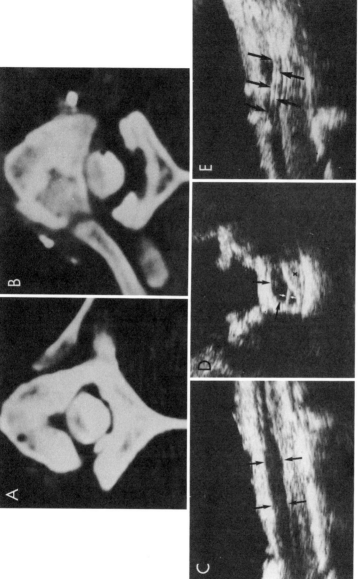

**Fig 18–6.**—Arachnoid cyst is seen after gunshot wound at T5. **A** and **B**, dorsal extramedullary collection of contrast material represents subarachnoid cyst deforming the spinal cord and pushing it anteriorly. No separate dense collection of contrast material was seen within the cord, but the poorly defined increased intramedullary density (best appreciated in **B**) was consistent with myelomalacia. **C**, sagittal intraoperative sonography (IOSS) shows arachnoid cyst *(arrows)* compressing the dorsal part of the spinal cord; more cephalad scans (not shown) disclosed a small unsuspected intramedullary cyst. **D**, transverse IOSS through the level of the maximum cord compression *(x)* shows arachnoid cyst *(black arrows)* within which septations were seen *(white arrows)*. **E**, after placement of the catheter *(arrows)*, the arachnoid cyst partially collapsed and the mass effect on the adjacent spinal cord lessened. (Courtesy of Quencer, R.M., et al.: AJR 142:593–601, March 1984.)

patients who had previous metrizamide-enhanced computed tomography (CT) or who were found on intraoperative sonography to have posttraumatic spinal cord cysts. Seven patients had cervical injuries and two had thoracic injuries; one probably had a thoracic cord contusion. The average interval from time of injury to presentation was 4½ years. Computed tomography scans were obtained in conjunction with metrizamide myelography preoperatively, and intraoperative sonography was done using a sector scanner having a 7.5-MHz transducer. Sonography was done after laminectomy in eight patients and after C7 corpectomy in two. In four patients sonography was used to locate the site at which a myelotomy should be done to reach the cyst most directly. Surgery was done within five days after CT with metrizamide enhancement in all but one patient.

A single cyst was found by CT in six patients, and two separate cysts were identified in two others. No cyst was found in one patient. In another, a posttraumatic subarachnoid cyst was identified (Fig 18–6). Areas of "myelomalacia" within the cord were identified in nine instances. The cysts were present in the dorsocentral area of the cord. The number of cysts present was overestimated by CT in four patients and underestimated in two. Intraoperative sonography was used on several occasions to confirm the proper position of a shunt catheter within a cord cyst or an arachnoid cyst. Cyst collapse was demonstrated after catheter placement. Five of six patients who had surgery aimed at directly decompressing an intramedullary or subarachnoid cyst via an indwelling shunt catheter improved clinically. Another patient improved without shunt surgery, and two improved after anterior cervical decompression and interbody fusion.

Intraoperative spinal sonography is helpful in the surgical management of posttraumatic spinal cord cysts. It provides a better picture of the number and location of cysts than does CT with metrizamide, and it aids a precisely positioned myelotomy. In some cases, unnecessary cord dissection can be avoided.

---

### The Choice of Contrast Agent for Myelography in Patients With Nonpenetrating Cervical Spine Trauma

Chat Virapongse, Franklin Wagner, Jr., Mohammad Sarwar, and E. Leon Kier (Yale Univ.)
Radiology 147:467–471, May 1983                                    18–10

The authors reviewed the findings in 40 patients with neurologic deficits from cervical spine trauma who underwent cervical myelography with iophendylate (Pantopaque), gas, metrizamide, or a combination of these. The 31 men and 9 women were aged 18–91 years. Most were evaluated within 24 hours after injury. There were 52 studies done, and two or more contrast agents were used in nine patients. All patients remained unchanged neurologically despite attempted closed reduction by skeletal traction, or had a reduction of less than 30% in the anteroposterior diameter of the spinal canal at the site of involvement.

Myelography was done by puncture at C1–C2. The dose of metrizamide used now is less than 1.25 gm of iodine. Only 2–3 ml of metrizamide (250

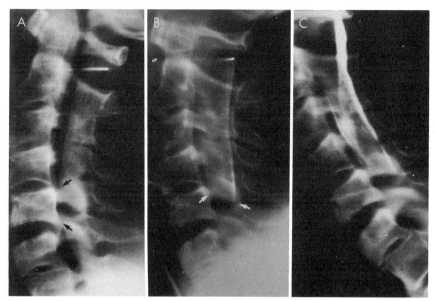

**Fig 18–7.**—Studies with gas, metrizamide, and iophendylate in a patient with subluxation of C5–C6. **A,** retrolisthesis is seen at C5–C6. Gas was instilled via C1–C2, but filled only the ventral subarachnoid space, leaving a so-called skip defect at C5 *(arrows)*. The canal is patent, with gas seen at C6–C7. Cord swelling or an anterior extradural lesion impinging on the cord was suspected, as the dorsal aspect of the cord was not seen. **B,** after 3 ml of metrizamide was added, complete blockage at C5 was seen as the result of compression by bone between the anteriorly positioned dorsal aspect of the C5 body and the lamina of C6 posteriorly *(arrows)*. **C,** the addition of 3 ml of iophendylate confirmed the findings of the metrizamide study. (Courtesy of Virapongse, C., et al.: Radiology 147:467–471, May 1983.)

mg of iodine/ml) is required in patients with complete block. The volume of iophendylate used generally is 3–8 ml. Usually, no more than three bolus injections of 7–10 ml of gas are made. Most diagnostic information is obtained from the lateral view. The findings in one patient are shown in Figure 18–7. Swelling of the cord was seen in 16 patients. In 11 patients bone impinged on the spinal cord, whereas 10 had complete block, 6 from bone and 4 from cord swelling. The cord was demonstrated better in patients with a block regardless of the contrast material used. Metrizamide gave the best results, whether or not the canal was blocked. All patients studied with metrizamide remained asymptomatic except for one who had nausea and vomiting.

Metrizamide appears to be superior to gas or iophendylate for use in demonstrating the injured spinal cord and associated problems. It is safe when administered in amounts less than 1.25 gm of iodine, using a C-arm or biplane fluoroscopic unit with tomographic capability. There is little need for computed tomography in these patients, even after intrathecal enhancement. Use of iophendylate should be discouraged because of the risk of arachnoiditis and the inferior radiographic outlining of the anterior aspect of the spinal cord in the supine position advocated by the authors.

▶ Drayer and colleagues carried out a double blind study on the comparison of iopamidol with metrizamide for lumbosacral myelography (*J. Neurosurg.* 58:531–537, 1983). There were 30 patients in each group. Some sort of adverse reaction occurred in 13 with iopamidol and in 20 with metrizamide. These chemically similar compounds gave uniformly good pictures. The most striking feature of the comparison was severe neurobehavioral reaction, seen in 17% of the metrizamide patients (6 of 30), whereas none occurred in the 30 iopamidol patients. This reaction group included disorientation, affective lability, dysarthria, asterixis, global aphasia, and visual field defects. Electroencephalogram was done in 11 of each group; four patients with metrizamide had abnormal records, but none of those with iopamidol did. Abnormal EEG was more likely to appear in patients with toxic confusional encephalopathy. Both compounds produced blush in sequential computed tomography scans.—O.S.

---

**The Indications for Metrizamide Myelography: Relationship With Complications After Myelography**
Harry N. Herkowitz, Richard L. Romeyn, and Richard H. Rothman
J. Bone Joint Surg. [Am.] 65-A:1144–1149, October 1983                    18–11

---

Metrizamide has replaced Pantopaque as the contrast medium of choice in lumbar myelography. The authors undertook a retrospective and prospective study of the effects of metrizamide myelography for suspected lumbar disk herniation in order to relate the occurrence of complications to objective clinical evidence of nerve root impingement. The retrospective series included 248 patients seen in 1980–1981 with suspected lumbar disk herniation. Another 110 patients were studied prospectively. There were 170 men with a mean age of 44 years and 188 women with a mean age of 41.5 years in the studies. The uniform myelographic procedure included removal of 5 ml of fluid through a 22-gauge needle inserted at the L3-L4 interspace, followed by injection of 12 ml of metrizamide solution. Patients were not allowed to lie flat for 12 hours.

Positive clinical and myelographic findings were present in 31% of cases, negative clinical and myelographic findings in 50%, positive clinical and negative myelographic findings in 13%, and negative clinical and positive myelographic findings in 6%. A total of 53% of patients had side effects after metrizamide myelography, headache being the most common. Five patients had a transient increase in pain, and three had transient disturbance in urination. Two patients, both alcoholics, had seizures after myelography. Complications occurred in 30% of patients with objective clinical and myelographic findings and in 70% of those with only subjective complaints and normal myelograms. In the prospective series, severe headache was much more prevalent in patients with subjective complaints than in those with objective clinical and positive myelographic findings.

Complications of metrizamide myelography were much more frequent in patients without objective abnormalities in this study than in those with positive clinical and myelographic findings. Myelography should, in general, be restricted to patients with objective physical findings who are being considered for the surgical treatment of herniated lumbar disk.

▶ The quantity of contrast material used in the case reported by Angiari et al. (*Neuroradiology* 26:61–63, 1984) was 15 ml of metrizamide for a concentration of 210 mg of iodine/ml—slightly higher than the maximal amount listed by the distributor in the United States. The lumbar injection for cervical myelography was followed by "extreme head-down position" (angle not given) at which time the patient flexed and rotated his neck to one side. He was immediately put foot down, and after a few minutes, examination proceeded, confirming the diagnosis of compression of several nerve roots. A jacksonian seizure was followed by right hemiplegia and global aphasia from which complete recovery had not taken place after six months. Computed tomography scan after the myelogram showed localization of contrast material in the left hemispheral sulci. The delay between the mishap and the onset of seizures was more than an hour. Prevention would appear to be most important, since no treatment (aside from anticonvulsants) is known. The authors apparently did not consider the phenomenon (still poorly understood, to be sure) of postictal Todd's paralysis, which is not always transient, after idiopathic seizures.

Macpherson et al. (*Clin. Radiol.* 34:325–326, 1983) analyzed the sequelae of allowing patients to be ambulatory vs. requiring bed rest after lumbar puncture for myelography, having used a 20-gauge needle. In 119 patients randomly allocated to these two groups, the authors found no significant difference in headache (52%–55%), nausea (25%–31%), vomiting (13%–14%), dizziness (18%–29%) between 61 ambulant and 58 bed-rest patients. Two ambulant patients had focal seizures (none with bed rest), and neither showed mental changes. There was some association between complications and dose of contrast medium (not specified in the article). The authors do think patients should stay in the hospital for 24 hours after lumbar myelography (radiculography) because of the possibility of mental changes or seizures.

A similar study for direct puncture cervical myelography, by Teasdale and Macpherson (*Neuroradiol.* 25:85–86, 1983) involved 120 patients. Headache was found in 60% of each group (ambulant or bed rest); slightly fewer of the bed-rest group had nausea, vomiting, and dizziness, but this was not of statistical import. Two bed-rest patients had seizures; four had mental changes, whereas only two of the ambulatory patients had changes. It should be noted that the bed-rest group had back and head elevation for the first six hours. In general, those in either group who received a larger dose of metrizamide (2,500–3,000 mg of iodine) compared with the standard 7 ml of 250 mg of iodine/ml) were apt to have more problems. The conclusion again is that after cervical puncture myelograms, bed rest is not particularly important.

Solti-Bohman and Bentson (*AJNR* 4:889–892, 1983) compared small-dose metrizamide myelography (3.75 gm of metrizamide) with use of larger amounts (6.75 gm). The latter were used for large obese patients and those in whom total spinal myelography was needed; the small dose, for small patients, children, and for seeing only one area of the spinal canal. In such instances, the injection was made as close to the area of interest as possible. There was little change in incidence of headache and vomiting, but a heartening decrease in psychoneurologic side effects with the small dose. Diagnostic quality was not impaired when the small dose was injected at the locus of interest, but the small dose was often inadequate for total canal study.

An interesting technique for introducing metrizamide into the cervical canal (for instance, for searching for acoustic tumors) is described by Anke (*Neuroradiology* 25:81–83, 1983). The patient is placed in lateral decubitus after 10 mg of diazepam for premedication. Puncture of the subarachnoid space is performed at C1–2 with vertical beam fluoroscopy. A connecting plastic tubing is fitted to the hub of the needle and filled with saline solution; the distal end of the tube is placed below the level of the needle. As soon as the subarachnoid space is entered, saline solution flows out of the distal end of the tube, and metrizamide can then be injected.

The prone position is preferred by McCormick et al. (*Australas. Radiol.* 27:119–131, 1983) for myelography either by lumbar or cervical puncture. For total inspection of the canal, prone lumbar injection of metrizamide of 10 ml of 250 mg of iodine/ml or 7 ml of 300 mg of iodine/ml is followed by turning the patient onto his or her side and then tilting head down. Flow is considerably easier in this position.—O.S.

---

### Anomalous Lumbosacral Nerve Roots: Myelographic Signs and Surgical Findings

E. Babin, G. Matge, and J. L. Dietemann
Ann. Radiol. (Paris) 26:295–305, April–May 1983                    18–12

The introduction of metrizamide to myelography has brought considerable improvement to the definition of images. The nerve roots, in particular, are much more clearly visible, which has led to the striking discovery of relatively frequent anomalies in the lumbar and sacral area. The authors report their observations in 45 cases in which the malformation consisted generally of conjoint roots, L5 and S1 roots being involved in most cases. Several myelographic patterns are described, and the malformations are occasionally bilateral or multileveled or both. The lateral surface of the dural sheath may be used to identify normal outlets.

The myelographic presentation of such anomalous roots should lead to further investigation such as discography, epidural venography, or computed tomography. Such root anomalies may be mistaken for a disk herniation, and conversely, an obvious disk hernia visible on myelography may conceal the presence of anomalous nerve roots. It is important to anticipate the presence of such an anomaly before deciding on incision site and surgical technique. Conjoint roots may be difficult to recognize on myelography in the presence of an ascendant hernia at the same level. The direct sign constituted by the shadow of the coupled roots above the anomalous outlet may be of help. The increasingly frequent use of tomodensitometry (computed tomography) in evaluation of a lumbar sciatica may well lead to failure to discover such anomalous nerve roots and may render surgery more difficult in certain cases.

---

### Differential CT Diagnosis of Extruded Nucleus Pulposus

Alan L. Williams, Victor M. Haughton, David L. Daniels, and John P. Grogan
Radiology 148:141–148, July 1983                                                        18–13

Most nucleus pulposus herniations may be identified on computed tomography (CT) images by the presence of a focal abnormality of the disk margin. The CT appearance of nuclear fragments that penetrate the posterior longitudinal ligament as well as the annulus is described. The authors reviewed preoperative CT scans of 57 patients in whom the diagnosis of an extruded nuclear fragment was made at laminectomy. Scans of another 31 patients with some CT findings similar to those of extruded disk fragment were also reviewed. Of the latter group, anomalous root sheaths were confirmed at myelography in 21 patients, and epidural tumors were diagnosed either at laminectomy or by the subsequent course in 10. In 20 of the 88 patients, tissue density within the spinal canal was measured using a computer program and region-of-interest cursor.

All CT scans in the 57 patients with surgically confirmed extruded disk fragments showed asymmetry of epidural fat and compression or displacement of a root sheath or dural sac. In 52 patients, an epidural soft-tissue mass, usually polypoid, was identified; in 27 cases this mass was contiguous with the disk, and in 25 it was separated from the posterior disk margin by epidural fat. The posterior disk margin protruded focally in 48 patients and was indistinct in 19. In 18, CT showed the disk fragment caudal to the intervertebral disk (14 patients), rostral to the disk (2), or lateral to the disk in the intervertebral foramen (2). In 3 patients, CT showed a virtually normal posterior disk margin despite an extruded fragment. The 21 patients with anomalous nerve root sheaths had either conjoined (15) or dilated (6) forms. The conjoined root sheaths showed asymmetric fat, dural sac, and root sheaths (Fig 18–8). The margins of the conjoined root sheaths were smooth and sharply marginated, and the density was similar to that of the dural sac. Asymmetry of the dural sac was usually apparent at multiple levels. Dilatation caused the root sheaths and the epidural fat to appear asymmetric; however, root-sheath density was homogeneous and similar to that of the dural sac. Tissue density measurements differed between the extruded disk fragments and root-sheath anomalies.

Extruded disk fragments have a varied appearance on CT. When a fragment is polypoid or far from the disk margin, the herniation can be recognized as extruded. However, in some instances a free fragment may not be differentiated by CT from a subligamentous herniation. Because extruded nuclear material can migrate substantially, a CT study must encompass the intervertebral foramen and all portions of the vertebral canal in which disk fragments may compress a nerve or root. A conjoined root sheath originating from the dural sac, without a contralateral root sheath at the same level, may simulate an extruded disk fragment on CT because the epidural fat appears asymmetric; however, the density measurements of the conjoined root sheath and the dural sac should be sufficiently similar to be diagnostic. A neurofibroma within the intervertebral foramen may simulate a lateral extruded disk fragment; however, these

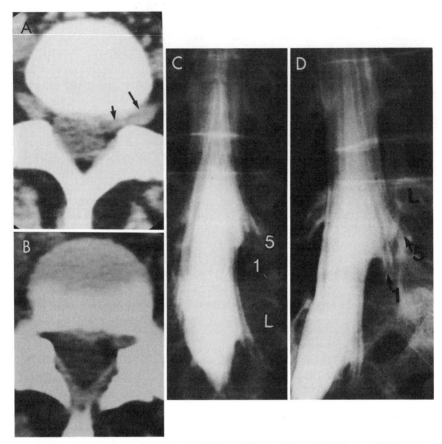

Fig 18–8.—Conjoined root sheath [density, 26 Hounsfield units (HU) and 42 HU]. **A,** axial CT section at L5–S1 shows the L5 ganglion *(large arrow)* in the left intervertebral foramen and the S1 nerve root sheath *(small arrow)* within the vertebral canal. Note the asymmetric dural sac (density, 16 HU) and epidural fat. **B,** asymmetry of the dural sac (density, 8 HU) and epidural fat are also seen in a section 5 mm caudal to the disk space. The left S1 root sheath *(arrow)* can be seen in the lateral recess. Densities of the conjoined root sheath are 26 HU and 42 HU. **C,** anteroposterior spot radiograph obtained during metrizamide myelography shows the L5 and S1 nerve roots exiting via a common root sheath. The asymmetric dural sac is seen caudal to the conjoined root sheath. **D,** oblique spot radiograph obtained during metrizamide myelography also shows the L5 and S1 nerve roots *(arrows)*. (Courtesy of Williams, A.L., et al.: Radiology 148:141–148, July 1983.)

tumors usually have smooth margins, unlike the irregular margins of a disk fragment.

▶ One must be careful not to ignore the fine print. The techniques used by these radiologists involve advanced computer programs which are not available everywhere, but the pictures are beautiful! Clarity of a totally different nature is shown in the article by Levitan and Wiens (*Radiology* 148:707–708, 1983) demonstrating the CT changes in chronic lumbar extradural hematoma which enable the authors to help distinguish such a hematoma from an extruded disk.

Such changes include tapered convex margins, length greater than 2 cm, and associated normal intervertebral disks. This rare entity should be considered in the CT differential diagnosis of lumbar extradural hematoma from extruded disk.

Recognition of an extruded disk by CT may obviate the use of chymopapain or otherwise alter the surgeon's approach to a disk herniation. Review of 40 surgically confirmed cases of extruded disks by Dillon et al. (*J. Comput. Assist. Tomogr.* 7:969–975, 1983) allowed diagnosis of the extruded disk material as lobulated soft tissue similar in attenuation to the material of the disk space; in 34 cases, the extrusion was 6 mm or more from the center of the parent disk. Calcification of the extruded portion was evident in five patients, in six, extruded free fragment was associated with a normal appearance of the parent disk material. The authors use the following differential diagnosis: enlarged nerve roots, calcification in posterior longitudinal ligament, calcified ligamentum flavum, basivertebral venous plexus, synovial cyst of facet joint, and epidural tumor.

The major differential diagnostic difficulty in CT scanning as well as in myelography is, according to Kieffer et al. (*JAMA* 251:1192–1195, 1984), the distinction of disk herniation from disk bulging. Bulging is a diffuse process, while herniation is focal. The major advantages of CT over myelography include demonstrations of abnormalities of the bony structures as well as thickening of the ligamentum flavum, far lateral disk herniations in the intervertebral foramen, and demonstration of fat. Unfortunately, CT does not demonstrate soft-tissue anatomy within the thecal sac, and it is more difficult (with CT than with myelogram) to demonstrate low thoracic spinal cord lesions, which may simulate lumbar disk herniation. Currently, these authors believe, the choice of diagnostic method for diagnosis of disk herniation is a matter of opinion and subjective preference.

The choice in the case of Firooznia et al. is for CT scanning, as indicated in the following abstract.—O.S.

---

**CT of Lumbar Spine Disk Herniation: Correlation With Surgical Findings**
Hossein Firooznia, Vallo Benjamin, Irvin I. Kricheff, Mahvash Rafii, and Cornelia Golimbu (New York Univ.)
AJR 142:587–592, March 1983                                    18–14

---

Lumbar spinal computed tomography (CT) findings were reviewed in 100 consecutive patients undergoing 116 surgical disk explorations. The 61 men and 39 women had a mean age of 49 years. The indications were back pain or radiculopathy, usually recurrent or of several years' duration. Each disk level was evaluated from the top of the neural foramen to the pedicle of the next caudad vertebra with axial cross-sections 5 mm thick. Six slices of each interspace were obtained, usually from the L3–L4 level to the S1 segment.

There were 97 true-positive preoperative predictions of herniated nucleus pulposus by CT. Seven true-negative, 8 false-negative, and 4 false-positive CT results were obtained. Two of 12 discrepancies between the

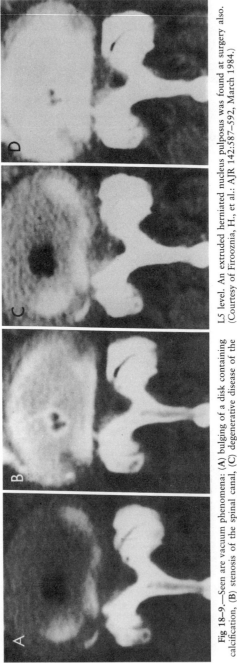

Fig 18–9.—Seen are vacuum phenomena: (A) bulging of a disk containing calcification, (B) stenosis of the spinal canal, (C) degenerative disease of the apophyseal joints, and (D) stenosis of the right neural foramen, all at the L4– L5 level. An extruded herniated nucleus pulposus was found at surgery also. (Courtesy of Firooznia, H., et al.: AJR 142:587–592, March 1984.)

CT and operative findings in 11 patients were the result of incorrect interpretations, and 5 were in previously operated-on patients. Three discrepancies occurred in patients with spondylolisthesis and 2 in patients with spinal stenosis (Fig 18–9).

Scanning with CT is the best available means of evaluating lumbar disk herniation, especially in patients not previously operated on. The study was accurate in 93% of the present patients when those previously operated on were excluded. Both conventional and CT myelography may be necessary when the CT findings are inconclusive, especially in surgically treated patients and those with spinal stenosis or spondylolisthesis.

---

**Pitfalls in the Computed Tomographic Evaluation of the Lumbar Spine in Disk Disease**
Ira F. Braun, J. P. Lin, A. E. George, I. I. Kricheff, and J. C. Hoffman, Jr.
Neuroradiology 26:15–20, January 1984                18–15

---

CT is an accepted noninvasive means of evaluating the lumbar spine in patients suspected of having disk disease. A high-resolution scanner and localizing digital scout imaging system are used. In studies done at Emory Univ., a tilted gantry was used to obtain slices parallel to the interspaces and adjacent vertebral body end plates. The nonangled technique may be helpful in assessing the osseous spinal canal. Five to 7 parallel 5-mm slices are obtained through each interspace and the adjacent vertebral bodies, with an overlap of 2 mm. The patient is examined in the supine position. When gantry tilt cannot be made parallel to the lumbosacral oblique axis reformatting is used for clarity.

Migration of herniated disk fragments may not be detected if slices are obtained only through the interspace. Contiguous slices may clarify a finding in a single slice which might be ascribed to an artifact or to partial volume averaging. Symmetric features cannot be used to diagnose disk herniation in the tilted, poorly positioned, or scoliotic patient. Even a gentle scoliosis can render CT findings difficult to interpret. Vertebral body misalignment, as in spondylolisthesis, alters the course of the dural tube and distorts the adjacent anatomy, changing the anatomical relationships used to diagnose disk disease. If patient motion occurs either rostrally or caudally after the scout image is obtained, the final images may not correspond accurately to those on the scout film. Postoperative changes also may be a problem, and recurrent disk herniation should be diagnosed only when there is close clinical correlation.

Accurate CT scanning of the lumbar spine requires considerable care in setting up the examination, positioning the patient, and interpreting the results. The scan findings should always be correlated with the clinical presentation and physical findings.

▶ This article bears careful assimilation. With the current interest in chymopapain injection and the current requirements that the patient selection be made on the basis of positive myelogram *or* positive CT scan, the importance of exact diagnosis matching the clinical syndrome is paramount. And it reemphasizes the need for neuroradiologic knowledge on the part of neurosurgeons, so intelligent interaction with the radiologists can be undertaken.

Osborne et al. (*Neurosurgery* 14:147–153, 1984) have put together a very useful directory of lesions that produce foraminal nerve entrapment in the absence of lesions seen in water-soluble contrast myelography. The computerized scans were taken with 5-mm contiguous slices 3 or 4 hours after intrathecal water-soluble contrast material. Samples are shown of entrapment due to lateral prolapse of the disk, superior articular hypertrophy, lateral recess stenosis, posterolateral vertebral bone lipping, tumors, postoperative scarring, spondylolisthesis and synovial cysts.

Computed tomographic findings may be inconclusive or misleading in cases of "conjoined" nerve roots, as exemplified by the case of Gebarski and Mc-Gillicuddy (*Neurosurgery* 14:66–68, 1984). When herniated nucleus pulposus is present in this situation, the affected nerve root may be the unsuspected one (e.g., syndrome of the L5 root with a disk protrusion at L5-S1). A combination of CT and metrizamide myelography may be necessary to avoid confusion in such a case.

See also Babin et al. (abstract 18–12) for myelographic findings and surgical findings in cases of anomalous lumbosacral nerve roots.—O.S.

---

### Computed Tomography of the Postoperative Lumbar Spine
J. George Teplick and Marvin E. Haskin (Hahnemann Univ.)
AJNR 4:1053–1072, September–October 1983                18–16

As many as a third of patients having lumbar spine surgery for herniated disk, spondylolisthesis, or spinal stenosis have unsatisfactory results, and determination of the cause is important. The authors reviewed the findings in about 750 patients with previous lumbar laminectomy who had computed tomographic (CT) scanning in a 28-month period. Most of them were patients with postoperative failed-back syndrome who had persistent or recurrent radiculopathy. Fifteen patients were examined within two weeks after operation to determine the early appearances of the postoperative spine. Contrast enhancement studies were done in 23 patients. Twelve patients were reoperated on after CT examination. Reformatting was rarely necessary.

The only clue to a minilaminotomy may be the absence of part or most of the ligamentum flavum. Some extradural scarring was seen in about 75% of the laminectomy patients, and about 40% had sizeable scars, seen as soft-tissue densities in the spinal canal and having a greater CT density than the thecal sac. The distinction between a diskectomy scar and recurrent disk herniation is outlined in the table. Extradural hematomas appeared as soft-tissue densities at the operative site in diskectomy patients. The postlaminectomy pseudomeningocele results from an inadvertent dural tear and the posterior escape of cerebrospinal fluid to form a rounded collection of low CT density at or near the midline. Bony overgrowth or spur formation of a facet or vertebral body can be secondary to surgical resection. Focal thickening of the dural sac near the operative site may be

DIFFERENTIAL FEATURES OF DISKECTOMY SCAR AND RECURRENT
HERNIATED DISK

| CT Characteristics | Diskectomy Scar | Recurrent Disk Hernation |
|---|---|---|
| Shape | From strands to mass, often irregular, but can be regular; often contours around thecal sac | Masslike density; does not follow sac contours |
| Location | Frequently extends well above or below the interspace; largest part may not be at interspace | Usually limited to interspace (rarely, fragment may migrate above or below) |
| Relation to thecal sac | Often retracts sac; often conforms to contour of sac; rarely compresses sac | Never causes sac retraction; may compress or deform sac |
| Associated scars | May be solitary or continuous with canal wall scar | Very infrequently associated with sizable scarring; if associated usually appears somewhat denser than adjacent scar |
| Free border into canal | Either sharp or indistinct | Free border usually sharp and distinct |
| Anterior (vertebral body) border | May not appear to be direct extension of anulus | Usually appears to be direct extension of anulus |
| Intravenous contrast enhancement | Shows marked enhancement | Little or no enhancement |
| CT density (Hounsfield units) | Usually less dense than disk herniation (50 to 75 H) | Generally denser than scar (90 to 120 H) |

(Courtesy of Teplick, J.G., and Haskin, M.E.: AJNR 4:1053–1072, September-October 1983.)

a manifestation of arachnoiditis. In complex cases, areas of lack of enhancement within a zone of marked enhancement may suggest the presence of residual disk fragments within a scar or area of fibrosis. Miscellaneous postoperative findings have included a "vacuum disk" phenomenon caused by removal of degenerated disk material through a defect in the anulus fibrosis, air in the thecal sac, and a fat graft. This last appears as a densely black area with little scar nearby.

Computed tomographic studies of the postoperative spine can help determine the cause of recurrent or new back pain and radiculopathy. Many aspects of incomplete or incorrect surgery are clarified by CT scanning postoperatively.

▶ The CT features of postoperative lumbar spine changes in asymptomatic subjects are listed by Braun et al. (*AJR* 142:149–152, 1984): eccentric vacuum phenomenon, gas within spinal canal, dural tube retracted toward surgical side in nonstenotic canal, intra- and extraspinal tissue accumulation, efface-ment of epidural fat, loss of distinction of ipsilateral nerve root, decrease in height of surgically violated disk space, and loss of definition of intraspinal contents. The authors note that these same sorts of changes are also to be seen in symptomatic patients; they concur with others that CT differentiation of symptomatic scarring from asymptomatic fibrosis and from small, clinically significant recurrent disk herniation is usually extremely difficult. They are cur-rently investigating the diagnostic advantages of CT myelography with water-soluble contrast material in differentiation between small recurrent disk hernia-tions and scar.

## Computed Tomography of the Spine: Curved Coronal Reformations From Serial Images

Stephen L. G. Rothman, Glen D. Dobben, Michael L. Rhodes, William V. Glenn, Jr., and Yu-Ming Azzawi
Radiology 150:185–190, January 1984                                                    18–17

Limited visibility of anatomical structures by standard axial computed tomography (CT) has increased interest in more flexible image orientations. The authors used a "curved coronal" image that is three-dimensional in its description but flat in its presentation and that follows the structural shape of anatomy. A set of regularly spaced axial CT images is required to generate a curved coronal reformation. An image is generated to act as reference to select a curved coronal reformation by choosing several pixels along the desired curvature. A complex polynomial equation representing a smooth curve is then used to extract pixels from the axial CT data to

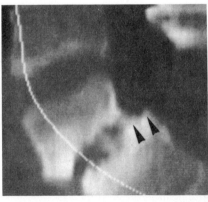
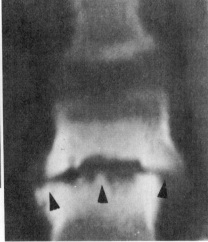

**Fig 18–10.**—Sagittal and curved coronal refor-mations produce planes perpendicular to the pa-thology and thus also show forward and lateral sub-luxation of L5 on the sacrum. This is not recognized on planar reformations. (Courtesy of Rothman, S.L.G., et al.: Radiology 150:185–190, January 1984.)

form the coronal image curved along the polynomial. It is also possible to generate a family of curved coronals separated by a standard distance between curved sections.

More than 150 patients were scanned with the use of curved coronal reformation as well as routine planar coronal reformation. The method has been used in both cervical and lumbar spinal CT. It is most useful in patients having steep lordotic curvatures. The findings in a patient with severe back pain that developed after interbody fusion are shown in Figure 18–10. Only the curved coronal image made it clear that there was a large amount of lateral subluxation.

The curved coronal reformation makes it possible to display the frontal view in any orientation. It functionally straightens the spinal lordotic curve, allowing all of the exiting nerve roots to be visualized out to their foramina on a single image. The plane of reformation can be angled so that it parallels oblique structures (e.g., the facet joints or the L5–S1 articulation) for better evaluation of actual anatomical relationships. Comparable advantages are obtained when using this technique to image the cervical spine.

▶ The coronal images of the spine are produced by plotting along the posterior aspects of the vertebral bodies, as seen in a midsagittal image generated from 24 scans, using 5-mm thick CT sections overlapping every 3 mm. Examples are shown of conjoined nerve trunks, asymmetric origin of nerve roots, asymmetric termination of the dural sac, facet fractures, and a tethered split spinal cord. This type of reformation requires a set of axial images parallel to one another, and hence cannot be obtained from a set which is angled at each disk space.—O.S.

---

**Evoked Potentials From the Motor Tracts in Humans**
Walter J. Levy, Jr., and Donald H. York (Univ. of Missouri)
Neurosurgery 12:422–429, April 1983                                    18–18

---

Previous systems for monitoring evoked potentials in order to detect cord damage at a reversible stage have utilized sensory functions. The authors evaluated 11 patients with the use of a technique developed in cats, which was based on direct stimulation of the area overlying the motor tract between the intermediolateral sulcus and the dentate ligament to produce a 100-m/second signal. In cat studies, the signal was abolished by section of the motor area but not by section of the dorsal columns or of the anterior quadrant of the spinal cord. Movement was produced when the correct frequency of stimulation was used.

Stimulation was done both at open surgery and percutaneously. In surgical cases, the electrode was placed at a site where there were no dorsal roots directly beneath the point of stimulation. The percutaneous electrode was inserted like a cordotomy needle to make contact with the surface of the cord just posterior to the dentate ligament. In both instances, recordings were from epidural electrodes placed through spinal needles in the low thoracic region. Movements were produced by a 1–5-mamp stimulus last-

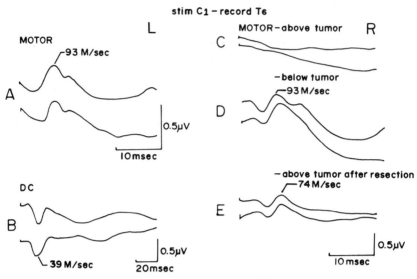

Fig 18–11.—Recording during the removal of a spinal cord meningioma. **A,** The motor tract on the normal side is present at 93 m/second. **B,** Dorsal column stimulation on the tumor side is slowed but present at 39 m/second. **C,** Motor potential on the tumor side is absent. **D,** The motor potential with stimulation at C5 and recording at T6, both below the tumor, is present at 93 m/second. **E,** Stimulation above the tumor and recording below, 15 minutes after its removal, show some return of the signal. (Courtesy of Levy, W.J., and York, D.H.: Neurosurgery 12:422–429, April 1983.)

ing 200 microseconds, in trains of 3–10/second, starting at a rate of 7 Hz. Studies were done in conjunction with nitrous oxide and narcotic anesthesia. Distal limb movements were elicited by stimulation of the motor tract area, but not by stimulation of the dorsal column area. The findings during removal of a cord meningioma are shown in Figure 18–11. The patient who had hemiparesis preoperatively had improved strength and better subjective sensation after tumor removal.

This technique can be helpful in assessing spinal cord function whether used at open surgery or percutaneously. The monitoring system may simplify evoked potential monitoring during surgery to a substantial degree. The method is a direct one, and there are no synapses in the pathway, as with somatosensory evoked potential recording. The system therefore should be less susceptible to anesthetic-induced changes. Further work is needed to define the exact role of the motor tract evoked potential.

▶ For those relatively rare instances in which it is important to know where the primary somatosensory area is, Lueders et al. (*J. Neurosurg.* 58:885–894, 1983) suggest that it is possible to localize this area by using direct pickup from subdural electrodes with stimulation of the median nerve. Evaluation of the various waveforms of the evoked potential permits differentiation of primary sensory cortex from the evoked potentials produced in the precentral motor cortex.—O.S.

## Detection of Brachial Plexus Dysfunction by Somatosensory Evoked Potential Monitoring: A Report of Two Cases

Michael E. Mahla, Donlin M. Long, Joy McKennett, Carol Green, and Robert W. McPherson (Johns Hopkins Med. Insts.)
Anesthesiology 60:248–252, March 1984                    18–19

The authors used somatosensory evoked potential (SEP) recordings from stimulation of the median nerves to monitor two patients for neurologic dysfunction during posterior fossa surgery performed in the park bench position. In this variation of the lateral decubitus position, the lower leg is straightened, allowing the trunk to roll forward on a cushion until a three-quarters prone position is attained. A towel roll is placed under the upper torso, *not* in the axilla where it could compress neurovascular structures. The dependent arm is rotated forward no more than 90 degrees.

Man, 67, had a right cerebellar mass extending into the foramen magnum as well as inoperable three-vessel coronary artery disease, past myocardial infarction with ventricular aneurysm, and recurrent congestive failure. On CT scanning, another lesion was seen deep in the right temporal lobe. Surgery was done in the park bench, or three-quarters prone, position under thiopental-induced anesthesia and controlled ventilation. The initial amplitude of the response to left median

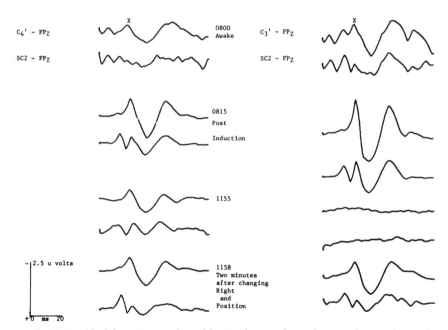

Fig 18–12.—The left tracing was obtained by stimulation and recording over the second cervical vertebrae (SC2-FP$_z$) and contralateral cortex (C4'-FP$_z$). The right tracing was obtained by stimulating the right median nerve and recording over the contralateral cortex (C3'-FP$_z$) and second cervical vertebrae (SC2-FP$_z$). A 2-msec delay was included so that waves are displayed between 2 and 82 msec after stimulus. (Courtesy of Mahla, M.E., et al.: Anesthesiology 60:248–252, March 1984.)

nerve stimulation was about 60% of that of right median nerve stimulation. This was reversed about an hour later, and subsequently the response to right median nerve stimulation disappeared (Fig 18–12). The right arm was adducted at the patient's side and extended at the elbow. The response reappeared within 3 minutes of repositioning the arm, and no further SEP changes were observed. No neurologic deficit was present postoperatively.

Hemodynamic instability and air emoblism occur less frequently during surgery in the park bench position than with the patient sitting. The risk of neurologic injury from positioning should be similar in the two positions. The park bench position would seem to place considerable stretch on the nondependent brachial plexus. Injury also can result from peripheral nerve ischemia. Monitoring the SEP can identify neurologic injury while simultaneously evaluating brain stem function. Ascending sites proximal to the cortex (e.g., the second cervical vertebra and Erb's point) should be monitored.

▶ One of the major problems in dealing with peripheral nerve tumors has been the difficulty of access to those parts of the nerves which have not yet reached the extremities so that tumors may grow to considerable size before detection. Computed tomography offers considerable help in this regard, according to Powers et al. (*J. Neurosurg.* 59:131–136, 1983). They describe the useful information given by CT in eight of nine patients with peripheral nerve lesions. A patient with schwannoma of the brachial plexus was the only one in whom the CT was unhelpful.—O.S.

# 19 Techniques

▶ ↓ The new journal *Microsurgery* appeared in 1983, as volume 4 number 1! It replaces the *Journal of Microsurgery* as well as the *International Journal of Microsurgery*. Julius H. Jacobson and Leonard I. Malis are the editors. Any field of medicine that employs microsurgery may be represented. Of particular interest to neurosurgeons in this issue is the article, "Immediate Total Scalp and Skull Reconstruction," by Smith et al., which deals with a man with basal cell carcinoma of the head necessitating use of a large free latissimus dorsi flap with overlying skin to replace 23 × 23 cm of scalp; fascia under the muscle was used as dural replacement, and titanium strips were criss-crossed to provide support for the scalp.

After resection of invasive neoplasms or trauma, there may be large defects in the scalp, cranium, and dura mater. In the nine cases cited by Barrow et al. (*J. Neurosurg.* 60:305–311, 1984) omental free flaps were taken by celiotomy, and the vascular supply to the omentum was anastomosed to branches of the external carotid artery and to internal or external jugular veins. The cases described involved gunshot wounds of the head, orbit, and face; chronic cavitating frontal sinus infections; resections of scalp invaded by tumor or badly infected and not healing. In some cases, omentum was used to form a base for rib grafts over exposed dura mater. Split-thickness skin grafts used to cover the omentum are not hair bearing, so the patient must use a hairpiece. No complications from laparotomy occurred in these cases.—O.S.

---

**Effects of Mannitol on Blood Volume and Central Hemodynamics in Patients Undergoing Cerebral Aneurysm Surgery**
Anders Rudehill, Michael Lagerkranser, Christer Lindquist, and Emeric Gordon (Karolinska Hosp., Stockholm)
Anesth. Analg. 62:875–880, October 1983                          19–1

---

Mannitol is used to reduce brain volume and intracranial pressure during cerebral aneurysm surgery. It was suggested recently that patients with subarachnoid hemorrhage (SAH) may have low blood volumes. Because SAH can cause disturbances of cerebral autoregulation and the blood-brain barrier, the effects of mannitol infusion on serum osmolality, systemic hemodynamics, and blood volume could affect cerebral hemodynamics unfavorably.

After a mean interval of 12 ± 5 days from SAH diagnosis, 10 patients with a mean age of 47 ± 15 years underwent intracranial aneurysm surgery. A volume of 500 ml of 20% mannitol (100 gm) was infused in 15 minutes after establishment of a circulatory steady state. Observations were made and samples taken for 1 hour at 15-minute intervals. Blood volume was measured prior to mannitol infusion and at intervals I, II, and III. Mannitol dosage varied between 1.0 gm/kg and 2.0 gm/kg. Blood loss during surgery was minimal.

Mean arterial pressure did not change during the investigation. During the 15 minutes between the control period and interval I (end of infusion), pulmonary capillary wedge pressure increased significantly (48%), but at intervals III and IV it was decreased significantly below control values. A significant increase in cardiac index (CI) occurred between the control period and interval I (25%). At intervals III and IV, the CI decreased to levels significantly below control values. No changes in pH, $Pa_{CO_2}$, or $Pa_{O_2}$ occurred; the arterial-mixed venous oxygen content difference varied inversely with CI, resulting in unchanged oxygen uptake. Prior to mannitol infusion, the blood volume was lower than normal (72.3 ± 8.7 ml/kg); it increased significantly to 75.6 ± 14.8 ml/kg at interval I but returned to control levels at interval III. The serum sodium concentration decreased from 135 ± 3 mmol/L to 125 ± 4 mmol/L between control and interval I, and was 129 ± 3 mmol/L at interval IV. Serum osmolality increased from 289 ± 10 mOsm/L to 312 ± 14 mOsm/L between control and interval I, and remained elevated.

There was no correlation between dose and increases in CI. The transient increase in blood volume after mannitol infusion produced a slightly hyperkinetic circulation. After 45 minutes, however, when blood volume returned to less than the preinfusion value, cardiac filling pressures and output were reduced, probably owing to peripheral pooling of blood. An additional decrease in central blood volume that results in further preload reduction could lead to inadequate organ perfusion. This is of concern as postoperative intravascular volume expansion has been advocated in prevention of ischemic complications associated with SAH. Mannitol infusion in intracranial aneurysm surgery should be followed immediately by administration of a plasma expander to achieve and maintain adequate blood volume and cardiac output; use of controlled hypotension later during aneurysm surgery makes this recommendation even more valid.

---

### Reappraisal of Cardiopulmonary Bypass With Deep Hypothermia and Circulatory Arrest for Complex Neurosurgical Operations

William A. Baumgartner, Gerald D. Silverberg, Allen K. Ream, Stuart W. Jamieson, Jean Tarabek, and Bruce A. Reitz (Stanford Univ.)
Surgery 94:242–249, August 1983                    19–2

---

Cardiopulmonary bypass with hypothermia and circulatory arrest can facilitate certain complex neurosurgical procedures for otherwise inoperable lesions such as giant aneurysms and medullary hemangioblastomas. The authors reviewed the results of 15 operations done with cardiopulmonary bypass in 14 patients in a four-year period. The eight women and six men had an average age of 48 years. Most aneurysms arose from the middle cerebral artery. Two patients had medullary hemangioblastomas. Prebypass cooling with a thermal blanket and infusion of cold normal saline is followed by bypass using an oxygenator primed with Ringer's lactate and packed red blood cells. Bypass is begun at flow rates of 40–50 ml/kg/minute. The target temperature is 20 C. Total circulatory arrest is begun when the vascular abnormality is to be attacked. Bypass is resumed at completion of the neurosurgical procedure, with the priming solution at about 20 C, to identify significant bleeding points.

The average cardiopulmonary bypass time was 146 minutes, and the average circulatory arrest time was 21 minutes. Total operating time averaged 7–9 hours. There were no operative deaths, and the intended procedure was achieved in all instances. Permanent complications included hemorrhagic infarction in the posterior fossa and a hemianopsia, after clipping of middle cerebral aneurysms, as well as a stroke due to thrombosis of the residual sac of an aneurysm six months after operation. Seven other complications were transient. The rate of thromboembolism was 29%, ascribed to cessation of circulation and cannulation of iliac veins; current modifications in bypass technique may minimize this type of complication.

The use of deep hypothermia and cardiac arrest permits the neurosurgeon to assess the pathology adequately and promotes the removal of otherwise inoperable lesions. The chief disadvantage of this approach is its effect on coagulation. Thrombocytopenia, probably due to sequestration, occurs in the cooling phase, and platelet dysfunction results from passage through the oxygenator. Bleeding has been controlled by administering cryoprecipitate and factor IX complex after the infusion of platelets, fresh plasma, and protamine sulfate. Closed peripheral cannulation is referable to thoracotomy in these cases.

▶ Intravenous nitroglycerine has been used for controlled hypotension in neurosurgery. Studies by Ghani et al. (*J. Neurosurg.* 58:562–565, 1983) indicate dangers of significant increase in intracranial pressure and decrease in intracranial compliance from use of this drug, which is commonly believed to be predominantly a vasodilator.—O.S.

---

**Hemodilution Anesthesia: A Valuable Aid to Major Cancer Surgery in Children**
Robert T. Schaller, Jr., Joanne Schaller, Alan Morgan, and Eric B. Furman (Univ. of Washington)
Am. J. Surg. 146:79–84, July 1983                                        19–3

---

The authors reviewed results in more than 300 children who were operated on under normovolemic hemodilution anesthesia. The method was developed for use in Jehovah's Witnesses who required major surgery but who refused blood products. Since 1974 it has been used in pediatric cardiac surgery and in spinal surgery for scoliosis. It is considered when loss of more than half the blood volume is anticipated.

The body temperature is lowered to 32 C to reduce metabolic demands. Blood is removed to reduce the hematocrit value to 20%, and each milliliter is replaced with 3 ml of Ringer's lactate containing magnesium, 2 mEq/L. Hypotensive anesthesia is achieved using halothane. Blood lost during surgery is replaced with equal volumes of Ringer's lactate to a hematocrit value of 14%, and donor red blood cells are subsequently used to keep the hematocrit value at this level. When blood loss ceases, the patient's own fresh blood is returned before closing the incision.

Twenty-five pediatric patients had 27 operations for presumed malignant disease using this technique. The mean anesthetic time was 5 hours. Eighteen patients presently were alive without disease at follow-up, but seven had died of their primary tumors. Six patients received packed red blood cells during surgery. The lowest intraoperative hematocrit value was a mean value of 14.3%. Urine excretion was stimulated by furosemide postoperatively. There were only two major anesthetic complications.

The relative lack of complications in these cases supports the safety of hemodilution anesthesia in children. Normovolemic hemodilution can make very difficult operations easier and in some cases might make it possible to perform an operation that otherwise would not be attempted. Most Jehovah's Witnesses will accept the method if the blood is kept moving and in direct contact with the vascular system, and in such cases a special closed-circuit, continuous-flow system is used after reduction of hematocrit to 15%. Donor blood is not given.

▶ Although none of the children operated on in this series had neurosurgical procedures, it seems to me that the technique described could easily be of value in neurosurgery. One of the times when it could be useful, perhaps, would be in operating on children with arteriovenous malformations, especially to avoid the disastrous hypervolemia which occurs after correction of voluminous arteriovenous shunts. In the discussion, Schaller spoke of comparisons with hypotension alone which are in progress. Such information should be most valuable, for the latter is being widely used, especially for aneurysm surgery. Lam and Gelb (*Anesth. Analg.* 62:742–748, 1983) describe a technique for the use of isoflurane, which decreases peripheral resistance while maintaining cardiac output. Desired levels of hypotension (mean ± SEM, 40 ± 1 mm Hg) were reached in about 5 minutes and recovery took little more than 6 minutes. When blood flow studies were carried out in two patients, it was found that cerebral flow increased slightly with intermediate hypotension, decreased 12%–16% during extreme hypotension, and returned to control values with return of normal pressures. All 13 patients had their aneurysms successfully clipped. This new anesthetic agent avoids the myocardial depression associated with halothane and the overshooting of pressures with sodium nitroprusside.—O.S.

---

**Prevention of Air Embolism With Positive End-Expiratory Pressure**
Rand M. Voorhies, Richard A. R. Fraser, and Alan Van Poznak (New York Hosp.-Cornell Med. Center, New York)
Neurosurgery 12:503–506, May 1983                                    19–4

---

Pulmonary air embolism is a potentially life-threatening complication of neurosurgical procedures done with the patient sitting. Positive end-expiratory pressure (PEEP) may be a useful means of preventing pulmonary air embolism in this setting, along with precordial Doppler monitoring, measurements of end-expiratory $CO_2$, and use of the semireclining position. Eighty-one patients, aged 3–76 years were managed in this way during suboccipital craniectomy or cervical spine surgery in 1976–1981. A right atrial catheter was not used. A baseline level of 5 cm $H_2O$ of PEEP was instituted when the patients were positioned. The level of PEEP was monitored by observing an airway pressure meter; levels exceeding 20 cm $H_2O$ were not required. Peak airway pressures did not exceed 35 cm $H_2O$. Blood pressure reductions were managed by volume expansion with 5% dextrose in Ringer's lactate.

Abnormal Doppler signals occurred during surgery in 41 cases, but all cases except one were transient and disappeared when the PEEP was increased. There was no evidence of barotrauma or systemic air embolization in any case, and no intracranial pressure elevations occurred. One patient had a 50% fall in end-tidal $CO_2$ when the abnormal Doppler signal was detected, followed by multiple premature atrial complexes and profound hypotension. The wound was packed with saline-soaked gauze, and the head was lowered. The patient recovered rapidly. Foamy blood was irrigated from the wound when the patient was prone, and a bleeding vein was coagulated.

Positive end-expiratory pressure can be used during neurosurgery to recreate the hemodynamic equivalent of the prone position and reduce the risk of air embolism. The need for right heart catheterization can also be decreased. Administration of PEEP to semireclining patients appears to be safe.

▶ Had the patient with premature atrial complexes and profound hypotension *not* recovered, it might have been difficult for the surgeon to justify *not* emplacing a right atrial catheter! An article by Albin et al. (*Neurosurgery* 3:380–384, 1978), which is mentioned in their references, contends that there are dangers of pulmonary embolism even in the prone position, so the argument that PEEP induces hemodynamic changes mimicking those in the prone position might not convince a jury.

An analysis of the cardiovascular responses in the seated position has been carried out by Marshall et al. (*Anesth. Analg.* 62:648–653, 1983). Anesthesia was induced with 60% nitrous oxide in oxygen supplemented with pancuronium 0.1 mg/kg intravenously: Supplemental anesthesia was administered to four groups of six subjects as follows: enflurane 0.7% end-tidal, halothane 0.4% end-tidal, innovar 0.1 ml/kg, and morphine 0.5 mg/kg. The authors found that morphine–nitrous oxide technique resulted in the least impairment of cardiovascular performance when patients were placed in the seated position before surgical stimulation. The legs were wrapped from toes to groins with elastic bandages, and knees were elevated to heart level. Measurements were taken when the patients were supine, in the position for operation, and an hour after skin incision. The changes that may have occurred after more prolonged surgery were not discussed.

High-dose fentanyl-oxygen anesthesia is well established in cardiac surgery and is proposed by Shupak et al. (*Anesthesiology* 58:579–582, 1983) for use in neurosurgery as well. The 10 patients studied were operated on in the sitting position for suboccipital craniectomies. Radial artery catheter, Doppler applied to the precordium, thermodilution balloon-tipped catheter in the pulmonary artery, ulnar nerve stimulation to test neuromuscular blockade, measurement of temperature and expired $CO_2$ levels, and a two-lead EEG were used in addition to the usual ECG and other monitoring. Intravenous fentanyl was given before tracheal intubation, and increased when systolic pressures increased more than 20% above preinduction levels. A single dose of 20 mg of furosemide was given intravenously during craniotomy. In the postoperative period, intravenous naloxone was used first by bolus injection and then by continuous infusion to maintain respiration at greater than 12 per minute. Absorption of epinephrine used in infiltration of the scalp could be detected by peripheral vasodilatation and was omitted in subsequent patients. On the whole, the technique provided satisfactory anesthesia and reliable reversibility without impairment of cardiovascular status in 10 neurosurgical patients (aged 35–65 years and without organic cardiac disease).

Du Toit et al. (*S. Afr. Med. J.* 63:378–379, 1983) ascribed quadriplegia during posterior fossa exploration to venous air embolism; certainly the latter did occur, as shown by sudden drop in blood pressure, elevation of central venous pressure, and drop of end-tidal $CO_2$ concentration. Aspiration yielded 130 ml of air from the central venous catheter. What they did not consider, apparently, was the possibility that the quadriplegia (which eventually improved for the legs but not the arms) may have been due to changes implicit in the sitting position for the removal of vermis hemangioblastoma. Certainly, similar problems with the cervical spinal cord have been reported without the air embolism and are very possibly due to compression of the spinal cord by osteophytes, especially in the presence of a narrowed spinal canal.—O.S.

---

### Precision Resection of Intra-Axial CNS Lesions by CT-Based Stereotactic Craniotomy and Computer Monitored $CO_2$ Laser

P. J. Kelly, B. Kall, S. Goerss, and G. J. Alker Jr. (SUNY, Buffalo)
Acta Neurochir. (Wien) 68:1–9, 1983　　　　　　　　　　　　19–5

---

An open stereotactic method was developed for reconstructing a tumor volume in stereotactic space from computed tomographic (CT) data and removing the tumor by $CO_2$ laser vaporization. The position of the laser beam in relation to the tumor is monitored by computer and displayed on a terminal in the operating room. Contrast-enhanced CT scanning is carried out with the patient's head in a stereotactic device, and the tumor volume is reconstructed from the digitized CT contours (Fig 19–1). Surgery is carried out after CT scanning as the CT slices are displayed. The tumor volume can be sliced orthogonal to any specified surgical view line. The tumor is vaporized slice by slice using 65–85 W of defocused laser power in a continuous mode.

Twenty-four patients underwent 26 computer-assisted stereotactic laser microsurgical procedures. Twenty-three patients had deep-seated tumors, and one had an arteriovenous malformation. The tumors were in such poorly accessible sites as the thalamus, basal ganglia, and third ventricle.

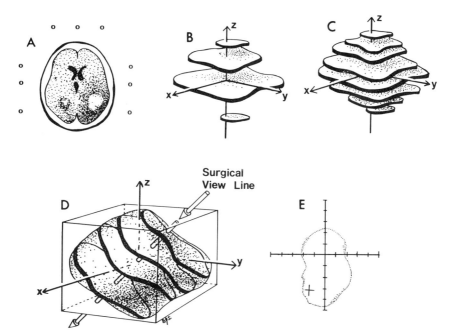

**Fig 19–1.**—Creation of tumor volume in stereotactic space from digitized computed tomographic contours. **A,** computed tomographic scan with reference artifacts and tumor outline digitized by surgeon. **B,** digitized tumor outlines are suspended in stereotactic space. **C,** interpolation program creates intermediate slices at 1-mm intervals. **D,** tumor solid is sliced in plane orthogonal to specified surgical view line. **E,** tumor slices are displayed on graphics terminal in operating room; position of laser beam is indicated by cursor *(cross).* (Courtesy of Kelly, P.J., et al.: Acta Neurochir. [Wien] 68:1–9, 1983.)

Twelve patients were improved a week after surgery, and seven were unchanged. Five of 23 patients had CT evidence of residual tumor. No patient with metastatic tumor or meningioma has had a local recurrence.

This method has proved useful in maintaining a three-dimensional surgical orientation for resecting intra-axial neoplasms from neurologically important regions of the brain. Lesions can be approached through relatively nonessential tissue. The $CO_2$ laser provides a precise, selective means of removing the lesions. The initial long-term results in cases of primary glial neoplasia have been disappointing. Aggressive adjuvant therapy, such as photoradiation, may be helpful in these cases. The best results have been obtained in treating tumors with distinct histologic boundaries.

▶ There are other stereotactic apparatuses for use with CT scanners, of course. The same issue contains a description of a modified Riechert-Mundinger device for this purpose (Sturm et al.: *Acta Neurochir.* [*Wien*] 68:11–17, 1983) as well as Patil's technical note on a rotary stereotactic system to be used with CT (ibid. 68:19–26, 1983).

Kelly et al. (*Neurosurgery* 14:172–177, 1984) describe a technique for putting data into a three-dimensional computer matrix corresponding to the coordinate system of a stereotactic frame located in the operating room. The data are derived from stereotactic computerized tomography and from digitized stereotactic angiographic data. Under local anesthesia, an incision in the scalp is made before inserting a guide tube resting on the skull, followed by a twist drill hole and insertion of an insulated biopsy cannula. A 1-mm cup forceps is inserted to obtain the biopsy. Bleeding within is managed by unipolar coagulation applied to biopsy forceps or to the uninsulated stylet. The most numerous tumor diagnoses were glioblastoma (23), astrocytoma (25), metastasis (13), meningioma (6), and infarction (4). Twenty tumors were in the thalamus; 9 in basal ganglia, and 20 in central areas of the brain. The advantages to the described system include the ability to do the biopsy in the sterile arena of the operating room, not in the radiography suite.

In the 1984 YEAR BOOK, articles appeared on $CO_2$ and Nd:YAG lasers. Wharen et al. published two articles on the latter in the *Journal of Neurosurgery* (60:531–539 and 540–547, 1984). There is a selective absorption of Nd:YAG light by hemoglobin, so it can selectively heat blood vessels rather than brain. Experiments showed that when short intermittent pulses were used, surrounding brain was not damaged, which permitted use of the laser as an adjunct in hemostasis for many neurosurgical procedures. It was used to help in resection of 10 cases of arteriovenous malformation, especially to define the plane between malformation and brain, coagulation of dural components, and achieving hemostasis of the bed after the malformation was removed. It was not effective in controlling high-flow bleeding from thin-walled vessels in the deep portion. The fiber-optic cable light delivery system allows excellent mobility of the handpiece, but the protective laser-light filters reduce light available to the surgeon. The Nd:YAG laser can be useful and it can be used safely, but its overall benefit in the resection of arteriovenous malformations awaits further refinements and experience. Analysis of the use of the argon laser is made in the following abstract.—O.S.

---

### Use of the Argon Surgical Laser in Neurosurgery

Stephen K. Powers, Michael S. B. Edwards, James E. Boggan, Lawrence H. Pitts, Philip H. Gutin, Yoshio Hosobuchi, John E. Adams, and Charles B. Wilson

J. Neurosurg. 60:523–530, March 1984                    19–6

---

The authors reviewed the results of neurosurgery done with the surgical argon laser in 68 patients. The laser was used when a brain or cord tumor grew in a location that made a surgical approach difficult (e.g., the brain base) or was hypervascular. The laser also was used to make dorsal root entry zone lesions and to produce spinal cord fenestration for syringomyelia. Advantages of the argon laser include the availability of a fiber-optic delivery system, a spot size that can be varied continuously between 0.15 and 1.5 mm, a single aiming and treatment beam, transmission of laser light through aqueous media (e.g., irrigating fluid and cerebrospinal fluid), and better hemostasis than is obtained by conventional methods. Protective eyewear must be worn by operating room personnel, but not when looking through the surgical microscope.

The argon laser was used to resect 16 extra-axial supratentorial and infratentorial tumors that were close or attached to important neural structures. The tumors were readily removed with minimal manipulation and retraction by alternate gutting of the interior with high-power density and irradiating the capsule with low-power density. Residual tumor attached to cranial nerves was vaporized using short pulses and a beam having a small diameter. Intra-axial tumors were removed with less manipulation of surrounding brain tissue than is necessary during tumor excision. In the treatment of intraspinal tumors, pial surface vessels were rapidly and efficiently coagulated with the argon laser before performing myelotomy with the laser. The creation of dorsal root entry zone lesions relieved pain in most patients. Also, the laser was effectively used to perform syringotomy in patients with syringomyelia.

The argon laser is limited chiefly by a relatively low power output, making excision of large tumors difficult; it has not been helpful in malignant gliomas or with arteriovenous malformations. The $CO_2$ laser can be applied in these patients, and the argon laser used for fine microsurgical work not requiring high-power densities.

▶ A fine review of the subject of lasers in neurological surgery by Edwards et al. appeared in the *Journal of Neurosurgery* (59:555–566, 1983). Particularly useful for the neophyte are the diagrams of the changes in focus needed for incision, vaporization, and coagulation. A table summarizes well the characteristics of the three major types of lasers discussed: $CO_2$, Nd:YAG, and argon, with regard to wavelength, power range, portability, maintenance record, cost, and types of delivery systems. Of interest is a table comparing experience with the $CO_2$ and argon lasers with regard to benefits derived; the $CO_2$ laser is considered very helpful (results better than conventional microsurgical technique) for acoustic neuromas and meningiomas, helpful for gliomas and metastases (results equivalent to those expected with standard techniques), unhelpful for dorsal root entry zones, and of dubious benefit for an axillary neuroma. In contrast, the argon laser is very helpful for dorsal root entry zone lesions, spinal intramedullary tumors, meningiomas; helpful for syringomyelia and cerebral metastases; not helpful for malignant gliomas and an arteriovenous malformation. The authors stress the need for proper training and experience before the laser can be used to its fullest advantage.

A comparison of laser systems has been made by Clark et al. (*Otolaryngol. Head Neck Surg.* 92:73–79, 1984). Selection should be based on principles of power density, radiant exposure, and selective absorption. The effect of the $CO_2$ laser is purely thermal at the tissue surface. Both argon and Nd:YAG lasers are pigment dependent and may penetrate tissues to variable levels before absorption and conversion to thermal energy. The $CO_2$ laser can achieve much higher power densities than the other two. Since there is a discrepancy between focused spot size and actual lesion size, the resulting lesions are essentially equal in size. The $CO_2$ beam requires a relatively dry field; the argon beam does not. Hemostasis is enhanced with the latter. No one laser is best for *all* procedures.

Jain, who has written a book (*Handbook of Laser Neurosurgery*, Springfield,

III., Charles C Thomas, 1983) also has contributed a chapter on the Nd:YAG laser in neurosurgery to a book (*Neodymium-NAG Laser in Medicine and Surgery,* Joffe et al. [eds.] New York, Elsevier, 1983). He believes this laser is indicated for microvascular surgery (repair of blood vessels and sutureless anastomosis), vascular anomalies in the central nervous system, removal of meningiomas, and in ventriculoscopy with coagulation of the choroid plexus as well as third ventriculostomy for hydrocephalus. His review of the use of lasers in neurosurgery appears in *Lasers in Surgery and Medicine* (2:217–230, 1983).—O.S.

## Percutaneous Insertion of Peritoneal Shunt Catheters With Use of the Veress Needle
Curtis Lockhart, Warren Selman, Gerard Rodziewicz, and Robert F. Spetzler
J. Neurosurg. 60:444–446, February 1984                                                     19–7

The hazards of percutaneous introduction of peritoneal shunt catheters have prevented the widespread use of the procedure. The Veress needle, used to enter the peritoneal cavity for laparoscopy, was found to be readily adaptable to the percutaneous insertion of intraperitoneal shunts. The design of the needle, a cutting device having a blunt-tipped inner cannula, permits its advancement through the body wall tissues with minimal risk of bowel perforation. When the blunt end of the needle meets resistance, it is forced into the needle shaft, allowing the needle to cut tissue; the spring-loaded blunt end then readvances (Fig 19–2).

The bladder is emptied by a catheter before making an infraumbilical stab wound and tunneling the catheter subcutaneously to the abdomen. The Veress needle, covered with a no. 12 intravenous catheter, is then advanced to the linea alba and thrust through the fascia and peritoneum. A guide wire is advanced through the cannula; the intravenous catheter is replaced by 8-F peel-away catheter and obturator; the obturator is withdrawn, and the peritoneal tubing is placed in the abdomen. The peel-away catheter then is separated, leaving the shunt tubing in the abdomen. The incision is closed with a single subcutaneous suture.

The safety and efficacy of the Veress needle have been documented in

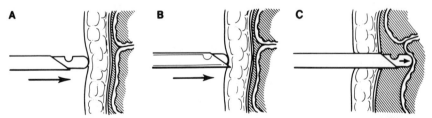

Fig 19–2.—Diagram shows Veress needle penetrating the abdominal wall. **A,** the needle is positioned against the skin above the linea alba. **B,** against the pressure and resistance of the skin and fascia, the outer cutting edge advances. **C,** after penetration of the peritoneum and loss of resistance, the blunt tip advances and protects the intraperitoneal contents from the cutting edge. (Courtesy of Lockhart, C., et al.: J. Neurosurg. 60:444–446, February 1984.)

large series. This technique of shunt placement has not been used in patients with abdominal scars, although percutaneous laparoscopy has been performed in patients who had previous abdominal surgery.

▶ The Veress needle has been used extensively to enter the peritoneal cavity for laparoscopy and also to enter for peritoneal lavage after blunt abdominal trauma.—O.S.

---

**Clinical Utility of Allogeneic Skull Disks in Human Craniotomy**
Donald J. Prolo, Robert V. Gutierrez, Jeffrey S. DeVine, and Sally A. Oklund
Neurosurgery 14:183–186, February 1984                                    19–8

An ideal material for cranioplasty would provide mechanical and biochemical properties equivalent to those of autogeneic skull, give an esthetically acceptable form, and provoke no sensitivity reactions. The authors evaluated the use of disks obtained from sterilized human cadaver skull in 45 patients requiring the repair of 115 burr hole defects. From 1 to 6 disks per patient were placed in all areas of the calvarium. The patients were followed up for six months to five years. Disks 15 mm in diameter were removed from cadavers aged 15–50 years who had died accidentally or of noncommunicable disease. The samples were reduced to thicknesses of 4–6 mm, washed with deionized water, and sterilized with "cold cycle" ethylene oxide gas before being lyophilized. A small ledge of bone near the dura mater is created to form a shelf on which the skull disk rests. It is secured in position with no. 28 stainless steel wire passed through opposing holes in the skull and adjacent skull flap.

The allogeneic disks were used in patients aged 10–88 years who underwent surgery for aneurysm, arteriovenous malformation, tumor, trauma, or infection. Frontal and right-sided operations predominated. Twenty-six patients with 64 implanted disks were followed for more than one year. No infections occurred, and none of the disks was rejected or resorbed. Formation of an osteoconductive matrix for revascularization was followed by new bone formation. On skull radiography the disks gradually became indistinguishable from the adjacent host cranium, and appositional new bone formation was seen within the disk in a patient who died three months after craniotomy.

Human cadaver allogeneic bone disks are useful and safe in filling burr hole defects after routine craniotomy. They are readily implanted during wound closure and eventually become living bone. The successful use of these small implants may be predictive of the likely biologic response to the use of larger sections of cadaver skull for supplanting skull defects.

---

**Hemispherectomy for Seizures Revisited**
Theodore Rasmussen (Montreal Neurological Inst. and Hosp.)
Can. J. Neurol. Sci. 10:71–78, May 1983                                    19–9

Superficial cerebral hemosiderosis develops in as many as a third of patients having hemispherectomy for seizures and has led to considerable reluctance to perform the operation even though it is highly effective in patients with medically refractory seizures associated with hemiplegia. Persistent intracranial bleeding presumably is involved in the late complications of hemispherectomy. Red blood cells may gradually seep into the operative cavity over a period of years from trivial jolts to the head or abrupt changes in intracranial pressure from coughing or sneezing. However, the author did not encounter the complication in 40 patients having two thirds or three fourths of a cerebral hemisphere removed who were followed up for four years or longer. A slight rise in intracranial pressure persisted in one patient, followed by cerebrospinal fluid (CSF) rhinorrhea, ventriculitis, and death. Another had a closed cyst in the removal cavity and died suddenly of brain stem herniation. Nine of 27 previous hemispherectomized patients had had superficial cerebral hemosiderosis on follow-up for a comparable period. The efficacy of the procedure, however, has been lessened; only 45% of patients were seizure free, compared with 59% of the patients in the hemispherectomy series.

In the present surgical procedure, the remaining segment of the involved hemisphere is disconnected from the rest of the brain by sectioning the white matter down to the medial pial surface, resulting in a functionally complete, but anatomically subtotal, hemispherectomy. Six of 8 patients have been free of seizures for two to six years after this operation. One of 72 other patients who have had a hemispherectomy carried out with preservation of about half of the bad hemisphere has possibly had minimal superficial cerebral hemosiderosis. A few patients have had a persistent increase in intracranial pressure due to inadequate absorption of CSF. Shunting is indicated if the effect lasts beyond the third or fourth postoperative week, even if the pressure rise is minimal. The surgery continues to be effective in reducing seizures.

The risk-benefit ratio of the functionally complete, anatomically subtotal hemispherectomy appears to be quite favorable, and the procedure seems indicated in seizure patients who have near-maximal or maximal hemiplegia and high-grade or complete homonymous hemianopia and whose seizures are a significant handicap despite appropriate drug therapy.

▶ See also the abstract below of the article on modification of hemispherectomy technique.—O.S.

---

### Hemispherectomy: A Modification
C. B. T. Adams (Radcliffe Infirm., Oxford, England)
J. Neurol. Neurosurg. Psychiatry 46:617–619, July 1983        19–10

---

Hemispherectomy probably is the best surgical treatment for epilepsy, but delayed hemorrhagic complications have stopped use of the procedure. Bleeding into the operative cavity presumably was the basic cause of complications. A subdural membrane may develop when blood is deposited on the inner dural surface, as in chronic subdural hematoma, and may bleed intermittently, spontaneously, or from minor trauma. Unlike other subdural hematomas, the cavity communicates with the ventricular system via an enlarged foramen of Monro, and the ependyma and subarachnoid spaces are subject to frequent minor bleeding. Iron is deposited in phagocytes in the ependyma and pia, producing granular ependymitis and superficial siderosis. This results in chronic meningeal irritation, elevated intracranial pressure from obstructive hydrocephalus, and cerebellar and cranial nerve abnormalities due to superficial siderosis.

It seems reasonable to attempt to prevent formation of a subdural hematoma in the operative cavity and to impede communication between the cavity and the ventricular system. Very careful hemostasis is necessary at the time of surgery. The dura can be mobilized and sutured down to the falx, tentorium, and the dura lining the floors of the middle and anterior fossae. The subdural cavity is insulated from the ventricular system by obstructing the ipsilateral foramen of Monro with a muscle plug. The septum pellucidum is kept intact. The remaining choroid plexus on the side operated on must be completely destroyed.

Four modified operations have been done since February 1980. All patients stopped having seizures and had improved behavior. Computed tomography scans gave evidence of effective insulation of the subdural cavity from the remaining ventricles. Further follow-up will show whether delayed hemorrhagic complications are avoided by this modified hemispherectomy.

► The late complications of hemispherectomy have given this procedure a bad name. Adams gives the short history of the development of the operation he is describing, starting with the work of P. J. E. Wilson (*Brain* 93:147, 1970). I mentioned this modification of hemispherectomy by Wilson and Ashley (*J. Neurol. Neurosurg. Psychiatry* 38:493–499, 1975) in the 1977 YEAR BOOK (pp. 438–439). Shortly thereafter I had the opportunity to do another hemispherectomy for uncontrollable epilepsy, and thought I would avoid some of the problems of stripping dura mater by using frozen dried dura mater sewed to the falx and the basal meninges to act as a barrier to movement of the cerebral hemisphere that remained. Alas, follow-up CT scanning showed eventual disappearance of this septum, presumably because it had not had the opportunity of being replaced by ingrowing cells because it was so large. I doubt very much that the muscle occludes the foramen of Monro for very long; it certainly doesn't stay long when used around an aneurysm.—O.S.

## Arthrography of the Cervical Facet Joints

Michel A. Dory (Clinique St. Pierre, Ottignies, Belgium)
Radiology 148:379–382, August 1983                                                     19–11

Disk and facet joint disorders can produce similar symptoms, and it often is difficult to determine the true origin of cervical pain. The author performed cervical facet joint arthrograpy, during steroid injection, on 21 joints in 14 patients with noninflammatory disorders. Three patients had repeated injections at intervals of 1–12 months. Medical and physical measures had failed to relieve pain in all cases. Significant disk disease was excluded by plain roentgenography, and severe nerve root compression was excluded by electromyography. A posterior approach was used, with a 22-gauge needle passed under fluoroscopic control. Passage of the needle through the joint capsule was usually felt, and injury to the vertebral artery or nerve root was avoided. Metrizamide was used in the first cases, but methylglucamine diatrizoate presently is used. Lidocaine is not necessary. Triamcinolone diacetate was injected after the reaspiration of contrast medium.

The distended facet joint capsule rarely ruptured after arthrography, but two patients had epidural leakage, and opacification of the foramen occurred in two others. The thickness of the joint cartilage could also be appreciated. Nine patients reported signficant pain relief, generally occurring within two days of the procedure and lasting for as long as 13 months.

Although clinical results of the steroid treatment are difficult to assess, the procedure has been helpful in positioning the needle for steroid injection and in confirming the presence of joint abnormality. Improvement may be likelier if pain is stimulated during distention of the facet joint. Injected steroids appear to be as useful in cervical facet syndrome as in lumbar facet syndrome.

▶ Dr. Ronald Pawl comments: "By the author's own admission, this is a hazardous approach to the joint, since the needle might penetrate through the joint and end up in the vertebral artery or the nerve root. My own experience has been that it is much simpler to anesthetize the joint from the lateral approach, coming in behind the vertebral artery, with the patient in the lateral decubitus position, and comfortable. My experience has also been quite variable as to patient response from this injection in the cervical region where relief is much less reliable than in patients who have had lumbar facet injections. Epidural steroid injections seem to be more effective, at least in relieving symptoms that appear to be coming from facet arthropathy." Dr. Pawl published a detailed description of his technique in *Surgery Annual* (9:391–408, 1977).—O.S.

---

**Bilateral Facet to Spinous Process Fusion: A New Technique for Posterior Spinal Fusion After Trauma**
David W. Cahill, Roberto Bellegarrigue, and Thomas B. Ducker (Univ. of Maryland)
Neurosurgery 13:1–4, July 1983                                                   19–12

---

Routine interspinous fusion is inadequate where one or both facets are fractured (Fig 19–3) or the posterior neural arch is disrupted in patients with fracture-dislocation of the cervical spine. The authors encountered four cases in which facet dislocation recurred after interspinous wiring

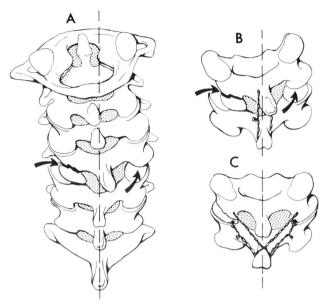

Fig 19–3.—**A,** artist's conception of unilateral facet fracture of C4 with rotational dislocation. **B,** routine interspinous wiring fails to provide adequate rotational stability, allowing redislocation despite intact fusion wires. **C,** bilateral facet to spinous process wiring of C4 to C5 provides excellent stability against rotational as well as anterior horizontal displacement. (Courtesy of Cahill, D.W., et al.: Neurosurgery 13:1–4, July 1983.)

and fusion and developed a new method for use in these cases. It is based on bilateral facet-to-spine wire loops. Loops of double-braided 22-gauge or 24-gauge steel wire are placed through perforations in the upper facets and through or beneath an intact spinous process one or two segments below. Routine interspinous wiring also may be useful in some cases. Pieces of corticocancellous bone are placed over the remaining posterior elements to assure bony fusion.

Twenty-five patients with facet dislocation or flexion-compression injury have had bilateral facet-to-spine wiring and fusion. The 18 having flexion-extension radiography three to four months postoperatively all showed stable fusion and excellent alignment. No patient deteriorated neurologically after fusion. The entire spectrum of deficits was represented in this series. No wound infections or hematomas have occurred, although prophylactic antibiotics and drains are not routinely used.

Facet-to-spinous process wiring preserves uninjured facet joint capsules below the level of injury, in contrast to interfacet wiring. The procedure can be combined with laminectomy without compromising the results of the fusion. The long-term results remain to be assessed, but early mobilization without a halo vest and ring apparatus and the assurance of a mechanically stable arthrodesis with alignment under direct visualization appear to be advantageous.

**Posterior Stabilization With an Interlaminar Clamp in Cervical Injuries: Technical Note and Review of the Long-Term Experience With the Method**
Renn O. Holness, William S. Huestis, William J. Howes, and Roland A. Langille (Dalhousie Univ., Halifax, Nova Scotia, Canada)
Neurosurgery 14:318–322, March 1984                                                   19–13

Early internal fixation with a stainless steel clamp was used to correct posterior cervical spine instability. The clamp is applied to the adjoining laminae of the involved vertebrae in patients with cervical subluxation or dislocation when there is significant radiologic evidence of posterior instability and minimal or no vertebral body involvement. The ideal situation is a dislocation caused by a ligamentous tear only; however, a linear fracture of the laminae or facets is not a contraindication as long as the pedicles are intact. Closed reduction usually is achieved with skull traction before surgery. Open reduction is done first if the facets are locked. If a nerve root deficit is present and subluxation is more marked on one side, a hemilaminotomy and root decompression can be done before applying the clamp. If a laminar or facet fracture is present, the clamp is applied to the nonfractured side. A cervical collar is used for three months postoperatively.

Fifty-one consecutive adults underwent this operation in a 10-year period. Most were injured in auto accidents and had posterior instability as the major skeletal defect. Twelve patients had bilateral dislocations with grade III–IV slippage. Seven had minor chip fractures of a vertebral body, but none had significant compression or vertebral body disruption. Twenty-two patients had linear fractures of the laminae or facet joints. Two early patients required reoperation for replacement of slipped clamps. No patient had neurologic deterioration after surgery. An elderly quadriplegic patient had fatal pulmonary embolism. No infections resulted from the presence of the clamps. No patient had recurrent instability because of delayed clamp slippage. Except for three quadriplegic patients, all of those followed up returned to work. Bony fusion was documented in all patients followed up for more than four years. No patient had delayed pain attributable to the clamp.

Posterior stabilization with the interlaminar steel clamp gives satisfactory long-term results in patients with cervical spine injuries. Reduction is maintained without the need for extensive external immobilization or for additional added bone, and fusion eventually occurs.

---

**Methyl Methacrylate Stabilization of the Cervical Spine**
Charles R. Clark, Kristaps J. Keggi, and Manobar M. Panjabi
J. Bone Joint Surg. (Am.) 66-A:40–46, January 1984                                    19–14

Methyl methacrylate is being used increasingly to stabilize the cervical spine. The authors reviewed results in 52 patients, mean age 57, who had

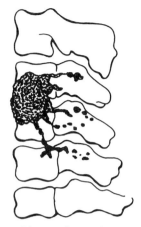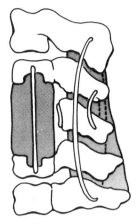

Fig 19–4.—Schematic diagram depicts metastatic carcinoma affecting the anterior and posterior elements of the cervical spine (producing an unstable, high-risk spine) and the construct to stabilize the spine. Posterior fusion, carried out first to provide stability, is followed by anterior decompression and fusion. (Courtesy of Clark, C.R., et al.: J. Bone Joint Surg. [Am.] 66-A:40–46, January 1984.)

cervical spine stabilization with methacrylate in a 10-year period. The most common diagnoses were malignant disease, fracture, and rheumatoid arthritis. Patients were followed up for an average of four years, excluding those who died within a year after surgery. All of the patients had significant neck pain preoperatively and many had neural symptoms. Twenty-four patients had objective neural deficits. The most common procedures were posterior cervical fusion and combined posterior cervical fusion, anterior vertebral body resection, and interbody fusion (Fig 19–4). No patient required rigid postoperative immobilization. Bone grafting was also done in most of the patients with fractures or rheumatoid arthritis.

Wound healing problems were avoided by use of a strong, interrupted closure of the ligamentum nuchae and by leaving the skin staples in place for about three weeks. No complications resulted from use of the methyl methacrylate itself. All patients had solid fixation, and no pseudarthroses occurred. One patient had an asymptomatic fracture of the methyl methacrylate mass without gross instability. All of the tumor patients who were followed up had a solid surgical construct clinically and radiographically, as did the fracture patients and those with rheumatoid arthritis. Most patients with cervical spondylosis had significant symptomatic improvement after surgery.

Methyl methacrylate can be used as an adjuvant to surgical stabilization of the cervical spine in patients with cord injury and bowel or bladder dysfunction or anesthesia who tolerate a halo vest or cast poorly. Cement also is used in elderly and debilitated patients who may not tolerate prolonged bed rest or the use of a halo vest. Such patients may be severely osteopenic, and conventional methods of stabilization may be inadequate. Alcoholic patients who are at risk of delirium tremens or who are non-compliant also can benefit from the internal stability provided by methyl methacrylate.

## Conservative Lumbar Laminectomy: Technique and Results
C. Gros, P. Frerebeau, J. M. Privat, J. Benezech, and M. Guillen
Neurochirurgie 29:207–209, 1983                                                    19–15

The authors introduce a procedure that is aimed at perfect reconstitution of lumbar musculature and is based on three years of experience with 200 cases.

With the patient lying on his or her left side, the paravertebral muscles of the right side are separated from the spinous processes and the right laminae. The spinous processes are then cut at their base, strong retractors providing wide exposure of the laminae (Fig 19–5). The resection must extend to the adjacent spinous processes above and below. Retraction allows as wide an exposure as necessary, and postoperative reconstruction is excellent. Reconstruction is achieved on two levels: on the aponeurotic level, silk sutures are used to bring the lumbar aponeurosis of the right side together with the intact left, which is reinforced by its spinous processes; this is followed by rejoining the left and right muscular masses by means of silk sutures passing between the spinous processes for support from the opposing side. The patient is generally ambulatory on the fourth or fifth day. The back retains its normal appearance, and the spinous processes seem to regain their normal position and stability.

▶ Unfortunately, I fail to find any practical justification for this unusual procedure in the text other than "to obtain a perfect reconstruction of the lumbar muscles." Some reduction in "dead space" occurs, since it is occupied instead

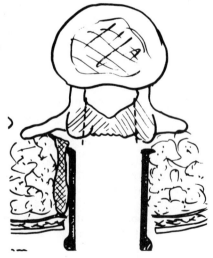

Fig 19–5.—Retractors provide wide exposure of the laminae. (Courtesy of Gros, C., et al.: Neurochirurgie 29:207–209, 1983.)

by the spinous process, securely attached to the paraspinal muscles on one side (and hence not likely to push on the dural sac, unless the latter protrudes posteriorly because of the laminectomy). Risks of later trauma that might impel the unattached bony spinous process against the dural sac and its contents are not discussed.—O.S.

## Combined Reconstruction of Vertebral and Carotid Artery in One Single Procedure

Fernando G. Diaz, James I. Ausman, R. A. de los Reyes, Jeffrey Pearce, Carl Shrontz, Bharat Mehta, Suresh Patel, and Manuel Dujovny (Henry Ford Hosp., Detroit)
Neurosurgery 12:629–635, June 1983                                    19–16

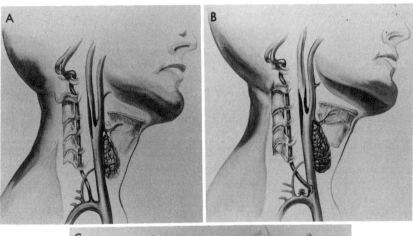

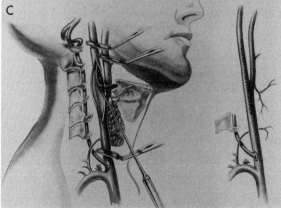

Fig 19–6.—Surgical procedure: **A,** stenotic lesions located at the origins of the internal carotid artery and the vertebral artery (VA). **B,** the proximal VA is ligated and clipped at its origin, and the detached VA reimplanted on the common carotid artery. **C,** the completed standard carotid endarterectomy maintains flow via the transposed VA. (Courtesy of Diaz, F.G., et al.: Neurosurgery 12:629–635, June 1983.)

Patients with vertebrobasilar insufficiency often have multiple areas of involvement of the extracranial circulation. The authors performed vertebral artery origin transposition and carotid endarterectomy ipsilaterally at the same session in eight patients. All had repeated episodes of vertebrobasilar insufficiency and angiographic evidence of internal carotid stenosis ipsilateral to the vertebral artery origin of stenosis. The five men and three women were aged 60–73 years. Seven patients had proximal vertebral artery lesions and one had severe bilateral subclavian artery stenosis proximal to the vertebral artery origins. The procedure is illustrated in Figure 19–6. Heparin was given before and during the operation. An end-to-side vertebral artery–common carotid anastomosis was completed before standard carotid endarterectomy was carried out.

Seven patients were completely relieved of symptoms. Dizziness persisted in a patient who also had a midbasilar stenosis, but his syncope and vertigo disappeared. Angiography showed complete restoration of flow through the vertebral system in all cases, with no evidence of stenosis. Only minor carotid artery changes were noted. All eight patients resumed their normal activities without restriction. Follow-up was for 3–24 months.

Simultaneous reconstruction of the vertebral and carotid circulations at a single operation can generally be completed within three hours and obviates the need for another operation in patients with lesions at both sites. No evidence of added surgical morbidity was observed. Blood flow is reestablished in both the anterior and posterior circulations simultaneously.

# 20 Pediatric and Congenital Disorders

▶ ↓ It is not possible to open these pages to a discussion of the topics addressed by the article, "Early Management and Decision Making for the Treatment of Myelomeningocele" (Gross et al.: *Pediatrics* 72:450–458, 1983). The opinions require so much space (at least two sides would have to be discussed) as to make the discussion endless. Clearly there is a group of doctors and their allies who believe that all such children should have immediate operation; Gross et al. consider that there is no emergency, that the sac can be closed after several days as well as on day 1, and that the extra time gives opportunity for a team approach to be employed before operation instead of after operation, as is commonly the case. The article by Gross et al. deals with evaluation of 69 infants in a five-year period. In my view, this is too short a period to make an evaluation of the process used; what is needed is a team evaluation after 15–20 years, to assess the impact on the growth and development of the child—and of the family. The Oklahoma group have had available a facility for the care of those children who were not operated on, and the 24 who received only supportive care all died by age 189 days. The authors refer, however, to a case in which the parents were influenced by a cousin who lived to age seven years with massive hydrocephalus, so clearly there are factors other than purely medical ones that vary from one part of the country to another. (These considerations, I am informed, include the fact that in some states untreated infants with hydrocephalus cannot be cared for by the state unless a shunt is put in place!) So the problems continue, and a resolution is not immediately apparent.

The ethical arguments concerning the treatment of spina bifida continue, as is evident from the so-called Baby Doe legislation. In consideration of 119 infants with operated cases of spina bifida, Lapras, and coworkers in Lyon, France (*Neurochirurgie* 29:125–127, 1983) found that a nondirective attitude towards the parents resulted in a total failure to recognize the risk of recurrence. A consequence of absence of special care for the next pregnancies was a recurrence of cases in four families. Since 1979, all parents have had genetic counseling, permitting the birth of 25 normal infants. In one instance, prenatal diagnosis revealed a fetal meningomyelocele and motivated a therapeutic abortion. The authors speak of a trial of polyvitamin therapy for two months before and at least two months after conception as a possible effective prophylaxis against spina bifida aperta; the evidence is not in as yet.

Early experience with ventriculoamniotic shunts appears to favor benefit to the fetus with hydrocephalus, according to Bland et al. (*Am. J. Obstet. Gynecol.* 147:781–784, 1983). They report a complication hitherto unreported: *Neisseria gonorrhoeae* ventriculitis. Based on their experience, the authors suggest close monitoring for pathogens of the cervix uteri, delivery prior to rupture of the amniotic sac, and cultures of shunt and ventricular fluid at delivery. The

infant was treated with penicillin successfully, and the hydrocephalus ultimately treated with ventriculoperitoneal shunt. Development at age four
months was said to be normal. The ethical aspects of such operations in utero
cannot, in my opinion, be adequately discussed without long-term follow-up
of not only the child but also of the family unit.

Injection of kaolin into the cisterna of fetal lambs and monkeys produced
enlarged heads with hydrocephalus, in experiments by Nakayama et al. (*J.
Pediatr. Surg.* 18:331–338, 1983). Fibrosis of the leptomeninges and subarachnoid spaces around the fourth ventricle were demonstrated at postmortem examination. Gray matter was relatively well preserved, while white matter was
severely attenuated. This model mimics the clinical and pathologic picture seen
in human infants and should permit experiments to demonstrate the possible
utility of ventricular drainage early in gestation of fetuses in whom hydrocephalus can be demonstrated by obstetrical sonography.—O.S.

---

### Serial Sonography of Posthemorrhagic Ventricular Dilatation and Poren-cephaly After Intracranial Hemorrhage in the Preterm Neonate

Arthur C. Fleischer, Alastair A. Hutchison, Albert L. Bundy, James E. Machin,
Gary A. Thieme, Mildred T. Stahlman, and A. Everette James, Jr.
AJNR 4:971–975, August 1983          20–1

---

The chronologic sequence of changes in the ventricular system and brain
parenchyma was documented after intracranial hemorrhage (ICH) to determine its utility in the therapeutic management of affected neonates.

During a two-year period, 136 preterm neonates were examined serially
with portable mechanical sector real-time sonography. Each neonate had
an average of 7 studies (range, 4–18) during an average of 36.5 days
(range, 20–97 days). Forty neonates (29.4%) had evidence of ICH, and
256 sonograms from this group were analyzed retrospectively. The gestational age averaged 29.8 weeks (range, 26–34 weeks), and birth weights
averaged 1,210 gm (range, 600–1,660 gm). The type of ICH was described
as follows: subependymal hemorrhage (SEH), hemorrhage localized to the
subependymal germinal matrix; SEH/intraventricular hemorrhage (IVH),
SEH with a small amount of IVH; IVH, hemorrhage occupying more than
50% of the ventricular lumen; and hemorrhage within the parenchyma of
the brain (IPH).

Only 1 of 19 neonates with SEH had ventricular dilatation, whereas 11
of 12 with SEH/IVH or IVH had moderate dilatation. Severe dilatation
occurred in six of nine infants with IPH. Of the 14 with moderate ventricular dilatation, diminution in ventricular size occurred spontaneously
in 4, and after serial ventricular aspiration in 2. Progressive dilatation
occurred in four of six infants with IVH and in six of nine with IPH. Thus,
progressive dilatation developed in 10 of 15 neonates with the more severe
form of ICH. Subependymal hemorrhage tended to occur in the latter half
of the first week of life, and mild dilatation typically occurred during the
next week. Moderate ventricular dilatation was seen during the second
week in infants with IVH, whereas severe dilatation occurred in the third

week of life. Diminution in ventricular size after IVH typically occurred near the end of the second week after ICH. The development of IPH was seen during the first week of life, with porencephaly at one month.

Current therapy for ventricular dilatation and porencephaly after ICH is directed toward minimizing compression and ischemia of brain parenchyma. The risk of progressive ventricular dilatation after ICH is related to the extent of the bleeding. Localized SEH/IVH tends to resolve, but extensive IVH and IPH are frequently associated with progressive dilatation. Once moderate or severe dilatation develops, it resolves spontaneously within three weeks in 33% of affected neonates; of the others, half remain unchanged and half experience progressive dilatation.

Documentation of progressive ventricular dilatation after three weeks is an indication for active medical or surgical therapy. Although knowing the extent of ICH may be helpful in prediction of posthemorrhagic hydrocephalus, serial sonographic examinations are necessary to determine when to undertake therapy. Serial lumbar punctures or external ventricular drainage are possible treatments whose long-term benefits remain to be determined.

▶ Dilatation of cerebral ventricles occurs in 22% of infants who have sustained intraventricular hemorrhage. Cisternography via lumbar injection of indium-111 diethylene triamine pentaacetic acid ($^{111}$InDPTA) has been used by Donn et al. (*Pediatrics* 72:670–676, 1983) to evaluate hydrocephalus in the preterm infant. When the dilatation follows bleeding, the ventricles fill promptly with radioactive material, but there is markedly delayed emptying with minimal flow over the cerebral convexities. Prompt filling of ventricles, delayed emptying, but with flow over the convexities is seen in infants after brain atrophy or periventricular leukomalacia. When the infant has noncommunicating hydrocephalus with Arnold-Chiari malformation, there is complete obstruction with no ventricular filling. Such a diagnostic tool has much to offer in understanding the cerebrospinal fluid dynamics in preterm infants.

Ultrasonic scanning demonstrates the occurrence of ventricular dilatation within days of intraventricular hemorrhage, prior to anticipated development of arachnoiditis. In a case described by Hill, Shackelford, and Volpe (*Pediatrics* 73:19–21, 1984) ventricular dilatation is conjected as being due to plugging of arachnoidal villi by small particulate matter seen within the dilated ventricles within a week of the hemorrhage.

In their analysis of cerebrospinal fluid cystic lesions in the neonatal brain, Chilton and Cremin (*Br. J. Radiol.* 56:613–620, 1983) adopted the classification of Harwood, Nash, and Fitz (*Neuroradiology in Infants and Children*, vol 3. St. Louis, Mosby, 1976, pp. 965–1053): encysted ventricle, arachnoid cyst, and porencephalic cyst (the last subdivided into schizencephalic clefts and encephaloclastic porencephaly due to acquired pre- or postnatal insult). Samples of each are shown, along with confirmatory CT scanning. Ultrasound may displace CT scanning in many instances for practical reasons (movement, radiation dosage, etc.) but limitations of each diagnostic technique must be dealt with.

A nicely illustrated article on real-time ultrasonography of the neonatal head by Rose and Wolfson appeared in *JAMA* (250:3212–3215, 1983). The final opinion is that ultrasonography is the primary screening examination of the unstable premature newborn because of its safety and ease of performance. However, for the stable infant, it is an adjunct to CT of the head, which is the primary diagnostic aid because of its clarity.

Perhaps it might be possible even in these preterm neonates to employ isosorbide solutions to help in management of posthemorrhagic ventricular dilatation. See abstract 20-4.—O.S.

---

**Intracranial Pressure Changes in Craniostenosis**
Ian R. Whittle, Ian H. Johnston, and Michael Besser
Surg. Neurol. 21:367–372, April 1984                                    20–2

---

Clinical and radiologic manifestations of intracranial hypertension frequently are an unsatisfactory basis for making decisions on management in patients with craniostenosis. Intracranial pressure was monitored continuously in 11 boys and 9 girls, mean age 4 years, with primary craniostenosis. Patients were seen at the Royal Alexandra Hospital for Children, Camperdown, Australia. No focal neurologic signs or evidence of intracranial hypertension were present in 17, but 3 of these had well-controlled seizure disorders. The most common indications for intracranial pressure monitoring were mild hydrocephalus and headaches. Eight children were treated previously. Nine had postoperative recordings to determine the efficacy of treatment. A lumbar subarachnoid catheter was usually used to monitor intracranial pressure. In all, 45 recordings were obtained. At least two sleep recordings were obtained in each child.

Most pretreatment recordings showed abnormal plateau or phasic pressure waves of high amplitude. Three of the eight children with clearly abnormal results on recordings had hydrocephalus. Five of the eight treated previously had abnormal findings on recordings. Initial intracranial pressure recordings were clearly abnormal in 65% of all children and mildly abnormal in another 15%. The findings were not related to age at initial recording or to number or location of prematurely fused sutures. Relatively slight effects of surgery on intracranial pressure were apparent in the early postoperative period, but seven of nine children experienced improvement in intracranial hypertension. Both children who failed to improve had lumbar peritoneal shunts for communicating hydrocephalus.

Many children with untreated craniostenosis have intracranial hypertension, whether or not the usual clinical or radiologic signs are present. In those treated previously, intracranial hypertension is likely to precede clinical abnormalities, if these occur at all. Conventional treatment may not lead to normalization of the intracranial pressure. When a substantial pressure reduction does occur, it may do so only after some time. Continuous monitoring of the intracranial pressure appears useful in assessing patients with craniosynostosis and in determining the efficacy of surgical treatment.

▶ The semantic value of the word *craniosynostosis,* used in Table 4 of this article (comparing the results of pressure monitoring in different series), should not be confused with the similar word used in the title: *craniostenosis.* I do not think that the situation inside the calvarium in a patient with linear synostosis of the sagittal suture can be compared with the interior of the head of a patient with Crouzon's disorder of multiple sutural closures. Hence there is no way one can really compare the different series quoted by these authors without the analysis of what type of synostosis was present in each series. Certainly Whittle et al. found increased intracranial pressures in 65% of their cases (20 in all), but 9 of the 13 with increased pressure were of the Crouzon or Apert type.

No arbitrary cutoff level for normal pressure was used; sustained pressure waves were regarded as pathognomonic of intracranial hypertension. Unfortunately, no control series could be ethically obtained, which leaves the criterion suspect. It is certainly against conventional concepts that patients with simple calvarial deformity (such as sagittal suture fusion) should have raised intracranial pressure (three of eight children). But then two of them also had hydrocephalus prior to operation, and that might imply that raised pressure (if it truly exists) may be related to the cause of the hydrocephalus and not to the suture fusion.—O.S.

---

**The Surgical Correction of Coronal and Metopic Craniosynostoses**
Jeffrey L. Marsh and Henry G. Schwartz (Washington Univ.)
J. Neurosurg. 59:245–251, August 1983                                      20–3

---

Several untoward sequelae were observed after the Hoffman procedure for unilateral coronal synostosis and the Marchac operation for metopic synostosis. Among these were induction of an additional synostosis, midline forehead ridging, lateral orbital wall step-off, and palpable fixation wires. Seven infants in a series of 21 operated on for craniosynostosis in the first 19 months of life had classic procedures, and the next 14 underwent modified procedures.

Unilateral coronal synostosis now is managed by bifrontal craniotomy to recontour both frontal bones. Cutting the medial "hinge" has replaced the medial greenstick fracture of the brow segment. The lateral orbital wall osteotomy is extended through the zygomaticofrontal suture into the body of the zygoma. A greenstick fracture rather than an osteotomy is made at the malar block. The supralateral orbit is lowered on the affected side as well by removing bone from the nasion and lateral orbital wall (Fig 20–1). The orbit and frontal bone are fixed with absorbable sutures rather than with wire. The supralateral orbital rim advancement is maintained with a calvarial bone graft fashioned as a tenon-in-mortise wedge. Similar procedures are performed bilaterally in infants with bilateral coronal synostosis. Differential advancement is used when the degree of orbital deformity is asymmetrical. The Marchac procedure is used to correct metopic synostosis, but the lateral orbital wall osteotomy is extended into

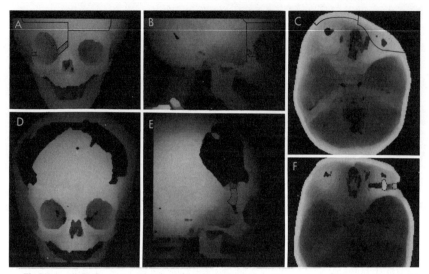

Fig 20–1.—A, B, C, preoperative three-dimensional osseous surface reconstructions in infant aged 5 months with right unilateral coronal synostosis. *Solid line* indicates the periorbital osteotomies, and bone resections are designated by *stippling*. Images were produced from standard axial CT scans. A, frontal projection shows verticalization of the orbital long axis and temporal bulging on right. The superior and inferior orbital fissures are seen in the left orbit (as in normal individuals), but the fissures are obscured on the right by incomplete mesial migration of the orbit because of the synostosis. B, right lateral projection. C, top view projection. Top of the calvaria is transparent, allowing inspection of the cranial base. Seen are recession of the right frontal bone, protrusion of the left frontal bone, compression of the right anterior cranial fossa, and ballooning of the right temporal fossa, D, E, F, bilateral frontal recontouring and right supralateral orbital advancement with caudal displacement seen two weeks after extended bicoronal craniectomies. D, frontal projection. The bicoronal craniectomies are observed between the triangular recontoured "frontal" plate and the unaltered midcranial vault. Note equalization of the orbital rim configuration. E, right lateral projection. The tenon-in-mortise self-retaining bone graft *(dashed line)* in the lateral orbital wall osteotomy maintains the orbital advancement. The osteotomy extends to the body of the zygoma. The brow contour is augmented with a calvarial onlay graft. F, top view projection shows expansion of the right anterior cranial fossa, equalization of the brow contour, and autogenous calvarial bone grafts *(dashed lines)* in the orbital roof and lateral orbital wall. (Courtesy of Marsh, J.L., and Schwartz, H.G.: J. Neurosurg. 59:245–251, August 1983.)

the body of the zygoma, and a self-retaining low lateral orbital wall calvarial graft buttress is used.

Adverse sequelae have been avoided using these modifications. A combined neurologic and plastic surgical approach to craniosynostosis successfully releases radial brain and calvarial growth vectors, permitting a more normal-appearing craniofacial configuration.

▶ The Hoffman procedure referred to was described by Hoffman and Mohr (*J. Neurosurg.* 45:642–652, 1976) and deals with lateral canthal advancement of the supraorbital margin. The coronal suture was released, and an artificial suture created in the anterior fossa. Marchac's procedure (*Plast. Reconstr. Surg.* 61:823–835, 1978) includes recontouring of the supralateral orbit and forehead to correct the deformities of metopic synostosis.

A detailed exposition of the principles for correction of craniosynostosis is presented by Marchac and Denier of the Hospital for Sick Children in Paris

(*Craniofacial Surgery for Craniosynostosis.* Boston, Little Brown, 1983). Each major variety is discussed. Separate chapters are given to Crouzon's and Apert's syndromes, and another to treatment of older children. The basic principle in infants has to do with the need to reform the supraorbital area ("floating forehead"), which is no longer needed after age 18 months; the differences in operation before and after this age are well illustrated. Facial advancement as a separate or combined procedure usually is delayed until age three to four years. Even if classic linear craniectomies (or even total cranial vault removals) fail, as they often do, in providing a solid, cosmetically proper cranium, secondary repairs can be made. The authors point out the need for doing something about cranial defects after age four years, whereafter the osteogenic properties of the dura mater may be lost. Marchac republishes some of his technique for using embedded, arching, split ribs to restore proper contours. Wire mesh and acrylic can be used if there is a lack of sufficient osteogenous bone. Early and late complications are described with the astounding statement that there have been no cases of postoperative epilepsy or visual or oculomotor problems. The book itself is well printed and has numerous excellent photographs and explicatory line drawings and an unusual number of pages in which a vertical half of the page is blank. Nonetheless, it is a book of such value that I commend it to any neurosurgeon who has to advise parents as to what can be done—and especially if he or she is to operate.—O.S.

---

### Isosorbide in the Management of Infantile Hydrocephalus

John Lorber, Stephen Salfield, and Tony Lonton (Univ. of Manchester, England)
Dev. Med. Child. Neurol. 25:502–511, 1983                                    20–4

---

It might be possible to reduce the number of hydrocephalic infants requiring surgery if the intracranial pressure could be controlled until spontaneous arrest took place. The authors evaluated isosorbide treatment in a series of 101 infants seen in a seven-year period with various types of hydrocephalus. Forty-seven infants had neural tube defects, 23 had primary congenital hydrocephalus, 17 had postmeningitic hydrocephalus, and 14 had posthemorrhagic disease. Isosorbide was administered orally or by nasogastric tube as a 50% solution in a standard dose of 8 gm/kg daily, in four daily doses. The dose sometimes was increased up to 12 gm/kg daily if the drug was well-tolerated but with suboptimal response. Fourteen patients with severe hydrocephalus were treated for less than a week before operation because of lack of control of pressure.

Forty-three infants in the series had a cerebral mantle with a thickness greater than 20 mm and had normal cerebrospinal fluid (CSF). Thirty-one of them remained shunt free, and nine others gained a worthwhile delay from isosorbide therapy. In the other 58 cases the goal was to reduce the intracranial pressure until it became clear whether shunting was necessary or until the infant was fit for surgery. Five of these patients were maintained without shunting, and a worthwhile delay was obtained in 30 other cases. Only 2 of 10 patients in whom delay was necessary because of abnormal

CSF were failures. Twenty-two infants with neural tube defects avoided shunting, as did nine of those with primary congenital hydrocephalus and five of those with acquired hydrocephalus. Six children died of shunt complications, and complications could not be excluded in six other cases. Shunting was more effective than isosorbide in controlling head size, but head size did not correlate with intelligence. Isosorbide was useful in a few shunted children who developed complications and required shunt removal. Most side effects (diarrhea, vomiting, and hypernatremia) from isosorbide were mild. Treatment was stopped in two patients with a serum sodium level greater than 150 mmol/L and one who vomited persistently.

Isosorbide (an osmotic diuretic) has precluded the need for shunting or allowed a delay in a substantial number of infants with hydrocephalus due to neural tube defects or primary congenital hydrocephalus. Its efficacy probably is due to the removal of intracerebral fluid resulting from the osmotic gradient produced between the serum and ventricular fluid. Close monitoring of the plasma electrolyte and urea levels is necessary.

---

**Critical Comments on Hydrocephalus Treatment, Based on So-Called "Arrested" Hydrocephalus**
R. Gruber
Z. Kinderchir. 38(Suppl.):33–35, April 1983                    20–5

---

The author conducted a comparative clinical and radiologic follow-up study of data on 109 hydrocephalic children to determine the criteria of shunt dependency. The patients were classified into the following four groups: 50 children with a normal functioning shunt; 34 children with an antisiphon device (ASD) shunt combination; 14 children with a nonfunctioning shunt which had not been revised for eight years and who were without pressure symptoms; and 11 children with the shunt removed at least five years earlier. None of the patients showed pressure symptoms at the time of investigation. From computed tomography findings a ventricle index was developed indicating the relationship of the width of the cella media to the transverse interior diameter of the skull. Patients who could attend a regular school and had an IQ of at least 85 were considered educable.

The high rate (30%) of nonfunctioning shunts and of shunts removed without difficulties and the amazingly similar findings in the group treated with ASD support the presumption that a shunt system without adequate ASD in an erect position is not only responsible for the high rate of preventable complications but also for the inability to use the natural compensation system.

The following conclusions were made. The smaller the ventricular system, the higher the complication rate was. The more effectively drained a ventricular system under shunt treatment appeared to be, the greater was the rate of chronic complaints and necessary revisions. The standard of well-being did not correspond with the amount of expansion of the compressed brain tissue after shunting. A normal appearing ventricular system was not necessarily a sign of adequate therapy, but was more apt to be a sign of a pathologic overdrainage. The widened ventricular appearance of the suction-protected ASD shunt resembled the findings of the arrested hydrocephalus and seemed to be closer to the goal of hydrocephalus therapy, namely, shunt independence. For the hydrocephalic child who is shunt-treated, a normal-appearing ventricular system is a pathologic finding and should not be considered a criterion of therapeutic success.

▶ One of the reasons for the author's conclusions may well be related to the disparity between head size and brain size at and after the time of shunting. Allied to this is the problem of postshunt synostosis of the separated calvarial bones. If the head is too large for the brain size, filling of the cranial cavity must be either by ventricular expansion or by extracerebral fluid accumulations. The former seems preferable!

In spite of great advances in technology, shunts still do not always work well. In the case reported by Jooma and Grant (*Surg. Neurol.* 20:231–234, 1983) a boy, 12 years of age, had a ventriculoperitoneal shunt for hydrocephalus ascribed to aqueductal stenosis. There was a multipurpose valve incorporating an on-off valve; but the valve was found on several occasions to be switched off, causing increased pressure and corresponding symptoms with irritability headache, drowsiness, etc. On one occasion, this was accompanied by cerebrospinal fluid rhinorrhea, and roentgenograms showed intraventricular pneumocephalus. Replacement of air by sterile saline solution brought prompt relief, and craniotomy allowed closure of the basifrontal skull and dural defect. The authors point out the potential dangers of pneumocephalus involved in trying to treat cerebrospinal fluid rhinorrhea if the computed tomography scan or ventriculogram shows a frontal porencephalic cyst (as was present in their case). They did not mention what they did with the capricious valve.

Assessment of shunt patency by lumbar spinal infusion of Elliott's solution A (an artificial cerebrospinal fluid) is described by Schultz et al. (*J. Neurosurg.* 58:553–556, 1983). If the shunt is working, infusion of fluid does not produce a rise in pressure (rate of infusion of 2.5 ml/minute for 10 minutes). In 12 patients so tested, the shunt was considered patent in 7, blocked in 4, and partially blocked in 1. Failure of ventricles to decrease in size after shunting need not mean the shunt is not working, as indicated by this test and confirmed by clinical improvement. Low-pressure valve systems were used in original shunts, and also in those who needed revision.

The flow of cerebrospinal fluid in shunts has also been measured by an electronic device implanted along the thoracic segment of the drainage tube. Hara et al. (ibid. 557–561, 1983) report rates varying from 0.05 to 0.78 ml/minute, with a suggestion of circadian rhythm (increased flow between midnight and 6 A.M.).

A number of young women with shunts placed for hydrocephalus have now reached the age for bearing children. Obstetricians can expect some of them to desire to bear children. A relatively small number of such pregnant women have been studied in the past, and Gast et al. (*Obstet. Gynecol.* 62[Suppl.]:29s–31s, 1983) present case reports of two such women. One had irradiation for inoperable posterior fossa tumor at age 21, needed a shunt a year later (when computed tomography showed hydrocephalus and no evidence of tumor). At 24 she became pregnant after use of endocrine substances. A normal, healthy full-term baby was delivered under epidural anesthesia for the mother. The second patient had a ventriculoatrial shunt at seven years of age; the last of three revisions took place at age 19. Pregnancy at 21 was complicated by apparent shunt malfunction, but shunt study failed to confirm this and eventual vaginal delivery took place. Eight months later, clinical and radiologic evidence of obstruction was followed by replacement of the obstructed atrial catheter, and new valve was also put in. The patient was pregnant at the time, and the second baby was delivered after use of pudendal anesthesia, without forceps, but with antibiotic prophylaxis.

The obstetrician faced with a pregnant woman who has had a ventricular shunt must be aware of the signs and symptoms of shunt failure; there is no special regimen for analgesia or anesthesia for the delivery; but antiobiotic prophylaxis is advocated because of the consequences of infection in the shunt. A single administration of antibiotics immediately before delivery should be sufficient, but they could be readministered 6–12 hours after delivery.—O.S.

---

## Abdominal Complications of Ventriculoperitoneal Shunts With Emphasis on the Role of Imaging Methods

Farooq P. Agha, Marco A. Amendola, Khalil K. Shirazi, Beatriz E. Amendola, and William F. Chandler (Univ. of Michigan)
Surg. Gynecol. Obstet. 156:473–478, April 1983                    20–6

---

The authors reviewed the imaging findings in 280 patients who had a total of 400 ventriculoperitoneal shunt procedures for various intracranial problems at two centers in 1976–1981. The 155 female and 125 male patients were aged 1 month to 52 years. All patients had computed tomography (CT) scans of the head and roentgenograms of the chest and abdomen. Some also had radionuclide clearance, ultrasonography, CT of the abdomen, contrast opacification of the shunt, and fine-needle aspiration of suspected cerebrospinal fluid (CSF) collections. The most common indications for shunting were congenital hydrocephalus and communicating hydrocephalus.

Complications relating to the abdominal end of the shunt occurred in 25% of procedures, and necessitated 120 surgical revisions; 40 patients required more than one. Common complications included mechanical malfunction (7%) and malfunction due to tip occlusion by fibrous encasement (10%). Twenty-five shunts (5%) became infected. Seven patients had CSF loculations and pseudocyst formation. Two had intestinal obstruction from adhesions, and one had a small bowel perforation by the shunt catheter tip.

One fourth of these ventriculoperitoneal shunt procedures were complicated, most often by mechanical shunt malfunction, catheter tip occlusion, and shunt infection. Other complications may include migration of the shunt and metastatic tumor spread by way of the shunt. Ventriculoperitoneal shunting remains the best long-term measure for relieving increased intracranial pressure. Computed tomography is useful in estimating the size and location of a cyst or fluid loculation and its relation to the shunt catheter. Fine-needle aspiration of loculated fluid collections with the use of ultrasonographic or CT guidance is a safe procedure with a high diagnostic yield and can also be therapeutic.

▶ It would be worthwhile to know how many of the patients were infants, since complications of shunting appear much more commonly in babies than in older patients. Curiosity impels me to ask how many revisions were needed in these 280 patients for trouble at the cranial end. And what do the authors suggest to help prevent these complications?

A hitherto unreported complication of ventriculoperitoneal shunting is obstruction of the ureter (in a woman, 36, who developed hydrocephalus secondary to tuberculous meningitis). Clarke, Paul, and Lye (*J. Neurosurg.* 59:542–544, 1983) were able to overcome the obstruction by shortening of the peritoneal catheter (of the low-pressure Raimondi variety), which was demonstrated by intravenous urography to overlie the obstruction that produced unilateral hydronephrosis. This type of obstruction has been reported previously with a lumboperitoneal shunt.

Among the complications of ventriculoperitoneal shunts are migration of the shunt tip into various abdominal and pelvic organs, especially if the shunt is rigid. The tip may also enter inguinal hernias, presumably aided by increased intra-abdominal pressure from fluid added via the shunt. Now Crofford and Balsam (*AJR* 141:369–371, 1983) report four instances of migration of the tip of the shunt through a patent processus vaginalis resulting in scrotal hydrocele. Three were in the neonatal period; the fourth was found in a boy, 4 years of age, whose shunt was placed for relief of hydrocephalus due to posterior fossa ependymoma. No mention is made of the type of tubing used. An earlier instance of this complication, by Ramani (*J. Neurosurg.* 40:772–773, 1974) was not included in their bibliography.

Abu-Dalu et al. (*Neurosurgery* 13:167–169, 1983) report three new instances of late perforation of the large bowel by the abdominal end of a ventriculoperitoneal shunt. Such a mischance should be suspected when a shunt infection harbors a gram-negative enteric organism; it may occur without peritonitis. The authors made the diagnosis by injection of contrast material into the distal end of the shunt. In the absence of evidence of peritonitis, the abdominal catheter can be extricated without incision (i.e., percutaneously) or, as in the cases of protrusion of the shunt tip through the anus, by pulling on the extruding part. In each case, the spring-reinforced distal catheter had been used.

What does a neurosurgeon do when the usual routes for shunting are no longer available? Try something different. Friedman and Gass (*Neurosurgery* 13:69–71, 1983) encountered a woman, 26, who had had subarachnoid-ureteral shunt at age 10 weeks for hydrocephalus. Reflux from a urinary tract infection led to meningitis in 1981, and the unvalved tubing was removed. The patient developed gross nystagmus, headache, and altered consciousness, and although there was increased lumbar puncture pressure, CT scanning did not show ventricular enlargement. Percutaneous lumboperitoneal shunting led to recovery sustained for four months, and recurrence of symptoms at that time was followed by shunt revision. This failed to give relief, although exteriorization of the shunt gave relief of symptoms. A two-stage procedure was then done to shunt from the lumbar subarachnoid space into the right atrium via the jugular vein. Immediate improvement after operation has persisted for the follow-up period of one year. Spetzler, in commenting, related two similar procedures when the peritoneal cavity refused to accept cerebrospinal fluid, and also described a rare instance of percutaneously inserted cisternoatrial shunt.

A new lumboperitoneal shunt catheter made of Silastic, which is kink-resistant without spring reinforcement, is described by Selman and Spetzler (*Surg. Neurol.* 21:58–60, 1984). It is inserted through a 14-gauge Touhy needle, held in place with subcutaneous fixation sleeves, and has multiple perforations at the lumbar end and three slit valves at the peritoneal end.—O.S.

---

### Dysgenesis of the Corpus Callosum

B. E. Kendall (The National Hospital, London)
Neuroradiology 25:239–256, August 1983                                    20–7

---

Dysgenesis of the corpus callosum comprises a range of malformations varying from total failure of commissuration of the telencephalon to minor degrees of deficiency usually involving the splenium. Isolated dysgensis can simulate the minor forms of lobar holoprosencephaly, but the lamina terminalis is not thickened, and the thalami are nearly always separated in dysgenesis. Demonstration of the fornices rules out holoprosencephaly. In simple dysgenesis the cortical axons that normally would cross in the corpus collosum are heterotopic and form thick bundles of myelinated fibers running ipsilaterally from the paraolfactory cortex and frontal lobes to the occipital and temporal lobes, ventral to the cingula. Loss of the supporting function of the corpus callosum presumably is responsible for separation of the hemispheres and widening of the third ventricle. Cavum septum pellucidi cysts often are present in association with partial dysgenesis and may depress the roof of the third ventricle. A cyst or lipoma or, rarely, another type of mesenchymal tumor may extend through the site of a dysgenetic corpus callosum. Various congenital malformations may be associated with dysgenesis of the corpus callosum.

Although the disorder is occasionally found incidentally, most patients with dysgenesis of the corpus callosum are symptomatic, having low intelligence and being subject to seizures. Disordered hypothalamic function has been described. Macrocrania is present in 20% of patients. Hydrocephalus may be the presenting feature in infants. Plain skull x-ray films may show hypertelorism or trigonocephaly. The chief angiographic abnormalities are related to the defective midline structures. They include an altered course of the pericallosal arteries, widely separated internal cerebral veins, and the negative image of the ventricular system in the capillary phase mirroring the abnormal anatomy. The complete anatomy usually is demonstrated on non-contrast-medium-enhanced axial CT sections, both in patients with isolated defects and in those with complex associated abnormalities. Heterotopic gray matter may cause focal nodular encroachment into the lateral ventricle and produce a picture resembling tuberous sclerosis.

▶ ↓ An editorial by Fulling and Naidich introduces a special number of *Neuroradiology* dealing with congenital malformations of the brain (25:177, 1983). There is a significant amount of embryology and pathology in this collection, in addition to what the authors term "derivative radiology," looking forward to use of radiology as a primary tool in the serial study of such congenital malformations. I regret the inability to put all of this information in the YEAR BOOK, but will content myself with offering the following abstract dealing with the hindbrain deformity in the Chiari II malformation and the preceding one on dysgenesis of the corpus callosum. A short summary of the other papers follows.

Diebler and Dulac (ibid. 25:199–216, 1983) review the literature and their own 31 personal observations on those hernias of brain through the defective cranium, termed cephaloceles. The most common locus, they find, is in the occipital region, but such sacs may contain occipital lobes or cysts of Dandy-Walker malformation. As one might surmise, the authors find computerized scanning a most valuable tool in elucidating the defects.

Occult cranium bifidum occurred in six cases described by Inoue et al. from Osaka (ibid. 25:217–223, 1983). The patients were children eight years old or younger, each of whom had been referred because of a midline subscalp "tumor" and who had no neurologic defect. The nodule consisted of arachnoid cells and fibrous tissue, with immature glial cells in one case. Operative removal of the mass was possible in each after proper radiologic study, which included CT and angiography. The bony defect was detected only on radiography. When there is no skin erosion or cosmetic problem, nor any possibility of infection, operation is unnecessary.

Holoprosencephaly (sometimes called arhinencephaly) is best considered a failure of cleavage of the forebrain, according to Fitz (ibid. 25:225–238, 1983). He has had experience with three cases with lobar holoprosencephaly (the most severe type), six with semilobar, and six with alobar disorder. Diagrams and pictures of children and their brains add to the radiologic information. Differential diagnostic considerations include agenesis of the corpus callosum, absence of the septum pellucidum, hydranencephaly, as well as a disorder of probably similar origin, septo-optic dysplasia.

Another collection of peculiar disorders are termed by Zimmerman et al. (ibid. 25:257–263, 1983) "migratory disorders" of human brain development. Depending on the type of disturbance of the nerve cells from the germinal matrix, the entity resulting may produce schizencephaly, agyria-pachygyria, heterotopias, or polymicrogyria. Examples of brains and radiographs clarify the problem of diagnosis, and the text gives clues as to the way these unfortunately not too rare malformations may arise.

Besides the foregoing anomalies of cleavage and migration, brains may be abnormal because parts may die. Such destructive lesions are described by Raybaud (ibid. 25:265–291, 1983). Agenetic porencephaly, lissencephaly, schizencephaly, micrencephaly, hydranencephaly, and multicystic encephalomalacia are described. Angiograms have been used to illustrate a number of these cases, as well as CT scans. The timing of the problem is used to separate agentic, encephaloclastic, and postnatal encephaloclastic lesions.

Probably more significant for most neurosurgeons, but also more readily encountered and written about, are the CT scans in the phakomatoses; some scans are displayed in the article by Gardeur et al. (ibid. 25:293–304, 1983). There were 17 normal scans in the 77 cases in their series. Sturge-Weber syndrome and von Hippel-Lindau disease are also discussed briefly.—O.S.

---

**The Chiari II Malformation: The Hindbrain Deformity**
T. P. Naidich, D. G. McLone, and K. H. Fulling
Neuroradiology 25:179–197, August 1983                                    20–8

---

The Chiari II malformation is a complex deformity almost always associated with myelomeningocele. It includes specific deformities of the hindbrain, the cervical spinal cord, and the craniovertebral junction. These deformities can be viewed as arising from the disproportionately rapid growth of brain tissue in what is initially too small a bony and dural posterior fossa that expands too slowly to accommodate the growing brain. The anatomical distortions eventually become "set" through myelination and remain fixed. Compression can cause secondary atrophy or pressure necrosis of the deformed structures. The embryogenesis of the hindbrain deformity is not understood, but hypotheses include traction by a myelomeningocele, a tissue-pressure gradient, and primary overgrowth of the rhombencephalon. Metrizamide computed tomography myelography delineates the major features of the Chiari II hindbrain malformation in vivo.

The bony posterior fossa is very small in Chiari II patients, and the dural roof of the fossa is hypoplastic. The foramen magnum usually is enlarged, as is the upper cervical spinal canal. The bony posterior arch of C1 is incomplete in most patients, but the defect is always closed by a fibroelastic band. The arch of C2 is always intact. Posterior spinal bifida with myelocele or myelomeningocele is nearly always present in the lower spine. The cord is displaced caudally for a variable distance and is compacted along its long axis by herniation of the hindbrain from above. The medulla and even the pons may be displaced into the cervical spinal canal, and the medulla buckles as it descends. The cerebellum is smaller than normal, and a "tongue" or "tail" of cerebellar tissue protrudes into the spinal canal behind the medulla and fourth ventricle. The fourth ventricle is elongated craniocaudally and narrowed transversely. Pressure on the inferior cerebellar vermis produces both acute and chronic changes. Hydromyelia is most marked in the lower cervical cord segments. Cervical syringomyelia is present in as many as 20% of patients. The entire vertebrobasilar arterial system may be displaced caudally.

Computed tomography, especially with metrizamide in the subarachnoid space, documents the deformities present in the Chiari II hindbrain malformation. It helps in determining the potential benefits of laminectomy of the upper cervical region.

▶ Based on 26 cases of arachnoidal cysts operated on at the Mayo Clinic from 1970 to 1980, Cilluffo et al. (*Acta Neurochir.* 67:215–229, 1983) conclude that the preferred treatment is direct surgical excision. Most of the nine children younger than eight years of age had enlarged heads; the other 17 were aged 16–63 and had headache, seizures, blurred vision among the more common symptoms. The primary diagnostic aid has been CT scanning. A number of patients had troublesome complications requiring shunting; one patient with posterior fossa midline cyst had ventriculoatrial shunt, cyst-ventricular shunt, and suboccipital craniectomy. Autopsy in this patient—the only one in the series who died—showed platybasia, Arnold-Chiari malformation, and thrombosed anterior spinal artery.—O.S.

---

**Chiari Malformation Presenting In Adults: A Surgical Experience in 127 Cases**
Walter Joseph Levy (Univ. of Missouri-Columbia), Laura Mason, and Joseph F. Hahn (Cleveland Clinic)
Neurosurgery 12:377–390, April 1983                    20–9

---

Findings were reviewed in 127 adult patients seen with Chiari malformation since 1946. The 72 women and 55 men had an average age of 41 years at presentation. The average duration of symptoms clearly related to the disease was about three years, but more vague symptoms such as headaches had been present longer. Pain in the cervical region or head was the predominant complaint, followed by various sensory changes and gait disturbance. Weakness, especially in the upper extremities, was a symptom in 53 patients. Physical examinations revealed hyperactive reflexes in the lower extremities in 66 cases, nystagmus in 60 cases, and gait disturbance in 54 cases. Other findings included cerebellar abnormalities, hand atrophy, and lower cranial nerve dysfunction.

Surgical operative notes showed that the foramen of Magendie was occluded in 55 cases. In 106 cases the tonsils were clearly below the foramen magnum. Arachnoid adhesions were present in 50 patients. Fifty-two patients had a syrinx. The basic operation consisted of decompression of the foramen magnum to at least C3 with an open dura mater plus exploration of the fourth ventricle and the opening of any membrane over the foramen of Magendie. In some cases a muscle plug was placed in the upper end of the central canal.

Six patients died postoperatively. Eighty-five patients with a follow-up of 6 months or longer were evaluated. Of 25 who had the basic operation, 11 were improved and 8 were unchanged, while of the 60 patients who had decompression plus muscle plug insertion, 29 improved and 16 were unchanged after operation.

Although overall results showed no clear difference with a plug, insertion of a muscle plug into the central canal appeared helpful in patients with progressive symptoms of Chiari malformation. Criteria for surgery should be conservative. Better treatment will require more knowledge of the pathophysiology of the disorder and its natural history.

▶ Among the findings in the 16-year-old youth with Arnold-Chiari malformation reported by Stone et al. (*Surg. Neurol.* 20:313–317, 1983) were headache, diplopia, ataxia, weakness of lower limbs, and enlarged head with massive hydrocephalus. Bilateral brain stem lesions were suggested by brain stem evoked potential study. Posterior fossa decompression confirmed the presence of the malformation, with cerebellar tonsils as low as C2 and C3 laminae. A plastic tube was placed in the newly opened fourth ventricle, the dura mater closed with a fascial graft, and the cranial decompression supplemented by upper cervical laminectomy (C1 to C5). After a somewhat stormy immediate postoperative course, the patient improved remarkably; six months later, the only residual neurologic finding was minimal nystagmus on lateral gaze. Intellectual functioning increased as indicated by Wechsler intelligence tests that were administered before and six months after operation. The evoked potential study also showed remarkable recovery, indicating the electrophysiologic reversibility despite congenital anatomic distortion.

Pecker et al. (*Neurochirurgie* 29:171–173, 1983) propose that evacuation of a syringomyelic cavity into the subarachnoid space is often ineffective because delivery of the fluid into the area around the spinal cord can cause variations in pressure with pulsations of the cord that may be inimical to the proper emptying of the cavity. They therefore have carried out syringoperitoneal shunts in four patients, hoping to obviate some of the difficulties of simple drainage. The longest follow-up is only two years, but the authors wish to present the procedure described in this technical note as a possible means of keeping the pressure in the syrinx low.—O.S.

---

## Experience With Surgical Decompression of the Arnold-Chiari Malformation in Young Infants With Myelomeningocele

Tae Sung Park, Harold J. Hoffman, E. Bruce Hendrick, and Robin P. Humphreys (Univ. of Toronto)
Neurosurgery 13:147–152, August 1983          20–10

---

The authors reviewed the surgical results in 45 infants seen before age three months with myelomeningocele and absent, or adequately controlled, hydrocephalus, who developed signs of Arnold-Chiari malformation and underwent laminectomy and opening of the dura mater for hindbrain decompression. The median age at presentation was 4 weeks. The myelomeningocele had been repaired surgically in 44 infants. All infants required insertion of a ventriculoperitoneal shunt, 42 before decompression. The most common presenting features were swallowing difficulty, apneic episodes, stridor, and bronchial aspiration. About one fourth of the patients had arm weakness, and eight patients had opisthotonus. Fourteen patients deteriorated dramatically after presentation.

Surgery revealed a transverse dural band constricting the dural sac at the C1 level in 41% of cases and mild arachnoid adhesion in 23%. The lowermost level of the cerebellar tongue or medullary kink was at the C1–C4 level in 29 cases and at C5–T1 in 16. Twenty-eight patients were alive when last followed up, all of whom had improved in their overall neurologic function. Twenty-four patients made a complete recovery. Most deaths were attributed to respiratory failure. About 71% of the patients who had developed cardiorespiratory arrest, vocal cord paralysis, or arm weakness within two weeks before decompression died, compared with 22.6% of those with more gradual neurologic deterioration.

Arnold-Chiari malformation is present in all patients with myelomeningocele, in whom it is a common cause of progressive neurologic deficit. Adequate decompression is achieved in affected infants by laminectomy with opening of the dura mater to below the tip of the cerebellar tongue and the medullary kink. Removal of the occipital bone and extension of the dural incision above the level of the foramen magnum are unnecessary and hazardous. Decompression should be done before rapid neurologic deterioration takes place, even if a functioning shunt is present.

---

## A New Understanding of Dorsal Dysraphism With Lipoma (Lipomyeloschisis): Radiologic Evaluation and Surgical Correction

Thomas P. Naidich, David G. McLone, and Saffet Mutluer (Northwestern Univ.)
AJR 140:1065–1078, June 1983                                         20–11

---

Both intradural lipoma and lipomyelomeningocele are forms of lipomyeloschisis, or dorsal dysraphism with lipoma. The spinal cord and conus are low and are split in the midline dorsally (Fig 20–2), and the caudal neural tissue therefore retains the shape of the embryonal neural placode. The authors reviewed the radiographic findings in 14 patients, six of them aged 1–12 months. The lipoma was in the midline in 2 of 12 evaluable patients. Five patients had undergone partial surgical correction of the superficial extradural component of the lipomyelomeningocele. All patients subsequently had definitive operative treatment. Metrizamide myelography and metrizamide computed tomographic myelography were carried out.

The final diagnosis was lipomyelomeningocele in seven cases, intradural lipoma in two, and lipomyeloschisis in the five patients who had previously undergone surgery. Spina bifida was present in all patients except one with intradural lipoma. The laminae were shorter on the side of the lipoma in seven cases, and three patients were scoliotic. Individual patterns of anomaly included skin-covered focal spina bifida; focal partial clefting of the dorsal half of the cord; continuity of the dorsal cleft with the central canal of the cord above, and occasionally below, the cleft; deficiency of the dura underlying the spina bifida; deep extension of subcutaneous lipoma to insert directly into the cleft on the dorsal half of the cord; and variable ballooning of the subarachnoid space to form an associated meningocele. A dorsal meningocele was present and continuous with the intracanalicular

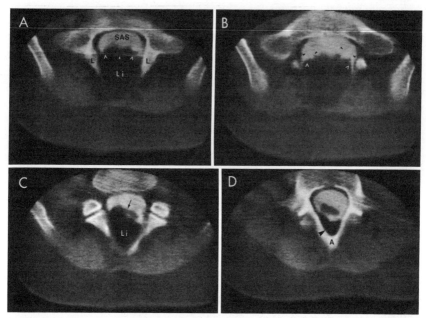

**Fig 20–2**—Lipomyeloschisis in a 10-year-old girl with previous purely extradural repair of lipomyeloschisis. **A** and **B**, axial-section metrizamide computed tomogram. Note bifid laminae *(L)*; lucent dorsal lipoma *(Li)*; ventral pial surface facing opacified subarachnoid space *(SAS)*; smooth, apparently distinct lipal-neural interface at dorsal surface of placode *(open white arrowheads)*; and junction of lateral borders of placode, lipoma, and subarachnoid space along dorsal root entry zones *(also open white arrowheads)*. Paired dorsal *(small black arrowheads)* and ventral *(large black arrowheads)* nerve roots arise from placode to course through subarachnoid space. Dorsal midline notch *(solid white arrowhead)* is believed to represent residual neural groove. Subarachnoid space bulges slightly posterolateral to dorsal root entry zones. **C**, lipoma *(Li)* ascends along posterior surface of placode and rotates placode *(arrow)*. **D**, lipoma separates from neural tissue to form extra-arachnoid fat pad *(arrowhead)* under intact arch *(A)* of next cephalic vertebra. Degree of rotation of cord and placode varies from level to level. (Courtesy of Naidich, T.P., et al.: AJR 140:1065–1078, June 1983.)

subarachnoid space in seven of the nine new cases and in none of the five patients who had undergone reoperation.

The precise nature of the lipal-neural interface in these cases remains unclear. Lipomyeloschisis presumably causes neurologic dysfunction through progressive deposition of fat, leading to increased intracanalicular mass effect, and also through tethering of the cord, resulting in stretching. High-resolution metrizamide computed tomographic myelography is helpful in planning surgical treatment.

Technique.—After identification of the most cephalic widely bifid lamina, the intralaminal fibrous band which tethers the placode is resected. Durotomy is done precisely over the meningocele, which is entered under direct vision, sparing the dorsal nerve roots at their entry into the placode. The lipoma is trimmed from the dorsal surface of the placode, and the dural tube reestablished to ensure lateral freedom from tethering.

Intraoperative monitoring of neural function by evoked potentials has so decreased operative morbidity that the authors now believe all lipomeningoceles should be treated in the neonatal period before onset of symptoms.

▶ Meningomyelocele was detected antenatally in four of nine neonates with this malformation delivered in a 24-month period in New Haven, Conn. Chervenak et al. (*Obstet. Gynecol.* 63:376–380, 1984) describe the discontinuity in the fetal spine and presence of a protruding sac as seen in ultrasound studies, undertaken primarily because of obstetric indications and not as part of a study with family history of congenital malformations. When fetal maturity was established, a low transverse cesarean section was carried out, with care to prevent pressure on the sac, so as not to rupture it. Repair of the meningomyelocele was done on day 1 in all four of these infants; and three later had ventriculoperitoneal shunts (days 5–18). One infant with recurrent apnea and bradycardia died. Optimal outcome for these congenital lesions appears to depend on a team approach.

The tethered conus is a congenital malformation of the spinal cord commonly in association with spinal dysraphia and intradural lipomas. It should be considered in any patient with dysraphism who has an unexplained progressive urologic, neurologic, or orthopedic disturbance. Merx et al. (*Diagnostic Imag.* 52:179–188, 1983) point out things to look for in lumbar myelograms in such patients. Injections should be done at the end of the lumbar canal to avoid injury to the spinal cord. All of the 16 patients in this series had bony deformities, ranging from simple occult spina bifida to severe forms of vertebral dysplasia. One had a tethered filum terminale alone; five had intradural lipomas, and the other nine had combinations of causes (lipoma, adhesions, spina bifida, diastematomyelia, rotation of the cord, scoliosis, etc.). The authors point out that all of the patients who had had myelomeningocele repair in the past showed an additional tethering filum terminale, which implies lack of very detailed analysis of the situation in the spinal canal before the original operation.

According to Skinner and Jacobson (*J. R. Coll. Surg. Edinburgh* 28:229–232, 1983), fewer than 100 cases of anterior sacral meningocele have been reported. Two cases are presented. One was detected in plain x-ray films of the pelvis in a man, 18, after accidental fracture of the right femur; he had previously been well. The second was found on examination of a woman, 19, complaining of lower abdominal discomfort. Laparotomy under the impression of ovarian cyst revealed the sac which was incompletely excised. Later neurosurgical operation through the bifid sacrum permitted ligation of communication between sac and sacral dura and drainage of the presacral sac. No neurologic deficits could be found in the lower extremities or sphincters two years later.—O.S.

---

**Intradural Spinal Cysts**
A. Fortuna and S. Mercuri (Univ. of Rome)
Acta Neurochir (Wien) 68:289–314, 1983                    20–12

---

The authors reviewed the findings in 18 cases of benign intradural spinal cyst and in 94 previously reported cases. There were 76 cases of arach-

noidal intradural cyst, 9 of neuroepithelial intradural cyst, and 27 of endodermal intradural cyst. Arachnoidal intradural cysts have been attributed to areas of low arachnoidal resistance; there is no evidence for
hereditary factor in humans. Proliferation of ectopic ependymal cells may
cause neuroepithelial cysts. A developmental origin of endodermal cysts

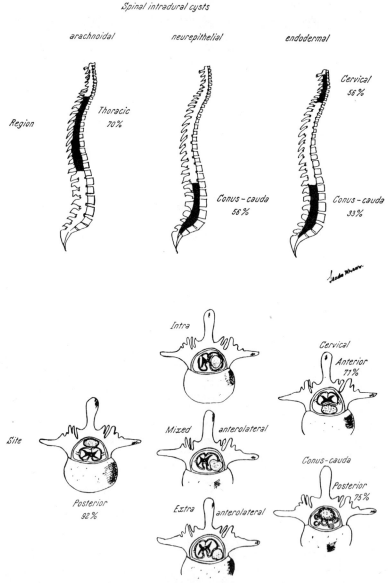

**Fig 20–3.**—Level and site of intradural cysts. (Courtesy of Fortuna, A., and Mercuri, S.: Acta Neurochir. [Wien] 68:289–314, 1983; Berlin-Heidelberg-New York; Springer.)

is accepted, and these cysts often are associated with severe neurovertebral abnormalities. Younger patients are more often affected by endodermal cysts than by other types, which tend to occur in the fourth to fifth decades of life. Neuroepithelial cysts tend to occur in women, and endodermal cysts in men. Sites of preference are shown in Figure 20–3.

The mean duration of symptoms in reported patients with arachnoidal cysts has been greater than in the other types of cyst. The symptoms are mostly those of root cord compression. The onset of arachnoidal cysts often is insidious, but they can have an acute onset and rapidly progressive course. The onset of neuroepithelial cysts often is acute with a rapid course. The onset of endodermal cysts tends to be insidious, with a long history, and the clinical course is typically slow. Cerebrospinal fluid blockade is more frequent in cases of neuroepithelial cyst than in arachnoidal cysts, and it is the rule in endodermal cysts. Myelography can be diagnostic of arachnoidal cysts, but a variety of nondiagnostic patterns are observed in cases of neuroepithelial cyst and endodermal cyst.

In cases of arachnoidal cyst, as much of the cyst wall as possible should be removed. The underlying cord is never very compressed. Intramedullary neuroepithelial cyst is best managed by posterior myelotomy with generous opening of the cyst. Partial removal may be adequate in extramedullary and mixed cases. Endodermal cysts are managed similarly. As in neuro-epithelial cysts, partial removal carries no risk of recurrence. Reported operative mortality has been about 3%, but mortality today is practically nil. Cyst removal and cord decompression are followed by rapid neurologic recovery except in some cases with a prolonged preoperative deficit. Only one of the authors' patients was left with a serious neurologic deficit and half of the patients have no neurologic problems.

# 21 Trauma

### Compound Frontobasal Skull Fractures: Surgical Management of Acute Phase
Robert H. Rosenwasser, Tomas E. Delgado, and William A. Buchheit (Temple Univ.)
South. Med. J. 77:347–350, March 1984                    21–1

The authors reviewed the management of five patients seen in a three-month period in 1982 with open frontal bone fractures, disruption of the frontobasal region, and fractures of the orbital roof extending posteriorly into the sphenoid bone. One or both frontal lobes and the frontobasal dura also were damaged. The age span was 11–34 years. Computed tomography (CT) is now the preferred method of evaluating these patients. Cervical spine x-ray films are obtained first, however, to ensure safety in the CT gantry.

The chief goal of surgery is to prevent infection by removing contaminated tissue and foreign material. Contused, devitalized skin margins often must be debrided. A tension-free closure usually is possible. A burr hole is placed in adjacent normal bone so that fragments need not be levered out. Bone fragments are not replaced because of gross contamination. All devitalized brain tissue is debrided. Meticulous hemostasis is necessary to prevent postoperative hematoma formation. An autogenous graft of fascia lata was necessary in all five patients. If the planum sphenoidale was disrupted, a fascial sling was attached superiorly over the frontal lobes and tucked underneath them back to the tuberculum sellae; fat was then packed outside of this (Fig 21–1). No patient had persistent cerebrospinal

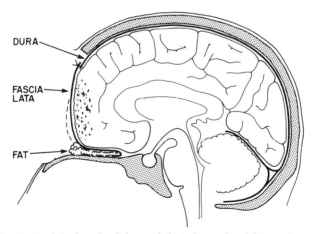

DURA

FASCIA LATA

FAT

Fig 21–1.—Repair of the frontobasal dura with fascia lata graft and fatty implants. (Courtesy of Rosenwasser, R.H., et al.: South. Med. J. 77:347–350, March 1984.)

fluid leakage postoperatively. Complete exenteration of the sinus mucosa was carried out, and all dead space was filled with autogenous fat. The supraorbital rims, if fractured, were wired laterally to the zygomatic processes and medially to one another.

Antibiotic prophylaxis with a combination of nafcillin, ticarcillin, and tobramycin was used in four of the five patients. A resistant gram-negative organism *(Serratia)* was isolated in the one patient in whom nafcillin and chloramphenicol were used prophylactically; this patient died of meningitis. Routine anticonvulsant prophylaxis is indicated in these patients. Complications associated with anticonvulsant therapy are infrequent.

▶ According to Alexandre et al. (*Zentralbl. Neurochir.* 44:169–173, 1983) basal skull fractures are associated with dural and cortical lacerations in an appreciable number of cases. Accordingly, surgical exploration is desirable, especially in frontal basal lesions. In a series of 115 cases of depressed frontal skull fractures, 85 involved the base. Preoperative cerebrospinal fluid leak was observed in 32 cases, associated with fractures into the frontal sinus in 12, ethmoid in 8, and to both and orbital roof in 8; no bony lesion was detected in the other 4. Skin wound was present over the fracture in 72 (62.6%). Cerebral lacerations were found in 50% of frontal vault fractures but in 59.5% of frontal basal fractures. Extra- and subdural hematomas were about twice as common in the basal fractures as in those of the vault. Operation on frontobasal regions was done through a bicoronal scalp flap and craniotomy, and intradural or extradural exploration to see the orbital roofs and basal dura and, as needed, the orbit. In operations on patients with hematoma, partial frontal lobectomy was done in 19, and frontal lobectomy to the sphenoid ridge in 3 of 52 operations. Maxillofacial surgeons cooperated in reconstituting the fractured maxilla and malar displacements. Suction drainage was not used; ordinary drains were removed in 24 hours. Pericranium was used for dural replacement; bone fragments were soaked in iodine solution until they were replaced in reconstituting the depressed areas. Infection requiring reintervention and local debridement occurred in only four cases.—O.S.

---

**Temporal Bone Fractures: Review of 90 Cases**
C. Ron Cannon and Robert A. Jahrsodoerfer (Univ. of Virginia)
Arch. Otolaryngol. 109:285–288, May 1983                    21–2

The presentation and course of 90 temporal bone fractures seen in 1975–1981 were reviewed. Motor vehicle accidents were the most common cause, accounting for 44% of cases. From 70% to 90% of all temporal bone fractures are longitudinal; they are usually caused by a blow to the temporoparietal region, and course lengthwise through to the petrous pyramid. Transverse fractures are usually caused by a frontoparietal blow, and they run perpendicular to the long axis of the petrous pyramid. Hemotympanum was noted on examination in 46 ears, and bleeding from the external ear canal in 27 ears. Thirteen patients had cerebrospinal fluid (CSF) otorrhea, and one had CSF rhinorrhea. Fourteen patients had facial paralysis, which in 10 cases was of delayed onset. Seventeen patients had surgery for repair of dislocated or fractured ossicles. In six cases the stapes superstructure was found to be fractured.

The status of the facial nerve must be documented at the time of initial examination. Prompt exploration is indicated if paralysis is definitely of immediate onset, but patients with paralysis of delayed onset have a better prognosis and can be followed with facial nerve testing. Exploration probably is not indicated in these cases, although some disagree. Facial nerve injury proximal to the geniculate ganglion may require exploration by the translabyrinthine route in patients with nonserviceable hearing, or by a middle fossa approach in patients who have retained hearing. The authors believe that antibiotic prophylaxis should not be used in CSF otorrhea because of poor penetration of normal meninges and because of possible antimicrobial resistance. Meningitis occurring months after head injury raises a question of slow CSF leakage. Vertigo can result from damage to the vestibular apparatus, a perilymphatic fistula, or labyrinthine concussion. Conductive, sensorineural, or mixed hearing loss can be present in patients with temporal bone fracture. The ossicular chain is most often disrupted at the incudostapedial joint.

---

**Risks of Intracranial Hematoma in Head Injured Adults**
A. D. Mendelow, G. Teasdale, B. Jennett, J. Bryden, C. Hessett, and G. Murray (Inst. of Neurological Sciences, Glasgow, Scotland)
Br. Med. J. 287:1173–1176, Oct. 22, 1983                     21–3

---

A traumatic intracranial hematoma is a major cause of preventable mortality and morbidity after head injury. Although traditional criteria emphasize deteriorating responsiveness as the classic clinical feature of a hematoma, the objective should be to identify patients at risk prior to deterioration. Patients in whom a hematoma develops commonly have either a skull fracture or impaired consciousness when first seen in a hospital.

The frequency of skull fracture and impaired consciousness in emergency room patients, patients admitted to primary surgical wards, and patients with surgically verified intracranial hematomas was calculated from samples of 545 patients with hematomas, 2,773 head-injured patients in emergency rooms, and 2,783 head-injured patients in surgical wards. The yearly number of patients older than 15 years of age who have these different features per million population was estimated as a basis for considering the advisability of routine computed tomographic (CT) scanning for the early detection of an intracranial hematoma.

With roentgenographic evidence of skull fracture and any impairment of consciousness (including disorientation), one of four patients in an emergency room or a surgical ward will develop a hematoma. With no skull fracture and preserved orientation, the risk to a patient in an emergency room is 1 in 6,000. The two intermediate situations, that of disorientation with no fracture and that of orientation with a skull fracture, showed risks of hematoma in 1 of 121 and in 1 of 32 patients, respectively. There is a consistent rank order of risks based on the presence of skull fracture, impairment of consciousness, or both. When both features are present, patients should be referred for CT without further delay after any necessary initial resuscitation.

Incidence of hematomas per million population in this study were: no skull fracture/oriented, 2 cases; no skull fracture/disoriented, 6; skull fracture/oriented, 3; and skull fracture/disoriented, 22. These data relate to surgically significant hematomas only. Many lesions seen on CT were managed conservatively and were excluded from the study. The rate of 36 patients (aged 15 years or older) per million with a hematoma is comparable to that calculated in two other Scottish neurosurgical units. The present work also confirms an earlier report that only 4% of patients who developed a hematoma lacked a skull fracture or neurologic signs at the time of hospital admission.

▶ All nine patients studied prospectively by Carlton and Saunders (*Neurosurgery* 13:153–159, 1983) for drainage of chronic and subacute subdural hematomas improved after twist-drill craniostomy and closed system drainage. Seven were cured by this method; two had to have trephinations when the improvement was insufficient. Thanks to the use of CT, most patients treated with twist drill drainage had this instituted within hours of arrival, compared with periods of more than four days in earlier years. Of importance medicolegally is the statement, "The patient with a subdural collection can become symptomatic at any time during its evolution"; similarly, once symptomatic, the patient may become worse at any time. The hospital stay for these patients was markedly shortened by the procedure, and follow-up CT scanning permitted early discharge when the majority of the collection was gone. The advantages of gradual drainage are also mentioned, including the avoidance of the rare but disastrous sudden decompression leading to brain stem hemorrhage.

In two patients described by Lesoin, et al. (*J. Neurol. Neurosurg. Psychiatry* 46:783–785, 1983) the clinical presentation was of a progressive quadriparesis, but the patients had bilateral chronic subdural hematomas! Actually, the first patient had persistent headache and change in behavior for some weeks before weakness of both legs developed; the second patient had right hemiparesis (arm and leg) before she developed quadriparesis (five days after onset). Intellect and behavior were normal. In neither case was a myelogram done, so it must have been evident to the medical attendants that the cause for the problem was in the head. Computed tomograms produced the evidence that led to evacuation of the hematomas.

Electron microscopy of bridging veins (from brain to sinus) in humans has been carried out by Yamashuma and Friede (*J. Neurol. Neurosurg. Psychiatry* 47:121–127, 1984). They found a lack of outer reinforcement of the venous walls by arachnoidal trabeculae when the veins cross out of the arachnoid. The difference may be marked; typical wall thickness in the subarachnoid space is 50–200 μm, while in the subdural space the thinnest part may be as little as 10 μm. Patterns of collagen arrangement including a tendency for circumferential fibers to predominate over longitudinal ones are considered to make the veins more resistent to distention while reducing resistence to traction. Cerebral atrophy accentuates the tendency to rupture in the subdural area. Rupture of bridging veins is also responsible, the authors believe, for chronic subdural hematomas, with formation of thin subdural membranes which tend to bleed more and thus make these hematomas larger.

As pointed out by Vydareny et al. (*Invest. Radiol.* 18:390–395, 1983), the debate concerning the radiographic evaluation of patients with head trauma now includes the problem of how and when to use CT. They have produced an algorithm for evaluation which starts with clinical evaluation. The CT scan is used for patients with an abnormal neurologic exam or with suspicion of serious head injury. Among those with normal clinical examination, if there is no palpable skull deformity the patient is sent home. If there is a penetrating injury or palpable deformity, skull films are taken, as is also done if there is suspicion of a basal skull fracture (as with otorrhea or rhinorrhea, blood in the middle ear, or hematoma over the mastoids [Battle's sign] or of the periorbital area [raccoon's eyes]). If the fracture crosses the middle meningeal vessels, a CT scan is obtained. The effectiveness of the algorithm was tested with a retrospective chart review of 608 consecutive patients. A financial savings of 65% would have been achieved, and no significant intracranial pathology would have been missed with the use of this algorithm.

On the basis of comparisons of plain and infused CT scans, Mauser et al. (*Neuroradiol.* 26:31–32, 1984) conclude that no incremental information was obtained in patients with acute head injury by infusions. Seventy patients were studied; 5.7% had an enhanced contusional focus after intravenous injection of contrast material. However, the plain CT had already suggested the presence and localization of the lesions. I disagree on the basis of their own pictures: one figure shows displaced ventricles compatible with a lesion (nonhemorrhagic) in the temporal lobe, whereas the infused scan actually shows the size, shape, and precise location of the lesion. Furthermore, as Langfitt has pointed out, the change in Hounsfield numbers can be useful in determining if there is swelling due to edema or due to hyperemia, and the treatment is, in part, dictated by that. Severely injured patients rarely have enhanced CT scans at the University of Pennsylvania, because (Dr. Langfitt writes) they are usually so sick that there is urgency about getting them either to the operating room or to the intensive care unit. He and his group are using nonradioactive xenon inhalations with CT in determining blood flow. Langfitt, incidentally, contends that the treatments of choice for acute brain swelling are hyperventilation and barbiturates.

Evaluation of possible overuse of skull films leads Bernard et al. (*Sem. Hop. Paris* 59:2567–2569, 1983) to consider that the presence of a skull fracture usually has no bearing on management. Medicolegal considerations, inadequate history, and insufficient physical examination are the chief reasons for unnecessary examinations. These authors believe that if neurologic signs are present, CT is the procedure of first choice.—O. S.

---

**Extradural Hematoma in Children: Primary and Secondary Lucid Intervals**
Peter E. Oatey, Trevor A. R. Dinning, and Donald A. Simpson
Med. J. Aust. 2:176–180, Aug. 20, 1983                                      21–4

Although the incidence of extradural hematoma in adults with head injuries has decreased, it continues to be an important complication after pediatric head injuries. Primary lucid intervals are well recognized in patients with extradural hematoma, but secondary lucid intervals are less widely appreciated. The authors studied the frequency of primary and delayed lucid intervals in children younger than 14 years of age.

Through a review of the case records of Adelaide Children's Hospital from July 1970 to June 1980, 26 children with extradural hematoma were identified. The temporal region was the most common site of injury (10 children), followed by the parietotemporal area (6) and the posterior fossa (3). In those with posterior fossa lesions the diagnosis was delayed because the onset of signs and symptoms was slow. No skull fracture was present in 6 children; however, fractures were visible both on x-ray films and at operation in 18 children; in 2 cases the skull fracture was not detectable on x-ray study. The absence of skull fracture after head injury is more common in children than in adults, probably owing to the greater flexibility of childrens' skulls. Symptoms developed within 3 hours in 35% of the children, within 6 hours in 58%, and within 24 hours in 73%. Scalp swelling (58% occurrence) was a common accompaniment of extradural hematoma, as was pupillary dilatation (50%). Papilledema occurred in six children (23%), within 3 hours in two and after 48 hours in four. Thus, the absence of papilledema does not preclude extradural hematoma. Three children had focal seizures, two within 24 hours of injury prior to surgery and one 24 hours after operation. Surgery was performed within 18 hours of trauma in 58% of those operated on. Full recovery was noted in 25 (96%) of 26 children; 1 child died within 12 hours of injury.

No initial loss of consciousness occurred in 16 (62%) children, and only a very brief loss in 5 (19%); in 5 others the loss of consciousness was prolonged. In 18 children (69%) there was a definite primary lucid interval, but in 3 there was no such interval; 5 others experienced deterioration in the level of consciousness but had been drowsy or unconscious since their accidents. A secondary lucid interval occurred in two children; in three others there was a second period of improvement in level of consciousness or of subsidence of clinical signs after a primary lucid interval and supervening unconsciousness. These events may lull the observer into believing that all is well, an attitude that is dangerous if the second period of deterioration develops rapidly.

---

**Nonsurgical Management of Extradural Hematomas in Children**
Dachling Pang, Joseph A. Horton, John M. Herron, James E. Wilberger, Jr., and John K. Vries (Univ. of Pittsburgh)
J. Neurosurg. 59:958–971, December 1983                    21–5

---

With the advent of computed tomography (CT), an increasing number of patients with head injury are scanned because of minor neurologic deficits or other disturbances. Some of these patients harbor an extradural hematoma (EH) of considerable size not threatening imminent brain herniation or focal cortical deficits. Although most of these patients still undergo craniotomy because of fear of delayed deterioration, the initial stable status of such patients warrants some rethinking about rational management—specifically, whether this particular category of EH always causes progressive brain compression and whether immediate surgery is mandatory.

From June 1978 to June 1982, 813 children were treated for head injury at Children's Hospital of Pittsburgh; 45 had medium to large EHs. Of these, 34 showed signs of focal cortical compression or acute brain stem herniation and underwent emergency evacuation of their hematomas. Eight boys and three girls, aged 2–14 years (mean age, 6.6), did not show evidence of focal cortical compression or acute herniation and were managed by close observation without immediate surgery. The interval between injury and initial diagnostic CT scans ranged from four hours to six days, with a mean delay of 2.9 days. Only three patients had initial symptoms requiring direct admission to the neurologic service.

With the use of CT, the hematomas were evaluated with respect to the size, location, density, and configuration of the clots. Locations were the posterior fossa (three cases), frontoparietal convexity (seven), and temporal fossa (one). Of the three posterior fossa hematomas, all extended above the tentorium and involved the occipital lobes. Only two clots were focal, one in the frontal region and one in the temporal fossa. Follow-up CT scans were done 5–11 days after injury and two to three weeks after injury, depending on symptoms. Particular attention was given to the volume and density of clots, degree of midline shift, and normalization of ventricular symmetry and cisternal patterns.

Recovery without surgery was observed in nine children 4–18 days after injury. Five displayed volume expansion 5–16 days after injury before final spontaneous clot resorption. Expansion correlated with persistence or increase in symptoms, whereas resorption correlated with improvement. Gradual uncal herniation was seen in one patient on day 6 and in another on day 8, presumably during the expansile phase of their clots; both had emergency craniotomy and recovered without morbidity. It is hypothesized that resorption dynamics of the subacute or chronic EH are similar to those of the chronic subdural hematoma, with predictable volume changes; and the outcome depends on intracranial pressure buffering capacity and rate of volume change. If subtle signs of brain dysfunction are monitored, selected patients with EHs may be safely managed without surgery. Factors influencing outcome of medical treatment include the size, location, configuration, and rapidity of accumulation of the clot, associated intradural lesions, extracranial decompression of blood through skull diastasis, and patient age. Urgent craniotomy is indicated if the patient shows decreasing level of consciousness, papillary abnormality, or cardiorespiratory instability. If signs of disabling raised pressure persist beyond three weeks or if CT scans show persistence of clot three months after injury, operation should be done.

▶ Most patients with extradural hematoma are seen within 24 hours of injury and usually show progressive deterioration of consciousness. Some present much later with a much better prognosis and much less urgency for operation.

With the advent of CT, these later lesions can be followed without operation, and if clinical symptoms improve, such serial follow-up may obviate operation completely. Three such patients are described by Illingworth and Shawdon (*J. Neurol. Neurosurg. Psychiatry* 46:558–560, 1983) to supplement the two cases presented by Weaver et al. (*J. Neurosurg.* 54:248–251, 1981). The three cases in the new article were managed mainly as outpatients. One must be really certain of adequate clinical observation in the hospital and of proper supervision outside of the hospital to justify such conservative therapy. A guardian angel probably would also help.—O. S.

---

**Extradural Hematoma: Toward Zero Mortality. A Prospective Study**
Albino P. Bricolo and Luisa M. Pasut (Univ. of Verona, Italy)
Neurosurg. 14:8–12, January 1984                                        21–6

---

Extradural hematoma is a common complication of head injury. It often is fatal if not treated soon enough to prevent irreversible damage from brain herniation and intracranial hypertension. The authors undertook a prospective study of findings in 107 consecutive patients with extradural hematoma treated in a three-year period. Several patients also had CT evidence of subdural hematoma or parenchymal damage, but extradural hemorrhage predominated. Two thirds of the patients were seen within 6 hours of injury, and 80% within 24 hours. In 75% of the patients the radiologic findings made it possible to evacuate the hematoma immediately in conjunction with mannitol administration. The mean patient age was 35 years, with a peak incidence at ages 11–20 years. Traffic accidents accounted for 50% of the injuries and falls for 42%.

Only 21% of the patients had a lucid interval. The temporal region was involved in 49% of the patients, the frontal region in 21%, and the parietal region in 23%. In 24% of the patients associated cerebral lesions were noted, most often focal brain contusions. Mortality was 5%. Overall, 89% had a good outcome when assessed six months after injury, based on the Glasgow criteria. All 25 patients who presented with no neurologic abnormality or with only one dilated pupil had a good outcome, as did 90% of hemiparetic patients who were operated on without delay. Impairment of consciousness was associated with a relatively poor outcome. Also, a poor outcome was more likely when the patient was transported from another hospital.

Zero mortality from extradural hematoma is a realistic goal for a modern hospital having suitable facilities for emergency neurosurgery. It must be recognized that in order to improve the outcome, deterioration must be prevented rather than being allowed to occur before a decision is made. The patient should not be taken initially to a hospital where immediate surgery cannot be carried out.

▶ Roda et al. (*Surg. Neurol.* 19:419–424, 1984) reported successful removal of epidural hematomas of the posterior fossa in males aged 6, 7, and 21 years. They have also analyzed 80 cases in the accessible literature. The hematomas resulted from a blow to the occipital region followed by a tear in a vessel (venous sinuses, meningeal arteries, or the diploetic and small dural arteries); rupture of bridging veins then complicated the growing hematoma. A classic lucid interval was reported in 23.1% of cases. A linear skull fracture, especially visible in Towne's projection, supports the diagnosis of posterior fossa epidural hematoma. Once the diagnosis has been made (now most readily with CT scan), operation is mandatory, with good prognosis if operation is promptly done.—O.S.

---

**Severe Head Injury Managed Without Intracranial Pressure Monitoring**
Gordon G. Stuart, Glen S. Merry, James A. Smith, and John D. N. Yelland
J. Neurosurg. 59:601–605, October 1983                                    21–7

---

Intracranial pressure (ICP) monitoring has become common practice in the management of patients with severe head injuries. Data on 100 consecutive cases of severe head injury seen in a 16-month period were reviewed. The patients did not open their eyes, respond verbally to voice, or obey commands for six hours, representing Glasgow Coma Scale scores of 8 or less. Gunshot wound cases were excluded. Intracranial pressure monitoring was not carried out. Forty-three patients received ventilatory assistance. Three fourths of the patients were males; nearly half were aged 11–30 years. Motor vehicle accidents accounted for 55% of cases and half the deaths.

Fifty-three patients were decerebrate or flaccid when admitted. Fifty-six had a skull fracture. Other major injuries were present in 24 cases. About half the patients had intracranial hematomas. Forty-four patients had craniotomy, and seven had repeated craniotomy. Dexamethasone was used in 56 cases, and manitol in 21. Barbiturate therapy was used in only one case. The mortality was 34%. Thirty-seven patients had a good outcome six months or longer after presentation, whereas 12 were moderately disabled and 11, severely disabled. Six patients were vegetative at follow-up.

Reasonable results can be achieved in cases of severe head injury without ICP monitoring, barbiturates, and dehydrating agents. Extradural hematoma is compatible with low morbidity and mortality if early decompression is carried out. Decompression sometimes must be done without previous computed tomography scanning.

▶ On the basis of study of 61 patients with closed head injury and raised intracranial pressure, McGraw and Howard (*Neurosurgery* 13:279–281, 1983) conclude that it is important to give more mannitol to reduce the pressure than is absolutely needed, for so doing makes it necessary to give subsequently increased doses to control the pressure. They decry the routine use of this very useful drug on a gram per kilogram, hourly, or serum osmolality basis for this reason. Treatment should instead be based on monitoring of the intracranial pressure. They believe the upper limit for tolerable pressure is 22 mm Hg (a level that causes collapse of the capillary venule junction). Enough mannitol should be used to lower the pressure to 22 mm Hg or below, and then no more until the pressure has been elevated to 25 mm Hg for 10 minutes or longer; maintaining the pressure at 15 mm Hg, for instance, may lead to administration of excessive amounts of mannitol. In comment, Muizelaar asks if it has been proved that mannitol acts by drawing water out of the brain; I think it has. However, the question is, From what part of the brain? I maintain it is from normal brain, not from edematous brain, and hence one must beware of causing brain shifts by excess mannitol.

Results of investigations in 11 patients with severe brain injury and associated intracranial hypertension induce Durward et al. (*J. Neurosurg.* 59:938–944, 1983) to propose that the best head position for such intubated patients is head up 15–30 degrees; elevations of 0 and 60 degrees produce detrimental changes in intracranial pressure, cerebral perfusion pressure, and cardiac output.

Arterial hypertension often accompanies severe head injury. Secondary injury to the brain from hypertension is feared sufficiently to warrant treating the hypertension. Robertson et al. (*J. Neurosurg.* 59:455–460, 1983) have analyzed the benefits and disadvantages of administration of hydralazine and propranolol to control such posttraumatic hypertension. The former increases heart rate and heart work and was accompanied by increased intracranial pressure. Propranolol, on the other hand, decreased heart rate, cardiac index, left cardiac work, pulmonary venous admixture and oxygen consumption. It also decreased circulating levels of catecholamines. The authors do not mean to imply that all hypertensive patients with head injury should be treated with propranolol, nor, indeed, that all patients with hypertension after head injury should have the blood pressure treated. If this is considered worthwhile, however, propranolol would appear to be a reasonable agent to use (in doses of no more than 1 mg/minute intravenously and continued at 20% of the loading dose per hour).

---

**Chart for Outcome Prediction in Severe Head Injury**
Sung C. Choi, John D. Ward, and Donald P. Becker (Med. College of Virginia)
J. Neurosurg. 59:294–297, August 1983                                    21–8

Head injury remains a major health problem in the United States. A reliable prognosis is important to both neurosurgeons and other physicians. The authors attempted to identify useful prognostic factors by reviewing the records of 264 patients seen from 1976 to 1981 with severe head injury who could not obey commands or speak intelligibly at admission. Patients with gunshot wounds of the head and those who were flaccid and apneic on arrival at the hospital were not included. The mean patient age was 31 years, and the mean Glasgow Coma Scale (GCS) score at hospital admission was 6.6. About 60% of patients had a moderate to good recovery. Surgery was done if emergency cranial computed tomogram showed a midline shift of more than 5 mm. All patients had intracranial pressure monitoring.

The GCS score, oculocephalic response, and age all were powerful predictive factors on both day 1 and day 4. Inclusion of other clinical and

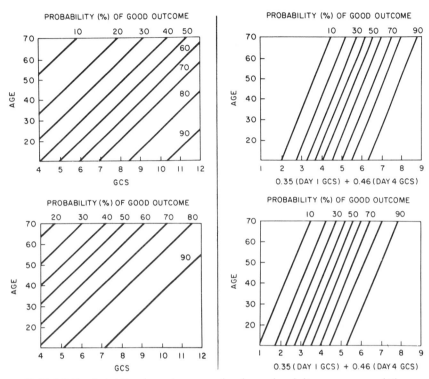

**Fig 21–2 (left).**—Probability of a good outcome as based on oculocephalic response, age, and Glasgow Coma Scale (GCS) score on day 1. Upper chart shows outcome probability for a patient with an absent or bilaterally impaired oculocephalic response, and lower chart shows outcome probability for a patient with a normal or unilaterally impaired response.

**Fig 21–3 (right).**—Probability of a good outcome based on oculocephalic response, age, and Glasgow Coma Scale (GCS) score on days 1 and 4. Upper chart shows outcome probability for a patient with an absent or bilaterally impaired oculocephalic response, and lower chart shows outcome probability for a patient with a normal or unilaterally impaired response.

(Courtesy of Choi, S.C., et al.: J. Neurosurg. 59:294–297, August 1983.)

laboratory parameters added only slightly to predictability of outcome. Predictive equations derived by the logistic regression method were plotted as charts (Figs 21–2 and 21–3). The accuracy of predictions made from the charts is expected to be 80% or more. The charts provide a measure of the severity of injury and of what might be the outcome if nothing drastic happens, but caution is needed in using them to make clinical decisions concerning whether or not to treat a given patient. The charts are based on the outcome of aggressively managed patients. Poorer outcomes could be expected if patients are allowed to become hypoxic or hypotensive, or if a delayed mass lesion or other serious complications develop.

▶ The Richmond group is one of those participating in the National Traumatic Coma Data Bank, concerning which there are two articles in the same number of the *Journal of Neurosurgery* (part I: "Design, Purpose, Goals, and Results" [pp. 276–284]; part 2: "Patients who Talk and Deteriorate: Implication for Treatment" [pp. 285–288]), both are by a group of authors headed by Lawrence Marshall. Thus far, data have been collected on 581 patients (443 males; 138 females). Glasgow Coma Scale scores of 8 or below were required to qualify for admission. Some of the patients talked on admission and then deteriorated to this level. Analysis indicates the high likelihood of subdural hematoma in this group, and since most have some shift, the authors strongly recommend early operative intervention before "inevitable deterioration" (clearly a different situation as contrasted with the opinions concerning the safety of waiting for some hematomas to resolve without operation—largely chronic subdurals, to be sure, but also with some epidural hematomas too).

The most important prognosticator of outcome of severe head injury in CT scanning is the state of the basal cisterns: obliterated cisterns have a worse prognosis. Additional help is obtained by seeing if there are lesions of the brain parenchyma. However, clinical findings are even more important in prognostication, according to van Dongen et al. (*J. Neurosurg.* 59:951–957, 1983). Clinical features included pupil reactions, best motor response, and age. Best predictions came, however, from a combination of these three factors plus state of ventricles and midline shift and lesions of the brain. It is a little difficult for me to understand how the state of the basal cisterns can be so useful when CT alone is used, yet not be important when clinical features are added. Perhaps the correlation of cisterns with pupillary size and reactivity takes care of this anomaly.

At the 1982 meeting of the Society of British Neurological Surgeons Braakman et al. (*J. Neurosurg.* 58:326–330, 1983) presented a prospective double-blind study assessing the effects of high doses of steroids in comatose patients after head injury. The criterion of one month mortality was used as a test. The dose used was 100 mg of dexamethasone given intravenously followed by a similar dose on each of the following four days. The trial ended after the entry of 159 patients, since no obvious benefit was discovered. There were significantly more pulmonary complications in the steroid group. The authors point out the problems of salvage and propose that in future trials of this sort those patients who are going to die or who are going to survive regardless of the treatment regimen should be excluded.

On the other hand, Dearden et al. (*Acta Neurochir.* 67:168–169, 1983) used a dose of 50 mg of dexamethasone given at once, followed by 100 mg/24 hours via constant intravenous infusion for three days, and reduction to 50 mg on day 4 and to 25 mg on day 5. Patients were entered into the study if the injury were severe enough to require intensive care with controlled ventilation. Intracranial pressure monitoring was used in all. Assessments were made in terms of duration of intensive care treatment and recovery status at one, three, and six months. Note the difference in criterion of usefulness compared with that of Braakman et al.

Creatine kinase isoenzyme activity in the serum and ventricular cerebrospinal fluid reflects the amount of primary brain damage after trauma, according to Hans et al. (*J. Neurosurg.* 58:689–692, 1983). When the levels are high at admission there will probably be a poor clinical outcome after six months. The activity in the serum falls off rapidly after the trauma, and hence is not so valuable as that determined in the cerebrospinal fluid.

Gunshot wounds in civilians are less likely than those in military personnel to be severe owing to the lesser energy associated with the lesser velocity. In the past, civilian gunshot victims with indications of brain stem malfunction (posturing) and a trajectory of bullet indicating passage through the geographical center of the brain have often been considered nonsalvageable. Kaufman et al. (*Acta Neurochir.* 67:115–125, 1983) report two such patients in whom the performance of multiple craniotomies to debride and evacuate hematomas led to useful survival. The authors emphasize debridement, dural closure, and postoperative monitoring of increased intracranial pressure; CT scanning has proved to be more valuable than angiography in these cases, especially in demonstrating the presence of clots.

Marshall et al. (*J. Neurosurg.* 58:566–568, 1983) reviewed data on 15 patients with oval pupil after injury to the head, and they conclude that this finding represents a transitional stage indicating transtentorial herniation with oculomotor compression.—O.S.

---

**Comparison of Outcome in Two Series of Patients With Severe Head Injuries**
Geert Jan Gelpke, Reinder Braakman, J. Dik F. Habbema, and Jørgen Hilden
J. Neurosurg. 59:745–750, November 1983                    21–9

---

The authors compared the outcomes in two Dutch series of severely head-injured patients, both covering the period 1974–1977. All patients had closed head injuries and were comatose for at least six hours, either immediately after injury or after a "lucid interval." The respective survival rates were 45% and 63% estimated one year after injury in most instances. The difference was due largely to that in the first 24 hours. An estimated 10.5% of the 18% difference in survival was attributed to differences in the severity of injury at admission. The rest could have been due to unmeasured variations in initial determinations of severity or to differences in the efficacy of management. The center with a more conservative management policy had the higher survival rate. Patients in both series had a lower survival rate if intracranial hematoma was present.

▶ The three determinants of the severity of brain damage used in the statistical analysis included age of the patient, total Glasgow Coma Scale Score (or motor response of the better arm), and pupillary reactions to light. The data are derived from a time when computed tomography was not available, but the authors do not consider that information from this form of study would have changed the outcome appreciably.

The less frequent use of certain "aggressive" treatment measures may partly explain the higher survival rate at one of the centers compared in this study. Although conclusive evidence from randomized trials is not available to assess the merits of aggressive treatment as a whole, a survey of the recent literature suggests that reports not finding "aggressive" treatment to be beneficial are more reliable in comparing series than are those that claim improved outcome after aggressive treatment of severely head-injured patients.

Among the therapies included as "aggressive" are routine artificial ventilation, administration of steroids (which other studies showed to be useful only in children), and tracheostomy. There seems to be more benefit from rapid evacuation of an intracranial hematoma than from prolonged intensive treatment thereafter.

There have been reports of disillusionment with the use of barbiturate therapy in patients with head trauma in whom pressure cannot readily be controlled. However, Rea and Rockswold (*Neurosurgery* 12:401–404, 1983) believe barbiturates can be effective in lowering intracranial pressure in such patients. In their analysis of patients with head injury, they found 27 whose pressure did not respond to hyperventilation, elevation of the head, fluid restriction, steroids, mannitol, and surgical decompression when indicated. If intracranial pressure still rose above 20 torr (slightly less than 300 mm $H_2O$), pentobarbital was given in doses of 3–5 mg/kg, followed by 1–3 mg/kg/hour. The barbiturate was continued until either the patient showed no cerebral blood flow or until intracranial pressure remained normal for 48–72 hours. Follow-up was at least six months for the surviving patients. Five of 15 who responded to barbiturate therapy died; 9 of 12 who did not respond to barbiturate therapy died (total mortality of 52% in the series of 27). Of the survivors, four had good recovery, five had moderate disability, two had severe disability, and two remained in a vegetative state.

There are obviously important problems with monitoring patients in barbiturate coma; in addition to studying the intracranial pressure and to taking repeated computed tomograms, one can use multimodality evoked potentials. Newlon et al. (*Neurosurgery* 12:613–619, 1983) report no change in brain stem potentials and suggest that only the first four peaks of the somatosensory evoked potential be used for analysis in patients with head injury who have received barbiturate therapy. Most of the effects on the somatosensory potentials are ascribed to the effect of the barbiturate on thermal regulation. Visual evoked potentials showed no change in wave form complexities and peak latencies, but amplitudes were generally depressed. The mean serum level of pentobarbital in the treatment group was 1.9 mg/100 ml.

In Oslo, Lundar et al. (*Crit. Care Med.* 11:559–562, 1983) have used epidural intracranial pressure, arterial blood pressure, serial electrogencephalography, somatosensory evoked potentials, and Doppler studies of carotid artery flow velocities for evaluation of seven patients under barbiturate coma that was induced for treatment of raised intracranial pressure. Full suppression of the EEG cannot be used for a guide when large doses of barbiturates are given; cortical and cervical sensory evoked potentials may, however, give an indication of whether or not an isoelectric EEG is due to brain damage or only to the drugs used. Cortical sensory evoked potential is invariably lost when brain tamponade develops (based on another series of more than 20 cases of verified tamponade). Determination of serum barbiturate levels appears to be of limited value, since the thiopental level resulting in an isoelectric EEG varied markedly among the patients.

Limitation of barbiturate therapy lies in the cardiodepressive effect of deep sustained barbiturate narcosis; further information about this can be obtained from central venous pressure monitoring. Central perfusion pressure (derived from intracranial and blood pressures), sensory evoked potential, and Doppler records offer valuable diagnostic and prognostic aid in management of patients with raised intracranial pressure. Typical changes in Doppler examination (of internal carotid blood flow) occur when the perfusion pressure is reduced toward zero and brain tamponade approaches.

The indications for barbiturate therapy in the series reported by Yano et al. (*Neurol. Med. Chir.* [Tokyo] 23:336–342, 1983) was intracranial pressure higher than 25 mm Hg. Follow-up after a year showed mortality of 100% for pressures over 60 mm Hg; 60.0% for pressures of 40–59 mm Hg, 53.8% for pressures of 30–39 mm Hg, and declining to 26.7% for those with intracranial pressures from 0–19 mm Hg.

The effects of thiopental and pentobarbital on heart rate, stroke volume per kilogram of body weight, cardiac output per kilogram systemic vascular resistance, mean arterial blood pressure, and central venous pressure were studied by Roesch and coworkers (*Anesth. Analg.* 62:749–753, 1983). In dogs having plasma concentrations of barbiturate ranging from 50% to 100% of the concentration producing EEG silence, these parameters were statistically indistinguishable for the two drugs. However, when given at concentrations of 45%–65% of dose causing EEG silence, thiopental produced ventricular bigeminy (reversed by lidocaine) in three of seven dogs. When thiopental was given in amounts more than that needed to cause a flat EEG, five of seven dogs died, whereas all dogs given pentobarbital survived. The authors conclude that pentobarbital may be a better choice for protecting the brain from ischemia when large doses are indicated.

On the other hand, prolonged intravenous infusion of thiopental sodium is credited for significant recovery of neurologic function in children aged 7 and 14 years, as reported by Sidi and co-workers (*Crit. Care Med.* 11:478–481, 1983). The barbiturates were given for 10 and 8 days, respectively, after failure of alveolar hyperventilation, osmotic and loop diuretics, and effective drainage of subdural catheters. Dexamethasone also failed to control the elevated intracranial pressure of over 20 mm Hg in each case.

Serial hemodynamic measurements were carried out by Traeger et al. (*Crit. Care Med.* 11:697–701, 1983) to try to evaluate the effects of pentobarbital therapy for posttraumatic intracranial hypertension. Heart rate, mean arterial pressure, and rectal temperatures were significantly reduced by pentothal given in loading doses of 4–7 mg/kg and maintenance doses of 1–4 mg/kg. When hemodynamic abnormalities occur, they are probably due to increases in venous capacitance, hypovolemia, and decreased barostatic reflexes rather than depression of myocardial function. Prevention of phenobarbital or other barbiturate hypotension is desirable since its appearance is related to an adverse effect on survival. The authors believe that patients with high dose barbiturate therapy should have right heart catheterization to monitor and treat changes in cardiac index and stroke volume index by volume expansion with pulmonary wedge pressure guidance.—O.S.

---

**Open Trial of Cimetidine in the Prevention of Upper Gastrointestinal Hemorrhage in Patients with Severe Intracranial Injury**
E. Mouawad, T. Deloof, F. Genette, and A. Vandesteene
Acta Neurochir. (Wien) 67:239–244, 1983                                        21–10

The authors examined the efficacy of cimetidine in preventing clinically significant gastrointestinal bleeding in 50 patients with severe intracranial trauma, 39 male subjects with a mean age of 34 years and 11 female subjects with a mean age of 40 years. Patients receiving anticoagulant therapy or nonsteroidal anti-inflammatory agents, pregnant women, and patients with a history of peptic ulcer disease were excluded. All but six patients were admitted within 48 hours of injury. All but one were comatose at admission. Cimetidine was given intramuscularly in a dose of 200 mg every four hours for 10 days, or orally or by nasogastric tube in a dose of 1 gm daily. A smaller dose was used if renal function was impaired.

Only 2 of the 46 patients who lived for 10 days had signs of upper gastrointestinal bleeding necessitating endoscopy. One patient had an esophageal ulcer and two gastric ulcerations on day 8, and the other had a duodenal ulcer on day 5. Both these patients had unfavorable arterial blood gas values from the outset. Cimetidine was continued, and antacids and iced saline lavage were also used.

Cimetidine appears to be useful in preventing upper gastrointestinal bleeding from stress ulceration in patients with severe intracranial trauma. This treatment is more practical in the intensive care setting than is the use of antacids and anticholinergic drugs.

▶ The authors did not have a placebo-treated group because they considered it to be unethical. I could not find any reference to the use of steroids although patients treated with aspirin or nonsteroidal anti-inflammatory medications were excluded. In at least one hospital in Chicago, the cost of oral cimetidine is $.35/300 mg, and the cost of intravenous or intramuscular cimetidine is $12.30/300 mg. The cost of one day in the intensive therapy unit is $735.00. If the results of this investigation are confirmed by others, the increased cost of cimetidine therapy would appear to be cost-effective, but the overall cost of treatment continues to rise. Now, try to justify compliance with the swell of regulatory criticism about keeping down the cost of medical care to a jury hearing a malpractice complaint of prolonged illness (or death?) as a result of gastrointestinal bleeding after head injury.

Both cimetidine and phenytoin are metabolized in the liver, and the enzyme systems appear to be related according to Salem et al. (*Epilepsia* 24:284–288, 1983). In nine patients with epilepsy who were not known to have liver disease or kidney problems, the early morning steady-state concentration of phenytoin was less than or equal to 15 μg/ml. Cimetidine was given in doses of 300 mg four times a day. Phenytoin levels thereafter were increased in six of the nine patients, and significantly so in five. Two patients developed signs and symptoms of phenytoin intoxication after receiving the cimetidine. No changes were noted in the levels of phenobarbital which three patients were also receiving, but there was some elevation—not considered significant—in the one patient who also was receiving carbamazepine.

Cimetidine (Tagamet®) is the most commonly used histamine $H_2$-receptor antagonist after head injury when corticosteroids are given simultaneously. A recent article by Mossman and Nightingale (*Infections in Surgery* 3:235–238, 1984) points out interactions of cimetidine with other drugs, based on changes in hepatic detoxification. Hepatic enzyme activity is inhibited, blood flow in the liver is reduced, and there are alterations in gastrointestinal pH. As a result, patients with benzodiazepines may become more drowsy, those with warfarin may have more bleeding problems, narcotic analgesics may become so powerful as to require use of naloxone, and elimination of phenytoin may be altered. Ranitidine (Zantac®) a newer $H_2$-antagonist, does not have the same interference with warfarin; whether it affects the other drugs is not yet clear.—O.S.

---

**Epilepsy Prophylaxis With Carbamazepine in Severe Brain Injuries**
F. L. Glötzner, I. Haubitz, F. Miltner, G. Kapp, and K. W. Pflughaupt (Univ. of Würzburg, Federal Republic of Germany)
Neurochirurgia (Stuttg.) 26:66–79, May 1983                     21–11

---

The authors tested the effectiveness of carbamazepine as a seizure prophylaxis in patients with severe head injuries and attempted to define conditions that have a high risk of seizures requiring a prophylactic regimen. One hundred thirty-nine patients older than 15 years with severe head injuries were randomly assigned to receive carbamazepine or placebo. During the acute stage of injury, concomitant medication of dexamethasone was given to 91%, phenobarbital to 61%, and diazepam to 59% of the patients. Dexamethasone had no apparent effect on the course of the investigation. Diazepam was given almost exclusively in combination with phenobarbital.

Prophylaxis was started immediately after the injuries were incurred and was continued for 1½ to 2 years. Carbamazepine dosage was adjusted individually to provide serum levels within therapeutic range. In case of a seizure all the necessary clinical management was initiated. Patients receiving carbamazepine showed a lower probability of posttraumatic seizures than did those receiving placebo ($P < .05$). This difference was statistically significant with regard to early seizures within the first week and with regard to the total follow-up time, but not regarding late seizures per se.

Brain lesions with a high risk of posttraumatic seizures were situated in the parietal and temporal areas and included acute subdural hematomas in all locations, temporal lobe and brain stem contusions, parietal epidural hematomas accompanied by other lesions, primary brain edema, penetrating injuries, and the deep stages of coma. Brain stem contusions were accompanied by a rather low probability of seizures. These various types and locations of brain lesions with the exception of brain stem contusions justify antiepileptic prophylaxis. The regimen consists of oral carbamazepine, 100 mg three times daily, given by gastric tube during the first two days and increasing to about 200 mg three times daily on the third day if warranted by the serum level. If oral medication is not possible within the initial 12 hours, phenytoin in a one-time dose of 750 mg of phenytoin infusion concentrate or a slow intravenous infusion of 500 mg of phenytoin per day is given until oral carbamazepine can be tolerated. Treatment should be continued for one year.

The authors emphasize that only persistent pathologic EEG findings indicate a high risk of seizures. Furthermore, in patients with subdural hematomas early paroxysms are significantly more likely to occur than late ones.

▶ There has been considerable variance of opinions as to the utility of preventive use of anticonvulsants after head injury. Pertinent to this is the finding by Desai and coworkers at the Cook County Hospital in Chicago (*Epilepsia* 24:289–296, 1983) that early seizures (within seven days of head injury) occurred in 4.1% of 702 patients. Children had a higher proportion of posttraumatic seizures than adults (8.7% vs. 3.1%). Obvious problems in such an analysis are discussed by the authors; these include early discharge from the emergency room without examination by a neurologist (hence implying lesser injury), severity of head injury (trivial injuries being those producing no loss of consciousness or posttraumatic amnesia; severe ones including loss of conciousness or amnesia or both for more than 24 hours, cerebral contusion, or intracranial hematoma), and need to control other variables (age, Glasgow Coma Scale, prior seizures, and use of alcohol).

A series of letters to the editor of the *Journal of Neurosurgery* (59:727–731, 1983) continues the uncertainty of the value of prophylactic use of phenytoin to prevent seizures after head injury. The original articles on the apparent lack of efficacy appeared in the *Journal* in February 1983 (58:231–235, 236–241). Criticism of the statistical data and of the therapeutic levels of drug indicates the unsettled nature of the situation and appears to call for a large cooperative trial.—O.S.

---

**Phenytoin and Postoperative Epilepsy: A Double-Blind Study**
J. Brian North, Robert K. Penhall, Ahmad Hanieh, Derek B. Frewin, and William B. Taylor
J. Neurosurg. 58:672–677, May 1983                          21–12

---

No pharmacologic regimen for postoperative seizure prophylaxis has been generally accepted. The authors undertook a double-blind trial of phenytoin in patients having supratentorial surgery at the Royal Adelaide Hospital, Australia. Patients who had previously received antiepileptic drugs and those with cerebral abscess were excluded. Treatment was begun in the recovery room with phenytoin in a dose of 250 mg, intravenously, twice daily, and continued with an initial oral dose of 100 mg three times daily for one year. Serum drug levels were monitored weekly by immunoassay in inpatients and every two months in outpatients, and dosage was adjusted to maintain a level of 10–20 mg/L. A total of 140 patients on phenytoin were compared with 141 placebo patients.

Eighteen seizures occurred in phenytoin-treated patients and 26 in placebo-treated patients. Life table analysis indicated no significant difference in risk between the two groups. Drug-treated patients had a lower incidence of seizures 7 to 72 days after operation. Compliance with treatment was apparent in 81% of patients. The average dose needed at one year was 5.35 mg/kg daily. Side effects required withdrawal from treatment in 12 cases. Phenytoin was not significantly protective in patients with high rates of epilepsy, those having surgery for metastasis, head injury with clot, and meningioma. Of nine study patients who had generalized seizures during treatment, eight had subtherapeutic phenytoin levels at the time, but most of those with focal seizures had therapeutic phenytoin levels.

Phenytoin reduces the risk of postcraniotomy epilepsy for about two to three months after operation, but not subsequently. Patients operated on for tumor, aneurysm, or head injury can be given 5–6 mg phenytoin/kg daily, orally, starting 7–10 days before operation, and treatment can be continued for one year. Other patients can be treated for two to three months postoperatively. Patients having shunt operations appear not to need phenytoin.

▶ Although Shaw et al. (*Acta Neurochir.* 69:253–258, 1983) state that their supratentorial operations carried a high incidence of postoperative seizures, these "high-risk" conditions included intracranial aneurysms other than those of the internal carotid artery, arteriovenous malformations (6), spontaneous hematoma (5), meningioma (15), and other benign pathologies (21). None had abscess. Six months of follow-up are reported for 102 patients who were treated either with phenytoin or carbamazepine. Sixteen (15.7%) patients have had seizures, and 11 of these had seizures within the first week after operation (9 while on carbamazepine). In the phenytoin group, 7 had seizures, 4 of them at three months or thereafter. An earlier retrospective seizure series had an incidence of seizures of 17%, from 92% of patients with abscess to 22% for those with aneurysm, arteriovenous malformation, or hematoma, and 50% for patients who had frontal explorations for pituitary tumors. A high incidence of side effects of medication was noted. I must admit to some inability to find a basis for the reported lack of benefit when there is no comparable series without anticonvulsants.—O.S.

---

**Halo-Thoracic Brace Immobilization in 188 Patients With Acute Cervical Spine Injuries**
Richard C. Chan, Joseph F. Schweigel, and Gordon B. Thompson (Univ. of British Columbia)
J. Neurosurg. 58:508–515, April 1983                                        21–13

---

The authors examined the effectiveness of halo-thoracic brace immobilization in achieving bone and ligamentous stability in 152 males and 36 female patients seen in 1975–1981 with acute traumatic cervical spine injury. Most patients were aged 15–40 years. The mean follow-up was 11 months. All but six patients were admitted within 24 hours after injury. Twenty-four patients initially had normal neurologic findings, 84 had incomplete cord lesions, and 80 had complete tetraplegia. The most common findings were locked facets and fracture-dislocation or complex fractures. A majority of patients with cervical fractures were initially managed by skull traction. The average time of halo immobilization was 10 weeks. A four-poster neck brace was fitted for two to four weeks after radiologic union was confirmed, and a soft cervical collar then was used when the patient was in bed.

Stability of bone or ligament or both was restored in 89% of cases. The average time to union was 11½ weeks. More than 80% of patients with locked facets eventually obtained stability following halo-thoracic immobilization. Eight patients exhibited cervical instability on x-ray study when the halo apparatus was removed 12 weeks after injury. Significant pain occurred only when the brace was poorly fitted or the Halo pins were loose. No deep infections occurred. Two patients developed cerebrospinal fluid leakage at a pin site, which resolved after a short period of immobilization. Four patients developed pressure sores over the buttocks. Another seven had scapular sores which were later minimized by cutting out part of the vest and using more padding. Fourteen of the 20 patients in whom stable union of cervical fractures was not obtained subsequently underwent posterior wiring and fusion.

Halo-thoracic immobilization provided adequate restoration of stability in nearly 90% of patients with cervical spine injury in this series, with few complications. No patient deteriorated neurologically. The brace permits early mobilization and rehabilitation, shortens the hospital stay, and is well accepted by patients. Halo immobilization also is an effective adjunct to cervical fusion. Complete tetraplegia does not contraindicate Halo immobilization. The method is recommended for all types of acute cervical spine injury, with or without cord trauma.

▶ The average time needed for fusion was about 12 weeks or three months. All four with hangman's fracture and all 22 with burst fractures healed without further incident. This is the first reported series of use of the halo-brace in a large number of patients with traumatic cervical fractures, 42% of whom had complete tetraplegia.

Dislocations of the cervical spine are missed in England as well as in the United States. Diagrams of how to take films to show the lower cervical spine appear in an article by Evans (*J. Bone Joint Surg.* 65B:124–127, 1983). This is familiar to neurosurgeons, of course. What is not, however, is the specific region of dislocation in this paper—the cervicothoracic junction. This is harder to visualize than the more common hidden area of C6-7. Evans also points out the need to do flexion and extension views (*after* routine lateral films fail to show obvious abnormality) to see subluxations which may be reduced in neutral positions. Even if the vertebral bodies are not clear in the usual lateral swimmer's view, an oblique view may show displacement of the "posterior facets." (Where are the "anterior facets"?). Evans describes a case material of 587 cervical injuries in which 14 patients had dislocation or fracture-dislocation at the C7-T1 level; only 5 had been correctly diagnosed before being referred to the Lodge Moor Spinal Injuries Unit in Sheffield. Eleven had complete lesions of the spinal cord; paralysis remained complete. Four died within seven weeks from massive pulmonary emboli. Three had incomplete lesions and made excellent neurologic recoveries although none of them had reduction of the dislocation! Evans concludes that operative reduction (needed if there is no fracture with the dislocation) is justified if the cord lesion is not complete (so nerve root recovery may be possible) and if the operation can be carried out soon after injury.

The absence of permanent neurologic sequelae from a complete fracture dislocation (C7 behind C6) was correlated by Baker and Grubb (*J. Neurosurg.* 58:760–762, 1983) with multiple neural arch and pedicle fractures which served to decompress the spinal cord from behind. Traction and manipulation after the computed tomography scan showed these fractures (and increased space available for movement) permitted reduction, which was maintained by traction for 18 days and a halo jacket for six months. Good alignment and fusion resulted without operative intervention.

An amazing lack of neurologic involvement followed an automobile accident in which the patient, age 29 years, incurred a complete dislocation of C2 in front of C3 with hangman's fracture of the arches of C2. Realignment under radioscopic control followed by halo cast fixation permitted completely normal alignment and healing of the fractures. Roda et al. (*J. Neurosurg.* 60:633–635, 1984) found three cases of complete fracture dislocation of the lower cervical spine, but no prior cases involving the upper cervical spine without neurologic disorder.

One might get the impression from the short article by Jordan (*Neurosurgery* 13:441–444, 1983) concerning migration of a metal pin in a patient with acrylic fusion of the neck that it was common knowledge of how such an operation is done ("a posterior cervical spine fusion from C3 to C5 utilizing metallic pins and methyl methacrylate was carried out"). I gather from Dunsker's comment that the pins or rods are placed through the spinous processes. I am not one to carp at the editorial urge to reduce the volume of words in scientific articles, but surely a brief description would have been a help in clarifying what was actually done. Six and Kelly are said to have "replaced most of the wiring with metallic pins inserted through drill holes in the base of the spinous processes." Did the authors do the same? What about "most of the wiring"? Was any wiring done in their case? (I didn't see any in the pictures.)—O.S.

---

**Efficacy of Methylprednisolone in Acute Spinal Cord Injury**
Michael B. Bracken, William F. Collins, Daniel F. Freeman, Mary Jo Shepard, Franklin W. Wagner, Robert M. Silten, Karen G. Hellenbrand, Joseph Ransohoff, William E. Hunt, Phaner L. Perot, Jr., Robert G. Grossman, Barth A. Green, Howard M. Eisenberg, Nathan Rifkinson, Joseph H. Goodman, John N. Meagher, Boguslav Fischer, Guy L. Clifton, Eugene S. Flamm, and Stephen E. Rawe
JAMA 251:45–52, Jan. 6, 1983                                              21–14

---

Although steroids are widely used in treating acute spinal cord injury, the rationale for this measure rests almost exclusively on animal studies. The authors report the results of a double-blind trial of high-dose methylprednisolone therapy involving 330 patients treated at nine centers for acute cord injury. All were admitted within 48 hours after injury, none had severe comorbidity. All were aged 13 years or older. Study patients received a bolus of 1 gm of methylprednisolone and the same dose daily for 10 days, whereas controls received a bolus and subsequent doses of 100 mg. All treatment was given intravenously. The study and control groups were neurologically comparable at admission.

No differences in recovery of either motor function or pinprick and light touch sensation were observed between the two treatment groups six weeks or six months after injury. The lack of an effect was independent of the severity of the initial deficit and the time between injury and the start of treatment. Deaths within a month of injury were nearly twice as frequent in the high-dose group, but differences in mortality were not significant. Infections of both the trauma and operative sites were more frequent in the high-dose group.

Patients with acute spinal cord injury who were given 1 gm of methylprednisolone daily did not do better than those given a standard dose of steroid. The findings conflict with those of many animal studies. It is possible that even the high dose of steroid used did not reach therapeutic levels, since in animals doses of 15–30 mg/kg of body weight were needed to lead to improvement in neural physiology.

▶ Following a series of articles on the apparent uselessness of steroids in treating severe head injury, comes the foregoing article on the lack of benefit of high doses of methylprednisolone compared with "standard" doses in acute spinal cord injury. Bracken et al. point out that their "study does not necessarily suggest that methylprednisolone is inefficacious in treating spinal cord injury, although this is a hypothesis that now requires testing."

The nonoperative treatment of spinal cord injury is still not standardized—nor is it often effective. Based on experiments on cats (caveat emptor!), Braughler and Hall (*J. Neurosurg.* 59:256–261, 1983) find that methylprednisolone has value in preventing the rise in tissue lactic acid associated with injury and also in improving blood flow. The dose needed is 30 mg/kg—and rigorous dosing after the initial injection would be necessary in view of the short action of this steroid. The authors point out that this dose is far above those currently in use for clinical management of trauma to the central nervous system.—O.S.

---

**Neurological Improvement Associated With Late Decompression of the Thoracolumbar Spinal Cord**
Dennis J. Maiman, Sanford J. Larson, and Edward C. Benzel
Neurosurgery 14:302–307, March 1984                                    21–15

---

The authors reviewed findings in 20 patients seen between 1975 and 1981 at the Medical College of Wisconsin Hospitals in Milwaukee. All had thoracolumbar cord injuries previously treated by laminectomy or spinal instrumentation. The most common sites of injury were L1, T10, and T12. Thirteen patients had a mass in the spinal canal causing cord compression. Seven had spinal angulation of 5–10 degrees with deformity of the spinal cord at the apex of the kyphos. Eight patients had had laminectomy only, eight had had laminectomy and insertion of Harrington distraction rods, and four had had rods placed as an isolated procedure.

A lateral extracavitary approach to the spine was used, with posterior stabilization when indicated. In 17 patients substantial neurologic improvement resulted. All seven patients with kyphosis regained the ability to walk, as did all but three initially nonambulatory patients with a spinal canal mass. Two other patients had improvement in sensation and in spasms. Eight of 14 patients had improved bladder and bowel control postoperatively. There were no deaths. Six patients had pneumothorax requiring closed thoracostomy, and one had a superficial wound infection. In one patient a late kyphotic deformity developed related to the premature removal of Harrington rods. No pseudarthrosis or late neurologic deterioration was observed on follow-up for two to eight years.

Restoration of normal anatomical relationships between the spinal cord and spinal canal in patients having previous surgery for thoracolumbar cord injury is frequently followed by significant improvement in neurologic function. A lateral extracavitary approach was used for anterior decompression and anterior interbody fusion of the thoracolumbar spine. Posterior element instrumentation can be done by this approach without repositioning the patient and under the same anesthesia. Morbidity is low after properly performed surgery.

▶ The prognostic limitations of somatosensory evoked cortical potentials in patients with spinal cord injury are discussed by York et al. (*Spine* 8:832–839, 1983). Absence of a sensory evoked potential after injury was always associated with no clinical recovery. However, the presence of a sensory evoked cortical potential was of little value in predicting the clinical state of the patient at the time of injury, or the potential for recovery. Acute respiratory distress or cardiovascular collapse or both in a patient with thoracic spine injury should suggest pleural hemorrhage, according to Freysz et al. (*Sem. Hop. Paris* 59:2229–2231, 1983).—O.S.

---

**Use of the Artificial Urinary Sphincter in Spinal Cord Injury Patients**
J. Keith Light and F. Brantley Scott (Baylor College of Medicine)
J. Urol. 130:1127–1129, December 1983                    21–16

---

Intermittent clean catheterization has improved the management of socially incontinent patients with spinal cord injury, and the artificial urinary sphincter now adds a further dimension to the rehabilitation of these patients. The authors reviewed data on patients with cord injury who had implantation of an artificial urinary sphincter. The 49 evaluable patients had a mean age of 35 years and were followed up for 3–60 months. There were 45 paraplegics and 4 incomplete quadriplegics in the study. Nearly all of the patients failed a trial of intermittent catheterization. The interval from injury to sphincter implantation ranged from 1 to 43 years.

Four of 20 patients with detrusor hyperreflexia had the sphincter removed because of infection. Twelve of the remaining 16 patients were totally continent. The overall success rate in this group was 70%. Seventeen of 20 patients with areflexia were totally continent after sphincter implantation, and another patient became continent when a tandem device was inserted, for an overall success rate of 90%. Three of six low-compliance patients were continent. Fifteen mechanical failures and 29 surgical failures occurred. The cuff continues to be the chief source of difficulty. In 12 patients the device was removed because of infection. No significant changes in renal function occurred, and the urographic appearances remained stable.

The artificial urinary sphincter produced total continence in more than two thirds of cord-injured patients in this series. The best results were obtained in highly compliant patients having detrusor areflexia, and the poorest results were in those with low bladder compliance. No clear-cut urodynamic criteria are available for accurately predicting the outcome of sphincter insertion. The only absolute contraindication to sphincter implantation is significant bladder fibrosis. Primary resection of the bladder neck is unnecessary in most patients with detrusor areflexia; sphincterotomy is sufficient, permitting placement of the cuff of the artifical sphincter around the bladder neck, the preferred position.

# 22 Disk Disease

▶ ↓ Discase® from Baxter Travenol Laboratories was approved by the Food and Drug Administration in 1984 and is now available for chymopapain injection. It still has the same vehicle; cysteine hydrochloride monohydrate is added as a reducing agent for the sulfur-containing chymopapain to keep the sulfur in the sulphydryl form. Sodium bisulfite and disodium edetate dihydrate are added to stabilize the solution. Chymodiactin has a different, "inactive" vehicle.

The Travenol brochure reports improvement rates of 68%–80% with a reported anaphylactic rate of about 0.4%. The material is to be used only in a hospital setting after certification that one or more members of the surgical staff have been trained in the technique of diskolysis and treatment of anaphylaxis. The prescribing information is very specific about assuring that chymopapain is not injected intrathecally. This point cannot be too highly emphasized, since there has been a flurry of recent reports of cases in which subarachnoid injection of Chymodiactin has been responsible for subarachnoid hemorrhage and inflammation of the spinal cord. To assist in safeguarding their product, the marketing arm of Baxter Travenol (Omnis Surgical) is offering seminars, monographs, and patient educational material to help in making Discase a safe and useful material.

To my surprise, the printed information states that Discase has been used in 2,000 patients who had prior surgical treatment for a lumbar or lumbosacral disorder. Half of these were said to be improved. Caution is advised because effectiveness in such patients has not been demonstrated in controlled studies. The text does not say whether the injections were made into the locus of a prior diskectomy or into adjacent, intact disks.

The recommended dose is 5.0 nanokatal (nkat) units per disk, since the maximal dose in a single patient is given as 10.0 nkat units, the implication is that no more than two disks should be injected (the vial contains only 12.5 units).

The use of local anesthesia in about 5,000 cases has not been associated with death due to anaphylaxis. Epinephrine, the most important drug to be used in treatment of anaphylaxis, may interact adversely with halothane, and hence the latter agent should not be used in general anesthesia for diskolysis.

A considerable amount of effort has now been directed to the possible determination of susceptibility to chymopapain, estimated at about 1% by the Mayo Clinic Medical Laboratories, where the Specific Antibody Laboratory has developed an immunoassay for IgE antibodies to chymopapain in serum. The time required for analysis is three days, and positive results are reported immediately by telephone to the referring physician.

Preoperative serum samples can also be tested by the Allergenetics Reference Laboratory, a division of Axonics, Inc., of Mountain View, California. Research is under way to compare chymopapain from various manufacturers, to prepare a quantitative chymopapain enzymatic activity test for use in the operating room, and to determine the role of chymopapain components in allergic reactions.

Hall and McCulloch (*J. Bone Joint Surg.* 65A:1215–1219, 1983) report 15 instances of anaphylactic reactions from intradiskal injection of chymopapain under local anesthesia in 4,282 patients (0.35%). Ten were women. The advantage of local anesthesia is that the patient can give early warning of subjective symptoms of anaphylaxis, as in 12 cases in this series. In only three patients was profound arterial hypotension noted before subjective warning symptoms. Anaphylaxis has not required endotracheal intubation in these authors' experience. All reported deaths due to anaphylaxis have occurred when chymopapain was injected while the patient was under general anesthesia.

The article on Chymodiactin by Javid et al. (*JAMA* 249:2489, 1983) falls in the time frame for the current YEAR BOOK but was reviewed at length in the 1984 YEAR BOOK (pp. 189–190) because of the intense interest in this new form of chymopapain suspension.

In the spring of 1984 there appeared the first issue of *Alternatives in Spinal Surgery,* written and edited by John A. McCulloch, M.D., formerly of Toronto and now at the Northeastern Ohio Universities College of Medicine in Rootstown, Ohio. The plan is to issue this bulletin as a quarterly, aiming to explore alternatives to major open spinal surgery. McCulloch emphasizes the lack of frequent adverse effects of chymopapain when injected into patients under local neuroleptic anesthesia. He repeats the warning not to inject the enzyme, directly or indirectly, into the spinal subarachnoid space. This is particularly troublesome when there is a connection between the nuclear space and the subarachnoid space, such as having had the needle pass through the latter on its way to the disk or after a myelogram or diskogram has traversed the subarachnoid space. He suggests that after passing through the skin, the stylet of the needle should be removed so that fluid may be recognized immediately if the spinal subarachnoid space is entered.—O.S.

---

**Late Results of Treatment of Intervertebral Disk Disease With Chymopapain**
Dwight Parkinson (Univ. of Manitoba, Winnipeg, Canada)
J. Neurosurg. 59:990–993, December 1983                              22–1

The author reports results in 33 patients studied according to a protocol acceptable to both the hospital ethics committee and to the manufacturers of Discase® (chymopapain). The protocol required that patients must be disabled by nerve root involvement, have a myelographic defect coinciding with the clinical picture, and have no other disease that could mimic presenting symptoms. Also, conservative measures must have been tried initially but without success. Myelography excludes the possibility of a silent tumor higher up. If swollen roots, cut-off roots, and angled takeoffs are noted carefully, laterally displaced disks are rarely missed. If more than one intervertebral disk deformity was seen, the only disk injected was that which would have been cut into had the patient been treated surgically;

an adjacent bulging disk was not injected simply because it was accessible. Diskography was avoided so as not to dilute the enzyme.

General anesthesia was not used because it would neither prevent nor modify anaphylaxis, but might delay recognition of its onset. The awake patient was given an intravenous infusion of Innovar; the anesthetist had epinephrine ready at the Y adapter of the intravenous line. At any suspicion of anaphylaxis, the patient was turned on his back, the legs were elevated, and epinephrine injected. Although no patient went into shock, there could have been two such incidents had this system of early recognition and action not been used. Patients were injected with chymopapain in the prone position, facilitating side-to side symmetry. The horizontal axis automatically becomes level, hence the vertical axis is perpendicular. Doses of 1–2 ml of 1:2,000 Discase were used according to the manufacturer's recommendation. A white reflux noted in 8% of the patients had no correlation with results. Most patients reported extensive back pain when the 1-ml volume was exceeded; although administration of the full 2-ml volume was attempted, no additional beneficial results were seen beyond those achieved with the 1-ml dose. After this procedure, patients were mobile the same day and were normally discharged on the next day. A test dose of chymopapain was not used, nor were preoperative cortisone or histamine blockers administered.

The patient consults a physician because of subjective complaints, and results were tabulated on this basis despite physician impressions. The outcome in 200 patients followed from 1 to 12 years was identical to that in the initial 33 patients treated and in a subsequent group of 105 patients. Approximately 1% reported worsening of symptoms; 65% reported complete absence of leg pain, and 15% noted complete absence of back pain. About 75% were able to conduct their normal activities. As the follow-up period approaches the 10-year mark, 96% report recovery; to a large extent, this is owing to the natural course of the disease. When chymopapain is properly used, the one specific risk is that of sensitivity reactions. To date, no evidence of delayed reaction, organ toxicity, autoimmune disease, carcinogenicity, or first-generation teratogenicity exists.

▶ The mechanism for the relief of sciatic pain by intradiskal injection of chymopapain is still disputed. Spencer and Miller (*Orthopedics* 6:1600–1603, 1983) contend that narrowing the disk reduces tension in the nerve root and, hence, pressure on the nerve root. They contend that disk narrowing is in itself a mechanism by which chemonucleolysis relieves sciatic pain. On the other hand, Dabezies et al. (ibid. 1621–1623, 1984) declare that disk space narrowing did not correlate with the end results.

Whisler (ibid. 1628–1630, 1984) points out that in a recent trial of Chymodiactin (the chymopapain preparation of Smith Laboratories), the total incidence of anaphylaxis was 2.05%, but only 0.20% in men. The erythrocyte sedimentation rate was elevated in some of the women, and there is also some apparent susceptibility of women during their menstrual periods. Pretreatment with cimetidine and diphenhydramine may be valuable in prophylaxis; certainly the most important drug for treatment is epinephrine (1:10,000). Intravenous diphenhydramine and 1 gm of hydrocortisone may then be used also.

Following chymopapain administration for disk herniation in humans, scanning electron microscopy shows a naked collagen network devoid of ground substance, according to Roggendorf et al. (J. Neurosurg. 60:518–522, 1984). Their series indicates that when chemonucleolysis fails, the reason is usually that the disk has been sequestered or the protrusion is very large in the vicinity of the intervertebral foramen. There was lack of evidence that the enzyme did not work—all cases showed signs of tissue digestion, both macro- and microscopically. At operation after failure of chemonucleolysis there is usually increased bleeding, which is ascribed to a local reaction to the enzyme. In this series, there was no histologic effect of chymopapain on the cartilage end plate.

Failures and complications of surgery for disk surgery led Cecile et al. (Ann. Radiol. 26:642–647, 1983) to offer chemonucleolysis as a valuable alternative. After four months, their patients (300 in all) had 75% very good and good results, while 25% reported average results or failures. Back pain was less well resolved than sciatica: resolution in 30%, improvement in 58%, and no change in 12%. Spondylitis is the chief drawback to chemonucleolysis. Substances that are better tolerated than chymopapain are needed; they may include collagenase.

Collagenase was employed in about 600 patients and chymopapain in about 40,000 cases, according to a review by Görge et al. (Dtsch. Med. Wochnschr. 109:68–72, 1984). They consider the success rate to be between 70% and 85% for the combined use of Discase and Chymodiactin. A footnote to the article says that because of histolytic injury from the use of collagenase in various clinics in Germany, this enzyme is no longer available.

Bromley and Gomez (Spine 8:322–323, 1983) studied 52 patients with herniated disks that were refractory to conservative therapy. The patients were treated by injection with lyophilized Nucleolysin (collagenase from Clostridium histolyticum) in Bogota, Columbia, and frozen Nucleolysin in New Jersey. Lumbar myelography showed a single level of disk protrusion; with the patient under local anesthesia and with an anesthesiologist in attendance, diskography was performed, followed by injection of 1 ml of Nucleolysin solution containing 300–600 units. Of the patients receiving doses of 500–600 units, 78% were relieved of their symptoms. There were no systemic or local toxic effects. Disk space narrowing was found in follow-up roentgenograms after injections of collagenase in those patients with successful results. There has been only one recurrence in follow-up of the successfully treated patients. About a fourth of the patients had increase in lumbosacral stiffness and spasm for as long as 10 days after injection. Most of the failures (no improvement after three to six weeks) had surgical exploration; most had sequestered pieces of disk, and one had spinal stenosis. A double-blind study was started in New Jersey in 1980 after this preliminary series was begun, and results are awaited.

The scheme of treatment proposed by Drouillard et al. (Ann. Radiol. 26:343–351, 1983) for sciatica unresponsive to medical therapy starts with computed tomography. If it is positive for disk (diagnostic accuracy in 34 patients with operation was 91.3%), treatment should follow—either chemonucleolysis or surgery. If the computed tomography (CT) gives negative results, myelography (radiculosaccography) should be carried out. If this study is positive, operation or enzyme injection should follow. If it is negative, clinical reevaluation is necessary. Most CT scans were done without contrast enhancement. The width of sections was 5 mm with a 3-mm increment (overlap) to ensure good resolution with density adequate for study of soft tissues. Parallel contiguous sections tangent to the disk allow reconstructions; when there is hyperlordosis, each section is directed at right angles to the axis or the spinal canal. When a section tangent to the disk at L5-S1 could not be made, a section tangent to the posterior edge was elected.—O.S.

---

**Percutaneous Diskectomy: An Alternative to Chemonucleolysis?**
William A. Friedman (Univ. of Florida)
Neurosurgery 13:542–547, November 1983                    22–2

---

A new method of lumbar disk removal was evaluated in patients with low back or extremity pain refractory to conservative measures and with neurologic or mechanical signs consistent with lumbar disk disease. An attempt was made to exclude patients having disk fragments no longer in continuity with the disk space. Lumbar computed tomography and metrizamide lumbar myelography were done in all cases.

TECHNIQUE.—Under general or local anesthesia, the patient is placed in lateral decubitus with the affected side down. Under fluoroscopy of the lumbar spine, a skin incision is made over the appropriate interspace. A special speculum is inserted to introduce a 40-F "chest tube" with trocar in place. The speculum and trocar are removed, and an 18-gauge K-wire is passed through the tube and popped through the anulus, then bent out of the way, thus fixing the tube in place. Through the tube the anulus is then incised, and the disk is removed piecemeal with pituitary rongeurs. The wound is thoroughly irrigated before withdrawing the "chest tube" and closing the incision in layers. Operative time ranges from 15 to 30 minutes.

Nine patients have had this procedure, one at L3-4 and the others at L4-5. All seven with sciatica were significantly relieved after the operation. One of the two patients with intractable low back pain and bilateral mechnical findings but normal neurologic findings was helped by the procedure. Three patients had paraspinal muscle spasm for as long as a week after operation. One patient had dysesthesia in the ipsilateral leg for several weeks. No other complications occurred.

Early experience with percutaneous diskectomy indicates that it is a technically easy procedure that may be a useful alternative to other methods of diskectomy in carefully selected cases. Postoperative discomfort is minimal, allowing a shorter hospital stay. The epidural space is not violated, and the nerve root is not directly manipulated. There is a risk of injuring the several structures present in the region, but no significant complications have occurred to date. Because of the height of the iliac crest, the technique is not used for diskopathy at L5-S1. The time needed for percutaneous diskectomy is considerably less than that needed for chemonucleolysis, and the risk of anaphylaxis is avoided.

---

**Lumbar Disk Herniation: A Controlled, Prospective Study With 10 Years of Observation**
Henrik Weber
Spine 8:131–140, 1983                                                      22–3

---

The treatment of ruptured lumbar and lumbosacral disks remains controversial with respect to indications for surgery in patients whose recovery is delayed. The author reviewed the long-term outcome in 280 patients with sciatica seen in 1970–1971 at Ullevaal Hospital, Oslo, and found to have lumbar disk herniation on radiculography. Sixty-seven patients had definite indications for surgery, while 87 remained on conservative management because of continuous improvement. A total of 126 patients still had radicular pain on sitting, moderate exercise, or increased abdominal pressure after two weeks in hospital. Treatment was randomized in this indeterminate group. Sixty-six patients were managed conservatively, whereas 60 were assigned to surgery.

Seventeen of the patients assigned to conservative treatment were referred for surgery in the first year of follow-up. The surgical results were better than those of conservative management, whether or not these patients were included in the analysis. A tendency toward better results from operation persisted at four years. There were fewer relapses in the surgical group in the first four years of follow-up, but the duration of recurrences was similar in the two groups. A slight increase in relapses was noted in the surgical group in the next six years. Fifteen patients eventually were considered permanently incapacitated. Five patients were operated on again, two of them twice; all but one had good to fair results. Only five patients had muscle weakness when last examined, but more than a third of the patients had sensory dysfunction. There was no difference in pain between the two treatment groups, and no difference in spinal mobility was noted. The only factor related to an unsatisfactory outcome at 10 years was older age.

Surgery is more effective than conservative management in relieving low back pain and sciatica due to disk herniation in the short term, and a similar tendency remains evident after 10 years of follow-up, although the difference is no longer significant. A delay of three months may be advisable before operating on patients with doubtful surgical indications. Temporary financial support for two to four years might be a reasonable approach to disablement benefits for these patients. The final outcome can be evaluated four years after presentation.

▶ The term *radiculography* does not appear in the index of the new fourth edition of Robert Shapiro's *Myelography* (Chicago, Year Book, 1984); in much of Europe it is the preferred term for contrast studies of the lumbosacral spinal canal. Since, in my opinion, such study is not complete without seeing the lower end of the spinal cord from which lumbosacral roots take their origin, and since very often the lumbar and cervical roots need to be seen in the same patient, I shall continue to use the general term myelography.

I am impressed by the thoroughness of the examinations of Weber's patients and the objective measurements of mobility (compass-measured distance between spinous processes of L1 and S1 in erect, flexed, and hyperextended positions, and for lateral flexion, measurement of the distance between a plumb line through the spinous process of L1 and through that of S1. The operation for herniated disk included small laminotomies and extradural removal of the disk hernia followed by "excochleation" (exenteration?) of the disk. There is no mention of foraminotomy, which I currently believe is essential to a long-term benefit from operation in view of the loss of disk height, approximation of the vertebrae, and displacement of the articular processes to impinge (in some cases) on the nerve root nearby.

It should be emphasized that these results occurred in patients who had radicular pains after a 14-day period in the hospital and in whom operation or conservative therapy was randomized. The conclusions are not based on the group of 67 patients with definite indications for surgery including scoliosis, intolerable pain, suddenly occurring or progressive weakness, or involvement of the sphincters. One thing I do miss from this study is the certainty that the surgeons all interpreted "herniated disk" the same way, and did not include "hidden disk," or "degenerated disk" or anything other than a definite bulge that compressed the nerve root and displaced it.

The author was unable to offer an explanation of the shift of the site of pain from the lower leg to the hip or sacroiliac joint, and the pain became permanent. Perhaps the article by Offierski and Macnab (abstract 22–6) may be related to this finding.

Pregnant women get herniated lumbar disks, and women with herniated disks become pregnant. What to do? LaBan et al. (*Arch. Phys. Med. Rehabil.* 64:319–321, 1983) found five pregnant women with evidence of herniated lumbosacral disk in a series of 48,760 consecutive deliveries at the William Beaumont Hospital. Average age was 28 years (range, 24–32). Each was placed in pelvic traction in the hospital and given thermotherapy; two were made comfortable with transcutaneous neurostimulation. Cesarian sections were done without complication. Myelograms then showed large herniated disks, which in subsequent three weeks failed to subside, and each came to lumbar laminectomy and diskectomy. Two of the patients had to have a foot drop brace temporarily, but otherwise the patients did very well.

Cesarian section was chosen as method of delivery to avoid possible consequences of increased intrathecal spinal fluid pressure during normal labor. The authors believe that postural and mechanical changes in ligaments undoubtedly do occur in the terminal stage of pregnancy but that they do not predispose the pregnant patient to disk rupture. (After all, the incidence was only 1:10,000!)

It is conventional to point out the values of psychological testing and the importance of psychological factors in the treatment and outcome of patients with low back pain. However, Lamontagne et al. (*Can. Fam. Physician*

29:1602–1604, 1983) have found no statistically valid differences between hospital workers with acute organic back pain and acute functional low back pain. Anxiety and depression were prominent in both, and perhaps more depression was evident in those with organic pain than those with functional pain. The Minnesota Multiphasic Personality Inventory was used to evaluate personality; anxiety was rated according to Spielberger's State-Trait Anxiety Inventory, and the Hamilton psychiatric rating scale was used for depression. Measurements were made by a clinical psychologist "blind to the experimental conditions." Twenty asymptomatic workers were used as controls. In view of these findings, the authors conclude it would be well to treat even those with organic back pain with psychotherapeutic means to hasten recovery. More accurate psychological instruments are needed to evaluate the large population of sufferers from low back pain.

Autogenous fat transplants have been used in 44 surgical procedures for diskogenic or spondylotic disease by Bryant et al. (*Neurosurgery* 13:367–370, 1983). Computed tomographic scanning has been used to follow the outcome, since the fat is clearly apparent because of its peculiar attenuation characteristics. The results confirm the occasional reports from reoperations in the lumbar epidural area that the fat does indeed survive and may serve as a barrier limiting growth of scar into the spinal canal.

A postlaminectomy pseudomeningocele is defined by Teplick et al. (*Am. J. Neuroradiol.* 4:179–182, 1983) as a spherical, fluid-filled space with fibrous capsule that occasionally develops after laminectomy and which lies dorsal to the thecal canal. They relate their experiences with 8 instances among 400 symptomatic postlaminectomy patients undergoing computerized tomographic examination. Whether these collections cause symptoms is conjectural; none of the eight have had surgical removal. Whether the arachnoid herniates through a dural tear to cause an arachnoid-lined cyst, or whether cerebrospinal fluid leaks through the dural and arachnoid tear and later becomes encysted is unclear. In four patients, myelograms were also done; in two, no communication between the pseudomeningocele and the lumbar subarachnoid space could be demonstrated.—O.S.

---

**The Knee-Elbow Position in Lumbar Disk Surgery: A Review of Complications**

Nils Eie, Torfinn Solgaard, and Hallvard Kleppe (Ullevaal Hosp., Oslo)
Spine 8:897–900, 1983                                                                22–4

---

The authors reviewed complications related to use of the knee-elbow position in 943 patients operated on for lumbar disk herniation. They represented 35% of all patients operated on between 1950 and 1981. Complication rates were 11% during surgery, 8% postoperatively, and 19% in the late postoperative phase. There were no postoperative deaths and no serious vascular injuries. Sepsis occurred in two patients. The rate of venous thrombosis fell from 10% in the 1950s to zero in the late 1970s. Reoperation or new physiotherapy was necessary in 11% of patients having fusion and in 24% of unfused patients.

An approach at the wrong level can be avoided if the correct level is identified by the lowest ligamentum flavum rather than by the lowest movable vertebra. Most dural tears were insignificant. A meningocele formed in three patients. Increased muscle weakness after surgery was rare and usually transient. Wound infection occurred postoperatively in 22 patients, disk and bone infection in 2, and aseptic vertebral necrosis in 1. Deep vein thrombosis occurred in 38 patients and pulmonary embolism in 14. Pseudarthrosis was the most common cause of pain in patients having fusion. Disk herniation and other causes were more prevalent in unfused patients.

Serious complications from lumbar disk surgery done with the patient in the knee-elbow position are rare and should be avoidable. Posterior spinal fusion appears to give better protection against recurrent pain than does simple removal of herniated disk material. The prevalence of thrombosis has decreased substantially in recent years; the decline is apparently correlated with the decrease in fusion operations but may also be related to active isometric exercises after operation.

▶ Most neurosurgeons are interested in the intercrestal (pelvic) line as an indication of where the spinous process of the fourth or fifth lumbar vertebrae may be located. Actually, according to Quinnell and Stockdale (*Spine* 8:305–307, 1983), it varies! There are L5-S1 disks that are well protected by high intercrestal lines, and in these, disk herniations are apt not to occur at L5-S1 but are more likely at L4-L5. The authors point to a fallacy which holds that a narrowed L5-S1 disk space cannot narrow further and hence that disk hernias are not apt to occur under these circumstances. Relative narrowing of the L5-S1 disk space implies a tendency to sacralization, according to these authors. "It is understood that diskographic evidence of disk degeneracy is no guarantee that the affected disk has been, is, or will be the origin of symptoms, but this is irrelevant to this study."

On the basis of studies in seven patients, Price et al. (*Radiology* 149:725–729, 1983) suggest computed tomography as the way of making the earliest diagnosis of diskitis, for the changes in ordinary radiographs are delayed and often obscured by accompanying degenerative disease of the spine.

Hutter (*Clin. Orthop.* 179:86–96, 1983) has reviewed results in 492 patients who were seen over a 25-year period and in whom a modified Cloward posterior lumbar interbody fusion was carried out. Fusion (with two blocks of iliac autogenous bone) resulted in 90% of the patients (aged 15–67 years; 60% males). The author emphasizes operation in a kneeling position so that the table can be straightened to lock the bone blocks in place; perioperative hypotension (usually 80–90 mm Hg systolic pressure) to control bleeding; exposure without rupture of the veins under the overhanging medial portion of the inferior articulating facet (followed by coagulation and division of the veins); and dissection of the cluneal nerves with ligation using nonabsorbable suture material to prevent the painful "cluneal syndrome." Fusion accompanied primary excision of the disk in 349 patients; 88 had one or more previous laminotomies, and 55 had congenital spondylolysis with spondylolisthesis. Excellent results were reported in 52%; 30% had good results. Fair results were found in 12% and poor results in 5%. Best results occurred in those with spondylo-listhesis, and next best occurred in those who had never before been operated on.

Intrathecal injection of iothalamate meglumine (60%) is to be avoided during diskography, which Hutter considers to be the most reliable diagnostic procedure for studying the disks. "The surgical treatment of lumbar pain and sciatica due to compression of spinal nerves should emphasize reconstruction of the neural spaces and stabilization rather than bone and soft tissue destructive procedures" (p. 96).—O.S.

---

**The Relationship of Complications to the Time Between Myelography and Diskectomy**
A. F. Lynch and R. A. Dickson
J. Bone Joint Surg. [Br.] 65–B:259–261, May 1983                    22–5

---

Contrast radiography commonly is carried out before diskectomy for prolapsed lumbar disk. A short interval between myelography and surgery seems to increase the risk of adhesive arachnoiditis. The authors examined the relation between the timing of spinal surgery after myelography and postmyelograhic symptoms in a prospective study of 22 patients with clinical evidence of lumbar disk prolapse, all of whom had failed to respond to conservative measures. Metrizamide myelography was administered using a dosage of 10 ml containing 170 mg of iodine per milliliter. Eight patients (group 1) were operated on 24–48 hours after myelography and 14 (group 2), more than a week after myelography.

Postmyelographic headache was comparably frequent in both patient groups, as was nausea. No patient had urinary retention. More patients had postdiskectomy headaches when surgery was done early after myelography. Groups 1 and 2 did not differ significantly in the amount of oral analgesics used. Significantly more group 1 patients had nausea one or two days postoperatively, and more metoclopramide was used in these patients. Six of the 8 patients in group 1 and 2 of the 14 in group 2 had urinary retention postoperatively.

Common postmyelographic symptoms are more frequent if diskectomy is done on the second day after metrizamide myelography than if it is done a week or more after myelography. At least a week should intervene between myelography and surgery in these cases.

---

**Hip-Spine Syndrome**
C. M. Offierski and I. Macnab (Univ. of Toronto)
Spine 8:316–321, 1983                    22–6

---

Both degenerative osteoarthrosis of the hip joint and degenerative disk changes in the lumbar spine increase with age, and they often occur together. Pain over the anterior aspect of the thigh is frequent in patients with hip disease, but it may also result from lumbar spinal disease. Most commonly there is a single source of disability, referred to as the "simple" hip-spine syndrome. Where hip pathology is suspected, local infiltration of lidocaine may clarify the source of disability. Infiltration of the fourth lumbar nerve root can indicate its contribution to the symptoms. "Secondary" hip-spine syndrome can occur where disease in the hip and spine are interrelated. Back pain from hyperlordosis in a patient with a flexion deformity of the hip and degenerating breakdown in the hip due to scoliosis with pelvic tilting are two examples. The failure to recognize concurrent hip and spine disease can lead to incorrect treatment.

Review was made of data on 35 patients with hip-spine syndrome: 30 women and 5 men with an average age of about 64 years. The primary sources of pain were hip disease in 24 patients and lumbar spinal disease in 11. Twenty-four patients had primary osteoarthrosis of the hip, four had secondary osteoarthrosis, four had a loose endoprosthesis, two had avascular necrosis, and one had nonunion of an osteotomy. Lumbar spine disease was due to degenerative disk disease in 34 cases and to a compression fracture of L4 in 1 patient. Simple hip-spine syndrome was present in 19 cases, a complex syndrome in 6, and secondary hip-spine syndrome in 6. In four cases the source of pain was incorrectly diagnosed. Two of them were treated with laminectomy and root decompression, although it was later recognized that their leg pain was due to osteoarthritis of the hip. Two failed to benefit from hip arthroplasty.

Concurrent disease in the lumbar spine and hip is not infrequent in older persons. In cases of complex or secondary hip-spine syndrome, injection of local anesthetic into the hip joint or the nerve root infiltration may help assess the causes of the patient's symptoms.

▶ Orthopedist Theodore Fox and I (who work together on complicated cases of low back and sciatic pain) have also been impressed by the co-incidence of back and hip pain syndromes and by their interaction, which sometimes accounts for persisting distress "in the hip" after operations on the back. They may coexist independently, or they may influence one another as shown in the article abstracted above.—O.S.

---

**Spondylosclerosis Hemispherica: Radiologic and Histologic Contributions to This Syndrome**
W. Dihlmann and G. Delling (University of Hamburg, Federal Republic of Germany)
ROFO 138:592–599, May 1983                                             22–7

---

Spondylosclerosis hemispherica (SSH) begins with back pain and shows a characteristic x-ray picture. The three lower lumbar vertebrae are the most frequent sites of the disease. The x-ray analysis of SSH from conventional lateral tomographs is shown in Figure 22–1. Infradiskal SSH is distinguished from pathognomonic supradiskal SSH by its multiple forms.

This lesion has multiple etiologies, including bacterial causes (florid or low-grade infections), stress due to scoliosis, ankylosing spondylitis, dorsal

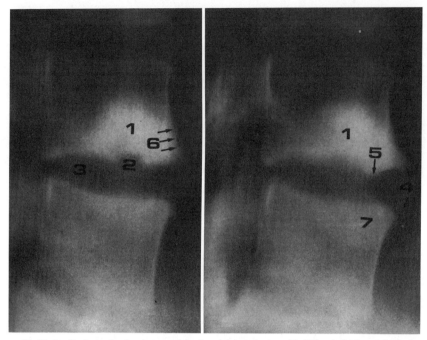

**Fig 22–1.**—Radiographs showing spondylosclerosis hemispherica with *(1)* hemispheric vertebral sclerosis, *(2)* small erosion on sclerotic base, *(3)* disk height reduction with or without spondyloretrolisthesis, *(4)* anterior intervertebral osteophytes, *(5)* socket or head-shaped diskopetal bone formation in anterior region of sclerotic base, *(6)* smooth or dentated periosteum reaction or vertical band ossification on anterior vertebra along sclerosis region, *(7)* multishaped sclerosis on adjoining caudal vertebra. (Courtesy of Dihlmann, V.W., and Delling, G.: ROFO 138:592–599, May 1983.)

disk prolapse, or diffuse disk degeneration. In most cases it is possible to ascertain the etiology from a consideration of the clinical and serologic findings, together with ordinary radiography, conventional tomography, or computed tomography. Appropriate treatment can be given after the cause of SSH has been determined.

The authors report data on 87 cases of SSH. Average age of women was 44 years and that of men 48.4 years. Women are affected twice as often as men. The sites of SSH were primarily in the fourth and fifth lumbar vertebrae. According to the x-ray pictures, the frequency of supradiskal hemispheric sclerosis was 100%, anterior intervertebral osteophyte 93%, disk height reduction without or without spondyloretrolisthesis 88%, periosteal reaction or longitudinal ligament ossification along the anterior contour of the SSH 81%, at least one erosion at the SSH base 77%, socket or head-shaped osteogenesis at the SSH base 74%, and infradiskal multiform sclerosis 67%. A summary of histologic findings in one patient examined at autopsy showed that the intervertebral disk was replaced with fibrous connective tissue. At the edges of the disk were remains of the cartilaginous end plate. The nearby marrow cavities were surrounded by sclerotic trabeculae. Within the marrow cavities fibrous tissue and scattered lymphocyte infiltrates were seen.

In one illustrated case it was discovered in 1980 that there, were at the edge of the sclerotic region, scattered calcium-rich foci which by 1982 became included into this region. Most probably such foci represent calcifications of marrow necrosis due to bacterial emboli. It cannot be explained why SSH is a relatively rare lesion while degenerative disk pathology is very frequent. The typical roentgenographic morphology is derived from the desiccation and breakdown of the nucleus pulposus; there is a significant reduction of the height of the disk. The missing disk buffer could cause the severe sclerosis of the spongiosa. The favorable prognosis of SSH due to low-grade infection justifies therapy by immobilization and analgesic-antirheumatic medication, and makes antibiotics superfluous.

▶ The problems of dealing with lesions found incidentally at examination are complex and have no uniform solution. A growing body of opinion has it that an incidental aneurysm probably should be attacked surgically, since the consequences of ignoring an aneurysm may be so dangerous. In the case of an incidentally found herniated lumbar disk, one can afford to temporize with close clinical follow-up and appropriate treatment if defects become symptomatic, according to Wilberger and Pang (*J. Neurosurg.* 59:137–141, 1983). They find a much higher incidence of painless root compression in these asymptomatic/incidental herniated disks than in classic herniated disk syndromes. They believe it possible that episodes of back or leg pain may be so fleeting as to have been forgotten or misconstrued as coming from another source, or that the bulging and subsequent rupture of the anulus are so gradual as to allow for slow adjustment of the nociceptive nerve endings. Finally, it is possible that subtle bulging causes repetitive neural injury to occur in such minute installments that ablative phenomena occur without the irritative phenomenon of pain.—O.S.

---

**Lumbosacral Spinal Fibrosis (Spinal Arachnoiditis): Diagnosis and Treatment by Spinal Cord Stimulation.**
Christian de la Porte and Jean Siegfried (Univ. of Zurich)
Spine 8:593–603, 1983                                      22–8

---

The authors reviewed data on 94 patients seen in 1973–1981 with low back pain, with or without spread into the lower extremities, who were candidates for therapeutic spinal cord stimulation. All had pain due to lumbosacral spinal fibrosis after multiple myelographies and operations on the lumbar spine. Operations were performed on 38 patients, with a mean age of 47 years and a mean of 3.5 previous operations and 5 myelograms. The mean duration of pain was more than 11 years. All patients had objective neurologic deficit. Nearly two thirds had paresis and one third had sphincter problems. Five patients had anesthesia dolorosa. A total of 88 procedures were done, not counting percutaneous test procedures, but 23 patients required only one procedure. Currently, one electrode is placed percutaneously into the spinal epidural space dorsal to the cord, at least 4 segments above the highest level of complaints. The receiver is placed in a subcutaneous pocket, usually in the right abdominal region.

Most patients use between 4 and 7 V, at 75–100 Hz stimulating three to six times a day.

The mean follow-up was about three years. There were no deaths, and no patient had neurologic deterioration or cerebrospinal fluid leakage after the procedure. Pain decreased in 60% of patients, and a substantial reduction in medication was possible in 40% of cases. Thirteen of the 38 patients returned to work, and patients worked for 26% of the total follow-up time.

A correct diagnosis of lumbosacral spinal fibrosis is very important. Classic surgical measures cannot be expected to lead to improvement in more than 30% of cases, and most successes are not long lasting. Spinal cord stimulation appears to be effective more often and has a low complication rate. Epidural stimulation should at least be tried before any destructive treatment method is considered.

▶ A prior issue of *Spine* deals with the clinical spectrum of spinal arachnoiditis (part I by G. S. Hoffman: *Spine* 8:538–540, 1983). Low back pain may be caused by this pathologic disorder, but often there is no clue as to the exact diagnosis, especially since there is a lack of significant data concerning early, mild, or moderate features of chronic arachnoiditis. Even myelography may not always demonstrate dural and arachnoidal abnormalities seen at operation (in about 30% cases). Better diagnosis may be in the offing with the combination of metrizamide myelography and computed tomographic scanning.

In beagle dogs it is possible to produce chronic adhesive arachnoiditis by intrathecal injection of iophendylate (Pantopaque) and autologous blood. Hoffman et al. (ibid. 8:541–551, 1983) have noted that in such a model, there is no good correlation between findings and the degree of arachnoiditis. Lesser degrees of arachnoiditis may be produced by this technique, and these may prove valuable in comparisons with human disorders.—O.S.

---

**Degenerative Spondylolisthesis With an Intact Neural Arch: A Review of 60 Cases With an Analysis of Clinical Findings and the Development of Surgical Management**
Nancy E. Epstein, Joseph A. Epstein, Robert Carras, and Leroy S. Lavine
Neurosurgery 13:555–561, November 1983                                    22–9

---

Results were reviewed in 40 women and 20 men aged 44–90 (average, 65) treated during a 12-year period. Lower extremity symptoms were present for 3 months to 10 years. Two thirds had signs of motor dysfunction, and sensory alterations and a positive Lasègue's sign were seen in 50% of those studied. All had advanced spondylosis and arthrosis, the latter to an advanced degree. Intermittent neurogenic claudication, present in 80%, contrasted sharply with the lesser neurologic changes; these patients required early surgical decompression. Electromyographic studies were performed in 33% of the patients, showing evidence of radiculopathy in all but two. Findings on x-ray examination included degenerative scoliosis in four patients, marked hyperlordosis in five, and a transitional L6 vertebra in three. Degenerative spondylolisthesis of approximately 1 cm was diagnosed in all patients; 40 had changes at L4–L5 alone, and 16 others had multiple levels of involvement in adjacent areas. Olisthesis was present in two patients at L3–L4 and in two at L5–S1. No patient had evidence of a neural arch defect.

Degenerative changes in the facet joints and canal size were seen on plain film but were better evaluated using computed tomographic (CT) scanning and myelography. A mistaken diagnosis of herniated and protruding disk was made in 50% of the patients based on CT findings, and similar errors were made in 40% based on myelograms; at present, both studies are used in a complementary fashion.

The procedure used in the last 40 patients included two-level laminectomy with foraminotomy and medial facetectomy. There was evidence of protruding disk in 16 patients, with herniation and sequestration in 2. Earlier patients had hemilaminectomy, interlaminar laminotomy, or coronal hemilaminectomy. At the typical L4–L5 level, the lower roots traversing the steplike defect were most severely involved. In more advanced disease the uppermost roots were also involved by the stenosing and arthrotic process. Medial facetectomy with undercutting of the facets assured decompression of the nerve roots far laterally through the foramina, the root being the primary guide. In the presence of spondylotic interbody fusion, which occurred in 60% of the patients, the facets could be sacrificed without causing further subluxation.

More than one operation was required in seven patients, all of whom improved significantly. Failure in another seven was associated with a history of disability, peripheral neuropathy, diabetes, hyperlordosis with obesity, and depression. Arthritis of the hips and knees was common, and it complicated recovery. Moderate postoperative discomfort that restricted function was noted in 12 patients. The remaining 41 had little or only minor disability relative to preoperative complaints. The sustained relief of intermittent neurogenic claudication was the most dramatic result. Patients were followed for as long as 7.5 years. Morbidity was minimal.

▶ I am somewhat surprised, as was Ehni (who discussed this article), at the absence of double-level disease in these patients. Recent cases I have encountered have had not only the spondylolisthesis without spondylolysis (In contrast to some orthopedists, I believe the term *pseudospondylolisthesis,* however it was originally defined, should be obliterated, for there is nothing "pseudo" about the slipping.) but also degenerative changes (spondylosis) at almost all lumbar levels, with resulting myelographic changes corresponding to problems at L2–3–4. Consequently, in addition to removal of the offending compression at the locus of the slipping, it has been considered proper to do a much longer laminectomy. The problem of what to do about the "weakening" of the back is unsolved; Cloward has described insertion of removed pieces of arch into the denuded disk space at the locus of spondylolisthesis. I believe it is possible that acrylic might be used (with appropriate metallic fixation) instead of Harrington and other rods when stability is a problem. I am suprised not to see a computed tomogram depicted. The use of a chairback brace in treating such patients, especially with intermittent claudication, should be mentioned because it may lead to considerable improvement, especially when the aging patient is not in good condition for an operation that cannot be called minor. Although Ehni did give some references to his earlier work (not included by Epstein et al.), he did not refer the reader to his part of a fine book dealing with *Lumbar Spondylosis* by Weinstein, Ehni, and Wilson (Chicago, Year Book, 1977).

Patients have a distressing habit of wanting reassurance that an operation will help them. Such predictions are difficult to make when the disorder concerns the back, particularly with that syndrome termed neurogenic intermittent claudication associated with lumbar spinal stenosis. A clue can be obtained from somatosensory evoked potentials picked up from parasagittal electrodes in the vicinity of the central sulcus following stimulation of median and peroneal nerves. Comparison of normal subjects with patients who had pain after walking (treadmill was used to mimic this activity) indicates that radiculopathy in those whose evoked potentials became abnormal after walking or after a change in posture (flexion or extension of the spine) had a mechanical cause, and operation to correct this was associated with a better result than in those patients in whom the evoked responses were unaffected by these maneuvers. The test can thus be helpful in determining neurogenic causes (compared with vascular ones) in claudication when clinical differentiation is unclear (Larson: *Surg. Gynecol. Obstet.* 157:191–196, 1983).

One of the most prominent symptoms with the complex of spondylosis and spondylolisthesis is neurogenic claudication. Porter and Hibbert (*Spine* 8:585–592, 1983) have tried the use of calcitonin in 41 patients with this disorder (not associated with Paget's disease) and in 10 control patients in a randomized double-blind study with crossover with a matching placebo. Considerable improvement in ability to walk without pain was deduced, and five patients have received the drug for more than a year without serious side effects. Two have not relapsed since discontinuing the drug. Patients who benefited were middle-aged men, formerly manual workers, who had pain extending below the upper calf limiting walking to under a mile. The beneficial effect is thought to be due to an arterial shunt mechanism whereby a reduction in skeletal blood flow provides for a deprived cauda equina. However, the authors concede that the mechanism of pain in neurogenic claudication is unclear and that the mechanism of action of calcitonin awaits hemodynamic and biochemical investigation.

Exum Walker (*J. Neurol. Orthop. Surg.* 4:109–117, 1983) believes that failure to provide adequate support and stability is probably the principal factor when surgery fails to relieve pain in chronic low back and sciatic disorders. His analysis of fusion procedures has led to suggestion for a two-stage procedure to provide support, stabilization, and decompression. Collapse of the disk leads to subluxation of joints and lordosis, most of which can be overcome by Harrington rod distraction. If there is considerable hypertrophic stenotic compression, the osseous canal and foramina need to be enlarged by thinning the appropriate elements with an air drill using a diamond bur. Posterior vertebral joints are exenterated, and osseous surface within and about the joints scarified in preparation for grafting. The inferior ends of the rods (which are now put in place) are supported by a transverse iliac bar. Bone grafts are then put in place in and around the joints and extended to include any of the dorsal osseous surfaces available. At the second stage, diskectomy is done by a transabdominal approach. Diamond burs are then used to reshape vertebral surfaces until they are plane and parallel. Anterior foraminotomies are done as needed. Metal wedges are then used to distract the vertebral bodies, and bone grafts put in place for fusion. The two-stage procedure eliminates iatrogenic arachnoradiculitis by avoiding exposure, manipulation, and retraction of the dura mater and nerve roots. Of 45 patients with adequate follow-up to date, pain relief has averaged 88%. The procedures have now been done in 67 patients, with striking relief of chronic back and sciatic pain. At first the two-stage procedure was done only in so-called failed back patients, but now Walker is using it as the initial attack on low back and sciatic pain.

A chapter in *Clinical Orthopaedics* (179:36–96, 1983) by C. G. Hutter relates his experiences over the last 25 years with 492 patients he has followed (average follow-up more than five years) following posterior lumbar intervertebral body fusion. His modification of Cloward's procedure includes, among others, use of only two iliac grafts for a given level with the widest part inserted anteriorly. Of 349 patients who had the operation for primary removal of disk and fusion, 56% had excellent and 29% had good results (85% beneficial results). In 88, his operation was a second one, and for these there were 34% excellent and 34% good results. For 55 with so-called congenital spondylolysis, 64% had excellent and 28% good results. Overall, 52% had excellent results (no pain, no limitations), 30% good (slight occasional pain working but not doing heavy labor), 12% fair (some pain, considerable limitation of motion, but not worse) and 5% poor results (failures). This is indeed an unusually large series—and from an orthopedist at that!

"The number of spinal stenosis cases that have occurred following primary laminectomy and secondary lumbar fusions has increased considerably during the past and present decade. Five such patients are added to the increasing literature, the beginning of which was started by Doctor Otto C. Kestler in 1966." So reads the abstract of an article by Cilento, a neurosurgeon, and Kestler, an orthopedic surgeon, (*J. Neurol. Orthopaed. Surg.* 4:119–123, 1983). In fact, four more patients are added, not five. "While it is true that stenosis can follow any spinal surgery, it has been more common with the *posterior fusions* [italics in original]. This type of arthrodesis should no longer be done anywhere in the world." Note that case 1 (of the 4) had cancellous bone grafts in the lateral gutters, and patient 2 is said to be exactly like patient 1. Patient 3 was achondroplastic with a gibbus at an L2 hemivertebra. Spinal fusion (type?) resulted in stenosis of the spinal canal. Patient 4 had had a post-diskectomy fusion over the spinal canal and its contents. Decompression should be done only after all conservative therapy fails, and arachnoidal scarring should not be operated on if at all possible. "Cerebrospinal fluid analysis may be essential in differential diagnosis of postoperative arachnoradiculitis (spinal stenosis) from other spinal maladies. Also it is very important to *carefully* remove (with a small-bore needle) whatever residual Pantopaque radiographic material that has been left in the dural sac." I must say that I have had great difficulty removing Pantopaque with a small-bore needle (e.g., 22G) even when it has been freshly introduced. Just how this is to be done in differential diagnosis *before* removing the bony fusion in such cases is unclear.—O.S.

---

**Microcervical Foraminotomy: A Surgical Alternative for Intractable Radicular Pain**
Robert Warren Williams (Univ. of Nevada)
Spine 8:708–716, 1983                                                                   22–10

During a 10-year period, the author performed microcervical foraminotomy in 235 patients who had 585 symptomatic cervical nerve roots. As many as six roots were decompressed at a single session. Ten patients had previous laminectomy or anterior diskectomy with interbody fusion. Foraminotomy was indicated for pain and neurologic deficit in a radicular distribution that failed to respond to thorough conservative management or previous surgery. Only clinical levels of radicular involvement were operated on without regard for abnormal radiodiagnostic results. The surgical microscope is used, and the foraminotomy is achieved with microrongeurs and microcurettes. The desired result of surgery is shown in Figure 22–2. An exact anatomical plane is produced between the perineural soft tissue and bone. The posterior and inferior foraminal walls are resculpted from inside out along this plane, avoiding mechanical pressure on the root. The amount of lamina removed is minimized by the use of microsurgical instruments.

Most of the patients operated on had radicular pain for months or years.

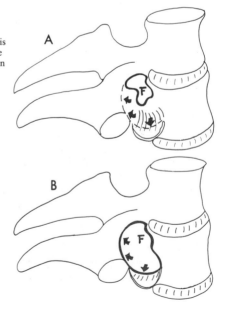

**Fig 22–2.—A,** a distorted foraminal tube *(F)* is shown with dotted line and arrows indicating the degree of decompression desired. **B,** at completion of the procedure, the posterior and inferior foraminal walls should be widely hollowed and smooth from entrance to outlet *(arrows)*. (Courtesy of Williams, R.W.: Spine 8:708–816, 1983.)

Myelographic defects were commonly present at asymptomatic levels. The 247 operations performed included 5 reoperations for recurrent unilateral radicular pain. The most common pathology was osteophytosis. Complications occurred in 10% of operations, including prolonged postoperative paresis in five patients. Radicular pain resolved within three days of operation in 96.5% of the patients, and all were relieved of pain ultimately. However, neurologic deficits remained essentially unchanged. Only five decompressed roots (0.9%) again became symptomatic; inadequate decompression may have been a factor in these cases. Radicular pain at a new level required further surgery in 4.3% of patients. The average postoperative stay was about four days.

Intractable radicular pain appears to result chiefly from nerve root irritation as the root passes through the cervical foramen. Thorough posterior and inferior foraminal decompression is effective treatment.

▶ Williams has reverted to a position espoused by Francis Murphey long ago; that is, that clinical localization was adequate for operations on nerve root compressions due to herniated disks in the neck, with few exceptions (Murphey et al.: *Neurosurgery* 38:679–683, 1973). The precise features on which localization is based are not detailed in Williams' article.

A complication rate of 10% seems unusually high, even if 7.7% cleared within six days. Prolonged postoperative paresis lasted less than one month in two patients and less than three months in three others. Even though the rongeurs were small, they still may have compressed the nerve root, especially in the presence of osteophytes. I find that using an air drill enables me to avoid this compression.

I wonder if Williams' failure to find the osteophytes so clearly seen in his figure 7 (not shown here) of an oblique view of the cervical spine might be related to the small exposure from behind? See comment to the following abstract, which reports a similar procedure using a larger incision.—O.S.

---

**Posterior-Lateral Foraminotomy as an Exclusive Operative Technique for Cervical Radiculopathy: A Review of 846 Consecutively Operated Cases**
Charles M. Henderson, Robert G. Hennessy, Henry M. Shuey, Jr., and
E. Grant Shackelford
Neurosurgery 13:504–512, November 1983                                   22–11

---

Between 1963 and 1980, one or more posterior-lateral foraminotomies were performed for simple cervical radiculopathy as the sole operative procedure in 305 men and 431 women (total procedures, 846). Males underwent 350 (41.4%) procedures and females, 496 (58.6%). Right-sided symptoms were present in 396 (46.8%) patients and left-sided symptoms in 450 (53.2%). Of the 736 patients, 283 (33.4%) had a history of surgically treated lumbar disk disease as well as cervical radicular disorders.

Preoperative symptoms included pain or paresthesia that was in a dermatomal pattern in 456 (53.9%) patients and was diffuse in 385 (45.5%). Five (0.6%) patients had no arm pain or paresthesia. Decreased pinprick sensation was apparent in 721 (85.2%) patients, and 576 (68%) had a motor deficit. In 835 (98.7%) instances, the preoperative diagnosis was either at C5, C6, or the C6-C7 interspace; on 449 (53.1%) occasions the diagnosis was at the C5-C6 interspace, and on 386 (45.6%) occasions it was at the C6-C7 interspace. Preoperative interpretations of the Pantopaque myelogram ranged from normal in 26 (3.1%) patients to severe spondylotic foraminal disease with central bar formation in 37 (4.4%). The mean duration of symptoms was 49.5 weeks, and the mean length of the follow-up was 145.9 weeks.

Technique.—Myelography is done to confirm clinical localization and to rule out other causes for symptoms. Electomyography was used very infrequently and discography not at all. Operation is done under general endotracheal anesthesia in the sitting position with legs wrapped. Central venous pressure lines are infrequently used since the complications of such insertions appears to be between 2.5% and 10%, whereas there have been no demonstrable air embolism difficulties as shown by Doppler or electrocardiographic monitoring or clinical evaluation. X-ray localization of the level of vertebra is done in the Operating Room. Small laminotomies of adjacent arches are done with small punches. The ligamentum flavum is not removed; the dura mater is rarely visualized. No disk material is removed. No postoperative immobilization with brace or collar is used.

Postoperatively, deep tendon reflex changes resolved in 96.9% of patients. A residual deficit was noted on sensory testing in 177 (20.9%) and a deficit in motor function in 12 (2.3%). Long-term results were evaluated similarly by patients and operating surgeon, with a "good-excellent" rating in 744 procedures (91.5%) and "fair-poor-failure" in 72 (8.5%). Recurrent signs were present in 172 (20.3%) patients. A second posterior procedure was required in 103 (13.9%) patients, the mean interval between procedures being 169.3 weeks. The true recurrence rate (same space and side) was 3.3%. A third posterior procedure was required in seven patients (0.1%), the mean interval between the second and third procedure being 156.6 weeks; four were ipsilateral and three contralateral.

There were no deaths. The complication rate was 1.5%, with wound infection in 10 (1.2%) patients and complications of wound separation in 3 (0.3%). Postoperatively, signs were present in 54 patients that were not noted preoperatively; 48 (5.7%) had sensory deficit, 3 (0.4%) had a motor deficit, and 1 patient had hypertonicity of the lower extremities. The mean time until return to work or other normal activities was 9.4 weeks.

▶ Fager (Neurosurgery 12:416–421, 1983) has had the unique experience of being able to compare pre- and postoperative myelograms in 72 patients who had had posterior or posterolateral operations for relief of nerve root or spinal cord compression. The intervals between the x-ray studies ranged from 3 to 26 years. The improvement in compressive syndromes can be demonstrated radiographically. Fager asserts that these results were achieved with none of the disadvantages or complications of cervical spine fusion, or of the removal of cervical disk tissue alone (also leading to fusion). Dunsker, in comment, commends Dr. Fager for taking the opportunity to evaluate his own performance and suggests that others do the same, regardless of what approach— anterior or posterior—is taken to problems in the neck.—O.S.

**Lateral Cervical Facetectomy: Surgical Pathology of Radicular Brachialgia**
C. Mosdal and J. Overgaard (Odense Univ., Denmark)
Acta Neurochir. (Wien) 70:199–205, 1984                                        22–12

The authors performed facetectomy and exposed the extrathecal part of the cervical roots from the axilla to the lateral border of the root canal in 113 patients with cervical osteochondrosis-disk herniation. Patients with unilateral radicular brachialgia and myelographic root pouch defects at one to three levels, without evident cord damage, were included as well as eight in whom operation was based on clinical or electromyographic findings. Facetectomy and removal of herniated disk fragments were carried out via a posterolateral approach. The average patient age was 50 years. Nineteen patients had previous interbody fusion.

In the 117 operations performed, disk herniation was found in 27 and uncovertebral exostosis in 43. In 59 patients a thick, fibrous periradicular cuff constricted the exposed nerve root. Thirty-five patients had facetectomy at more than one level. Four revision procedures were necessary. Seventy patients had significant or complete relief of radicular symptoms and signs. All but 1 of the 27 patients having removal of herniated disk tissue recovered, and 22 of them resumed their former work. Three of 10 patients in whom an isolated uncovertebral exostosis was left in place had a good outcome, as did 3 of 16 in whom it was ablated. Twenty-seven of 37 patients followed after removal of isolated fibrous tissue encircling the nerve root had a good operative result. Two of five patients without surgical pathology recovered. Only one patient benefited from a revision procedure. There were no serious complications, but nerve root lesions contributed to a poor outcome in two instances.

Decompression of the extrathecal part of the nerve root may be combined with removal of a fibrous cuff, when present, and lysis at the lateral border of the root canal. However, the overall efficacy of this procedure is difficult to determine.

► Operation was done in the sitting position, with unilateral exposure of the facet area. Total or subtotal facetectomy was done with an air drill under saline irrigation, using a flat-jawed rongeur to remove the inner compacta shell. The vascularized cuff around the nerve root was cut longitudinally and usually easily stripped from the nerve root and ganglion. Root mobility was considered reduced by the cuff which sometimes was 2 mm thick. I do not recall seeing such a cuff (or recognizing it, perhaps), but I think if I have unwittingly failed to remove such a cuff, the bony decompression apparently sufficed to give the patient relief from the radiculopathy. It would have been informative to have seen a picture of the microscopic findings.

The authors believe that this peculiar periradicular cuff would not have been found by an anterior approach—an operation with which they are quite familiar, as indicated in the same journal by Mosdal's article on 18 years' experience with Cloward's operation (interbody diskectomy and fusion) in 755 cases (*Acta Neurochir.* [Wien] 70:207–225, 1984). Kiel "surgibone" was used in almost all cases. After follow-up of from 1 to 13 years, 71% of patients reported relief from neck pain, brachialgia, and neuropathy. Only 42% of those with myelopathy were benefited. Complications (in 4%) included four wound hematomas, one wound infection, one donor site infection, one septicemia. Horner's syndrome occurred in 4 patients, and 17 patients had vocal cord paresis (persisting in 8 cases). Contralateral radicular signs occurred in two, root lesions in three, medullary contusion in three, and epidural hematoma in two. In two cases of quadriplegia, repeat myelogram was followed by laminectomy; in one case of Brown-Sequard syndrome, the graft was revised.

In Aarhus, Denmark, between 1965 and 1979, 1,106 patients were operated on for problems arising from cervical disk disease with the use of Cloward's method of diskectomy (Eriksen et al.: *Acta Neurochir.* [Wien] 70:181–197, 1984). Calf bone grafts were used for part of the series and were given up because they were followed by more reoperations than when other material was used for bone graft. Reoperation was less commonly needed when homografts (442) or autografts (631) were used. The end results seemed not to depend on whether herniated disk was found or the principal finding was osteochondrosis. Benefits were reported in 81% immediately after operation, with 63% reporting long-term benefits. Results did not vary according to whether the posterior longitudinal ligament was incised, excised, or left intact.

Nine patients (0.8%) had vertebral hemorrhage, and one of these developed tetraplegia. Four patients, two without medullary symptoms before operation, developed myelopathy; one died within three months, and one paraplegic and two tetraplegic patients survived. Two others had slight medullary symptoms. Laryngeal edema occurred in 18; 1 died. Four other deaths (for total of six) were due to cardiopulmonary failure. Twelve patients had recurrent nerve palsy, and six of these persisted for more than three months (exact permanence not given). The lesions of the paraplegic and tetraplegic patients are considered to be probably due to lesion of the anterior spinal artery.—O.S.

---

**Posterolateral Approach to Ruptured Median and Paramedian Cervical Disk**
Charles A. Fager (Lahey Clinic, Burlington, Mass.)
Surg. Neurol. 20:443–452, December 1983                                22–13

---

The author has long used a posterolateral approach to ruptured median and paramedian cervical disks that permits direct access to the lesions and satisfactory decompression of the spinal cord, especially where spondylosis is present, while avoiding the disadvantages of anterior disk surgery. Surgery is done with the patient sitting. Enough laminae are exposed to ensure adequate decompression when spondylosis or cervical canal stenosis is present. Removal of at least three laminae is always necessary. The entire facet on the opposite side need not be freed. Muscles are dissected using an electrodissecting device. Unilateral foraminotomy with wide lateral removal of bone provides for extradural exposure of the lateral wall of the spinal canal and posterolateral excision of the disk fragment. A dural incision above and below the nerve root allows lateral division of the stretched dentate attachments above and below the disk space. The operating microscope is used to release the fragment. The disk space is not entered, and movement of the cord has seldom been necessary. The anterior dural opening need not be closed.

Twenty-eight patients have been operated on since 1950, 26 for significant myelopathy or myeloradiculopathy. Two others had obvious cord compression and massive myelographic defects but no neurologic deficit. All patients improved after operation, and 16 of them recovered fully. Eight had minor residual symptoms or signs at follow-up. No patient had an increased deficit postoperatively. Postoperative contrast studies confirmed satisfactory excision of the lesions and decompression in the eight patients examined. No patient had instability of subluxation postoperatively.

The posterolateral approach to median and paramedian ruptured cervical disks is a useful one that avoids all the disadvantages of anterior cervical surgery and provides good access to the pathology. Atraumatic removal of compressive lesions is readily carried out by this approach.

▶ The description by Dr. Fager emphasizes the care with which he approaches this delicate area. Extension of the neck is avoided during intubation, and flexion is avoided during the operation. The paravertebral muscles are dissected beyond the lateral margin of the facet at the level of disk rupture on one side only. The lateral wall of the spinal canal is exposed extradurally on the side indicated by the preoperative myelogram, computed tomographic study, or both. Stretched dentates are cut, the dura mater incised over the bulge, and the soft disk removed. The disk space is *not* entered, and Dr. Fager has seen no recurrences. The anterior dura is not closed; the posterior dural incision is. It is uncommon to have to elevate or retract, even delicately, the spinal cord. No incidence of increased deficit has been encountered in these 28 patients, in contrast to the author's experience with spondylotic myelopathy. The operative technique bears considerable resemblance to that used by some neurosurgeons in removing herniated disks in the thoracic area.

Four different operative approaches have been used at the University of Pittsburgh for removal of thoracic disks. These are described by Sekhar and Janetta (*Neurosurgery* 12:303–305, 1983) as laminectomy (now given up as a primary approach), posterolateral extrapleural approach, transthoracic operation, and transpedicular operation. They prefer not to do the transthoracic procedure because of the need to collapse the lung, open the pleura, and mobilize tha aorta. Probably the best is the posterolateral approach. This is also the concurring opinion of Patterson (who also uses a transthoracic approach at times) and also of Epstein (who has found it sometimes beneficial to tilt the patient 15–20 degrees away from the surgeon).

"Expansive open-door laminoplasty" is the term used by Hirabayashi et al. (*Spine* 8:693–699, 1983) to describe the decompressive procedure they use in cases of cervical myelopathy due to spinal stenosis. It is a variant of earlier operations in which laminectomy has been done, the thickness of the arches reduced, and the bones replaced. The major feature of the Japanese authors' procedure is to remove about 4 mm of bone at the junction of lamina and facet (using an air drill to thin the bone and special rongeurs to take off the rest of the thinned bone). On the side of the major radiculopathy, the bone margins are lifted, and after most of the spinous processes have been removed, the laminae en masse are displaced backward and to one side as in opening a door. On the "hinge" side, a few sutures are used to prevent the "door" from being pushed closed when the deep neck muscles are resutured. Recovery rate is said to be 66%. "There was no case in which the symptoms were worsened postoperatively, although one case developed Brown-Sequard syndrome, and in three others, muscle weakness of the C5-C6 appeared transiently."—O.S.

## Spinal Cord Compression Due to Prolapse of Cervical Intervertebral Disk (Herniation of Nucleus Pulposus): Treatment in 26 Cases by Diskectomy Without Interbody Bone Graft

Sean A. O'Laoire and David G. T. Thomas
J. Neurosurg. 59:847–853, November 1983                                      22–14

In a four-year period, 17 men and 9 women aged 27–71 (mean, 47) were treated for spinal cord compression due to prolapsed cervical disk at the National Hospital for Nervous Diseases, Wimbledon, and Atkinson Morley's Hospital, London. Duration of symptoms varied from three weeks to 12 years, being less than three months in 50% of the patients. Signs of cord compression ranged from spasticity of the lower limbs alone to severe weakness and sensory loss in all four limbs and trunk. The most severe disabilities were often associated with loss of proprioception in the upper limbs. Disability was termed mild when the patient's activities were only minimally limited (3 patients), moderate when the patient was independent but unable to engage in normal activities (14), and severe when self-care was impossible (9).

Predisposing factors, present in nine patients, included prior cervical trauma in five and a preexisting cervical fusion in four (spontaneous in three). Other conditions that masked the development of spinal cord compression were present in four patients. Compression of the cord by a radiolucent extrathecal soft-tissue mass between the vertebrae was interpreted as a disk prolapse. Patients with compression by osteophytes alone were not included in this series. A single prolapse was noted in 20 patients, and 6 had prolapse at two adjacent spaces. The principal disk involved was at the C3-C4 space in 11 patients, the C4-C5 space in 5, the C5-C6 space in 9, and the C6-C7 space in 1.

Anterior diskectomy was performed in all patients. A transverse rectangular window was excised from the anterior aspect of the disk anulus, and the disk removed without excision of the cartilage plates. If no defects were present in the posterior aspect of the anulus, it was left intact; when a defect was present, it was enlarged, and the posterior anulus was excised together with any protruded disk fragment. Fragmented nucleus pulposus was present behind the line of the vertebral bodies in all cases. In 17 patients, no defect was present in the anulus, which bulged back into the spinal canal. A defect was seen in eight patients, fragmented nucleus pulposus lying behind the anulus in front of the posterior longitudinal ligament.

All but one patient improved postoperatively. Spasticity and dysdia-dochokinesia were often improved within hours; posterior column impairment and weakness often improved within days. Movement at the treated levels was abolished, and alignment was maintained in all cases. Bone fusion was noted in 15 patients and fibrous union in 3; alignment was maintained in all 18 three months postoperatively. Follow-up time was one to five years.

It is essential to differentiate compression of the spinal cord due to prolapsed cervical disk from that due to cervical spondylosis. Interpretation of some reports is difficult because of lack of differentiation between nerve root compression and cord compression in spondylosis. Other reports fail to distinguish root compression due to cervical disk prolapse from cord compression due to spondylosis. The present results reinforce the claims that relief of cord compression due to prolapsed intervertebral disk by excision of the disk carries an excellent prognosis.

▶ In a 15-year period, Lesoin et al. (*Sem. Hop. Paris* 59:2669–2677, 1983) have operated on 1,000 patients with myelopathy due to cervical spondylosis; 150 were treated by decompressive laminectomy, and 850 by anterior approach. There were four times as many men as women, and 80% of the patients were aged 50–70. Actually, analysis of the material indicates that 15% of the anterior operations were done for radiculopathy; 25% for myelopathy (and of these 60% were for paraplegia or tetraplegia and 30% for amyotrophy in the upper limbs with pyramidal tract disorders in the lower limbs; the other patients in this group had a syringomyelic syndrome or spastic-ataxic syndrome or Brown-Séquard syndrome). A radiculomyelopathy constituted the other 60% of the original 850 cases. Up to 1980, the anterior approach was that of Cloward with bone graft; after 1981, the approach was diskectomy without bone graft. The authors believe that for pure myelopathy laminectomy is indicated if there is a combination of spinal canal stenosis, multilevel osteophytes, rapid progression, and a patient older than 65. A normal or large spinal canal, monolevel or multilevel large osteophytes, patient age in the 50s, and spastic paralysis are arguments for an anterior approach, with complementary laminectomy to follow in case of incomplete benefit. If there is combined radicular and medullary involvement and if the symptoms can be explained by a single diskal protrusion, the anterior route is preferred. At times, it is possible to operate on several levels in this way, sometimes in several staged operations. If there is associated canal stenosis, one may prefer to combine laminectomy with anterior diskectomy. The results with simple diskectomy and removal of protrusions are slightly better (75%) than with the Cloward procedure (63%). It should be noted, of course, that technical aids now available were not available early in the Cloward series. Although radiologic results are better with the Cloward procedure, there are no correlations between the x-ray results and the clinical results.

It should also be noted that the follow-up with the nonfused cases operated by anterior approach is less than two years overall, in contrast with the longer follow-up with the fused cases.

About 80% of the cases with myelopathy were improved or stabilized. Benefits of anterior operation for motor root syndromes were less apparent than benefits for sensory root complaints. Progression with myelopathy is given, in another place, as 11% compared with 65% of those treated medically. I do not find any discussion or figures on complications.—O.S.

▶ The instrument-making company Aesculap has put out a brochure, "Anterior Cervical Fusion and Interbody Stabilization With the Trapezial Osteosynthetic Plate Technique," by Dr. Wolfhard Caspar of the Neurosurgical Clinic of the University of the Saar, at Hamburg (January 1984). This well-illustrated pamphlet is designed to describe the techniques and instrumentation for improved results in operations on disk disorders and spondylosis, pseudarthrosis after fusion operation, unstable cervical spine injuries, and tumors involving the vertebral bodies. Unusual elements involved include special screws placed into vertebral bodies to permit a vertebral body distraction system to separate the bodies without sacrificing space between the bodies. The instruments permit retracting bodies over two interspaces (i.e., three bodies) and permit use of bone grafts that are larger than those hitherto used and are taken from the iliac crest with a double-bladed reciprocating saw, permitting exact measurement of the graft. The author states that the vertebral plates should not be removed lest the graft herniate into or damage the vertebral bodies. Four-level fusions are, he says, readily carried out. In addition, a variety of perforated trapezoidal plates have been made to permit "osteosynthesis," that is, the holding together of vertebral bodies that are otherwise unstable or between which have been placed grafts that otherwise would not stay in place. The use of screws that go all the way through the anterior and into the posterior cortices of the bodies is deemed to be the primary improvement in the use of screws to hold plates in place. The screws can be removed after a year (following fusion) if desired. With the use of pre- and postoperative antibiotics for several days, there has been only one instance of osteomyelitis in 48 plating procedures. The plate fixations enable early ambulation without need for a halo cast sytem. Portions of this material may be read in German symposia, the abstract volume of the Seventh European Neurosurgical Congress of 1983, and in a forthcoming article in *Zeitschrift für Orthopädie und Ihre Grenzgebiete* (1984, in press).—O.S.

---

### Anterior Cervical Diskectomy With and Without Fusion: A Prospective Study

Jarl Rosenørn, Elisabeth Bech Hansen, and Mary-Ann Rosenørn (Copenhagen Municipal Hosp.)
J. Neurosurg. 59:252–255, August 1983                                    22–15

---

A generally good clinical outcome has been reported with both diskectomy (DE) and diskectomy with interbody fusion (DEF) in patients with cervical disk herniation, but most studies have been retrospective. The authors undertook a prospective study comparing these operations in 63 patients seen in 1978–1981 with herniated cervical disk confirmed by Pantopaque myelography. Only herniated disks related to the clinical and radiologic abnormalities were operated on. Patients with fracture, dislocation, or significant osteochondrosis producing narrowing were excluded. Twenty-four patients had acute symptoms of disk herniation. Thirty patients had evidence of involvement of more than one root, and six had bilateral symptoms. One patient had signs of medullary compression. The average duration of symptoms was one year. Thirty-two patients underwent DE and 31, DEF. The fusion operation was that of Cloward, using frozen-dried bone grafts.

Excellent and good results were significantly more frequent in the DE group at three months, and excellent results were more prevalent after DE at 12 months. In the DEF group, men had a better clinical outcome than women at 12 months. Women had a much longer sick-leave period than men after DEF. The mean hospitalization was six days after both operations. One patient required reoperation for a subfascial hematoma. No wound infections or cases of osteitis or diskitis occurred.

Soft herniated cervical disks are best managed by diskectomy alone, especially in women. The procedure is easier than diskectomy with interbody fusion, the period of postoperative sick leave is shorter, and the clinical outcome is better. The sex-related difference in prognosis after DEF is not understood, but the slighter bones, ligaments, and muscles present in women may be responsible, since they provide less resistance to the extension provided by the bone graft.

▶ The authors specifically state that they did not include patients "with significant osteochondrosis with narrowing of the intervertebral foramina or the spinal canal." The technical details of the operations are not given; it would be useful to know which patients (if any) had foraminal enlargement at operation. It seems almost incredible to me that with 54% of the patients older than age 51, foraminal narrowing (with herniated cervical disk, by definition of the protocol) should not have been a problem.

A long-term follow-up is clearly essential if for no other reason than to worry about what happens to intervertebral foramina when the disk is removed and the disk space collapses. A major difference with the analogous situation in the lumbar spine has to do with the orientation of the articular processes; in the lumbar spine, they may shift and compress the nerve root. Whether this ever occurs in the cervical spine remains to be shown.

Bollari et al. (*Surg. Neurol.* 19:329–333, 1983) report a series of 57 patients with cervical root syndromes or myelopathy treated by removal of the disk without fusion. The anterior inferior margin of the upper vertebral body was removed to allow better visualization of the entire disk. Cortical cartilaginous plates were also removed to improve visualization. With the microscope, visualization of the fibers of the posterior longitudinal ligament allowed determination of whether there was pressure from osteophytes, in which case these were removed (with pituitary rongeurs [sic!]); openings in the anulus were used to locate herniated disk material, which was also removed. The ligament was usually not removed when the disk was herniated but was removed when there was spondylosis. Anterior foraminotomy was done for radicular syndromes, taking care not to injure the vertebral artery.

Radicular syndromes were immediately improved in 19 patients, and others improved later so that 44 were clinically cured six months after operation. The other three complained of minor pains in the arms. Of 10 patients with myelopathy, 3 were greatly improved, 5 slightly improved, and 2 were unchanged.

Almost complete fixation of the joint is present in every case after one year, with reduction of the height of the interspace operated upon. The space above, or the space below, the operated level may become widened. It is the authors' opinion that radicular discomfort is almost always due to disk pathology and not to osteophytes.

At the 1983 meeting of the Congress of Neurological Surgeons, Richard C. Williams described a new method for anterior cervical fusion. This involves use of a special 1-mm side-cutting drill and specially designed instrumentation for removal of two small rectangular grafts from the vertebral bodies adjoining the pathologic disk space. After removal of the disk and posterolateral osteophytes, the two grafts are put together to form a single block graft which is inserted between the vertebral bodies, without impaction, "completely immobilizing the interspace." Satisfactory postoperative results in about 300 cases with involvement from one to four levels are reported.—O.S.

# 23 Infections

**Ventriculostomy-Related Infections: A Prospective Epidemiologic Study**
C. Glen Mayhall, Nancy H. Archer, V. Archer Lamb, Alice C. Spadora, Jane
W. Baggett, John D. Ward, and Raj K. Narayan (Med. College of Virginia)
N. Engl. J. Med. 310:553–559, Mar. 1, 1984                    23–1

Intraventricular catheterization is the best means of monitoring intracranial pressure in patients with neurologic disorders, but its use has been
limited by the risks of infection and hemorrhage. The authors undertook
a prospective study of ventriculostomy-related infections in 172 consecutive neurosurgical patients seen in a two-year period who underwent
ventriculostomy for monitoring intracranial pressure. The indications included head trauma, intraventricular hemorrhage, brain tumor, and subarachnoid hemorrhage. Catheterization was with a no. 5 pediatric feeding
tube using a twist drill hole at the coronal suture. Some patients received
four 1-gm doses of nafcillin intravenously as prophylaxis during the first
24 hours after catheterization. It is safe to carry out the procedure in the
intensive care unit.

Ventriculitis or meningitis developed in 19 patients (11%) in the course
of 213 ventriculostomies. The most common pathogen isolated was coagu-
lase-negative staphylococcus. Cerebrospinal fluid (CSF) pleocytosis was
associated more closely with the diagnosis of ventriculitis or meningitis
than were fever and leukocytosis. Risk factors for ventriculostomy-related
infection included intraventricular bleeding, neurosurgery, an intracranial
pressure of 20 mm Hg or more, ventricular catheterization for more than
5 days, and irrigation of the system. Previous ventriculostomy did not
increase the risk of infection after a subsequent procedure. Infection was
significantly associated with mortality.

In about 9% of 213 ventriculostomies in this series, infection developed
in relation to the procedure. The diagnosis should be based on the results
of culture of the CSF after aspiration through the ventricular catheter or
lumbar puncture. Ventricular catheters should be removed after five days
and reinserted at a new site if further monitoring is necessary. Every attempt should be made to limit irrigation of the system.

**Incidence of Postoperative Infection in 1,000 Neurosurgical Interventions
and Effect of Prophylactic Antibiotic Therapy**
J.-L. Raggueneau, J. Cophignon, A. Kind, A. Rey, A. Goldstein, C. Thurel,
C. Dematons, B. George, and F. X. Roux (Paris)
Neurochirurgie 29:229–233, 1983                    23–2

The authors studied prophylactic antibiotic therapy in neurosurgical
procedures carried out between December 1980 and March 1982, with

the objective of establishing the frequency of neurosurgical infectious complications, discerning factors favoring infection, and studying the effect of prophylactic perioperative antibiotic treatment in 37% of these interventions. Criteria for infection were those defined by Malis: local suppuration with positive cultures; bacterial meningitis; meningeal syndrome with inflammatory appearance of the scar and polynucleosis in the spinal fluid but with no bacterial isolate. The factors likely to favor an infection were considered to be: emergency surgery, opening of a paranasal sinus (traumatic preoperative or perioperative), the presence of a foreign body, perioperative corticotherapy, diabetes, duration of surgery, and age of patient.

It was found that an infectious surgical complication (cellulitis at the incision site, meningitis, or both) occurred in 5.1% of the entire group. Emergency surgery, opening of the sinus, and duration of surgery for more than five hours were found to elevate the risk of infection, but age of patient, diabetes, and corticotherapy seemed to have no significant influence. Similarly, the preventive administration of an antibiotic agent (Cefalotin) had no impact on the incidence of general infection, except in procedures lasting for more than five hours. The risk of infection was found to be high (7.8%) after craniotomies and even greater (14%) after ventricular shunts. For the latter procedure it was not possible to isolate factors promoting infection. Cervical operations led to infection in 2.8%, and spinal operations only in 1.4%.

In the absence of promoting factors, the risk of infection is minimal (1%) but increases considerably in patients with one or more intercurrent infections.

▶ Guidelines for prevention of surgical wound infections are proposed by Polk et al. (*Arch. Surg.* 118:1213–1217, 1983). The group of physicians convened by the Centers for Disease Control consider surveillance and classification, preparation of the patient, preparation of the surgical team, ventilation and air quality in the operating room, cleaning and culturing, operative technique, wound care, topical antibiotics, and prophylactic antibiotics. The latter are recommended for operations with life-threatening consequences if infections occur, including neurosurgical operations. Depilatory creams have long been preferable to razor preparation, which probably increases chances of infection. Preparation of the operative site with chlorhexidine, iodophors, or tincture of iodine is appropriate. Suture material should be monofilament, and of the smallest caliber compatible with accurate apposition and strength of closure. Failure to remove soaked dressings after operation increases bacterial contamination. Each time a drain is inserted a sound indication must be present; closed suction drains passed through separate stab wounds are probably best. A short preoperative stay in the hospital is safest, and nutrition should be maintained at all times. Antibiotics for prophylaxis must be started before operation and are given for short periods only. I urge all readers to read this article in its entirety—and to disseminate its important features.

The use of a reservoir in ventriculoperitoneal shunts is very much worthwhile as an entry for intraventricular antibiotic therapy in cases of cerebrospinal fluid shunt infections, according to Frame and McLaurin (*J. Neurosurg.* 60:354–

360, 1984). Two shunts were completely replaced (from ventriculoatrial to ventriculoperitoneal shunts). Nine of 10 evaluable cases were considered cured by a combination of oral (for systemic) administration and intraventricular (via shunt) injections done daily. The oral antibiotics were trimethoprim-sulfamethoxazole and rifampin; the intraventricular material was usually vancomycin. (Kanamycin and cephapirin were used in two cases.) Eight of the 11 patients had to have temporary externalization of the peritoneal end of the shunt. The authors suggest revisions be done during the antibiotic period.

The review by Forward et al. (*J. Neurosurg.* 59:389–394, 1983) of 35 infections in 32 patients with ventricular shunts is difficult to evaluate. Eight patients had relapses after apparent cure, which makes for 43 clinical episodes, but figure 3 deals with results of therapy in 34 clinical courses. Ventriculoatrial shunts were present in 15 patients and ventriculoperitoneal shunts in 17; but 3 patients had shunts of other types (2 ventriculosternal and 1 lumboperitoneal), and 3 patients had more than one type of shunt. Fourteen patients were over age 20. The number of the younger patients who had each type of shunt is not given, so we have no way of knowing if young patients with ventriculoatrial shunts get more infections than old patients with ventriculoperitoneal shunts (as some maintain). In fact, there is no information as to why the shunts were done in the first place, how many patients had them placed in infancy, whether the older patients (ages ranged from 2 months to 70 years) had shunts for hydrocephalus from tumor, from "normal pressure hydrocephalus," or whatever. What does seem to be clear is that in this group of patients, therapy with parenteral antibiotics and only partial shunt removal yields an unacceptably high failure rate for treatment of infections.

A double-blind placebo controlled study carried out by Wang et al. (*JAMA* 251:1174–1177, 1984) failed to show any benefit from prophylactic sulfamethoxazole and trimethoprim (Bactrim® and Septra®) in preventing infection after ventriculoperitoneal shunt surgery. Infections did occur in 4 of 55 patients in the treated group, and in 5 of 65 in the placebo-treated group. The incidence of shunt malfunction was about the same (18 of 51) in those receiving antibiotic prophylaxis as in those who did not (23 of 60).

Based on a double-blind study, Odio et al. (*Am. J. Dis. Child.* 138:17–19, 1984) have discontinued the use of vancomycin as a prophylactic antibiotic for cerebrospinal fluid shunt procedures. There were too many adverse reactions: rash occurred in 35%, and there was no obvious decrease in incidence of infections (17% as compared with 23% in the placebo group). Frame and McLaurin (*J. Neurosurg.* 60:354–360, 1984) describe no such problems with their use of vancomycin (given only intraventricularly) in the treatment of established infections of shunt systems.—O.S.

---

**Experience With Brain Biopsy for Suspected Herpes Encephalitis: A Review of Forty Consecutive Cases**
Richard B. Morawetz, Richard J. Whitley, and Dennis M. Murphy (Univ. of Alabama)
Neurosurgery 12:654–657, June 1983                                    23–3

The only definitive method available for diagnosing herpes simplex encephalitis at present is the isolation of herpes simplex virus (HSV) from brain biopsy tissue. The authors reviewed experience with 40 consecutive patients, clinically suspected of having herpes simplex encephalitis, who underwent diagnostic brain biopsy from 1973 to 1981. Biopsies were done as part of an experimental antiviral treatment program in patients with a tentative clinical diagnosis. The biopsy site was determined by the patient's localizing neurologic signs, the EEG, and the computed tomography scan changes but was ordinarily from the inferior temporal gyrus of the affected side. The 30 male and 10 female patients had a median age of 19 years. Idoxuridine treatment was used in early cases, and vidarabine or acyclovir was used in later cases.

Seventeen patients (42.5%) were ultimately diagnosed as having herpes simplex encephalitis by isolation of HSV in tissue culture. Biopsy specimens from two patients were negative, although HSV was grown from brain tissue obtained at autopsy. The overall mortality was 32.5%; no death was ascribable to the biopsy procedure. Eight of the 15 virus-positive patients survived: 3 of them were normal at follow-up, 3 were moderately impaired, and 2 were severely disabled. The prognosis worsened with an increasing interval between the onset of symptoms and the start of antiviral therapy, with increasingly severe neurologic impairment at the onset of therapy, and with abnormal computed tomography findings at the time of biopsy.

Brain biopsy remains the best means of establishing a diagnosis of herpes simplex encephalitis and allowing the initiation of antiviral therapy. There is interest in cerebrospinal fluid glycoprotein determination by radioimmunoassay, in the hope that glycoproteins produced during HSV replication and excreted into the cerebrospinal fluid can aid diagnosis.

---

**Clinical Stages of Human Brain Abscesses on Serial CT Scans After Contrast Infusion: CT, Neuropathological, and Clinical Correlations**
Richard H. Britt and Dieter R. Enzmann (Stanford Univ.)
J. Neurosurg. 59:972–989, December 1983                          23–4

The authors describe a classification of human brain abscesses into stages of development with the use of computed tomography (CT).

Brain abscesses were studied in 14 patients, 6 of whom had multiple sites. Brain CT scans were used to follow each lesion during the course of treatment. In nine patients, serial CT scans were performed after contrast infusion at time intervals of 0, 5, 10, 20, 30, 45, and 60 minutes. In three patients, the initial CT study included scans at 10–15 minutes and at 70 and 90 minutes. In staging the abscesses, the criteria used were the pattern and the time-density curve of contrast enhancement. The degree of ring-contrast enhancement was quantified by measuring the CT units above baseline. Baseline value for normal brain at the location of each abscess was obtained by measurement at the analogous location in the contralateral hemisphere.

On precontrast CT scans an area of low density was compatible with either cerebritis or early capsule stages. Findings for cerebritis classification were a thick diffuse ring of enhancement and further diffusion of contrast material into the central lumen and/or lack of significant decay in enhancement on scans 30–60 minutes after contrast infusion. If a faint rim was present on the precontrast scan, the lesion was placed into the capsule stage. On postcontrast scans an abscess was placed in the capsule stage if there was a relatively thin ring of enhancement and, more importantly, if the delayed scans showed a decrease in intensity of enhancement and minimal diffusion of contrast material. To verify the accuracy of CT staging, tissue obtained at surgery or autopsy was studied to determine the histologic stage of each brain abscess.

Initial CT staging was found to be accurate in all 14 patients. By combining CT scan findings, surgical observations, and histologic examination, it was possible to classify patients into one of four stages: early cerebritis, late cerebritis, early capsule formation, or late capsule formation. In early and late cerebritis the precontrast CT scans showed an ill-defined area of low density. The patterns of enhancement were greatly variable depending on the time course of the lesion. The density of the necrotic or lucent center was also variable in the cerebritis stage. In order to differentiate the cerebritis from the capsule stage, delayed CT scans following contrast infusion were obtained. In the cerebritis stage, ring enhancement intensity did not decrease at 60–90 minutes. In the early capsule formation stage, the precontrast scan showed a faint ring that had higher density than that of both the surrounding edematous brain and the necrotic center. In all five patients with well-enscapsulated abscesses, the collagen capsule was delineated on the precontrast scan owing to a low-density necrotic center and the surrounding edematous brain. Contrast enhancement showed a high-density thin ring in one case and a ring of moderate thickness in three cases. Corticosteroid administration greatly reduced contrast enhancement in the cerebritis stage but had little effect in the capsule stage.

Aspiration of the abscess is strongly favored for lesions in the cerebritis stage, while for lesions in the well-encapsulated stage there seems to be little difference between results of aspiration, aspiration followed by excision, or excision alone. Computed tomography after aspiration can be used to determine if repeated aspiration is warranted.

▶ The Rumanian neurosurgeons continue to analyze their series of cerebral and cerebellar abscesses: Arseni et al. (*Zentralbl. Neurochir.* 44:39–51, 1983) report finding 108 cases of abscess of unknown origin among the total of 810 cerebral abscesses hospitalized from 1936 to 1979. The overall mortality of the group was 29.7%. The sources are undetectable by ordinary means of investigation in vivo, and even the pathologists have been unable to discover the source of brain abscess each time. Arseni et al. believe these loci of infection in the brain are primarily metastatic via the hematogenic route. Even the modern era of antibiosis fails to give an increased cure rate. The surgical goal of this group of neurosurgeons has been total ablation. A particular feature of the recovery of many patients has been a high proportion of "neuropsychiatric" aftereffects, which include, in descending order of frequency, motor deficits, epilepsy, speech disturbances, hemianopia, cranial nerve palsies, and balance disturbances.

A review of the neurosurgery of otorhinologic sepsis by Williams (*Clin. Otolaryngol.* 8:121–133, 1983) emphasizes the need for accurate bacteriology as a prerequisite for medical treatment of the abscess; when antibiotics need to be given before sensitivities are known, chloramphenicol is the best choice. Subdural empyema and cerebellar abscess justify wide exploratory craniotomy or craniectomy. Dexamethasone and mannitol are used as antiedema measures, along with epilepsy control. The author believes a neurosurgeon may be of assistance to otorhinologic surgeons in the management of mucoceles and osteomas of the frontal sinuses, especially when cranioplasty is needed to complete a perfect cosmetic result.

The importance of obtaining cultures from suspected brain abscesses is stressed by Steinberg et al. (*J. Neurosurg.* 56:598–601, 1983). Their patient, aged 17 years, had an abscess in the area of the caudate nucleus. *Fusarium oxysporum* (a common soil saprophyte) was grown from the aspirate. The patient died in spite of intravenous and intraventricular amphotericin.

A man with meningitis from which no organism could be cultured later developed pulmonary densities, which a biopsy later proved were due to *Nocardia asteroides.* Norden et al. (*Arch. Neurol.* 40:594–595, 1983) treated the patient with sulfisoxazole and ampicillin; he became afebrile, and serial computed tomograms showed thickening of the capsule and decreasing edema. Lumbar puncture just prior to discharge showed only 10 lymphocytes/cu mm. Complete resolution of the abscess occurred, and the patient was to take the antibiotic for a year. The authors consider medical therapy for cerebral nocardiosis to be better than surgery if the patient responds initially. Most cases occur in immunocompromised patients; they usually involve many areas of infection, and most terminate fatally.

In the patient with basal ganglion abscess described by Chandrasekar et al. (*Infections in Surgery* 2:927–930, 1983) needle aspiration was not done in view of the strategic [sic] position of the abscess. It did not disappear after five weeks of penicillin, chloramphenicol, and antituberculosis therapy. The abscess increased in size (as shown by change in computed tomographic (CT) scan), and metronidazole was given intravenously for a week and thereafter orally. After one month, the patient was discharged but continued on the drug for another month. At the end of that time, the lesion had shrunk to a small compact density on CT scan, and the patient appeared well. The authors emphasize the need for early inclusion of metronidazole in treating brain abscess of unknown origin, in which anaerobes may play a role. I believe it might also be tried in cases in which aspiration yields no bacterial growth. (Cultures are not always successful.)

There is a wide variety of organisms that may invade patients whose immune system is suppressed. Occasionally, these may set up infections in the central nervous system. In the patient, age 34 years, described by Snow and Lavyne (Infections in Surgery 2:669–679, 1983) there was a brain abscess from which *Toxoplasma gondii* was identified by biopsy at open operation. Improvement followed use of pyrimethamine and clindamycin. (The latter was substituted for sulfadiazene because of sensitivity to sulfa drugs.) There is a brief review of other cases of infection of the brain with this organism; most of the patients have not survived. It thus behooves neurosurgeons to become familiar with acquired immune deficiency syndrome (AIDS) so that unusual organisms may be suspected.

From a total of 160 patients with AIDS Snider et al. (*Ann. Neurol.* 14:403–418, 1983) selected 50 with neurologic complications. These included 31 with infections of the central nervous system, 9 with neoplasms (cerebral, meningeal, and thoracic epidural lymphomas and 1 thoracic plasmacytoma), 6 with vascular complications (3 cerebral hemorrhages), 8 with peripheral neuropathy, and 18 with miscellaneous disorders. It behooves neurosurgeons to be aware of these involvements of the nervous system, some of which might well be confusing—and others might require surgical intervention.—O.S.

---

**Open Evacuation of Pus: A Satisfactory Surgical Approach to the Problem of Brain Abscess?**
R. S. Maurice Williams (Royal Free Hosp., London)
J. Neurol. Neurosurg. Psychiatry 46:697–703, August 1983          23–5

---

The proper operative management of intracerebral abscess remains unclear; both primary radical excision and repeated aspiration have been advocated. The author evaluated a procedure in which the abscess capsule is widely incised through a generous exposure, all pus is removed under direct vision, and the inside of the capsule is cleaned out with antibiotic solution. The capsule is left in place, and the wound is closed without drainage. Intravenous antibiotics in high dosages are begun when the diagnosis is suspected. Patients with evidence of marked cerebral compression or extensive brain edema around the abscess receive intravenous dexamethasone and mannitol. The abscess cavity is treated locally with penicillin and either gentamicin or streptomycin. Anticonvulsants are given prophylactically.

Fifteen patients with intracerebral abscesses were treated (during 1977–1982) by open evacuation, and two others by primary excision. The parieto-occipital region was the most common abscess site. Ten patients had blood-borne infection. The most common causative organisms were anaerobic streptococci. All the abscesses were encapsulated. Five had more than one loculus. One abscess had burst into the subarachnoid space by the time of operation. All but two patients had a focal neurologic deficit at the time of surgery. Five had signs of meningeal irritation. Four patients were very drowsy. No wound sepsis or meningitis occurred postoperatively. Ten patients had a rapid, uncomplicated recovery after a single operation. Five patients were operated on again. Twelve patients were normal when last seen. One recovered from the abscess but was permanently disabled by a carotid thrombosis. One patient had seizures only immediately after operation. Three others have had occasional seizures.

Open evacuation is the best surgical treatment for most cases of brain abscess. The problems of repeated aspiration are avoided. Leaving the empty abscess capsule within the brain does not cause wound sepsis or late recurrence of the abscess. The capsule may persist as a ring shadow for several weeks on computed tomography, but this should not lead to reexploration if the patient is improving.

▶ With the advent of computed tomography scanning it may well be possible to cure many cases of brain abscess associated with congenital heart disease by aspiration, in the opinion of Kagawa et al. (*J. Neurosurg.* 58:913–917, 1983). They review 62 cases of abscess with congenital cyanotic heart disease, of which 61.2% had tetralogy of Fallot and 10% had transposition of the great vessels. Most of the abscesses were supratentorial, chiefly in the frontal, temporal, and parietal lobes. Almost 20% had multiple abscesses. Although surgical removal after aspiration was very effective in the authors' hands, they believe the aspiration technique may be adequate.

The chief reasons given by E. A. Kahn (in Schneider et al. [eds.]: *Correlative Neurosurgery,* ed. 3. Springfield, Ill., Charles C Thomas, 1982, p. 419) for advocating removal of the entire abscess are avoidance of late epilepsy, minimization of recurrence from the retained capsule, and discovery of loculations.—O.S.

---

### Subdural Empyema: CT Findings
Robert D. Zimmerman, Norman E. Leeds, and Allan Danziger (Albert Einstein College of Medicine)
Radiology 150:417–422, February 1984                                    23–6

---

Before computed tomography (CT) was available, mortality from subdural empyema was as high as 50% despite administration of antimicrobial therapy and use of advanced neurosurgical methods. The authors reviewed the CT findings in 49 patients seen at three centers with surgically proved subdural empyema. The 28 males and 21 females had an average age of 21 years. Both plain and contrast-enhanced scans were obtained in 45 patients, and 29 were evaluated serially. Frontal sinusitis was the most common cause of empyema, followed by postoperative infection, meningitis, and trauma. No obvious source of infection was identified in four patients.

An extra-axial hypodense collection was identified prospectively in 44 patients. In three patients a small extracerebral collection was seen only on careful review, and in two no empyema could be identified even retrospectively. Of these five patients, four had serial studies that showed an empyema. Five prospectively identified empyemas were very small. All lesions were unilateral, and most were over the convexity. The contour of convexity lesions depended on the degree of localization and age of the collection. The configuration of the lesions did not distinguish subdural from epidural empyemas. A well-defined rim opacification (Fig 23–1) was a consistent finding. The cortex adjacent to the empyema commonly was involved. Mass effect with compression and displacement of the ventricles

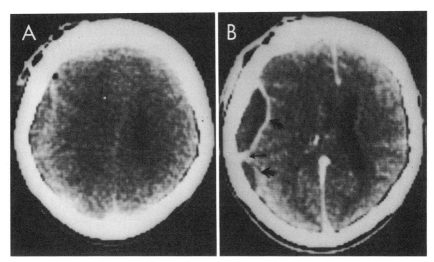

**Fig 23–1.**—Scans in patient with a ten-day history of progressive right hemiparesis. **A,** unenhanced, and **B,** enhanced, scans show a crescentic hypodense subdural collection next to the right cerebral hemisphere. A small amount of air is present in the antidependent portion of the collection. The cortex adjacent to the empyema is hyperdense, and there is white matter edema and a midline ventricular shift. After infusion of contrast material (**B**), there is well-defined discrete medial rim enhancement *(curved arrowheads)*. Also, the membranes are seen beginning to wall off the collection into two separate but contiguous collections *(small arrow)*. (Courtesy of Zimmerman, R.D., et al.: Radiology 150:417–422, February 1984.)

was apparent in all patients. Infusion of contrast material was followed by moderate diffuse enhancement of the adjacent cortex or, less frequently, focal gyral enhancement or areas of ring enhancement. The postoperative empyemas exhibited more marked rim enhancement than did the more acute lesions due to otorhinologic disease.

The improved prognosis of subdural empyema since the advent of CT is a result of earlier, more accurate diagnosis and timely intervention; this examination is the most sensitive and specific test for subdural empyema. If no lesion is apparent, a repeat enhanced scan should be obtained within 24 hours, especially if neurologic deterioration continues.

---

**Surgical Considerations in Treatment of Intraventricular Cysticercosis: An Analysis of 45 Cases**
Michael L. J. Apuzzo, William R. Dobkin, Chi-Shing Zee, James C. Chan, Steven L. Giannotta, and Martin H. Weiss (Univ. of Southern California)
J. Neurosurg. 60:400–407, February 1984          23–7

---

Infestation of the human brain with the larvae of *Taenia solium* is becoming more frequent with increasing immigration of persons from endemic areas. The authors reviewed the management of 45 patients seen in 5 years primarily with isolated intraventricular involvement. Isolated cyst formation, ependymitis, and combinations of both were observed.

Associated parenchymatous involvement was evident in 20% of the patients. The most common ventricular sites of infection were the fourth and the third ventricles. In nearly all cases positive contrast ventriculography was needed for proper preoperative diagnosis. The mean posttreatment follow-up exceeded three years.

Several patients with fourth ventricular cysts had an acutely progressive course and required urgent ventriculostomy. Most underwent primary excision of cystic lesions. Patients with evidence of ependymitis required cerebrospinal fluid (CSF) diversion. A transcallosal approach to third ventricular cysts was used in six of eight patients. Most had successful cyst excision without complications and remained asymptomatic during the follow-up period. Patients with aqueductal infestation were successfully managed by ventriculoperitoneal shunting. All five lateral ventricular lesions were excised successfully, most via a transcallosal approach.

Direct excision is the best management of ventricular cystic lesions caused by cysticercosis. Diversion of the CSF may be necessary if complete cyst excision is not feasible. Primary direct surgical management has succeeded in patients with solitary lesions who lacked ependymitis and evidence of focal ventricular obstruction; permanent CSF diversion is not necessary in these patients. Stereotaxic endoscopic cyst excision is a possibility in some. Administration of praziquantel may prove to be effective, especially in patients with parenchymatous involvement.

▶ Salazar et al. (*J. Neurosurg.* 59:660–663, 1983) note that one of the forms of neurocysticercosis for which surgery is indicated is that in which a cyst in the fourth ventricle occludes the outflow of cerebrospinal fluid. If the cyst remains after the lateral ventricles are shunted, the diagnosis of cysticercosis is highly suggested. The possibility of this disorder is not excluded by negative complement-fixation results in the cerebrospinal fluid.

The symposium on C*ysticercosis of the Central Nervous System* edited by Palacios et al. (Springfield, Ill., Charles C Thomas, 1983) indicates that operations are rarely of value except when ventricular obstruction is present. Immunotherapy is mentioned in a few words and without detail.

Pranziquantel is effective against a broad range of parasitic flukes (Trematoda) and tapeworm (Cestoda) infections and was approved for marketing in the United States in 1983 by the FDA; it is currently labeled for use in schistosomiasis. "Pranziquantel is uniquely effective for killing tissue-encysted larvae (cysticerci) of *Taenia solium,* the pork tapeworm. Cerebral cysticercosis, frequently a life-threatening illness, has been diagnosed with increased frequency in the United States among Latin American and other immigrants from endemic regions. Although recent reports suggest benefit from pranziquantel, treatment of cerebral cysticercosis is complex and potentially dangerous, and controlled clinical trials are needed" (Weniger and Schantz: *JAMA* 251:2391–2392, 1984).

Physicians considering the use of pranziquantel for unlabeled indications should contact the drug licencees. For cysticercosis, this would be EM Industries, Hawthorne, N.Y. Weniger and Schantz remind us that the FDA does not restrict the manner in which a physician may use an available drug. Such "unlabeled'' uses may reflect approaches to drug therapy that have been extensively reported in medical literature. They must, however, be submitted by the manufacturer to the FDA before approval for such use can be acted upon, so there is good reason to keep in touch with the manufacturer (from whom further information is to be obtained).—O.S.

# 24 Tumors

► ↓ Twelve years after his death, Georg Merrem, onetime chief of Neurosurgery at the Karl Marx University in Leipzig was honored by articles in the *Zentralblatt für Neurochirurgica* (44:185–280, 1983). Most deal with tumors of the fourth ventricle and craniovertebral junction. Niebeling (Merrem's successor) and co-workers found medulloblastoma to be the most common of the 167 tumors of the region of the fourth ventricle (out of 1,028 infratentorial tumors). If tumors infiltrated into the right cerebellar hemisphere they were likely to be medulloblastomas; if infiltration from the fourth ventricle was into the left cerebellar hemisphere, they were most likely to be spongioblastoma! Adult patients studied by Goldhahn et al. (ibid. p. 235–240) were more apt to have ependymomas than medulloblastomas, with better end results of operation than in children, especially if diagnosis was made early. A different Goldhahn (ibid. p. 241–243) emphasized clinical pictures of these tumors to encourage earlier diagnosis; Fried and colleagues (ibid. p. 245–249) also emphasized utility of early diagnosis and radical removal of these tumors, usually medulloblastomas, in children. Marked difference in outcome depends in large part on localization to the fourth ventricle area as compared to spread to the hemispheres or the brain stem.

Craniospinal tumors may present as transverse cervical myelopathy or as cerebellar dysfunction, according to Skrzypczak et al. (ibid. p. 251–254). From more than 1,000 infratentorial and 400 spinal tumors, they have found 34 craniospinal tumors: ependymoma (10), meningioma (9), astrocytoma (7), and lesser numbers of neurinomas, spongioblastomas, angioblastomas, and even 1 medulloblastoma. The EEG findings in craniospinal and posterior fossa tumors were described by Geikler (ibid. p. 255–256). Normal records were found in only 12 of 238 patients with tumors of posterior fossa and craniospinal junction. The role of edema might be deduced from the improvement in EEG that followed steroid therapy.

Presumptive histologic diagnosis of tumors of the fourth ventricle and spinal spaces cannot be made from computed tomography (CT), according to Dietrich et al. (ibid. p. 257–260). Angiography is worthwhile in clarifying blood supply of angiomatous tumors; ventriculography is useful when there are questions of patency of aqueduct and relation of tumor to the rhomboid fossa of the fourth ventricle. Anesthetic problems are considered by Woschick (ibid. p. 261–265); difficulties with autonomic regulation are related to outcome, but overall improvements in outcome of operations on tumors of the posterior fossa are related to better anesthesia, microsurgical techniques, and intensive care facilities. Brachmann and Fried (ibid. p. 267–273) illustrate the help that can come from direct instillation of iodinated contrast material into the third ventricle via catheterization through a frontal burr hole, even acknowledging the manifest values of CT scanning. Eichler (ibid. p. 275–278) believes the best results with medulloblastomas (while imperfect) come from combinations of operation, radiotherapy, and chemotherapy.

Clinically, it is difficult to predict the histologic nature of a posterior fossa tumor in a child. Of 129 verified tumors at the Children's Hospital in Los Angeles in the years 1964–1981, 52 were medulloblastomas, 33 were astrocytomas of the cerebellum and fourth ventricle, and 16 were verified (and 16 more presumed) brain stem astrocytomas. There were 16 ependymomas. Zee et al. (*Surg. Neurol.* 20:221–226, 1983) studied CT scans of 10 children with verified ependymomas; calcifications were found in 5, a much higher percentage than in any other type of tumor, especially a midline one. One case of calcified brain stem ependymoma was found, the first studied with CT.

The experience of neurosurgeons with medulloblastoma in 144 children at the Hospital for Sick Children, Toronto, over the years 1950 to 1980 is reviewed by Park et al. (*J. Neurosurg.* 58:543–552, 1983). The vermis was the principal location of tumor in 93%, but 32% also had involvement of the brain stem. Desmoplastic medulloblastomas (distinguished by an abundant stroma with reticulin fibers) (15% of the total) were found in younger children (20 of 21 who were nine years of age or younger) and had a poorer prognosis than classic medulloblastoma, distributed with almost equal frequency in five-year intervals to age 16. Metastases were supratentorial in 14.6%, to the spinal cord in 12.5%, and systemic in 9% of the 144 cases. Overall survival was 47% for five years and 42% for 10 years. Substantial complications of radiotherapy included intellectual retardation and delayed hypopituitarism. The relatively better results in patients treated in the last five years (60% five year survival) may be explained by more aggressive surgery, decrease (to only 60% of cases) in use of ventricular shunts, and incorporation of millipore filters when shunts are used (to prevent systemic spread). There is an exchange of letters to the editor of the *Journal of Neurosurgery* (59:364–365, 1983) in which Hoffman asserts that if a shunt must be used for children with posterior fossa tumors, it should be with a filter (an undescribed malleable filter material which is not prone to breakage). Guthkelch and Taylor expressed their lack of conviction that filters are valuable in such shunts.

A summary of experiences with 57 cases of cerebellar astrocytoma in children is reported by Lapras et al. (*Neurochirurgie* 29:241–246, 1983). Computed tomographic scanning in use since 1977 defines three types of cerebellar astrocytomas: a cystic form with mural nodule but without enhancement of the cyst wall, a cystic form with both nodule and wall enhancement, and a massive (more or less solid) form. Only six patients had a ventriculoatrial shunt before operation. Removal of tumor was macroscopically total in 48. When the cyst wall was not enhanced, only the nodule was removed; the wall was removed when it was enhanced. In nine patients, restoration of cerebrospinal pathways by cannulation of the aqueduct by a silastic tube was undertaken. Mortality in this series was 5.2% (operations done between 1964 and 1982). Three patients had recurrence. Radiation therapy was used in six. There were 30 girls and 27 boys, aged 1–14 years (average age at onset, six years). One third were between ages 2 and 10. All operations were done in the sitting position, without adverse effect. Five children had postoperative "meningocele" at the operative site, which did not require reoperation, nor was shunting necessary. Four instances of meningitis subsided with antibiotic therapy.

Of 234 verified neoplasms seen at the Children's Hospital of Philadelphia since 1975, 10 (4.3%) were gangliogliomas of the cerebral hemispheres. Sutton et al. (*Neurosurgery* 13:124–128, 1983) found that learning disturbances and behavioral disturbances were common in the children whose presenting problem was seizures, usually poorly controlled. The characteristic CT appearance was of a low-density (similar to cerebrospinal fluid) area without contrast enhancement. Biopsy only was done in one thalamic tumor; the child died. Radiation therapy was given for those who had subtotal removal and in one with presumed total removal. Improved seizure control after treatment is considered responsible for improved intellectual activities and behavior. The authors, and Sklar in comment, consider aggressive surgical therapy appropriate for this type of tumor.—O.S.

---

**Intracranial Tumors in Neonates: A Report of Seventeen Cases**
Rashid Jooma, Brian E. Kendall, and Richard D. Hayward (Hosp. for Sick Children, London)
Surg. Neurol. 21:165–170, February 1984                                    24–1

---

Previous reports on the surgical treatment of intracranial neoplasms in neonates have indicated poor results. The authors reviewed the outcome in 17 children with intracranial neoplasms who were symptomatic within the first two months of life. The average age at onset of symptoms was 2.4 weeks, and the average delay until diagnosis was 6 weeks. The most common abnormalities were alteration of behavior, anorexia, irritability, or unusual quietness. Vomiting was frequent and was prominent in several infants. Four neonates were symptomatic at birth. Ten had macrocrania and other features of infantile hydrocephalus. Rotary nystagmus was noted in two infants and a bruit over the skull in two. Findings on skull radiographs were abnormal in 14 infants. All five tumors studied angiographically were vascular. There were 12 supratentorial and 5 infratentorial tumors in the series. Nine of the 13 verified tumors were neuroectodermal in origin.

Ten infants were operated on, two of them after cerebrospinal fluid shunting. Two were irradiated postoperatively. The operative mortality was 40%, and the total case mortality was 80%. The two survivors had, respectively, an intraventricular cavernous angioma and a medulloblastoma. Only one of the four infants not operated on who had an unverified suprasellar tumor is alive four years after radiotherapy for a chiasmal glioma. Thus, only 3 of the 17 children are alive. Death occurred at an average of 45 weeks after presentation. Two of the surviving infants were severely retarded.

Only a few histologic types of neonatal brain tumor (e.g., cavernous angioma, choroid-plexus papilloma, and teratomatous cyst) can be expected to respond significantly to treatment. Angiography and CT are helpful in the preoperative evaluation of neonates with brain tumors and in selecting those with tumors suitable for excision. An aggressive approach to most of these tumors is not warranted at present. The radiation dose used is limited by the increased sensitivity of the immature brain.

▶ Intracranial tumors in newborn infants have such poor prognosis for life and for intellectual growth that the authors are reluctant to advise any sort of aggressive approach at present. Nevertheless, I believe it necessary to determine the type of tumor by obtaining a piece of it. (Occasionally there is an operable meningioma!) It may well be that intracavitary radiation would so limit the adverse effect of radiation on the noninvolved brain as to make it worthwhile.—O.S.

---

**Isodense Colloid Cysts of the Third Ventricle: A Diagnostic and Therapeutic Problem Resolved by Ventriculoscopy**
Michael P. Powell, Michael J. Torrens, J. L. Gordon Thomson, and J. Gerard Horgan (Bristol, England)
Neurosurgery 13:234–237, September 1983                    24–2

---

Colloid cysts of the third ventricle can cause morbidity and even sudden death; although uncommon, they are of neurosurgical importance because they are benign and surgically accessible. The authors reviewed experience with 18 patients seen since 1976 with colloid cysts of the third ventricle. All presented with headaches and vomiting. Four patients had had lumbar puncture despite papilledema at the referring hospital, leading to cardiopulmonary arrest and subsequently death in one case. Only two of the nine isodense cysts were diagnosed correctly by computed tomography (CT). Metrizamide ventriculography was helpful in one of the three cases. All but one of the patients had significant hydrocephalus, despite an average cyst size of only 11.1 mm. No shunt procedure was needed after definitive operation.

Ventriculoscopy led to a correct diagnosis in five cases. It was carried out through a coronal right frontal burr hole using a forward-viewing endoscope 2.6 mm in diameter. In three other cases diagnostic ventriculoscopy confirmed a CT diagnosis of colloid cyst. In one case the cyst was not identified after dimer ventriculography. Therapeutic ventriculoscopy was successful in five of six cases. Two cysts were aspirated endoscopically, but the surgeon elected formal craniotomy for cyst wall removal. One large hyperdense cyst was too solid and large to be removed endoscopically. Craniotomies were done using a transcortical approach with the operating microscope. Forniceal splitting was never necessary. All patients improved after cyst ablation and were well at follow-up. One patient who was in coma when admitted has a short-term memory deficit, but the follow-up is relatively short and he is continuing to improve.

Ventriculoscopy is a useful means of managing isodense anterior third ventricular lesions. Further study of lesions at this site identified by CT is essential, even if the cyst is small, and especially if ventricular dilatation is present. Ventriculoscopic aspiration of the colloid cyst was successful in several of the present cases.

► The lack of photographs is a detriment to clarity in this article. Although the authors declare they are presenting case details of nine isodense cysts, they mix in cases of other types of cysts at unexpected times, e.g., "In view of the relatively avascular wall, it is not surprising that only four cysts in our series enhanced, both iso- and hyperdense cysts." Do these isodense cysts with enhancement still qualify as isodense? I assume (without evidence) that contrast enhancement was searched for in all nine isodense cysts. A similar difficulty has arisen in the past with the question of isodense subdural hematomas, which are not so isodense when contrast enhancement is used. I have no doubt that increased use of magnetic resonance scans will solve many uncertainties about third ventricular masses. Perhaps I would have had less cause for nitpicking if the title had been something about ventriculoscopy of third ventricular masses, instead of specifically isodense cysts. I think it would be informative to know if the authors have done ventriculoscopy in cases of proven tumors of the third ventricle. (Six of the nine isodense cysts were suspected of being tumors before operation.)—O.S.

---

### Diagnosis and Management of Pineal Tumors
Rashid Jooma and Brian E. Kendall
J. Neurosurg. 58:654–665, May 1983                                  24–3

---

Some have advocated radiotherapy for the management of tumors of the pineal region, especially germinomas, but others have found direct surgery to be safe. The authors reviewed 35 cases of pineal region tumor, in most of which neuroradiologic studies included computed tomography (CT). The 26 men and 9 women had a mean age of 17 years. Symptoms were present for a mean of eight months before diagnosis. There were 17 germinomas, 6 malignant (all in males) and 2 benign teratomas, 5 pineoblastomas, 1 pineocytoma, 3 astrocytomas, and 1 subependymoma in the series. The most common symptoms were those secondary to hydrocephalus. Visual abnormalities also were frequent. Ten patients presented with changes in behavior, personality, or memory. Nine patients had diabetes insipidus. Papilledema was the most consistent finding, followed by the ocular features of a tectal plate lesion. Two patients, both with teratomas, had precocious puberty. Human chorionic gonadotropin and α-fetoprotein levels were assayed in 11 patients.

In CT scans, germinomas tend to be well defined and slightly hyperdense, with increased calcification in the pineal gland but rarely in the tumor; enhancement is generally homogeneous, and if there is diffuse periventricular enhancement, diagnosis of germinoma is virtually diagnostic.

Calcification within the tumor itself is strongly suggestive of teratoma especially if there is fat within. Ill-defined margins and surrounding edema usually indicate malignancy. Pineoblastomas are hyperdense, with marked contrast enhancement. The gland itself has not been found to have increased calcification in the authors' experience.

Twenty-six patients had surgical treatment, most of them by an occipital transtentorial approach. There were no operative deaths. One patient died with malignant teratoma after reexploration for rapidly recurrent disease, and one died with malignant astrocytoma. Postoperative morbidity has been minimal. All surviving patients but one, a retarded child, are functionally independent. Twenty-one of the operations were for a pineal mass, and six were for ectopic germinoma or metastasis.

A combination of CT, cerebrospinal fluid cytology, tumor markers, and the response to 1,000 rad in five tractions of irradiation will usually permit the selection of germinomas for further radiotherapy, whereas tumors of the pineal region that are less likely to respond to irradiation can be operated on primarily. Operation is indicated if a tumor fails to respond to a dose of 3,000 rad. Teratomas and pineal parenchymal tumors should be operated on early, because they generally respond unsatisfactorily to irradiation.

▶ Over a 50 year period, 45 patients with tumor in the region of the pineal body were encountered at the University of Iowa and the V.A. Medical Centers. In an analysis of these, Hitchon et al. (*Neurosurgery* 13:248–253, 1983) found 34 with papilledema, 27 with Parinaud's syndrome, and 2 with precocious puberty. Diagnosis of pineal tumor was established by roentgenologic studies in 43, and by autopsy in 2. As Neuwelt comments, the therapeutic approach used is at one end of a spectrum, i.e., radiologic presumptive diagnosis, shunting, and radiotherapy, whereas his is at the other end, i.e., an aggressive direct approach to obtain a tissue diagnosis and, in many cases, gross resection of the tumor. In contrast to the Iowa authors, he has been disappointed in the use of hormonal markers in improving the accuracy of preoperative diagnosis. The former followed the course of their 45 patients, of whom 21 are still alive and 18 are not. They emphasize the value of CT in predicting the histologic characteristics of the tumor, an emphasis that is decried by Neuwelt. Craniotomy, done in four of those who still survive, yielded three tissue samples: germinoma in two and epidermoid in one. Diagnosis of nonsurvivors included glioma (7), pineoblastoma (3), germinoma (1), metastasis (1), teratoma (1), and unknown (5). (The diagnosis in 18 survivors is unknown.) Neuwelt is unhappy with the idea of giving radiotherapy when the diagnosis is unknown; perhaps the compromise of giving a trial dose first, followed by CT scan, and operating if the tumor doesn't shrink is a valid one—or the one with which the French have had more experience, that is, the performance of stereotactic biopsy before definitive treatment, which should be more widely practiced.

The mechanism whereby pineal tumors produce precocious puberty is still controversial according to Ventureyra and Badejo (*Surg. Neurol.* 21:45–48, 1984). Their discussion is based on a case in which a boy, age nine years, was demonstrated to have an arteriovenous malformation in the region of the posterior part of the third ventricle and pineal body and had been investigated at age six because of precocious puberty. Hydrocephalus required ventriculoperitoneal shunt, but before radiosurgical therapy could be carried out, the boy died of intraventricular hemorrhage. The authors believe that the early puberty was a combination of mechanical effect of the malformation and ischemia secondary to steal phenomena. Thalamic extension of the malformation is considered responsible for the endocrine dysfunction arising from the hypothalamus.—O.S.

## Disappearance of Plasma Melatonin After Removal of a Neoplastic Pineal Gland

Edward A. Neuwelt and Alfred J. Lewy (Oregon Health Sciences Univ.)
N. Engl. J. Med. 308:1132–1135, May 12, 1983                    24–4

A marker of pineal tumors would be very helpful if complete pinealectomy is attempted microsurgically. The authors describe a male patient with a typical tumor of the pineal region in whom melatonin disappeared from the plasma after total resection of the tumor.

Boy, 17 years, presented with progressively severe nocturnal headaches and was found on computed tomography to have a partially cystic, enhancing tumor containing calcium in the pineal region. Computed tomography ventriculography indicated obstructive hydrocephalus. A normal circadian rhythm of plasma melatonin was documented. A total gross excision of an encapsulated tumor of the pineal gland was achieved four weeks after insertion of a ventriculoperitoneal shunt. A predominantly low-grade astrocytoma was diagnosed; the tumor contained what seemed to be rests of pineoblastoma; and postoperative radiotherapy was given. No plasma melatonin was detected postoperatively. The patient was well 16 months after the operation except for some diplopia on far lateral gaze.

This patient was thought preoperatively to have a germinoma. Tumors of the pineal gland can have mixed histologic findings. Stereotactic needle biopsy may be dangerous because of the proximity of the deep venous system and also may fail to provide an adequate tissue sample. Plasma melatonin may prove to be a useful marker of pineal gland neoplasms and other lesions. The pineal gland appears to be the sole source of plasma melatonin in human beings.

▶ The authors stress the need for specificity in the assay of melatonin to make sure that it arises from the pineal body. They believe that the gas chromatography–negative chemical ionization mass spectrometry technique is better for this purpose than the more commonly used radioimmunoassay.—O.S.

## Preoperative Embolization of Intracranial Meningiomas

Hans-Peter Richter and Walter Schachenmayr (Univ. of Ulm, Federal Republic of Germany)
Neurosurgery 13:261–268, September 1983                    24–5

The authors reviewed experience with the preoperative embolization of intracranial meningiomas in 31 patients, 18 women and 13 men with an average age of 51.5 years, who had suspicious computed tomography findings. Diagnostic transfemoral angiography was done with local anesthesia, using less painful low-osmolality contrast mediums such as ioxi-thalamate in all but four patients. This was followed directly by emboli-zation in 30 cases. The tip of the 5-F catheter was placed as close as possible to the tumor-feeding branches of the external carotid artery, generally in the distal internal maxillary artery. Strips of gelatin foam were used as emboli in 19 cases, lyophilized dura in 10, and both mate-rials in 2.

Branches of both internal and external carotid arteries contributed to the vascular supply of the meningioma in 20 cases; branches of the external carotid artery alone supplied the tumor in 11. All but two patients were operated on less than 10 days after embolization. Most of the tumors were larger than 4 cm in diameter. Convexity, parasagittal area, and falx were locations in 23 cases, skull base in 6, and posterior fossa in 2. Areas of recent or fresh ischemic or hemorrhagic infarction were seen in 18 tumor specimens. Five patients had complications from embolization, none of lasting importance. Embolization completely occluded tumor vessels aris-ing from the external carotid artery in 24 cases. The tumors with a purely external carotid arterial supply were nearly avascular and were easily removed with minimal blood loss. Two patients with tumors having dom-inant feeders from the internal carotid had significant blood loss at op-eration. Preoperative embolization clearly facilitated tumor removal in cases with a sole or dominant external carotid supply to the tumor.

Embolization is a useful preoperative measure in patients with intra-cranial meningioma. It can be safely carried out in the same session as diagnostic angiography. Embolization is especially useful in cases of highly vascular tumors and where the feeding vessels can be reached only after tumor removal, as in meningiomas of the skull base. Embolization is now done whenever possible and is followed by operation within a week.

▶ Subselective embolization of meningiomas is considered simple, safe, and effective in producing tumor necrosis and intraoperative hemostasis by Teas-dale et al. (*J. Neurosurg.* 60:506–511, 1984). Patients (36) shown by computed tomography (CT) to have meningiomas underwent selective carotid angiogra-phy; significant external carotid feeders were embolized in 27 cases. No reli-able measures of vascularity were obtained before or after embolization by CT or dynamic radioisotope scan findings. Gelfoam was used in 14 patients; "Lyo-dura" in 12. The particles were 0.5/0.5 mm to 1/1 mm in size. No patients had cranial nerve palsies; one did have a 2 × 2–cm area of scalp necrosis requiring plastic surgery. Operations were carried out 2–21 days after embolization in 26 cases. (Permission was withdrawn in one.) Surgeons considered that emboli-zation had facilitated surgery in 13, of whom 9 had purely external feeders. No effect was found in three, and the tumor bled profusely in spite of emboliza-tion in four. No remarks were made about the other six. The authors did not consider their study primarily intended to determine if embolization was help-ful. However, no patient had a postoperative neurologic deficit, and none died.

I presume that "Lyo-dura" is a trade name for frozen-dried human dura ma-ter. Strikingly absent from the article is an analysis of the differences, if any, between the two embolizing materials and of the time between the embolization and operation as a function of the different materials. A gap of 10–20 days between use of Gelfoam and operation would appear to lend some doubt as to the possible efficacy of the procedure, whereas the more permanent dural fragments might be expected to last longer.

One might believe that neurosurgeons are well acquainted with the signs and symptoms of olfactory groove meningiomas and could leaf rapidly through the recent article on this subject by L. Bakay (*JAMA* 251:53–55, 1983). Yet, the lesson illustrated is one that has not been emphasized by neurosurgeons in their talks to other doctors—and one that is more honored verbally than in the performance. How many clinically active neurosurgeons actually take the trouble to test for the sense of smell, much less inquire about anosmia as a symptom? So thanks to Dr. Bakay for his review of 36 cases and his admission that the only early one operated on was one found incidentally by CT scan. He makes an excellent analogy with the early diagnosis of acoustic tumors by paying attention to early complaints of hearing loss, and he suggests early investigation of patients whose difficulty in smelling is not clearly due to trauma, other diseases (including temporary obstructive anosmia), or surgical procedures. Clearly neurologists and neurosurgeons need to emphasize the importance of proper neurologic examination—it does not take very long to test for smell. (Although, to be sure, tests should not be made using odor from packs of cigarettes which, one hopes, will not be readily available to physicians who regard their own health with some interest.)—O.S.

### 105 Patients Operated Upon for Cerebellopontine Angle Tumors: Experience Using Combined Approach and $CO_2$ Laser

Gale Gardner, Jon H. Robertson, and W. Craig Clark (Univ. of Tennessee)
Laryngoscope 93:1049–1055, August 1983                                   24–6

The authors reviewed the results of surgery for cerebellopontine angle tumors in 105 patients; the mean age was 51 years. One patient had bilateral tumors but was operated on only once. A histologic diagnosis of acoustic neuroma was made in 91% of patients. Three lesions were removed by a middle fossa approach, 14 by a suboccipital approach, 23 by a combined suboccipital-translabyrinthine approach, and 65 by a translabyrinthine approach. Only 30% of patients required blood replacement. The carbon dioxide laser was used in 14 operations. Most operations were single-stage procedures.

Adjacent structures, predominantly the facial nerve, were injured in 17% of cases. Six patients died as a direct result of surgery or resulting complications. Two thirds of the patients eventually had a return of 90% or more of facial nerve function. Nearly half the patients had postoperative complications. All but six patients had total or nearly complete removal of their tumors. Eighty-nine of 97 evaluable patients returned to their preoperative activities, and 5 others resumed limited activities. All operative deaths were in patients with large tumors, but mortality was less in those having translabyrinthine or combined surgery than in those treated by the suboccipital approach alone. Bacterial meningitis, long-term facial nerve dysfunction, fifth nerve dysfunction, hemiparesis, and hydrocephalus all were most frequent in patients with larger tumors. Most of these complications were less frequent when the translabyrinthine approach was used. Forty-four patients have had 89 revision procedures, most of which were tarsorrhaphy and wound revision, and 11 have had facial nerve anastomosis.

Early diagnosis enhances the results of surgery for cerebellopontine angle tumors. Proplast (a porous implant material from Dow Corning) now is packed into the aditus during closure to prevent persistent cerebrospinal fluid leakage when the mastoid air cell system is widely opened. No recurrences have been noted in patients having total tumor removal, but long-term follow-up is necessary. A combined approach through the labyrinth and subocciput appears to be useful. The carbon dioxide laser can be used to rapidly reduce the tumor mass with minimal manipulation of the tumor and adjacent neurovascular structures. Its advantages over other lasers lie in the lack of pigment dependence and virtual absence of scatter and coagulation necrosis.

▶ Facial nerve paralysis after removal of an acoustic tumor may be permanent or may last many months. During this period, some method of helping the eye to close for protection as well as appearance would be a boon to the patient. Such a procedure is described by Jelks and Ransohoff (*Neurosurgery* 12:318–320, 1983); it consists in encircling the eye by insertion of Silastic bands under the skin of the upper and lower eyelids to give dynamic closure for the eye. The prosthesis has been removed in 9 of the 15 patients in whom it was installed because of recovery of facial nerve function; it is still in place, well tolerated, in the other six while they await return of spontaneous function of the facial nerve.

After appropriate animal experimentation, Rubin et al. (*Plast. Reconstr. Surg.* 73:184–192, 1984) have carried out a Z-plasty of the human tongue in two patients who had had hypoglossal-facial anastomosis for peripheral facial paralysis. Each had had "the usual problems with food and speech," for 18 and 24 months respectively. It took more than four months in the first, and two months in the second for normal tongue movement to occur, presumably from reneurotization of the paralyzed muscle. Tracheostomy was not needed in either case, although extensive edema of the tongue persisted for some weeks.

The clinical findings in patients with acoustic neurinomas are detailed by Harner (*Mayo Clin. Proc.* 58:721–728, 1983). Earliest are unilateral hearing loss, tinnitus, and dysequilibrium. Decreased corneal reflex, nystagmus, and facial hypoesthesia are the most frequent physical findings. Special audiometric tests are needed in those patients with residual hearing. Most information currently is being obtained from acoustic reflex tests and the brain stem evoked response. The most accurate roentgenographic test is CT with dye enhancement, with or without the use of air contrast. Early diagnosis is essential for early safe operation leaving minimal deficits.

Comparisons of radiologic, clinical, and otologic examinations have been made by Heller et al. (*ROFO* 139:48–55, 1983). Hearing loss, tinnitus, and dizziness are the most common problems of 190 patients seen in a 32-month period. Comparisons of tumor patients and those who had other posterior fossa problems emphasize the loss of hearing and the change in corneal reflexes with tumors. These authors believe the CT scan is more reliable than tomography or measurements of the canals in Stenvers views. Contrast enhancement is obligatory. If an intracanalicular tumor is suspected, CT with air injection should follow the ordinary CT with enhancement.

Nuclear magnetic resonance (NMR) imaging of posterior fossa tumors is discussed by Randell et al. (*AJNR* 4:1027–1034, 1983). These authors found that NMR was more sensitive overall and in detection of tumors and that it displayed mass effects more clearly; CT was better for demonstrating calcification and bony changes, as well as the margin between tumor and edema in some instances. Hence there is not yet a distinct advantage of one technique over the other, except possibly the superiority of NMR for malignant tumors.

In a woman with neurofibromatosis, bilateral acoustic neuromas caused deafness on the right and severe hearing loss on the left. After the left tumor was removed, Hitselberger et al. (*Otolaryngol. Head Neck Surg.* 92:52–54, 1984) implanted a depth electrode in the cochlear nucleus. After two months it failed, and a depth electrode was devised and put in place after 18 months of total deafness. Platinum pads on a Dacron mesh were put in place over the junction of the eighth nerve root and the cochlear nucleus, and wires that were attached thereto led out of the cranium through the scalp over the ear. A wearable analogue stimulator was connected, permitting the patient to hear many environmental sounds well; speech reading has improved, and her own speech is very modulated, unlike the loud unmodulated speech of deaf persons. The implant has allowed her to function independently in her environment.

The good results in the excision of cerebellopontine angle meningiomas (14 completely, 8 subtotally) in the series presented by Sekhar and Jannetta (*J. Neurosurg.* 60:500–505, 1984) is ascribed to good neuroanesthesia, use of a surgical microscope, and understanding of the pathologic relationships. Vascular relations were determined in all cases by vertebral angiography before operation. Carotid angiograms in 18 patients allowed visualization of enlarged meningohypophyseal trunk in 8, and enlarged posterior branch of middle meningeal artery in 2. Most tumors (19 of 22) were more than 2.5 cm in diameter. Retromastoid approach in 19 was made with the patient in lounging position. Subtemporal approach is better for the tumor in the tentorial notch and around the upper end of the basilar artery. Postoperative radiation is recommended for angioblastic and malignant meningiomas; for incompletely removed benign tumors, the use of radiation is controversial.—O.S.

---

**Stereotactic Radiosurgery in Cases of Acoustic Neurinoma: Further Experiences**

Georg Norén, Jürgen Arndt, and Tomas Hindmarsh (Karolinska Hosp., Stockholm)

Neurosurgery 13:12–22, July 1983                                    24–7

---

Stereotactically directed, single-dose gamma radiation can arrest the growth of acoustic tumors and even initiate their shrinkage. The authors reviewed their experience with this method in 14 consecutive patients with acoustic neurinomas 7–30 mm in size. The 10 women and 4 men had a mean age at treatment of 49 years and were followed up for 4 years. In 2 cases, the intracranial component of the tumor had been removed at open operation. The radiologic workup included contrast computed tomography (CT), metrizamide cisternography, CT cisternography with metrizamide, and, in three cases, pneumoencephalography. The highest target dose delivered was 125 Gy.

Eight tumors decreased in size after radiosurgery, two were unchanged, and three were larger. One of the last tumors subsequently decreased in size. One completely deaf patient regained some hearing, but most patients who were not deaf at the time of treatment continued to deteriorate in terms of speech discrimination scores. Five patients had transient facial weakness after treatment. Two developed facial hypesthesia, which in one case was transient. Thirteen patients were in good or excellent general condition at follow-up. One patient died of intercurrent disease six months after radiosurgery and exhibited extensive central tumor necrosis at autopsy.

Stereotactic radiosurgery is worth considering as an alternative to open operation for acoustic neurinoma, particularly in poor-risk patients and those with bilateral tumors. Extremely accurate tumor localization is essential, and improvements in CT techniques have been most helpful in this regard.

---

### Clinical and Pathological Effects of Bromocriptine on Prolactin-Secreting and Other Pituitary Tumors

Daniel L. Barrow, George T. Tindall, Kalman Kovacs, Michael O. Thorner, Eva Horvath, and James C. Hoffman, Jr. (Emory Univ.)
J. Neurosurg. 60:1–7, January 1984                                   24–8

---

The effect of bromocriptine on pituitary adenomas other than prolactinomas is not clear. The authors undertook a prospective study of bromocriptine, given for six weeks before transsphenoidal surgery, in 12 patients with pituitary macroadenomas confirmed by computed tomography (CT) and endocrine studies. Treatment began with 2.5 mg daily and was increased to 2.5 mg three times daily after two weeks. In two patients drug treatment was discontinued several days before transsphenoidal microsurgical tumor removal.

Excluding a patient who also received high-dose dexamethasone therapy, five patients had a significant reduction in tumor size during bromocriptine therapy, whereas six had no change. All of the former patients had lower prolactin levels and some relief of symptoms while taking bromocriptine. Four of five patients in this group had prolactinomas, and one had an acidophil stem-cell adenoma containing prolactin granules. All tumors in the patients who failed to respond lacked prolactin granules. Both responsive patients who stopped using bromocriptine because of side effects subsequently had an increase in tumor size. Most patients in both groups had a decreased serum prolactin level during bromocriptine administration.

Bromocriptine is not a tumoricidal agent and cannot yet be recommended as primary treatment, but it may hold potential as a preoperative adjunct to shrink prolactinomas, possibly making their excision easier and more complete. No size reduction was observed in nonfunctional pituitary tumors in the present series. The authors believe the effect of bromocriptine is not on tumor vascularity but possibly by its inhibition of hormonal synthesis in tumor cells. Bromocriptine treatment should be continued up to the time of operation in patients with prolactinoma. It is possible that treatment for too long a time can produce fibrosis and make excision difficult.

▶ On the other hand, from the endocrinologist's viewpoint, bromocriptine therapy of macroadenomas seems well worthwhile. Ayers (*Fertil. Steril.* 40:846–848, 1983) reports a case of resolution of pituitary insufficiency and radiologic resolution of a 14-mm adenoma with suprasellar extension after six months of bromocriptine therapy. He proposes two groups of macroadenoma patients without visual or neurologic contraindications who might be especially suited for carefully monitored medical therapy: those with associated hypothalamic dysfunction and those with fertility as an immediate goal. Aggressive surgical therapy may result in pituitary insufficiency, and conservative debulking procedures may require bromocriptine therapy for residual therapy and hyperprolactinemic anovulation.

There is no doubt that bromocriptine therapy can reduce the size of pituitary prolactinomas—sometimes even to the extent of creating a "secondary empty sella syndrome," as in two cases reported by Weiss et al. (*Neurosurgery* 12:640–642, 1983). These authors are dubious about the outcome of expensive long term-bromocriptine therapy and believe the current best therapy for large prolactin-secreting tumors is reduction of the size with bromocriptine therapy, followed by surgical resection.

Amenorrhea-galactorrhea occurred in a woman, 40, who also had left visual difficulty and left-sided weakness. This was traced to an intra- and extrasellar tumor which proved to be a craniopharyngioma. Arem et al. (*Surg. Neurol.* 20:109–112, 1983) found that subtotal removal of the tumor resulted in disappearance of the elevated prolactin level and clinical symptoms. In this case, at least, encroachment by the tumor on the hypothalamus or pituitary stalk produced interference with the prolactin-inhibiting factor and led to the syndrome usually associated with prolactin-producing adenoma of the pituitary gland.

Follow-up of patients with transsphenoidal adenomectomy for hyperprolactinemia 5–10 years after surgery is reported by Serri et al. (*N. Engl. J. Med.* 309:280–283, 1983). Recovery of menses, cessation of galactorrhea, and normal plasma prolactin levels occurred after operation in 85% of 28 patients with microprolactinomas, but only in 31% of 16 with macroprolactinomas. Recurrence of elevated prolactin levels took place in 12 of 24 with small tumors and in 4 of the 5 with large tumors who had had initial normal values after operation. No sign of recurrent tumor was radiologically evident in either group. The authors conclude that recurrence of hyperprolactinemia after successful surgery is frequent but delayed and that the lower the postoperative level, the better the chances of maintained improvement.

The rat is one of the animals in which spontaneous pituitary adenomas develop. In a study with female Wistar rats, Yamagami et al. (*Surg. Neurol.* 20:323–331, 1983) found that oral administration of caffeine caused decreased body weight and increased weight of the pituitary glands; pituitary adenomas were found in 27 of 40 rats, compared with only 9 of 30 in the control group. The pituitary tumors appeared to be endocrinologically nonfunctioning. The authors stress the concept that some environmental factors, including caffeine, may induce pituitary tumors!—O.S.

---

### Transsphenoidal Microsurgical Management of Cushing's Disease: Report of 100 Cases

James E. Boggan, J. Blake Tyrrell and, Charles B. Wilson (Univ. of California, San Francisco)

J. Neurosurg. 59:195–200, August 1983                                    24–9

The authors reviewed data on 104 patients who underwent transsphenoidal microsurgical exploration of the sella turcica for diagnosed Cushing's disease in 1974–1981. The 86 female patients and 18 male patients had an average age at operation of 35 years. Thirteen patients were operated on before age 20 years. Nine patients had failed to respond to pituitary irradiation, and three had recurrent Cushing's disease after adrenalectomy. The average duration of disease was five years. One hundred patients have been followed up for an average of 4.6 years. Surgery was performed under coverage of exogenous steroids.

In five patients, there were technical treatment failures because bleeding from the dural venous sinus prevented exposure of the pituitary. One of them was included in the analysis after having a second operation. Eighty-five selective adenomectomies and 12 total hypophysectomies were carried out. Three patients showed no abnormality at operation, and all had persistent Cushing's disease. Nine patients had a second transsphenoidal operation. Sixty of the 82 patients with histologically confirmed tumors had microadenomas. Seventy-one patients responded to selective microsurgery and 7, to total hypophysectomy. Four had recurrent disease after selective surgery. Four of the 22 patients who failed to respond now are thought to have an ectopic source of ACTH. Ninety-two percent of patients with confirmed microadenoma have had long-term remissions. Forty-eight percent of the 25 patients with extrasellar extension of disease responded to surgery. Morbidity has been minimal, but two patients died postoperatively of myocardial infarction. One patient whose tumor invaded the pituitary stalk developed permanent diabetes insipidus. Two previously irradiated patients required surgical repair of a cerebrospinal fluid leak. One of these patients had meningitis. Two patients had postoperative visual symptoms.

Transsphenoidal microsurgical exploration of the pituitary is the suggested primary treatment for all patients with Cushing's disease. If patients in whom total hypophysectomy is not an option and patients whose diagnosis did not meet strict endocrinologic criteria are excluded, more than

90% can be expected to have a lasting remission after transsphenoidal microsurgery.

▶ At times neurosurgeons are put in a position which requires that they be able to give information as to the relative merits of bilateral adrenalectomy and of pituitary surgery for amelioration of Cushing's disease. Supplementum 251 to volume 102 of *Acta Endocrinologica* (1983) contains a series of papers by co-workers of Bror-Axel Lamberg on the occasion of his 60th birthday. One article, by Pelkonen et al. (pp. 38–46) deals with the results of adrenal and pituitary surgery and concludes that there are indeed drawbacks to the bilateral adrenal operation, including the development of Nelson's syndrome (pigmentation and enlargement of the pituitary) after adrenalectomy. Short-term results of pituitary surgery are very good in microadenomas, but not as good with macroadenomas. "Whether the many shortcomings associated with adrenalectomy can be overcome by pituitary surgery remains to be established by long-term follow-up investigations."

There is sometimes great difficulty in differentiating the origin of excess ACTH production. In patients with Cushing's disease (ACTH-secreting pituitary adenoma), a bolus injection of ovine corticotropin-releasing factor will cause further increase in already elevated levels of ACTH and cortisol, according to Chrousos et al. (*N. Engl. J. Med.* 310:622–626, 1984). No such response is seen in patients in whom the origin of the ACTH excess is ectopic, so this test may be valuable in determining if transsphenoidal adenomectomy should be advised.

For those who use the transsphenoidal approach to the sella and its contents, variations in septation of the sphenoidal sinus and its pneumatization may be of some importance. These changes are described by Banna and Olutola (*J. Can. Assoc. Radiol.* 34:291–293, 1983). In cadaver specimens without pituitary adenoma, a single septum was found in 61%, two septa in 14%, and more than two in 12.8%—11.4% had no septa. Insertion of the septum was the lowest point in the sellar floor only in half of the specimens; when it was inserted to one or the other side of the midline, this point was not the lowest point in the floor.

A nice review of the surgical anatomy of the sphenoid sinus, particularly in relation to the sella turcica, is to be found in the *Journal of Laryngology and Otology* (97:227–241, 1983). Elwany et al. from Alexandria, Egypt, used cadavers, dried skulls, and living subjects (50, 100, and 100 instances, respectively). There are presentations of measurements of the sinus, intercarotid distances, locations of the ostium, and discussion of the two major types: presellar and postsellar sinuses. (The former may present numerous difficulties during transsphenoidal hypophysectomy.) A completely central intersinus septum was encountered only in 27% of cases, implying that it should never be used as a guide to the midline during hypophysectomy; the vomer is a better guide.

There are a number of technical difficulties with the sublabial rhinoseptal approach to the hypophysis, and it is in the hope of avoiding these that Hoyt, et al. (*J. Neurosurg.* 59:1102–1104, 1983) have modified a transantral approach described in 1961 by Hamberger et al. (*Arch. Otolaryngol.* 74:2–8,

1961). Incision is made in the gingivobuccal fold, a special self-retaining retractor is put in place to permit resection of the nasoantral wall, whereafter the ethmoidal labyrinth is exposed. This is exenterated to permit entry into the sphenoid sinus. The anterior wall is removed, exposing the floor of the sella turcica. The angle of approach is about 25 degrees off the midline. The nasantral bone plate removed in the exposure is used to occlude the anterior sellar wall. The sella is 2–3 cm closer to the gingival incision as compared to the usual rhino-septal approach, and there is no risk of causing nasal deformity. Repeat operations are much more easily accomplished than with rhinoseptal surgery. Injury to the inferior orbital nerve should be avoided, and the sphenopalatine artery may be interrupted.

Leclerq and Grisoli say that after they showed the relative importance of the inferior hypophyseal artery in supplying the structures involved in production, transportation, and storage of the antidiuretic hormone (*J. Neurosurg.* 58:678–681, 1983), it occurred to them that it might be possible to avoid diabetes insipidus in transsphenoidal hypophysectomy (ibid. 58:682–684, 1983). After a window is made in the anterior wall of the sphenoid, the dura mater is opened and the arachnoid pushed upward to permit piecemeal removal of the anterior lobe without disturbing the pituitary stalk, the posterior lobe, and the inferior hypophyseal artery. The sella need not be packed with fat or muscle, since the arachnoidal space has not been entered. Diabetes insipidus has not been seen in a series of 15 patients operated on with this technique (whereas the ordinary method has produced 5 instances of permanent, and 10 of transient, diabetes insipidus).

In the Hungarian approach to pituitary adenomas with suprasellar extensions, Pásztor et al. (*Acta Neurochir.* 67:11–17, 1983) used a transnasal, transseptal, transsphenoidal technique which is quicker than the sublabial approach and avoids the denervation of the upper incisor teeth. Of 278 tumors approached in this manner, 55% (154) had suprasellar extensions. Results failed to improve when air was injected by the lumbar route (in the hope of forcing the capsule to drop and making more tumor accessible). Apparently, the diaphragm will drop spontaneously if the tumor is soft, whereas even a thin layer of firm, solid tumor will prevent this. If a high suprasellar or pararetrosellar residuum persists after transsphenoidal operation, a second operation (transcranial) is considered after a delay of two months. In elderly patients, radiation therapy may permit delay until regrowth from the residuum is demonstrated on computed tomographic scan or until new visual symptoms appear. The authors believe that patients with normal appearance of the optic disks (regardless of degree of clinical visual difficulty) had an excellent prognosis for vision after operation; full recovery did not occur if the disk was very pale or atrophic. Operative mortality was 7 (2.5%) of 278 patients, and in 5, autopsy revealed hemorrhage into high suprasellar residual tumor. Two died of meningitis. In the last two years, mortality has fallen to 1.9%.

In a series of 100 consecutive patients with pituitary tumors surgically treated at the University of Florida, there were 10 with pathologically verifiable hemorrhagic necrosis. Six of these had classic apoplectic onset; four had asymptomatic lesions. Kaplan et al. (*Surg. Neurol.* 20:280–287, 1983) found that the asymptomatic hemorrhages occurred in intrasellar tumors of younger patients with prior endocrine disturbances. The larger tumors of symptomatic patients had supra- and parasellar extensions, and all were chromophobic adenomas with very prominent vascularity. Significant neurologic improvement followed prompt surgical intervention (usually transsphenoidal approach) in each of the symptomatic patients. This was followed by endocrine replacement and radiation therapy in this group.

Klibanski et al. (*J. Neurosurg.* 59:585–589, 1983) describe six patients with pituitary macroadenomas secreting only the α subunit of glycoprotein hormone. Previously, these patients were considered to have "nonfunctioning chromophobe adenomas." After operation (usually transsphenoidal) and radiation therapy, the α subunit levels decreased. All the patients had evidence of partial hypopituitarism; four of the five men had some hypogonadism. Determination of α subunit hypersecretion may help identify some patients with pituitary tumors, and it certainly would be an easier way to monitor postoperative course than waiting for visual deterioration to bring the patient to attention.

The experience of Fraioli et al. (*J. Neurosurg.* 59:590–595, 1983) indicates that most pituitary adenomas arising in puberty are or will become invasive. These authors studied nine patients with symptoms beginning between ages 11 and 15; seven had invasive tumors. Encapsulated tumors, on the other hand, were found in 8 of 9 with symptoms beginning between 16 and 20; and in 152 of 189 with symptom onset after age 20. The authors stress the need to differentiate between childhood, puberty, and adolescence.

It does not take long for analysis to show whether acromegaly will be helped by transsphenoidal hypophysectomy. Growth hormone levels were tested during operation and in the early period thereafter by Bynke et al. (*Acta Endocrinol.* 103:158–182, 1983). In 11 of 14 patients (2 at reoperation) the serum human growth hormone concentrations were normalized within three hours after completion of surgery. In five patients only partial restoration of levels was obtained, and it was in two of these that reoperation made the levels normal again. These levels proved to predict the subsequent benign course of the patients during the follow-up which averaged 27 months.—O.S.

---

### Vascular Studies in the Preoperative Evaluation of Pituitary Adenomas Before Transsphenoidal Surgery

Krishna C. V. G. Rao, Harry A. Allen, Phillip J. Haney, Robin Yu, and Harvey Levine
Surg. Neurol. 21:175–181, February 1984                    24–10

---

The transsphenoidal approach to pituitary microadenomas is being used increasingly, but even with high-resolution and dynamic computed tomographic (CT) scanning, subtle vascular variants and anomalies involving the parasellar carotid arteries cannot always be clearly defined. Review was made of findings in 62 patients seen between 1978 and 1982 with a probable sellar mass who underwent CT examination with a third-generation or fourth-generation scanner. Most studies were done both with and without enhancement with contrast material. Dynamic CT in the coronal plane was done in a few recent patients. Vascular studies were carried out whenever surgery was decided on. Digital subtraction angiography was used in more recently treated patients. Digital intravenous subtraction angiography or standard carotid arteriography provided useful preoperative information in five instances.

Focal bony erosion may be apparent only on thin-section pluridirectional tomography. A microadenoma may not be located at the site of focal erosion. Most small lesions can be demonstrated by direct coronal CT scanning alone or in combination with metrizamide cisternography. An ectatic carotid artery or proximal intracerebral artery may loop into the confines of the sella, and angiography can define its relationship to the adenoma. An intrasellar carotid anastomosis can cause focal sellar erosion, and a contiguous cavernous carotid artery can cause sellar enlargement. These variants must be identified when transsphenoidal surgery is planned. Vascular studies will be necessary until present dynamic CT techniques are refined and are available routinely. Digital intravenous subtraction angiography can be used in place of standard cerebral arteriography.

---

### Surgical Treatment of Brain Metastases From Lung Cancer

Narayan Sundaresan, Joseph H. Galicich, and Edward J. Beattie, Jr. (Meml. Sloan-Kettering Cancer Center, New York)
J. Neurosurg. 58:666–671, May 1983                    24–11

---

Brain metastasis is the most significant form of systemic relapse in lung cancer. Resection followed by irradiation is an important option in cases with a single metastasis. The authors reviewed the results of surgery in 23 male and 12 female patients, median age 51, who had resection of brain metastases of non-oat-cell lung cancer in 1978–1981. One patient had two brain metastases. Adenocarcinoma was present in 29 patients, squamous cell cancer in 5, and bronchiolar carcinoma in 1. Brain metastasis occurred synchronously in 14 cases and metachronously in 21. The overall median interval between primary diagnosis and the recognition of brain metastasis was four months. Twenty-one patients had metastatic disease limited to the brain. Seven of the other 14 had metastases to bone or liver as well as chest disease.

Thirty-two patients had elective craniotomy under steroid therapy, and three had emergency craniotomy. Twenty-nine patients received radiotherapy postoperatively, usually to the whole brain. Steroids were continued during radiotherapy. One patient died postoperatively of pulmonary embolism. Two others had postoperative clots evacuated. Three patients had an increased neurologic deficit after surgery, but all improved, one of them completely. The overall median survival was 14 months. The one-year survival was 53% and the two-year rate, 25%. Patients with disease limited to the brain and those having aggressive surgical treatment of the primary tumor did the best. Only three patients had computed tomography (CT) evidence of recurrence at the site of the initial brain metastasis. Two patients had radiation-induced complications. Three fourths of all patients were neurologically stable or improved for 6 months or more after operation, and 65% remained improved for 14 months.

The results of surgery and radiotherapy for brain metastasis of lung cancer are improving. Most patients have had useful neurologic palliation. The proportion of patients who are candidates for removal of solitary brain metastases should increase in the future. Patients who are symptomatic from a large mass lesion often can have palliation by resection of the mass even if the prospect of long-term survival appears to be poor. Tissue diagnosis of the lung lesion prior to surgery on the metastasis is important to exclude oat-cell carcinoma.

▶ There continues to be discussion of the role of radiotherapy in the prophylactic treatment of the head for patients with known small-cell lung cancer. At one time, it was considered proper to irradiate the head of such patients, even though no metastases were known to be present. Rosen et al. (*Am. J. Med.* 74:615–624, 1983) have analyzed the records of 330 patients with small-cell lung cancer treated at the National Cancer Institute or other hospitals using the same protocol between 1970 and 1980. Prophylactic cranial irradiation was associated with a significant reduction in metastases to the central nervous system. The benefits appeared to be primarily in those who had a complete response to the treatment of the primary tumor following systemic combination chemotherapy with or without chest irradiation. A prospective study would appear to be useful in removing the technical imperfections of this retrospective study. However, there is no evidence that cranial irradiation would be of value for prevention of cerebral metastases in patients who do not attain a complete response to initial therapy.

Jerome Posner spoke on treatment of metastatic tumors to the brain at the February 24, 1984, meeting of the Interurban Neurosurgical Society. Of 201 cases at Memorial Sloan-Kettering Cancer Center, 72 were from lung, 38 from breast, 26 from melanoma, 11 from colon, 11 from kidney, and 11 from testis. Computed tomographic scanning indicated 51% were solitary and 85% were supratentorial. Responses to radiation and steroid were best with lymphoma, testicle tumor, and oat-cell carcinoma of lung; 75% of breast carcinomas responded, 33% of those from colon, and none of those from melanoma. There was little evidence that misonidazole sensitization was helpful in radiation. In view of the disputes concerning operation, radiation before or after operation, chemotherapy, etc., Posner offered the following: If the brain lesion is of uncertain nature (e.g., breast carcinoma metastasis in a woman may be confused with meningioma), it is best to get a look at it by operation. If the primary carcinoma is radio-sensitive, use radiation. If the tumor is accessible (e.g., lobar), one may either radiate or operate. If the tumor metastasis is "inaccessible" (in a sensitive part of the brain or in the brain stem), radiation is probably best.—O.S.

---

**Computed Tomography–Guided Stereotactic Interstitial Therapy for Cerebral Tumors by Means of Temporary or Permanent Implantation of $^{125}$Iodine Seeds**

H. J. Thiel, W. J. Huk, R. Müller, and R. Sauer (Univ. of Erlangen-Nürnberg, Federal Republic of Germany)
ROFO 138:348–355, March 1983                    24–12

---

The resistance to therapy of inoperable malignant gliomas is a serious problem. Less than 20% of patients with glioblastoma multiforme are suited for tumor resection. Postoperative high-dose radiation therapy can lengthen survival by 18–42 weeks; however, no effect on the total survival time can be observed. Increase of radiation sensitivity through hyperoxygenation and whole body hypothermia, chemical radiosensitizer, intraoperative radiation therapy, local hyperthermia, and chemotherapy did not bring about any changes.

The prognosis in general or technically inoperable tumors is even less favorable, which can be attributed to the biologic features of malignant gliomas. These tumors have a high rate of growth and a tendency to local recurrence. They also have a tendency to extensive infiltration and are resistant to loose ionized rays.

Brachytherapy through new technical developments has recently received increased attention as a treatment of cerebral tumors. Computed tomography (CT) provides a diagnostic target area; an exact topographic anatomical coordination of the tumor may be determined as well as its shape and volume. Through the development of a new targeting device, stereotactic intervention combined with the CT scanner under CT visual control is possible and stereotaxic surgery is significantly simplified. This computer-supported radiation plan permits, using CT cross-sections and orthogonal x-ray pictures as a base, the provision of three-dimensional isodose distributions. The afterloading principle improves the radiation protection for operator and personnel. The patient wears a leaded rubber hood until no radioactivity is present at a distance of 1 m.

The combination of interstitial therapy and percutaneous high-voltage therapy described here should improve the prognosis of brain tumors. After examination of the biopsy material and establishing the diagnosis of a brain tumor, [125]I seeds are implanted. The seeds are placed either in the point of the catheter or are distributed chainlike within the puncture canal. For tumors of low malignancy the authors recommend the permanent implantation of [125]I seeds of low activity (10–60 mCi, at 6–10 rad/hour) as the primary form of treatment, possibly supplemented by external high-voltage therapy. For tumors of greater malignancy, temporary implantation of high activity [125]I is indicated (more than 200 mCi, at 25–100 rad/hour) as a local boost before or after total volume irradiation of the brain.

▶ A lecture on diagnosis and treatment of craniopharyngiomas by I. Granholm of Stockholm was presented at the 31st Annual Meeting of the Italian Society of Neurosurgery, Rome, in October 1982 (*Acta Neurochir.* 69:152–153, 1983). He repeated Cushing's proposition that mortality would continue to be high unless the usually multilocular lesion can be destroyed in situ; however, he pointed out the adverse effects of the panhypopituitarism that results in children and the far from satisfactory quality of life even when the tumor is removed. Intracavitary treatment with a radioactive isotope may well be the treatment of choice for cystic craniopharyngiomas. Another useful technique is the stereotactically directed irradiation of the remaining solid tumors (a third of all craniopharyngiomas).—O.S.

### Brachytherapy of Recurrent Malignant Brain Tumors With Removable High-Activity Iodine-125 Sources

Philip H. Gutin, Theodore L. Phillips, William M. Wara, Steven A. Leibel, Yoshio Hosobuchi, Victor A. Levin, Keith A. Weaver, and Sharon Lamb (Univ. of California, San Francisco)

J. Neurosurg. 60:61–68, January 1984                                    24–13

The authors reviewed the results of 40 implants of high-activity [125]I sources in 37 patients with recurrent malignant primary or metastatic brain tumors. Patients who had solitary lesions of as much as 6 cm in largest dimension with distinct margins on computed tomography (CT) were treated. The age range was 3–68 years. All tumors recurred after surgery and irradiation, and 26 patients had received chemotherapy. Most patients had primary anaplastic astrocytomas or glioblastomas. Implantations were done using a CT-directed stereotaxic technique, with the sources held in afterloaded catheters that were removed after the desired dose was delivered. The minimum tumor dose ranged from 3,000 to 12,000 rad delivered from 44–282 mCi of [125]I divided among one to three implanted sources. The energy of the emission from [125]I is lower than that from [192]iridium and [198]gold, accentuating the sparing of normal tissues during brachytherapy (as contrasted with the effect on intervening tissues such as occurs with teletherapy with [60]cobalt). The diminished energy permits shielding of surgeons, nurses, and other personnel by leaded aprons, useless for the more penetrating radiation from gold and iridium.

Thirty-one patients receiving 34 implantations were evaluable. Eighteen treatments produced documented tumor regression lasting for 4 to more than 13 months; five others stabilized the disease for 4–12 months. The overall response rate was 68%. Focal radiation necrosis was seen at exploration 5–12 months after implantation in two patients whose tumors responded initially and then progressed, and in three whose disease progressed after treatment. Tumor was identified in two of the latter patients. All improved after resection of the necrotic mass, and only one subsequently had evidence of tumor regrowth. About half of the patients with malignant glioma are alive after a median follow-up of nine months; two still are alive more than 24 months after implantation. Four patients had complications, including brain abscess, bacterial meningitis, and severe operative edema.

The results obtained with interstitial brachytherapy in this series probably are superior to those obtained using chemotherapy in patients with recurrent malignant brain tumors. Focal radiation necrosis appears to be surgically manageable. The extent of the neurologic deficit that might be produced in a given patient cannot be predicted.

▶ It would be wise to pay more attention to this technique of getting more radiation into the place where it is needed. One might thereby obviate the problem described by Safdari et al. (*Surg. Neurol.* 21:35–41, 1984) of multifocal, bilateral brain radionecrosis masquerading as tumor dissemination. The 36-year-old North African woman involved had had subtotal removal of a partially intraventricular oligodendroglioma, for which she received 3,600 rad of cobalt irradiation to the whole brain, and 1,600 rad to the frontal lobe through which access to the tumor was obtained. The postradiation problems started some four to five weeks after conclusion of the radiotherapy; CT scanning did not reveal the nodules until some seven months after that. The effect of chemotherapy in producing or aggravating response to radiation is still unclear.

Delayed radiation necrosis has not hitherto been successfully treated medically, according to Rizzoli and Pagnanelli (*J. Neurosurg.* 60:589–594, 1984). Two patients with such lesions following radiation for metastatic carcinoma from the thyroid and for astrocytoma were treated with heparin followed by warfarin, with marked improvement. The effects of these drugs other than their anticoagulant properties are discussed with reference to the benefits from their use.—O.S.

---

**Intraarterial 1,3-Bis(2-Chloroethyl)-1-Nitrosourea (BCNU) and Systemic Chemotherapy for Malignant Gliomas: A Follow-Up Study**
Charles R. West, Anthony M. Avellanosa, Nilou R. Barua, Arun Patel, and Chung I. Hong (Roswell Park Meml. Inst., Buffalo)
Neurosurgery 13:420–426, October 1983                                   24–14

---

The authors reviewed the results of combination chemotherapy in 25 adults seen in 1978–1980 with malignant gliomas who survived the first induction treatment. Cases of medulloblastoma were excluded. Chemotherapy was begun two to four weeks after recurrence or progression of disease, or after initial surgery in most patients with newly diagnosed tumor. A total of 72 courses of intraarterial 1,3-bis(2-chloroethyl)-1-nitrosourea (BCNU) and 67 courses of systemic vincristine and procarbazine (BVP) were used as induction therapy. This was followed by 106 courses of systemic 1-(2-chloroethyl)-3-(4-methylcyclohexl)-1-nitrosourea (methyl-CCNU), vincristine, and procarbazine (MVP) as maintenance therapy. A median of three courses of each regimen were given, with six-week intervals between each treatment.

Fifteen (60%) patients responded to both BVP and MVP, while 10 did not. The overall median survival was 12.7 months. Seven of 10 unirradiated patients responded and lived for 9–22 months. Two of three patients with recurrent glioma responded. All four patients with anaplastic astrocytoma that was not irradiated responded. The patients who failed to respond all died within eight months. One patient had seizures during the intraarterial infusion of BCNU, and about half the patients had seizures between treatments. Six patients required dose reductions of MVP therapy because of leukopenia or thrombocytopenia or both.

A majority of patients in this study with malignant glioma responded to combination chemotherapy. It is feasible to administer BCNU by arterial infusion, but further work is needed to establish the optimal dose regimens. The epileptogenic effects of BCNU have been the most troublesome side effects. Myelotoxicity was the chief side effect of long-term maintenance MVP therapy. Since reactive edema occurs after intraarterial injection of BCNU, as much tumor as possible should be removed to avoid problems with raised intracranial pressure.

▶ There is a problem with intraarterial injections of chemicals, not only for glioma therapy but also to dissolve intraarterial clots. Perhaps the authors might take a page from the article by Zeumer et al. (abstract 26–6) on fibrinolysis by means of a catheter with balloon to block off sensitive areas such as the ophthalmic circulation; one could certainly occlude the carotid above the ophthalmic artery and then infuse BCNU—providing there was good collateral flow from the other side!

Use of a new device for supraophthalmic carotid infusion of chemotherapeutic agents is reported by Kapp et al. (*J. Neurosurg.* 58:616–618, 1983). It is a flexible, flow-directed single-lumen catheter which does not depend on a balloon tip to negotiate the carotid siphon.

The main complication of intraarterial chemotherapy with blood-brain barrier change for brain tumors has been seizures, according to Neuwelt et al. (*AJR* 141:829–835, 1983). They present data to indicate that these are related to use of meglumine iothalamate to monitor barrier modification in enhanced CT. Subsequent data indicate the relative safety (although not with the same clarity) of use of radionuclide scanning. Intraarterial administration of 25% mannitol solution has been used to produce a transient breakdown in the blood-brain barrier and hence to produce better entry of chemotherapeutic agents into the region of the brain tumor. It is admitted that the barrier is not intact in brain tumors, but it is also apparent that some residual barrier does exist and that it prevents chemotherapeutic agents from exerting their maximum benefit. Metrizamide has been used in a canine model but appears to have a short period of enhancement so that it is difficult to document modification of the barrier.

On the basis of experiments in dogs, Neuwelt et al. (*Ann. Neurol.* 14:316–324, 1983) conclude that cyclophosphamide appears to be safe enough to warrant evaluation in clinical studies that utilize blood-brain barrier modification to enhance drug delivery. Doxorubicin hydrochloride (Adriamycin), 5-fluorouracil, *cis*-platinum, and bleomycin are not safe to use with osmotic blood-brain barrier modification. *Cis*-platinum, in fact, when injected into the carotid artery, damages the blood-brain barrier and produces marked neurotoxicity in the absence of additional barrier modification. Exact relevance to human use is unclear, since earlier studies have shown that carmustine (BCNU) given intraarterially is more neurotoxic in dogs than in humans.

The systemic toxicity of chemotherapeutic agents limits their use. Dedrick et al. (*Cancer Treat. Rep.* 68:373–380, 1984) suggest that if the agent is injected intraarterially to attain the best concentration near the tumor, then it might be possible to pass the returning venous blood through a suitable extracorporeal device to remove the drug before returning the venous blood to the body. The pharmacodynamics are discussed in this provocative article.

The administration of ACNU (an aminonitrosourea) is an effective treatment for brain tumors, but it is very toxic for bone marrow cells. Phenobarbital is reputed to reduce this toxicity, so Yumitori et al. (*Acta Neurochir* 70:155–168, 1984) have combined ACNU with phenobarbital therapy in 13 patients with malignant brain tumors. Phenobarbital was given twice a day starting two days before the intraarterial infusion of ACNU (over 31 minutes). Mannitol was given before the ACNU to reduce brain edema so the drug would not be too diluted around tumor cells; urokinase was given (intravenously?) to reduce embolic complications, and in some patients hydrocortisone was given daily for five days before the ACNU. (I fear I do not know that mannitol reduces brain edema around tumor cells, whereas I do know it takes fluid from normal regions of the brain.) Computed tomograms show that at least in some cases, masses within the brain shrank or disappeared. Clinical as well as marked radiologic improvement occurred in five patients; some improvement occurred in another five, and none in three. No complications were experienced. The authors believe their technique is useful in treatment of patients with brain tumors, especially as a supplement to radiation or when there is recurrence and more radiation cannot be given.—O.S.

---

**Comparison of Postoperative Radiotherapy and Combined Postoperative Radiotherapy and Chemotherapy in the Multidisciplinary Management of Malignant Gliomas: A Joint Radiation Therapy Oncology Group and Eastern Cooperative Oncology Group Study**
C. H. Chang, J. Horton, D. Schoenfeld, O. Salazer, R. Perez-Tamayo, S. Kramer, A. Weinstein, J. S. Nelson, and Y. Tsukada
Cancer 52:997–1007, Sept. 15, 1983                                                  24–15

---

Malignant gliomas are not consistently cured by present surgical and radiotherapeutic measures. The authors evaluated chemotherapy in a joint study of 626 patients seen with malignant glioma from 1974 to 1979. Two thirds of the 554 evaluable patients have died. All patients had biopsy-proved supratentorial malignant glioma and were operated on within four weeks. They were randomly assigned to receive control radiotherapy with 6,000 rad to the whole brain in 7 weeks, the same radiotherapy with a booster dose of 1,000 rad to the tumor, whole brain irradiation plus 1,3-bis(2-chloroethyl)-1-nitrosourea (BCNU) or control radiation plus combination chemotherapy with 1-(2-chloroethyl)-3-(4-methylcyclohexl)-1-nitrosourea (methyl-CCNU) and imidazole-4-carboxamide. Steroids were used to control cerebral edema postoperatively and during radiotherapy and initial chemotherapy.

Age was the chief prognostic factor in this study. The 18-month survival was best in patients younger than age 40 years. Patients with anaplastic astrocytoma did better than those with glioblastoma. Other significant prognostic factors were initial performance status, the time since the onset of symptoms, and the presence or absence of seizures. Among patients aged 40–60 years, those given BCNU appeared to have better survival than controls, but no treatment option exhibited overall superiority. Both chemotherapeutic regimens produced some toxicity. Combination chemotherapy produced more severe thrombocytopenia than did treatment with BCNU alone.

Further study is needed of the value of booster irradiation in the postoperative treatment of patients with malignant glioma. A small but significant beneficial effect of combined BCNU and irradiation was noted in patients aged 40–60 years in the present study. No treatment option was better than control therapy of radiotherapy alone.

▶ Contrary to some other recent reports, Levin and co-workers from the University of California, San Francisco (*Cancer* 51:1364–1370, 1983) believe there is improvement in the prognosis of patients with recurrent medulloblastoma as a result of sequential therapies which they describe. In 36 children and adults aggressive treatment for recurrence included systemic, intraventricular, and intrathecal chemotherapy and in some instances, reirradiation with the radiosensitizing agent misonidazole. Results were evaluated with the patient on steady or decreasing doses of steroids because of the mimicking of improvement due to cytotoxic agents by the use of steroids. More males had recurrences than did females, and the recurrences in males were usually earlier in onset. Most recurrent tumors were in the posterior fossa. Because of marrow effects of earlier irradiation, chemotherapy doses were usually smaller than those given to patients with brain tumors without prior spinal radiation.

All patients received vincristine, followed by one of the hexitol epoxides (dianhydrogalactitol [DAG] or dibromodulcitol [DBD]) given into the ventricles if there were malignant cells in the cerebrospinal fluid. Reirradiation with misonidazole was used when all else failed. In all patients, the presence of subarachnoid or spinal cord disease was a negative prognostic factor. In no patient were the authors able to reverse positive cytologic findings in the spinal fluid or elevated cerebrospinal putrescine levels. Adriamycin, bleomycin, *cis*-platinum, and cyclophosphamide were given when no alternative agents were available, especially in the presence of myelosuppression, and the tumor was progressing rapidly. New treatment approaches are needed, especially in patients in whom gross tumor removal could not be accomplished.

Dibromodulcitol is a derivative of hexitol used by Afra co-workers at the National Institutes of Neurosurgery and Oncology in Budapest (*J. Neurosurg.* 59:106–110, 1983) in conjunction with surgery and radiation in patients with supratentorial glioblastomas. Median survival time in patients with radiation alone was 40 weeks; with radiation and DBD, it was 57 weeks; and it was 60 weeks with radiation, DBD during radiation, and DBD plus CCNU thereafter. Transient myelosuppression resulted at times with this last combination. How the DBD acts to improve survival is unknown, but it appears to be a useful agent deserving of further investigation.

For all histologic grades of malignant brain tumors (supratentorial) in children, the therapy described by Phuphanich et al. (*J. Neurosurg.* 60:495–499, 1984) produced a mean time-to-tumor-progression for first recurrence of 75 weeks; the mean survival time was 180 weeks. All had initial subtotal removal or biopsy, followed by radiation therapy. Chemotherapy was added in 12 of the 27 children; only 7 had recurrence (mean progression time of 130 weeks). Age at initial diagnosis was significant in prognosis: those younger than age 10 years survived longer than those older than 10. The authors suggest that chemotherapy be used routinely with radiation therapy at first treatment and that aggressive chemotherapy be used at recurrence. Only two of the children had implanted radioactive materials, at the time of recurrence, and, indeed, because all of the numbers are small, there is a need for a cooperative trial to determine the optimum treatment for these tumors (4, glioblastoma; 14, anaplastic astrocytoma; and 9, malignant glioma).

Although children with malignant brain tumors need both radiation and chemotherapy, they often cannot tolerate the chemotherapy in this sequence. Allen et al. (*Cancer* 52:2001–2006, 1984) believe results may improve if the chemotherapy is given before the radiation, particularly if the nature of the tumor is such that complete neuraxis radiotherapy will be needed.

At a meeting of the Wisconsin Neurosurgical Society, Dr. Glenn Meyer of Milwaukee discussed treatment of recurrent tumors that had failed to respond to surgery or radiation. There is an available treatment protocol that uses bone marrow collection, with reinfusion after administration of high doses of AZQ, a radiation sensitizer which appears more potent than those hitherto used.

Review of 12 cases of biopsy-proved reticulum-cell sarcoma (microglioma) of the central nervous system (a rare tumor) by Sagerman et al. (*Radiology* 149:567–570, 1983) indicates that radiation therapy alone (at least in doses of 3,000–5,000 rad [30–50 Gy] has little to offer.) (Only one patient has remained free of recurrence for 79 months; the others are dead.) Initial management should probably combine a higher dose of radiation with chemotherapy.

In the 20 patients with malignant gliomas studied by Mahaley et al. (*J. Neurosurg.* 59:201–207, 1983), subcutaneous inoculations with one of two human glioma tissue culture cell lines plus cell wall component of the bacillus Calmette-Guérin were given. In addition, levamisole was given. Radiation and chemotherapy with BCNU were started after the first month of immunization. Patients inoculated with a cell line termed D-54MG have had a longer survival than those treated with the U-25MG cell line; survival times have also been longer than those of 58 patients with glioma given the same sort of postsurgical radiation and chemotherapy without immunization. Three patients who came to autopsy showed no evidence of allergic encephalitis. Therapeutic efficiency cannot, the authors say, be determined in this uncontrolled and nonrandomized group.

Human interferon-α prepared from human blood leukocytes was administered to 12 patients with verified diagnosis of glioblastoma multiforme. In 1 of 12 patients, Boëthius and colleagues (*Acta Neurochir.* 68:239–251, 1983) considered that the interferon produced some benefit. It may be that if the tumor burden was smaller, the interferon might have been more effective. Problems obviously exist concerning doses and schedules of drug administration, and it is possible that other types of interferons might have a more pronounced antitumor effect.—O.S.

---

**Necrotizing Myelopathy Associated With Malignancy: A Clinicopathologic Study of Two Cases and Literature Review**
Victor J. Ojeda (Queen Elizabeth II Med. Centre, Nedlands, Western Australia)
Cancer 53:1115–1123, Mar. 1, 1984                                                   24–16

Necrotizing myelopathy is the least frequent neurologic paraneoplastic syndrome. Two patients were found at autopsy to have extensive spinal cord necrosis associated with breast cancer and lung cancer, respectively. The gray and white matter were affected along most of the extent of the spinal cord in both cases. No local or systemic causes of cord necrosis were identified. The patient with breast cancer was treated by mastectomy, administration of cyclic systemic chemotherapy, and cranial irradiation, as well as intrathecal methotrexate after onset of weakness and areflexia of lower limbs. Only local irradiation to the upper chest and supraclavicular region was used in the patient with lung cancer; progressive paraplegia was thought to be due to carcinomatous metastases to the spinal cord. The cord vessels were normal in both patients despite the widespread presence of necrosis and hemorrhage. One patient had focal cerebellar necrosis as well.

Twenty-two patients with paraneoplastic necrotizing myelopathy have been reported in the English language medical literature since 1903. The pathogenesis of this disorder remains unclear. Carcinomas and lymphoid malignancies are the most common associated neoplasms. The association could be coincidental, because necrotizing myelopathy usually occurs in patients without cancer. In some patients the disease is associated with vascular abnormalities of the spinal cord. The paraneoplastic syndrome constitutes a minority of the nonvascular, idiopathic type of necrotizing myelopathy.

---

### Spinal Metastases With Neurological Manifestations: Review of 600 Cases

Jean Paul Constans, Enrico de Divitiis, Renato Donzelli, Renato Spaziante, Jean Francois Meder, and Christine Haye
J. Neurosurg. 59:111–118, July 1983                24–17

---

The authors reviewed the findings and treatment in 600 cases of spinal metastasis causing a neurologic syndrome, seen at Ste.-Anne Hospital, Paris, and the Institute of Neurosurgery, Naples, in 1965–1980. The most common site of primary tumors was the breast in female patients and the lung in male patients. Purely intradural lesions were present in 1.2% of cases, purely epidural lesions in 5%, purely bone lesions in 10.3%, and associated or complex lesions in the rest. The means by which vertebral metastases can cause neurologic disorder are illustrated in Figure 24–1. An acute onset was present in about one fourth of cases; an insidious onset, in 11% of cases. Most patients presented with central or root pain; more than a third, with a motor deficit. Isolated sphincter disturbance was rarely the presenting feature. Myelography was done in all but 20 cases.

All but seven patients were treated, 78% of them by both surgery and radiotherapy. Surgery alone was used in 20 cases; radiotherapy alone, in 108 cases. The goal of surgery was to decompress the cord and nerve roots, not to attempt a radical cure. Radiotherapy consisted of a total dose of 4,500 rad to the lesion and the adjoining vertebrae. Forty-four percent of patients improved after treatment, and progressive symptoms were controlled in another 41% of cases. The outcome was clearly related to the preoperative state. Patients who had early and complete treatment were benefited in a high proportion of cases. The best results were obtained in patients who received both operative treatment and radiotherapy.

Spinal metastases should always be treated, preferably by both surgery

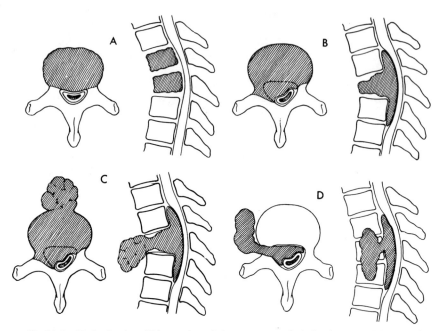

**Fig 24–1.**—Mechanism by which pure bone lesions cause neurologic involvement originates with vertebral "collapse" *(A)*. Various mechanisms may cause associated lesions, including expansion within spinal canal of primary bone lesion, with plugging or sleeve-like effect *(B);* direct invasion by adjacent paravertebral focus *(C);* or extension of paravertebral lesion (usually from a lymph node) via connecting foramen *(D)*. (Courtesy of Constans, J.P., et al.: J. Neurosurg. 59:111–118, July 1983.)

and radiotherapy. Surgery should be as rapid and simple as possible and should cause little trauma. The goal is to improve the quality of life and relieve pain, not to alter the final outcome.

▶ It is obvious that the authors have a relationship different from that of many American neurosurgeons with their medical colleagues. It is rare, at least in academic centers, that we could say, "Neurosurgery was carried out at the onset of the earliest metastatic manifestations." I would agree that there is still controversy concerning the use of radiotherapy alone as the most effective treatment. In most cases in this series, both surgery and radiotherapy were used. The authors believe there cannot be consistent improvement after 24 hours or even less of the onset of paraplegia.

Myelograms are usually done in patients with cancer who may have epidural compression of the spinal cord or cauda equina. In a significant number of cases, the myelogram fails to confirm the clinical impression of compression of spinal contents. In an attempt to elucidate this problem, Bernat et al. (*Cancer* 51:1953–1957, 1983) studied data from 133 patients who had malignant disease and myelography. Of 71 patients who did not have myelographic evidence of compression, 35% had vertebral metastases, 24% carcinomatous meningitis, 21% plexopathy or neuropathy, and 21% had miscellaneous diagnoses including radiation myelopathy, herpes zoster, subacute necrotic myelopathy, chronic low back pain, anterior spinal artery occlusion, and other single causes of trouble. The myelograms did pick up three instances of myelopathy from cervical spondylosis and one case each of spondylolisthesis, intramedullary metastasis, and epidural varix. The 62 verified cases of metastatic disease of the spinal contents were similar to those in other series with regard to such factors as age, sex, and primary source of tumor.

The authors stress the desirability of making a diagnosis when metastasis is present, but also the desirability of avoiding this potentially onerous test if there is no metastasis—or if the clinical condition of the patient is such that removal of a metastasis is not worthwhile (owing to the parlous situation).

The possibility that computed tomographic scanning will replace myelography in similar cases is discussed, with attention paid to the 9% of patients with carcinomatous metastasis of the spinal contents who turned out to have two areas of compression.

A review of the treatment of spinal metastases with myelographic block has been carried out by Tomita et al. (*Acta Radiol. Oncol.* 22:139–143, 1983) using a series of 78 patients seen in a single year at the Memorial Sloan-Kettering Cancer Center. Both lumbar and cervical punctures were used to determine the extent of the block. Patients were given dexamethasone (100 mg intravenously) before or after myelography, followed by tapering doses. Radiation consisted of 5 Gy (500 rad) daily for three days, a four-day rest, then 3 Gy daily for five consecutive days; radiation was centered on the site of the block, extending two vertebral levels above and below. Patients who could not walk before treatment did not recover this ability, and paraplegic patients benefited the least. Only 2 patients improved neurologically; 11 became paraplegic. The authors believe that radiation therapy may be indicated for patients with stable neurologic condition, compression due to tumor, subtle or no bony spinal changes, and tumors responsive to radiation (hematopoetic, breast, and prostatic tumors). Patients who have acute progressive disease but are not paraplegic, especially those who have tumors not sensitive to radiation and who are in good systemic condition, are candidates for surgical decompression. Patients who deteriorate during radiation therapy (or thereafter) are also candidates for operation if prolonged survival is anticipated. The spinal cord should be extensively decompressed if operation is done, and spinal stabilization, often using Harrington rods, should be performed. The authors advocate inclusion of diseased articular facets, pedicles, and part of the vertebral bodies with the laminectomy. Underlying spinal nerve roots should be decompressed. At times transthoracic vertebral body resection may be used. If the patient has systemic metastases, prognosis is generally poor, and extensive surgical procedures may then be unacceptable.—O.S.

---

**Distraction Rod Stabilization in the Treatment of Metastatic Carcinoma**
Joseph F. Cusick, Sanford J. Larson, Patrick R. Walsh, and Robert E. Steiner (Med. College of Wisconsin)
J. Neurosurg. 59:861–866, November 1983                    24–18

---

Investigations of surgical management of metastatic tumor involvement of the spinal column have generally been limited to evaluation of the relative merits of laminectomy and radiation therapy. Surgical procedures to excise a ventrally located epidural tumor or dorsally displaced vertebral body may be effective and avoid the complications of laminectomy; however, the patient's general medical condition may contraindicate such operative risks. Some patients with metastases of the thoracic and upper lumbar spinal column have gained good palliation through posterior fixation devices and concurrent methyl methacrylate fusion.

During a two-year period, seven patients have undergone dorsal mechanical stabilization of the spinal column. Indications for this procedure included intractable pain, absent or minimal neurologic deficit, and clinical and radiologic verification that the major tumor involvement was in the ventral portion (vertebral body and adjoining structures) of the thoracic or upper lumbar levels. The operative technique consisted of bilateral insertion of Harrington distraction rods with hook placement 2 or 3 vertebral segments above and below the involved vertebral body. Prior to final rod positioning, no. 20 stainless steel wires (six cases) or Steinmann pins (one case) were passed through drill holes in the base of the spinous processes of the vertebral segments spanned by the rods. The wires were woven about the spinous process, or the pins were positioned to form a matrix for the acrylic fusion which included both wires and rods.

All patients had almost total and sustained relief of preoperative pain and were able to perform activities with full weight bearing within the first postoperative week. The two patients who had shown signs of mild spinal cord compression failed to improve clinically. None of the other patients exhibited neurologic impairment.

Distraction rod stabilization at the thoracic and thoracolumbar regions in the present study supports the observation that local mechanical stability is important in reducing pain in metastatic carcinoma of the thoracic spine. The restoration of vertebral body height and the positioning of supportive beams between the spinous processes and facet joints may reduce the translational deformity in the anterior components of the spinal column and impart a resistance to bending rotational forces originating in the posterior elements. This form of stabilization reduces stresses on the anterior spinal column from axial compressive loads, thereby lessening the risk of fracture-dislocation of a vertebral body that has been compromised by metastatic tumor involvement. In this series, dorsal acrylic fusion was used as a supplement to the distraction rod stabilization. The reduction of tensile forces almost completely protects against rod fracture or disengagement that may occur when flexion causes elongation of the dorsal aspect of the vertebral column.

▶ Ninety patients have been treated by J. P. Kostuik (*Spine* 8:512–532, 1983) by anterior spinal cord decompression for lesions of thoracic and lumbar spine due to primary and metastatic tumor (13 cases), spinal deformity (15), pyogenic infection (15), burst fractures (32), and thoracic disks (4). Fresh neurologic deficits were present in 51. Although levels that were decompressed ranged from T5 to L5, the majority occurred at L1. Various plates, rods, and cables were used, along with a variety of techniques for bone grafting (ribs, iliac blocks, and both combined). The greater correction of kyphotic deformities and more rigid internal fixation was produced by anterior Harrington distraction systems, as compared with other systems. Posterior fixation was not used after the anterior fixation devices were developed. No patient was made worse from a neurologic standpoint. Only 3 of 79 cases developed nonunion, and 2 of these had not had fixation devices.

On the other hand, Bryant and Sullivan (ibid. 8:532–537, 1983) believe excellent results with unstable fractures of the thoracolumbar spine can be obtained with posteriorly placed Harrington distraction rods, supplemented with segmental sublaminar wiring. They used autogenous iliac bone packed into the lateral recesses after destruction of facet joints and decortication. All 15 of their patients who were followed 12–27 months (average, 19) attained fusion; none required a second procedure for pseudarthrosis, broken wires, broken rods, or displaced hooks. The patients with spinal cord injury were placed in a Jewett brace when rehabilitation was begun; these were worn only when the patient was up, for six to eight weeks. Patients without neurologic defects were placed in an underarm cast for six to eight weeks.

---

**Paraplegia and Prostatic Cancer**
R. M. Jameson (Royal Liverpool Hosp., England)
Eur. Urol. 9:267–269, September–October 1983                    24–19

---

Paraplegia in patients with malignancy often is an indication that survival for more than a year is unlikely, but prostatic malignancy is an exception. The author reviewed data on 24 men with prostatic cancer and paraplegia, 20 of whom lived for more than five years after the onset of paralysis. Eighteen of them were rehabilitated and had a good quality of life. Paralysis often began rapidly in these patients, after signs of nerve root irritation. Emergency laminectomy was done in 10 cases to decompress the spinal cord. The preferred management of the malignancy was orchidectomy. Outflow urinary tract obstruction was managed by transurethral resection, and patients received low-dose Premarin therapy. Ongoing high-dose synthetic estrogen therapy was withdrawn. Testosterone and serum acid phosphatase levels decreased on treatment with the conjugated estrogens. Recent studies suggest that subcapsular orchidectomy is as effective as total orchidectomy in the control of prostatic cancer.

The cause of paraplegia is not always obvious in patients with prostatic cancer. The serum acid phosphatase concentration was elevated in several of the present patients. Laminectomy is recommended only in patients with rapidly advancing neurologic signs or symptoms. The treatment of choice for elderly patients is orchidectomy, since high-dose estrogen therapy can cause cardiovascular complications. Most patients with prostatic cancer and paraplegia can be rehabilitated and can survive for many years.

▶ The author states that delay in surgical decompression is contraindicated when there is advancing paraplegia. Radiation therapy is not even discussed. No problems with instability of the spine are mentioned, nor is the exact location (epidural space, vertebral body, etc.) of the metastases indicated.

Prostatic metastatic carcinoma was the type of metastatic carcinoma found in 2.4% of all metastases in an investigation of the autopsies in Geneva reported by Demierre and Berney (*Neurochirurgie* 29:143–149, 1983). In a seven-year period, 7,592 autopsies revealed 159 cases of prostatic cancer. Of these, 10 had intracranial metastases, always associated with spread to other parts of the body. Only 3 of 21 patients with intracranial prostatic metastasis were admitted to a neurologic or neurosurgical ward, and no intracranial operation was done. Such statistics indicate the rarity of intracranial metastases from prostatic carcinoma.—O.S.

---

**Neuroblastoma With Intraspinal (Dumbbell) Extension**
Leif O. Holgersen, Thomas V. Santulli, John N. Schullinger, and Walter E. Berdon
J. Pediatr. Surg. 18:406–411, August 1983.                                   24–20

---

Preoperative evaluation of paraspinal tumor should include intravenous urogram, chest x-ray study, skeletal survey, bone and liver scan, bone marrow aspirate, and ultrasonography. In a child requiring urgent spinal cord decompression, these procedures are frequently completed following laminectomy.

During a 30-year period, 23 patients were treated for paraspinal tumors with extradural extension (dumbbell) tumors. With the exception of one patient, aged 29 years, all were younger than age 12 (9 younger than age 1 year and 13 between ages 2 and 12) at diagnosis; 11 were boys and 12, girls. Ganglioneuromas were present in 3 cases, ganglioneuroblastomas in 6, and neuroblastomas in 14. No neurologic symptoms were seen in the 3 patients with ganglioneuroma; 19 of the 20 patients with malignant tumors had symptoms of spinal cord compression. Early symptoms in patients younger than age one year included regression in motor development and diminished lower extremity movement in three each. Early symptoms in patients older than age two were also usually motor deficits (7 of 14 cases). Pain referred to the back, buttock, posterior thigh, or leg preceded motor and sensory symptoms in five patients.

Delays in diagnosis were from six weeks to three years in 10 patients. At diagnosis, varying degrees of lower-extremity motor deficit were present in 18 cases, with paralysis in 8. Involvement of the anal sphincter and urinary bladder was seen in 8 patients and Horner's syndrome in 2. Roentgenograms revealed increased interpediculate distance, enlarged intervertebral foramina, and other spinal abnormalities in 16 of 23 patients. All patients with malignant tumors had positive myelograms.

The 3 patients with ganglioneuroma and 13 with malignant tumors are alive and free of disease. Of the seven patients with malignant tumors who died, five were in stage IV and one in stage III; one patient with stage II disease died during laminectomy. Age and stage were important prognostic factors; location was not. Treatment consisted basically of excision and radiation or only radiation. Patients receiving lower dose radiation (less than 2,000 rad) did as well as those given larger doses. Chemotherapy in those with stages III and IV tumors has not yet been proved to increase survival. Morbidity in patients with malignant tumors was high: four have spinal deformity and eight have neurologic deficits. The higher survival rate in patients with neuroblastoma having extradural extension is notable; however, the high morbidity associated with the disease and treatment is of concern.

▶ On the other hand, when vertebral tomography or computed tomographic scanning reveals enlargement of a spinal foramen in advance of operation and when myelography confirms the probable presence of an intraspinal component, a single-stage approach to surgery is advocated by Grillo et al. (*Ann. Thorac. Surg.* 36:402–407, 1983). They present results in three cases of schwannoma and one of neurofibroma, all in adults. The patient is placed in the lateral thoracotomy position. Incision has a vertical component in the line with spinous processes, then curves laterally about 5 cm below the presumed tumor site to become a posterolateral thoracotomy incision at the tip of the scapula. Thoracotomy is done with rib removal if necessary, and the intrathoracic tumor is mobilized so that it is attached only by its intraforaminal isthmus. The neurosurgeon then does a laminectomy to expose the tumor and to cut the nerve root to which it is attached; if the dura mater permits, it is closed. A pleural flap is used to seal the foramen to prevent cerebrospinal fluid leak. In one patient, the laminectomy was not necessary, for the tumor could be removed by cutting the nerve at the foramen, which was enlarged. The discussing thoracic surgeons (at the meeting where the paper was presented) concurred with thoracic and neurologic surgeons in the concept of single-stage approach. The authors speak of serious neurologic complications from a two-stage approach. I do not see any a priori reason why this should be true if the same kind of care is used; it has not been the case in those patients with dumbbell tumor who have been operated on in two stages at the University of Illinois.

Neurosurgeons are much more familiar with paragangliomas of the head and neck than with those of the spinal canal. Seven cases added to the 11 previously reported are presented by Böker et al. (*Surg. Neurol.* 19:461–468, 1983). There is no specific clinical diagnosis in presentation of these spinal masses, usually in the cauda equina, with the exceptions being the three epidural tumors in the thoracic spine in the present series. At times, histologic diagnosis is difficult, with some appearing much like ependymoma or even angioblastic meningioma. History of flushing and persistence of elevated urinary excretion of noradrenalin favored the diagnosis of paraganglioma.

The preservation of stability of the spine in considering operation on extramedullary spinal tumors is the basic reason for a unilateral microsurgical approach proposed by Eggert et al. (*Acta Neurochir.* 67:245–253, 1983). As compared with patients with laminectomy, those with hemilaminectomy had fewer levels operated on; the exposure included only unilateral subperiosteal detachment of muscles. A high-speed drill was used to remove the hemilamina; at times part of the spinous process, articular process, or pedicle was also removed, creating a space 10–15 mm wide. The dura was opened only over tumor. The tumor was eviscerated before clarification of relation to vessels, roots, and spinal cord to avoid pressure on the spinal cord. Adherent remnants were cut away with scissors. Epidural suction drain was used after tight closure of the dura. (Just how this was managed after excision of the dural attachment of a meningioma is not made clear.) At any time this unilateral approach can be converted into a full laminectomy. However, I find it difficult to accept the statement that "exposure of the dorsal parts of the spinal cord after hemilaminectomy is equivalent to that after laminectomy." In the laminectomy series 21 patients were aged 30–80; in the unilateral series, 21 patients were aged 14–78. Evidence that there was or would be anticipated spinal instability is not presented. There is also no detail of how many operations were done at the various levels of the spine, which I believe is important in assessment of stability. (In general, this article applies to meningiomas and neurinomas; the former are usually in the thoracic spine where full laminectomy should not produce much instability.)—O.S.

---

**Neurogenic Tumors of the Sciatic Nerve: Clinicopathologic Study of 35 Cases**
Juergen E. Thomas, David G. Piepgras, Bernd Scheithauer, Burton M. Onofrio, and Thomas C. Shives (Mayo Clinic and Found.)
Mayo Clin. Proc. 58:640–647, October 1983                    24–21

---

The authors reviewed findings in 35 patients with neurogenic sciatic nerve tumors seen in the past six decades; there were 21 neurofibrosarcomas, 7 neurilemomas, and 7 neurofibromas. A wide age range was represented; patients with neurilemoma were the oldest and those with neurofibroma the youngest. Pain or dysesthesia was the initial feature in nearly all of the patients, and pain was progressive in all. About a third of each group had numbness or paresthesias. The neurologic deficit generally was mild in patients with both neurilemoma and neurofibroma, but some of those with neurofibrosarcoma had marked deficits. One patient with neurofibroma had von Recklinghausen's disease. Computed tomography consistently detected the tumors (Fig 24–2).

Six of seven neurilemomas were readily excised totally, and complete resection of neurofibroma was possible in 3 patients. In all, 42 operations were done for neurofibrosarcoma. Potentially curative surgery was delayed or refused for various reasons in seven patients. Twelve patients with neurofibrosarcoma received radiotherapy. No recurrence of neurilemoma was observed during a mean follow-up of nine years. One patient had recurrent neurofibroma. Eleven of 20 patients with neurofibrosarcoma, followed up for a mean of 10½ years after onset of symptoms, died as an immediate result of the tumor. Four of the six known survivors were well when last seen; one had locally recurrent disease and one had metastatic disease. Three of the 4 who were well had hindquarter amputation, as did 5 of 13 patients who died or had locally recurrent or metastatic disease.

Computed tomography of the pelvis and thighs is the best means of diagnosing sciatic nerve tumors. Surgery is the only acceptable treatment of these neoplasms. Cure of neurofibrosarcoma may require disarticulation

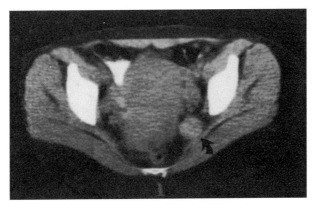

**Fig 24–2.**—Neurofibrosarcoma *(curved arrow)* in intrapelvic portion of left sciatic nerve as seen on CT scanning. (Courtesy of Thomas, J.E., et al.: Mayo Clin. Proc. 58:640–647, October 1983.)

of the hip or hindquarter amputation. Wide resection is the best alternative but is clearly suboptimal. Some patients with neurofibrosarcoma survive for some years after onset of symptoms.

▶ It is possible that the increasingly widespread use of somatosensory evoked potentials in studying back and leg pain will permit diagnosis to be made earlier and with avoidance of the possibility (discussed in the article abstracted above) of transformation of a benign into a maligant tumor. The problem of where along the course of the sciatic nerve the mass may be located may well yield to magnetic scans by which the entire extremity might be visualized.—O.S.

# 25 Hemorrhages

▶ ↓ In the Notes and Letters section of the *Annals of Neurology* (14:696–699, 1983) is an exchange of opinions concerning aneurysms and third-nerve palsies, with pupil sparing as the bone of contention. For instance, Keane, from Los Angeles—USC Medical Center, believes that the risks of angiography for patients with isolated pupil-sparing third-nerve palsies "appears likely to exceed any benefits." Serdau et al. from Hôpital de la Salpétrière advise dim-light examination and pharmacologic tests including cocaine when apparent pupil sparing is associated with third-nerve palsy, since this may reveal involvement of pupillary fibers and allow visualization by angiography of an aneurysm of the posterior communicating area. What the text has to do with the title, which includes pupil sparing in Claude Bernard Horner syndrome, is unclear. Boghen (Hôtel-Dieu de Montréal) contends that aneurysm must be considered in the· differential diagnosis of even partial third-nerve palsy regardless of the state of the pupil, referring to such an occurrence in a case. These letters were in response to an article (ibid. 13:149–154, 1983) by Kissel et al. (Washington University) whose reply reiterates their opinion that at least five days should elapse, with observations, before deciding that a patient with pupil-sparing third-nerve palsy does not need an angiogram. Their basic concept is that relative pupil sparing is not uncommon with aneurysms. Trobe and Nadeau (Gainesville, Fla.) confirm pupil sparing in intracavernous aneurysms, but they deny that berry aneurysms at the junction of posterior communicating and internal carotid arteries cause total third-nerve palsy but with complete pupil sparing.

If there is to be any significant decrease in mortality in patients with aneurysms, it must come from early diagnosis. I must disagree heartily with the waiting attitude when there is third-nerve palsy with apparent pupil sparing. I have seen patients with total third-nerve palsy including the pupil with normal angiograms (especially in diabetics), and I have seen aneurysms in patients with pupil sparing as part of incomplete third-nerve palsy due to aneurysm—which has later ruptured! It seems to me that the risks of angiography are not so great (especially using digital subtraction arteriography, to say nothing of digital subtraction venous angiography), even in a diabetic arteriosclerotic patient, as to validate omission of angiography.

The arguments concerning the origins of aneurysm have not yet ceased; the occasional finding of aneurysm in very young patients is difficult to reconcile with the increasing occurrence of rupture as patients get older and more atherosclerotic. Neil-Dwyer et al. (*J. Neurosurg.* 59:16–20, 1983) present evidence that type III collagen deficiency is associated with ruptured intracranial aneurysms, but they are unable to pinpoint how the deficiency allows the formation of aneurysms. The inherent weakness of the branching points where aneurysms appear may be involved. Obvious points of interest include inheritance of type III collagen levels in relatives of aneurysm patients. The authors have also been involved in studies of other somatic aneurysms and also of the

Ehlers-Danlos syndrome type IV, which also is related to deficiency in type III collagen deficiency.

Kristensen (*Acta Neurochir.* 67:37–43, 1983) compared the incidence of bleeding intracranial aneurysms in Greenlandic Eskimos (9.3 per 100,000 population per year) to that in Caucasian Danes (3.1 per 100,000 per year). About half of the Eskimos were younger than age 20 compared with 27.2% of the Eastern Danes. Aneurysmal rupture occurred in 436 Danes in the period 1976–1981; for the same period there were 27 Greenlandic Eskimos with such diagnosis. Even considering the small numbers of cases, the author has found a significantly greater incidence in aneurysmal subarachnoid hemorrhage in Greenlandic Eskimos ($P < .001$). Pope et al. (*Lancet* 1:973–975, 1981) found that some patients with aneurysm are deficient in type III collagen, and Kristensen wonders if there might be differences in connective tissue properties between her two populations.

An elaborate family tree has been drawn up by Patrick and Appleby (*Neuroradiol* 25:329–334, 1983) to illustrate their case report of familial intracranial aneurysm and infundibular widening. Four patients presented with subarachnoid hemorrhage, proved by angiography to be from aneurysmal rupture; all were clipped successfully, but one patient was left with hemiplegia and epilepsy. Two relatives investigated electively were found to have aneurysms which were successfully clipped; two others were found to have infundibular widening, and they developed transient cortical blindness after angiography. One more elective investigation in a patient, age 11, was without abnormal finding or complication. Four members of the generation next older than the original four mentioned above (including the father of 11 children who had aneurysms clipped) had died, at ages from the 20s to the 40s, of cerebral hemorrhage! In all, this family had a 30% incidence of aneurysm and a 20% incidence of infundibular widening—and this same high incidence of infundibular widening was also found in other reports of families with aneurysms.

---

### The "Warning Leak" in Spontaneous Subarachnoid Hemorrhage
Graeme P. Duffy (Hobart, Australia)
Med. J. Aust. 1:514–516, May 28, 1983                    25–1

Although the sudden onset of severe headache may make subarachnoid hemorrhage (SAH) obvious, the implications of a less catastrophic onset may not be recognized. The author reviewed the presentation of 102 patients seen in a two-year period with symptoms of SAH. Sixty-three were proved to have SAH. Forty-six of these 63 patients had bleeding from a ruptured intracranial aneurysm. Thirteen of these 63 had a history suggesting a warning leak in the preceding four weeks, and all of these had a ruptured aneurysm. Eight had seen a physician at the time of the warning leak, and three had been admitted to hospital. Three patients with a warning leak and later aneurysmal rupture died, five were left with significant neurologic disability, and five made a good recovery. Computed tomography (CT) failed to distinguish prospectively between clinical grade I–II patients who bled from an intracranial lesion and those who did not.

More than a quarter of patients in this series with ruptured intracranial aneurysm and SAH had symptoms of a warning leak. The actual incidence probably is higher, since only patients who sought medical help for the symptoms of a warning leak were included in the present series. Forty percent of the patients with a warning leak were in clinical grade III or worse at admission for the subsequent hemorrhage, and their eventual morbidity and mortality were much higher than in patients who were in better condition after initial bleeding. Some patients with clinical features suggesting a warning leak have not bled. A negative CT scan should not preclude lumbar puncture, but if both tests are negative within a week of the onset of symptoms, angiography should not be necessary.

▶ Jomin et al. (*Surg. Neurol.* 21:13–18, 1984) report results with 500 ruptured and operated aneurysms in 486 patients encountered in a six-year period ending December 31, 1982. All multiple aneurysms were approached surgically at the same operation as the one that bled. In 102 patients there was a history of prior meningeal hemorrhage. None of the patients developed secondary hydrocephalus, presumably because of the use of postoperative lumbar punctures and systematic corticosteroid injections. Spasm was recorded in only 31 patients, always in patients younger than age 50, during the first week after rupture. Mortality was highest in patients aged 70–79 (40% of 10 patients), but the spontaneous mortality and morbidity after bleeding is so great the authors believe operation is indicated. Overall, there was a cure rate of 74.8%, death rate of 13.5%, and poor results in 13.3%. The only real contraindications to surgery are arterial spasm and cerebral ischemia downstream from the aneurysm.

In his editorial note after this article, Bucy complains that because of the lack of access of academic neurosurgeons to medical students, the latter do not learn the warning signs of aneurysmal rupture. "Failure to diagnose" is still a potent source of malpractice suits.

A variety of causes lead to failure to visualize an aneurysm after subarachnoid hemorrhage. Among these causes are: vasospasm, inadequate projections, poor quality of films, lack of attention to the aneurysm of note in case of multiple aneurysms, and no evidence of aneurysm even in retrospect. In 10 patients studied by Ishii, et al. of Niigata, Japan (*Neurol. Med. Chir.* [*Tokyo*] 23:471–477, 1983) 8 of the hidden ruptured aneurysms were disclosed by repeat angiograms, and 2 by autopsy; the anterior communicating area was involved in 5, middle cerebral in 3, and internal carotid in 2. The size of nine aneurysms ranged from 1.5 × 2.5 mm to 4.0 × 4.5 mm (average 3 mm in length and 2.5 mm in diameter). The conclusion appears to be that if you don't find the cause by angiography, repeat the angiogram—and pay particular attention to the region of the anterior communicating artery with special views.—O.S.

---

**Timing of Surgery for Intracerebral Hematomas Due to Aneurysm Rupture**
Brian Wheelock, Bryce Weir, Reginald Watts, Gerard Mohr, Moe Khan, Michael Hunter, Derek Fewer, Gary Ferguson, Felix Durity, Douglas Cochrane, and Brien Benoit
J. Neurosurg. 58:476–481, April 1983                                    25–2

Intracerebral hematoma from ruptured intracranial aneurysm is not rare, and can be readily diagnosed by computed tomography (CT). The authors reviewed the outcome in 132 such cases collected from 11 centers in Canada. An intracerebral hematoma was demonstrated by CT adjacent to a ruptured aneurysm without antecedent sugery in these cases. The overall mortality was 38% (43% for patients admitted on the day of the bleeding or the following day). Only 9% of patients were discharged without a significant neurologic deficit. About half the patients who were operated on and survived were discharged directly to home.

Survival correlated inversely with the blood pressure on admission. Brain herniation was significantly associated with a poorer neurologic grade at all times in hospital, with a larger hematoma and with higher mortality. Neurologic grade correlated with morbidity and mortality in the overall series. About one fourth of patients had ischemic deterioration from vasospasm, and this was associated with a poor outcome after surgery. Poor-grade patients were apt to have most prompt admission, and this short interval between clinical onset and admission was significantly related to longer hospitalization and a poorer status at discharge. Parietal hematomas were particularly dangerous; temporal ones were associated with best outcome.

There would appear to be no advantage to delaying operation if a patient with intracerebral hematoma is deteriorating. The aneurysm should be clipped at the time the hematoma is evacuated. The mortality in patients who had evacuation of hematoma without aneurysmal clipping was 75% compared with 29% in patients who had clipping after removal of the clot. About half of patients admitted shortly after aneurysmal rupture will survive if operated on early. If they survive the first few days without brain herniation, the timing of surgery is not critically important, but morbidity may be marginally less with earlier operation. The best approach to patients with poor prognostic signs includes clot evacuation, simultaneous clipping of the aneurysm, and control of the elevated intracranial pressure.

▶ It seems possible that results might be better now that calcium blockers can be used to mitigate vasospasm.

The same multicenter cooperative program has also dealt with results from intraventricular hemorrhage due to aneurysm rupture. The mortality was 64%. The ratio of width of ventricles (between the caudate nuclei) to the width of the brain (ventriculocranial ratio or VCR) as seen in CT scans was the most sensitive indicator of prognosis: if the VCR was higher than 0.25 (1:4), no patient survived. Upper limit of normal is 0.155. Reduction of intracranial pressure would appear to be mandatory, although shunting does not always accomplish this purpose.—O.S.

---

**Hydrocephalus Following Aneurysmal SAH**
A. Spallone and F. M. Gagliardi (Univ. of Rome)
Zentralbl. Neurochir. 44:141–150, 1983                    25–3

---

The pathophysiology of hydrocephalus after subarachnoid hemorrhage

(SAH) remains incompletely understood. The authors assessed the occurrence of hydrocephalus following SAH from ruptured intracranial aneurysm in 137 patients who received antifibrinolytic therapy within three days of the ictus and continued on treatment for at least six days. Ninety-one patients (group A) received 3 gm of tranexamic acid or aminomethylcyclohexanecarboxylic acid (AMCA) daily along with 300,000–400,000 KIU of aprotinin daily, and 46 (group B) received 6 gm of AMCA daily only. The two groups were clinically comparable. The mean interval from SAH to operation was about 13 days.

Twelve patients were considered to have clinically significant ventricular enlargement. All but one of them underwent shunt operation and eventually improved clinically. The incidence of hydrocephalus was 6.6% in group A patients and 13% in group B. Group B patients also had a higher rate of severe cerebral ischemic complications, and hydrocephalus was likelier to develop in patients with such complications. Antihypertensive drug therapy correlated with ischemic complications, but not with posthemorrhagic hydrocephalus. Three patients were operated on for hydrocephalus without having had direct surgery for their aneurysms; none of them rebled during follow-up for as long as three years. One patient with hydrocephalus rebled after removal of the shunt because of infection. Shunt revision was necessary in another case, also because of meningeal infection.

Symptomatic hydrocephalus followed SAH in about 9% of patients in this series. Computed tomography provides guidelines to management in these cases. Repeated lumbar puncture no longer is indicated as a therapeutic measure. Shunt surgery is nearly always helpful when there are clear indications for treatment of hydrocephalus. All shunted patients in the present study eventually improved. The findings do not support a role for periventricular ischemia as the cause of clinically significant hydrocephalus after SAH.

▶ The statement in the text of the article abstracted above that "the incidence of hydrocephalus was strikingly different in differently treated patients . . . although not in a statistically significant manner" (p. 143) is difficult to reconcile with the statement in the summary: "Group A showed significantly less formation of hydrocephalus and ischemic complications" (p. 141). There is a peculiar lack of discussion of the apparent benefit of adding aprotonin (an extract from pancreas) to the tranexamic acid (AMCA). Also missing (because of the nature of the study) is a comparative analysis in the authors' patients of incidence of hydrocephalus without treatment with AMCA. The most reasonable conclusion to which I can come is one the authors also reached: both ischemic complications and hydrocephalus after subarachnoid hemorrhage are probably results of breakdown products of the blood.—O.S.

---

**Causes of Unfavorable Outcome After Early Aneurysm Operation**
Bengt Ljunggren, Hans Säveland, and Lennart Brandt (Univ. of Lund, Sweden)
Neurosurgery 13:629–633, December 1983                                25–4

The authors reviewed data on 160 consecutive patients in grades I–III operated on in the acute stage for a ruptured supratentorial aneurysm and attempted to determine the causes of an unfavorable outcome in the 42 patients (26%) who did not make a good recovery. Fourteen of these patients died within a month after operation. Ten survivors had major deficit at follow-up, whereas 18 others were classified as having fair results, with minor to moderate neurologic or mental deficits or impaired cerebrospinal fluid (CSF) outflow necessitating a shunt operation.

In 18 cases a delayed ischemic deficit appeared more than three days postoperatively and persisted. One third of patients who were hypertensive before subarachnoid hemorrhage were in this group. Eleven patients had deficits due to surgical trauma. Three of them had anatomically complex aneurysms. A persistent hemorrhagic deficit occurred in six patients in grade III who did not recover completely from the effects of initial subarachnoid bleeding. Three patients required shunt surgery for impaired CSF outflow. Rebleeding occurred in two cases. One death was due to a postoperative intracerebral hematoma. The outcome in patients in grades I–II could not be related to whether operation was done on the first, second, or third day after bleeding. Preoperative grade itself was an important factor in the final outcome.

The condition of the patient in the acute phase after subarachnoid bleeding from ruptured intracranial aneurysm appears to be the chief determinant of the outcome after early aneurysm surgery. A favorable outcome is much less likely in patients in grade III because of both late cerebral dysfunction and persistent hemorrhagic deficit. Late cerebral dysfunction accounts for about 40%–45% of unfavorable results when operation is done on all patients in grades I–III within 72 hours of aneurysm rupture.

▶ Some of the unfavorable outcomes after operation proved to be unrelated to the operation, but were due to the original hemorrhage (e.g., vitreous hemorrhages, hydrocephalus from impaired outflow of cerebrospinal fluid). Delayed ischemic deficit appeared to be the chief single adverse condition, but it apparently could be obviated, at least in most cases, by use of nimodipine treatment, inasmuch as 23 patients so treated did not have permanent delayed ischemic deficit. It seems clear that early operation is warranted in patients with grades I and II classification. Whether it is justified in grade III patients is unclear.

The mortality for operations done in the first 24 hours after subarachnoid hemorrhage obviously varies with the grade of the patient. In a series of 223 cases operated by the same surgeon, 69 were done within 24 hours. Sano and colleagues from Aichi, Japan (*Neurol. Med. Chir.* [*Tokyo*] 23:355–360, 1983) found total mortality including grade V was 39%, but only 6.7% when only cases in grades II and III were analyzed. Mortalities in late surgery (mainly grades I and II) were only 2.4%. Vasospasm occurred in only 10.6% of those operated acutely, whereas it was found in more than 40% of those operated from days 2–14. Mortality in grade IV cases was 6 of 22 for acute stage operation, and 19 of 23 in grade V died with only 1 good recovery. The authors conclude that acute stage surgery (within 24 hours) should be done when computed tomography (CT) showed a packed hematoma in the basal cistern.

In the ongoing debate on timing of operation on aneurysm, Bolander et al. (*Acta Neurochir.* [*Wien*] 70:31–41, 1984) present statistics to indicate benefits of early operation. In 62 patients graded (Botterell) I and II, early operation was done within 72 hours, with mortality of 5% compared with 13% for those operated on later. There was no difference in morbidity between the two groups.

In the series of 500 aneurysms (in 486 patients) operated on by Jomin et al. (*Surg. Neurol.* 21:13–18, 1984) 232 were conscious, 109 were obnubilated, 63 were obnubilated and had discrete neurologic deficit, 33 were in coma with considerable neurologic deficit, and 49 were in coma with evidence of brain stem involvement. Anterior communicating artery aneurysms were most common (166 cases); 145 aneurysms were from the carotid, with 106 at the origin of the posterior communicating artery, 26 at the bifurcation, and 13 at the ophthalmic artery. Four aneurysms involved the upper tip of the basilar artery, and 10 arose at the origin of the posterior inferior cerebellar artery. All eight aneurysms larger than 2.5 cm in diameter were in the anterior circulation. Ten patients had two aneurysms, and two had three; all the multiple aneurysm cases had the aneurysms operated on at the same session. There were 75% cures, 13% poor results, and 12% deaths. The authors state that 56 patients (11.5%) had considerable sequelae (poor results) and 13.5% died within a month of operation. The 61 patients operated on within 48 hours as emergencies had large compressive hematomas; 37 died, 22 had considerable sequelae, and only two had good results. The authors conclude that the best time to operate is within the first week although an associated arterial spasm and cerebral ischemia "downstream" "represent the only real absolute contraindications to neurosurgery."—O.S.

---

**Cerebral Vasospasm After Subarachnoid Hemorrhage: An Update**
Roberto C. Heros, Nicholas T. Zervas, and Vassilios Varsos (Harvard Med. School)
Ann. Neurol. 14:599–608, December 1983                 25–5

---

Cerebral ischemia is the most likely cause of neurologic deterioration occurring a few days after subarachnoid hemorrhage when other obvious causes (e.g., rebleeding) are ruled out. Deterioration is nearly always associated with severe regional or generalized vasopasm. About half of these patients die or are left with a serious deficit. Vasospasm is at least as important a cause of morbidity and mortality after aneurysmal bleeding as is rebleeding. The clinical status on hospital admission is the chief clinical predictor of vasospasm. Plain computed tomography (CT) done within three days of onset of bleeding is the best means of determining the severity and distribution of vasospasm. Vasospasm correlates directly with the amount of blood in the subarachnoid space, and the blood may be directly responsible for the spasm. Many endogenous substances have been implicated, and neurogenic factors may become significant under certain pathologic conditions, e.g., acute subarachnoid hemorrhage. Both intrinsic structural changes and extrinsic vessel wall infiltration by inflammatory cells and red cells may lead to persistent luminal constriction.

The ideal approach to vasospasm is a preventive one. Induced hypotension is used less frequently today, because increased cerebral perfusion pressure is beneficial once clinical vasospasm develops. Daily infusions of colloid may help prevent vasospasm in patients at risk. Careful attention to electrolyte balance is necessary to prevent significant hyponatremia. Antifibrinolytic agents may worsen the vasospasm, but the evidence is inconclusive. Most pharmacologic attempts to prevent vasospasm have been disappointing; however, results of recent studies of calcium channel blockers (e.g., nimodipine) are more encouraging. Some surgeons believe that the early removal of as much blood as possible from the subarachnoid cisterns will prevent vasospasm. Once ischemic symptoms develop, the cerebral perfusion pressure should be raised by decreasing the intracranial pressure, if elevated, or increasing the systemic pressure with vasopressors or with cardiotonic agents and volume expansion. The authors are reluctant to raise the systolic pressure much above 200 mm Hg under any circumstances. Caution is needed in using vasopressin in order not to induce or exacerbate hyponatremia.

▶ The review is excellent (using 109 references); the conclusions are depressing: "After many years of intensive research, the only therapy of substantial value currently available for vasospasm is symptomatic—namely, improvement of cerebral perfusion pressure. New avenues of research must be explored to determine whether specific remedies for vasospasm can be found. Better understanding of both the normal physiology of smooth muscle contraction and relaxation and the pathophysiology of vasospasm are necessary to direct these research efforts." The treatment with reserpine and kanamycin proposed by Heros et al., given for several days before operation in patients in good condition, appears to prevent postoperative vasospasm. It does not seem to prevent preoperative vasospasm. Nimodipine is not yet available in the United States, but caution is advised until the value of this and other calcium channel blockers can be proved in studies with large numbers of patients.

Volume expansion as a technique for overcoming the bad effects of cerebral vasospasm after subarachnoid hemorrhage has come to be accepted therapy. However, there are numerous complications, and the technique is not always effective. In order to increase the assurance that the proper amounts of fluids are being maintained, Pritz (*Surg. Neurol.* 21:239–244, 1984) has used a triple lumen thermodilution Swan-Ganz catheter in determination of what mean pulmonary artery wedge pressure would generate the greatest cardiac output. In the two cases described, the neurologic problems after clipping (one case) or after bleeding without angiographic evidence of a source (one case) were greatly ameliorated by administration of electrolyte solutions, salt-poor albumin, or blood. Neither patient developed pulmonary hypoxia, congestive heart failure, pulmonary edema, myocardial infarction, or symptoms of intracranial hypertension.

Although Trémoulet et al. (*Neurochirurgie* 29:235–240, 1983) were unable to find a correlation between vasospasm and cerebral blood flow as measured by the xenon-133 technique, they did find a decreased mean cerebral blood flow in the first two weeks after subarachnoid hemorrhage in those patients who had an uncomplicated course. This was particularly true if the flow in the cortex was higher than 70 ml/100 gm per minute. Having seen the variance in brain size with age and sex, and without obvious reason, in brain-cutting experiences over the past 35 years, I am still distressed about the theoretical calculation of the brain weight. An interesting illustration and case history is included, dealing with a woman, 56, whose blood flow study on day 10 showed reduction in flow in the territory supplied by the left middle cerebral artery, on whose trunk was an aneurysm (at the bifurcation). Five days after the flow study, the patient became aphasic. Operation was deferred until day 33 when the flow became normal again, but the patient had aphasic sequelae. The authors believe the scheduling of operation should await the appearance of a blood flow rate higher than 60 ml/100 gm per minute.

In dogs, chronic vasospasm produced by injections of autologous blood into the cisterna magna on two occasions mimics clinical posthemorrhage spasm, according to Chyatte et al. (*J. Neurosurg.* 59:925–932, 1983). Before the second blood injection, dogs were given ibuprofen (Motrin) or Solumedrol (methylprednisolone) or both in doses of 30 mg/kg. These dogs had a much shortened time for meningeal reaction compared with control dogs without drugs. There were toxic effects from the combined drug therapy as compared with either drug alone. Severe vasospasm was prevented from appearing by the use of either drug alone, and the authors consider this as evidence in favor of the inflammatory nature of "vasospasm." Because of antiplatelet effects, ibuprofen should be reserved for postoperative use when the risk of additional bleeding has been eliminated. High-dose methylprednisolone has significantly less antihemostatic effect but causes more metabolic disturbance, and it should be more appropriate for short-term preoperative use. Histologic studies of the "vasospastic" arteries in dogs suggest functional or histologic derangement of smooth muscle cell contractile elements; the arteries in vivo respond better to vasoactive agonists and do not show the myonecrotic changes seen in chronically "spastic" arteries.

In one of the patients with pituitary apoplexy described by Cardoso and Peterson (*Surg. Neurol.* 20:391–395, 1983), there was blood found in the subarachnoid cisterns when operation was done. In the other, vasospasm was found by preoperative angiography—but the spinal fluid on that day, seven days after onset of sudden headache and photophobia, was xanthochromic and had increased protein. Both patients thus may have had spasm due to bleeding from the pituitary apoplexy instead of from an aneurysm.

Migraine is not usually considered a "neurosurgical disease," but it may at times mimic the distress of subarachnoid hemorrhage from aneurysm and is hence of interest. The migrainous patient (with "cluster" variant type) described by Garnic and Shellinger (*Neuroradiology* 24:273–276, 1983) was a medical student, 33, who had angiography as a last step in evaluation. One injection into the right internal carotid (after a four-vessel angiogram had shown nothing of importance) precipitated an attack typical for her headaches, and the films showed spasm of the anterior and middle cerebral arteries. The headache remitted after administration of Tylenol with codeine; the patient was discharged to take propranolol (10 mg four times per day).

The next article (ibid. 24:277–281, 1983) by Masuzawa and colleagues also deals with angiography in migraine; during an attack, angiography showed dilatation of all secondary and tertiary intracranial branches of the internal carotid artery without changes in the external carotid. When the migraine subsided, all branches of the intracranial vessels (including the basilar artery) showed abnormal segmental narrowing or vasospasm! Some of the narrowings persisted in a left carotid and vertebral angiography six weeks later when the patient was asymptomatic.—O.S.

---

**Acute Surgery of Cerebral Aneurysms and Prevention of Symptomatic Vasospasm**
L. M. Auer (Graz Univ., Austria)
Acta Neurochir. (Wien) 69:273–281, 1983                                      25–6

---

Vasospasm is a prognostic factor when it occurs after subarachnoid hemorrhage due to ruptured cerebral aneurysm; it is considered a result of blood degradation products. The author undertook a study of the calcium antagonist nimodipine in clinical grade I–III (Hunt-Hess) patients aged 15–70; all were operated on within 72 hours of subarachnoid bleeding from a ruptured cerebral aneurysm. Grade III patients were operated on within 48 hours of onset. Patients with a preoperative focal neurologic deficit were excluded. Nimodipine solution was applied locally after aneurysm clipping and was infused at a rate of 0.25–0.5 μg/kg per minute for as long as two weeks after subarachnoid bleeding. Patients then received 60 mg of nimodipine four times daily, orally.

The 25 patients having uncomplicated surgery had no mortality or severe, irreversible morbidity and no severe, symptomatic vasospasm. One patient had two brief transient ischemic attacks 11 days postoperatively, without associated vasospasm; the other 24 had an uneventful course. Six additional patients had intraoperative complications and resultant neurologic deterioration. Four recovered within two weeks of operation. Twenty-two of the 25 patients followed up at six months were fully recovered, whereas three had a minimal deficit.

These preliminary results suggest that acute surgery need not worsen the prognosis of patients with subarachnoid bleeding from ruptured intracranial aneurysm. Severe vasospasm does not appear to occur with early surgery and administration of local and systemic nimodipine therapy. Some narrowing of large vessels may still occur, but vasospasm seems to develop only at a subcritical level.

▶ Of 619 consecutive cases of subarachnoid hemorrhage admitted to the Teikyo Hospital in Tokyo, 527 were submitted to microsurgery; operative mortality was 5.6%, while overall mortality for all admissions was 12%. Keiji Sano ("Microsurgery of Intracranial Aneurysms," in M. Mizukami et al. [eds.]: *Hypertensive Intracerebral Hemorrhage.* New York, Raven Press, 1983, pp. 62–76) gives the following principles. Microsurgery of aneurysms with removal of subarachnoid blood clots is indicated in the first three days of subarachnoid hemorrhage in grades I–III in patients under age 60. After day 3, surgery is indicated for cases in grades I and II, but for higher grades operation is not done unless there is neurologic improvement. Any case with neurologic deterioration to a higher grade should have computed tomographic (CT) scan and angiography to determine if vasospasm, the most probable cause of deterioration, is present. If it is, surgery is postponed until vasospasm begins to subside and disturbances of consciousness improve. A long waiting time is dangerous because rebleeding may occur when vasospasm subsides; usually the optimal period is the second week after onset of vasospasm. If CT shows an intracerebral hematoma due to a ruptured aneurysm, immediate removal of hematoma and clipping of aneurysm is indicated (as in 25 of the 32 patients with hematoma found in this series). Three died, 12 are well and working, 6 care for themselves, and 4 are bedridden; so almost 50% achieved useful social function.

Contrast-enhanced CT scans done in the first three days after subarachnoid hemorrhage may show prominent cisternal enhancement. In the series studied by Tazawa et al. (*Neurosurgery* 12:643–648, 1983), if the hematoma in the subarachnoid space was not removed within three days, severe vasospasm was found in the locus of the remaining hemorrhage. There was no obvious relationship between enhancement found after day 3 and subsequent vasospasm. If these findings are confirmed, then it will be possible (theoretically) to operate safely on aneurysms at an early date if there is no cisternal enhancement. It seems from the foregoing that one should operate early to remove hemorrhage, or if there isn't much enhanced area, one should operate early anyhow. Hmmm....

Experiments in dogs induced Yoshida et al. (*Neurol. Med. Chir.* [*Tokyo*] 23:659–666, 1983) to try to prevent angiospasm after early operation for ruptured aneurysm by intrathecal irrigation with the plasminogen activator urokinase. Continuous irrigation with urokinase was started on the second postoperative day and carried out for 2–13 days (average, 8.3 days). From 500 to 2,500 ml of irrigation fluid containing 12–36 units of urokinase were used daily. In many cases, postoperative clinical course was better than anticipated from the preoperative neurologic condition. There was one case of severe meningitis but no undesirable reaction of the central nervous system. Even better results may occur when the total dose and concentration of urokinase are properly modified. Fifteen patients showed full recovery; 4 had partial restriction; 2 were homebound; 3 needed further nursing but were not vegetative; and 3 died.—O.S.

## Aneurysmal Rebleeding: A Preliminary Report From the Cooperative Aneurysm Study

Neal F. Kassell and James C. Torner (Univ. of Iowa Hosp., Iowa City)
Neurosurgery 13:479–481, November 1983                    25–7

Rebleeding is a major cause of mortality and morbidity after aneurysmal subarachnoid hemorrhage. Traditionally it has been considered that the peak time of rebleeding is one week after aneurysm rupture. Recent data obtained from the Cooperative Aneurysm Study challenge this notion.

Between January 1981 and September 1982, 2,265 patients were admitted within three days after their first subarachnoid hemorrhage to the 68 centers participating in the International Cooperative Study of Timing of Aneurysm Surgery. Patients with intracerebral hematomas requiring emergency evacuation were excluded from this series. Patients were treated according to local practice; for 45%, operation was planned on days 0–3. Overall, 43% received antifibrinolytic agents; 69% of those patients whose operations were planned seven days or later after the initial hemorrhage received these drugs. The daily and cumulative rebleeding rates for the first 14 days after subarachnoid hemorrhage were calculated.

Within 48 hours of the initial rupture, 79% of the patients had been admitted to the hospital. Within 14 days of the initial hemorrhage, 127 (5.6%) rebled. The peak interval for rebleeding was within the first 24 hours after initial hemorrhage when approximately 4.1% of the patients rebled. The rebleed rate dropped sharply until the end of 48 hours to approximately 1.5% per day and declined gradually thereafter. The cumulative rebleed rate was 19% at 14 days. No increased incidence of rebleeding was noted at end of week 1 or beginning of week 2. Patients on antifibrinolytics had a cumulative 14-day rebleeding risk of 14.1%, whereas the risk was 26.5% for those not given these agents.

In this study the cumulative two-week rebleed rate (excluding the first day) was 19%, which agrees closely with other reports. However, the pattern of rebleeding was different in that the maximal rebleeding risk occurred within 24 hours of initial hemorrhage and then declined rapidly to a relatively constant level (irrespective of antifibrinolytic therapy). A major hypothetical advantage of early operation is the prevention of rebleeding. However, these data suggest that in approximately 1 of 25 cases, the aneurysm will rerupture before diagnostic studies are completed and operation can be accomplished. Since emergency surgery is usually not possible, medical means to minimize rebleeding, such as pharmacologically induced systemic arterial hypotension, during the first 48 hours after subarachnoid hemorrhage should be considered. Antifibrinolytic agents may not be effective as there is usually a delay of 24–48 hours before adequate levels can be attained in the cerebrospinal fluid and perianeurysmal clot.

▶ This is such a deviation from commonly accepted concepts that the figures deserve careful scrutiny. In the section on methods, the bald statement is made, "These patients were treated according to local practice." Perhaps, as suggested by the authors, pharmacologically induced systemic hypotension *was* used in the first 48 hours or thereafter, and if so, this might account for results differing from earlier reports of peak rebleeding during the first two weeks. In a comment following the article, Jane et al. noted that the paper confirmed their own findings of maximum rebleeding on day 1 and a gradual decrease thereafter. Another point of some confusion lies in the lack of definition of "rebleeding"! Before the advent of CT scanning, and hence implied in some earlier reports, rebleeding was not always confirmed by lumbar puncture. Sometimes a sudden worsening of the patient's condition was used as criterion, and this may well be mimicked by sudden ischemia due to "vasospasm." I think future analyses should state what criteria for "rebleeding" have been used.

Review of long-term outcome in 182 patients with multiple intracranial aneurysms who had bled at least once was carried out by Winn et al. (J. Neurosurg. 59:642–651, 1983). The minimal risk of rupture of a hitherto intact aneurysm is about 1% per year, but it is higher in the presence of hypertension. The hemorrhage rate is about the same as that observed in patients with a single aneurysm and is not insignificant.—O.S.

---

**Temporary Clipping During Early Operation for Ruptured Aneurysm: Preliminary Report**
Bengt Ljunggren, Hans Säveland, Lennart Brandt, Erik Kågström, Stig Rehncrona, and Per-Erik Nilsson (Lund Univ. Hosp., Sweden)
Neurosurgery 12:525–530, May 1983                                          25–8

---

Little is known of patient tolerance for temporary arterial clipping during aneurysm surgery done within the first days after subarachnoid bleeding. The authors reviewed experience with 16 patients who were subjected to temporary arterial clipping during operation for ruptured supratentorial aneurysm. All but two were operated on within three days after subarachnoid hemorrhage. Ten patients had a ruptured middle cerebral artery aneurysm and 6, a ruptured anterior communicating artery aneurysm. All patients were in at least fairly good condition preoperatively. Temporary clips were used because of premature aneurysmal rupture in 10 cases. The clips were used to facilitate dissection in five cases and to properly clip a broad-based aneurysm in one case. Yaşargil clips were used in most cases. The occlusion times ranged from 4½ to 30 minutes. Induced hypotension was not used.

Temporary clipping did not appear to lead to angiographically detectable arterial wall changes or an increase in thromboembolic complications in these cases. None of the patients who had clipping for rupture of a middle cerebral artery aneurysm had a worse neurologic deficit postoperatively, but two patients with ruptured anterior communicating artery aneurysms developed severe late angiographic vasospasm, and one of them developed delayed focal deficits. No permanent new deficits resulted from temporary clipping done to facilitate the dissection of middle cerebral artery aneurysms. Both pericallosal arteries were clipped in one patient with no permanent adverse effects.

Temporary clipping of the middle cerebral artery may be well tolerated for as long as 20 minutes in early aneurysm operations and can facilitate proper clipping of the aneurysm with minimal arterial trauma in difficult cases. One or both anterior cerebral arteries or the pericallosal arteries can be clipped safely if necessary during aneurysm operations performed in the acute stage.

▶ Temporary clips are only seldom used in cases of aneurysm surgery. Eighteen cases have been analyzed by Kourtopoulos et al. (*Acta Neurochir. [Wien]*

70:59–64, 1984). Duration of occlusion appears not to be a factor in the outcome. The location of the temporary clip does appear to be important; all patients with distal placement of the clip on the middle cerebral artery (i.e., beyond the perforating branches) made good recovery, whereas none of the ones with proximal clipping (which causes hypoperfusion in the lenticulostriate and other perforating vessels) had a good outcome.

The possible adverse effects of temporary clips during surgery for aneurysms can also be monitored by somatosensory evoked potentials. Wang et al. (*J. Neurosurg.* 60:264–268, 1984) and Symon et al. (ibid. 60:269–275, 1984) describe the technique and discuss the use of such potentials during and after operation. Central conduction time was not affected in 9 of 15 patients; in 6 others, there was immediate prolongation of this parameter, with immediate recovery within 15 minutes in 5 patients and within 40 minutes in the sixth. The study of these potentials before operation is also valuable; no prolongation of conduction time was found in patients in clinical grades I–III, but in grade IV it was markedly lengthened. Difference in conduction time in the two hemispheres after surgery were also apparent in some cases and had prognostic significance.

A brief discussion of evoked potentials in aneurysms is a part of a longer article on perioperative evoked potentials in a variety of neurosurgical conditions by Valencak and colleagues from Austria (*Neurochirurgie* 29:349–357, 1983).

It is convenient to reduce the systemic blood pressure during operation on intracranial aneurysms. There is a distinct hazard in this as is pointed out by Hitchcock et al. (*Acta Neurochir.* [*Wien*] 70:235–241, 1984). There is possible risk for both immediate and delayed neurologic deficit, and this is increased when the systolic pressure is reduced below 60 mm Hg. The longer the period of the lowered pressure, the more the risk. Some patients are more prone to this complication than others, and the authors propose the possibility that bedside tests of cerebral blood flow and other monitoring procedures may permit identification of such patients.—O.S.

---

**Ophthalmic Artery Aneurysms**
A. Huber and M. G. Yaşargil (Univ. of Zürich)
Klin. Monatsbl. Augenheilkd. 182:537–543, June 1983                    25–9

---

True saccular aneurysms of the ophthalmic artery are extremely rare events that may produce severe conduction disorders of the optic nerve by compression or hemorrhage. Although echography and computed tomography (CT) are valuable additional diagnostic procedures, carotid angiography is the best method for diagnosis of a saccular aneurysm of the ophthalmic artery. Angiography and CT also solve problems of differential diagnosis. Surgical treatment is recommended for all cerebral aneurysms. With today's microsurgical technique, frontotemporal craniotomy, unroofing of the optic canal, and direct clipping of the aneurysm or the whole ophthalmic artery proximal to the aneurysm is the preferred approach.

For a clearly intraorbital aneurysm, a lateral orbitotomy must be used as the alternative to the transfrontal access. Carotid-ophthalmic artery aneurysms, which originate on the medial or superomedial surface of the internal carotid artery at or near the origin of the ophthalmic artery, are more frequent.

The authors report the results obtained in a group of 33 patients with a total of 40 carotid-ophthalmic artery aneurysms. Sixteen patients had multiple and seven had bilateral carotid-ophthalmic aneurysms. Nine patients had aneurysms on the other sites of the circle of Willis. Furthermore, 11 patients had asymptomatic aneurysms which were discovered and clipped along with the symptomatic aneurysms. The incidences were significantly higher in women (90.9%) than in men. The most frequent initial sign was subarachnoid hemorrhage with or without localized neurologic deficiencies. Endocrine disturbances were not observed preoperatively. Considering the close relationship between the carotid-ophthalmic aneurysm, the optical nerve, and the chiasm, it is surprising that only 21.2% of patients showed visual symptoms preoperatively. The authors found in most cases a definite correlation between the size of the aneurysm and the functional visual disturbances. When general clinical symptoms, such as recurrent intense headaches or signs of subarachnoid hemorrhage, accompany unilateral progressive loss of vision, the possibility of an aneurysm should be considered and four-vessel angiography is an absolute necessity, in part because of multiplicity of aneurysms.

Twenty-seven patients were treated by direct clipping, and all but one (with temporary postoperative diabetes insipidus) had a complete recovery without significant neurologic problems. Temporary postoperative impairment of the visual fields were observed in four patients (12%). Postoperative permanent amaurosis on the basis of an occluded ophthalmic artery was not observed during this study. Aneurysms unsuitable for clipping were handled by encasement with muscle and Aron-Alpha glue. Bilateral carotid-ophthalmic aneurysms (7 cases in 33 patients) were taken care of at the same sitting through the same unilateral approach.

▶ Of 312 giant intracranial aneurysms treated in London, Ontario, 93 were located between the intracavernous portion and the bifurcation of the internal carotid artery. In the analysis carried out by Viñuela et al. (*Neuroradiology* 26:93–99, 1984), it was found that 65 were carotid-ophthalmic, 12 in the region of the posterior communicating and anterior choroidal arteries and 16 at the bifurcation. Most presented with evidence of compression of neighboring structures; only 14 had subarachnoid hemorrhage. The large size (more than 2.5 cm) and the presence of partial thrombosis or calcifications or both do not preclude bleeding. The authors emphasize the need to identify the aneurysm neck without superimposition of surrounding vessels to detect calcification in or near the neck, to assess the morphology and dynamics of the circle of Willis in cases requiring occlusion of the parent artery, and to document progressive thrombosis within the aneurysmal sac after therapy.—O.S.

## Management of Aneurysms of the Petrous Portion of the Internal Carotid Artery by Resection and Primary Anastomosis

Michael E. Glassock III, Peter G. Smith, Arthur G. Bond, Samuel R. Whitaker, and Loren J. Bartels

Laryngoscope 93:1445–1452, November 1983                25–10

Experience with exposure of the petrous part of the internal carotid artery in removing extensive glomus tumors has made resection and repair of aneurysms at this site a technical possibility. The symptoms of an intrapetrosal internal carotid aneurysm are quite variable and often nonspecific. The clinical signs are equally variable. Pulsation of the mass is not necessarily a prominent feature. The differential diagnosis includes a high jugular bulb, a cholesterol granuloma, an aberrant but otherwise normal carotid artery, and glomus tumor. Biopsy should be deferred until after definitive neuroradiographic study. Both computed tomography and retrograde jugulography may be helpful, but cerebral angiography remains the decisive procedure for diagnosing intrapetrosal aneurysm. An aneurysm may appear smaller than it actually is if a large part of it is filled with thrombus.

The approach to resection of these aneurysms is illustrated in Figure 25–1. Aneurysmectomy with restoration of arterial continuity is the best

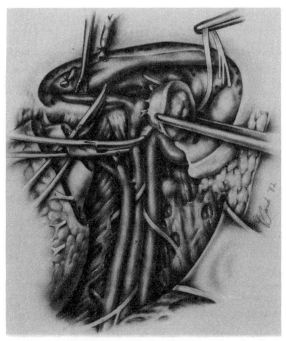

Fig 25–1.—Resection of the pseudoaneurysm, following exposure of the petrous part of the ICA. Removal of the bony sleeve lateral to the artery exposes the arterial laceration and surrounding arteritis. Unaffected portions of the proximal and distal artery are atraumatically occluded.
(Courtesy of Glassock, M.E., III, et al.: Laryngoscope 93:1445–1452, November 1983.)

approach where clinically feasible. The risks of permanent conductive hearing loss and temporary facial paralysis from the infratemporal fossa approach are warranted by the potential morbidity from less definitive treatments. Full-thickness defects are best repaired by end-to-end anastomosis via rerouting of the arterial segments. Temporary internal shunting is the simplest means of protecting against cerebral ischemia or infarction during operation. Temporary occlusion of the arterial segments should be done with the use of hypothermic anesthesia, with or without barbiturate augmentation, even if an adequate cross-circulation is present. Active, poorly controlled bleeding calls for immediate carotid ligation. Aneurysmal extension to the level of the foramen lacerum precludes direct repair of an intrapertrosal aneurysm. Common carotid ligation appears to be safer than internal carotid ligation. Trapping is a more definitive procedure than simple proximal ligation. It is useful to wrap the dehiscent part of the asymptomatic intrapetrosal aneurysm or the laterally displaced internal carotid artery with muscle or fascia to induce fibrosis. Observation of a petrosal aneurysm is rarely indicated, even if symptoms are absent.

▶ The basic approach here is that of Ugo Fisch, the otologist from the University of Zurich. His infratemporal approach for tumors of the skull base and lesions of the petrous portion of the carotid artery was described in an article he wrote with Pillsbury (*Arch. Otolaryngol.* 105:99–107, 1979) and in several other articles, including his chapter "Carotid Lesions at the Skull Base" in Brackmann, D. F. (ed.): *Neurological Surgery of the Ear and Skull Base.* New York, Raven Press, 1982. Recently Batzdorf and Gregorius (*Neurosurgery* 13:657–661, 1983) have described an experimentally based technique for surgical exposure of the high cervical carotid artery that involves mandibular osteotomies.

Some years ago, Ernest Sachs, Jr., clearly showed the lack of benefit from wrapping aneurysms with muscle (although this is a procedure of hallowed history). The muscle simply does not survive, nor does it evoke the reactions that fine-mesh gauze does (with apparent improvement in results). The search for better "glues" continues; perhaps the manufacturers of "Biobond" (from Japan) could now apply for consideration as makers of an "orphan drug."—O.S.

---

**Intraoperative Use of Real Time Ultrasonography Applied to Aneurysm Surgery**
Akio Hyodo, Masahiro Mizukami, Toshiaki Tazawa, and Osamu Togashi (Mihara Meml. Hosp., Gunma, Japan)
Neurosurgery 13:642–645, December 1983                     25–11

---

The authors report experience with intraoperative real-time ultrasonography done during 13 aneurysm operations in 1982–1983. Five patients had middle cerebral artery aneurysms, four had anterior communicating artery aneurysms, and two each had internal carotid and distal anterior cerebral artery aneurysms. An ATL mechanical sector scanner was used, with the scan head wrapped with a sterile rubber bag placed on the dura after the craniotomy. In two cases the aneurysm was detected by real-time ultrasonic imaging. In one case of a large aneurysm, the thick and thin parts of the aneurysm wall were detected. Accompanying abnormalities such as intracerebral hematoma, massive subarachnoid hemorrhage, and hydrocephalus were consistently detected. In three cases with mild subarachnoid bleeding, only normal structures were noted on ultrasonic imaging.

Intraoperative real-time ultrasonography provided information concerning the aneurysm itself in 2 of these 13 cases and, in several instances, coexisting abnormalities. It is expected that intraoperative ultrasonography will prove helpful during surgery on giant aneurysms and thrombosed aneurysms.

---

### Transvascular Treatment of Giant Aneurysms of the Cavernous Carotid and Vertebral Arteries: Functional Investigation and Embolization

Alex Berenstein, Joseph Ransohoff, Mark Kupersmith, Eugene Flamm, and Douglas Graeb

Surg. Neurol. 21:3–12, January 1984                    25–12

---

The management of giant aneurysms of the carotid and vertebral systems remains a challenge. The authors used detachable balloons, placed percutaneously, to treat nine carotid cavernous aneurysms, three petrous aneurysms, one giant vertebral aneurysm, and an aneurysm of the posterior inferior cerebellar artery with repeated subarachnoid hemorrhages. A double-lumen balloon catheter was used to assess tolerance to acute occlusion of the carotid or vertebral artery under systemic heparinization and local perfusion or heparinized saline proximal and distal to the occlusion. Debrun detachable balloons were used.

Occlusion was successful in eight of the nine cases of cavernous aneurysm, in the three cases of petrous aneurysm, and the case of giant vertebral aneurysm. It failed in one case of cavernous aneurysm with associated fibromuscular hyperplasia of the internal carotid, which prevented a percutaneous approach. The arterial lumen was occluded in all cases. Trapping of the aneurysm, the preferred method, was possible in all except four instances. The patient with a posterior inferior cerebellar artery aneurysm was managed by occlusion of the vertebral artery and did well before dying six weeks later of aspiration pneumonia. All the patients who were successfully treated improved clinically, with relief of retro-orbital pain and, usually improvement or resolution of ocular cranial nerve palsies. The only complication was a delayed, transient ophthalmic embolic episode.

Tolerance to acute occlusion of the internal carotid can be reliably tested before transvascular balloon occlusion of a giant aneurysm. Balloon occlusion may prevent delayed embolic complications if the cavernous segment can be trapped, excluding the C4 and C5 branches of the artery from the circulation. The results have been at least as good as those of superficial temporal bypass and better than those reported with ligation of the cervical carotid artery.

▶ A quite similar article by Kupersmith et al. appeared in *Neurology* (34:328–335, 1984). It gives somewhat more detailed information on the neuro-ophthalmologic findings before and after treatment primarily by embolization with detachable balloons.

Delayed embolic complications after carotid artery occlusion are related by Berenstein et al. to collateral vessels to the C4 and C5 segments of the artery, while balloon trapping decreases the length of the thrombosed segment and prevents retrograde filling of the aneurysm. Heros (*Surg. Neurol.* 21:75–79, 1984) has summarized 12 cases of probable embolic complications during or after therapeutic occlusion of the internal carotid artery. Three were personal cases (Heros et al.: *Neurosurgery* 12:153–163, 1983), and the others were collected from inquiry of 30 other neurosurgeons. The cases involved combined internal carotid ligation and extracranial-to-intracranial bypass for treatment of giant intracranial aneurysms. The danger appears to be greater with occlusion of the internal than with occlusion of the common carotid artery. Heros believes the risk of embolization may be sufficient to warrant reconsideration of the probable benefits of ligation of the common rather than the internal carotid artery. He also suggests the propriety of using major anticoagulation whenever carotid ligation is undertaken unless there has been a recent subarachnoid hemorrhage or craniotomy.

Therapeutic occlusion of the basilar artery or of both vertebral arteries represents a different type of therapy for these lesions. Collateral blood flow to the brain stem in these cases, described by Pelz et al. (*J. Neurosurg.* 560–565, 1984) is supplied by the posterior communicating arteries. Angiographic morphology must be known before deciding whether the patient can withstand such procedures. Vertebral angiograms with carotid artery compression are often needed to supply this information. At least one large posterior communicating artery appears to be necessary for vascular occlusion to be successful. Placement of a tourniquet on the basilar artery, which has some risks of its own, appears to be a very useful test for determining the ability of the patient to withstand basilar occlusion.

A cadaver study of the posterior communicating arteries in 126 cranial cavities is reported by Bisaria (ibid. 60:572–576, 1984). Two arteries on one side and three on another were found along with funnel-shaped junctional dilatations in 6.3%. (One cadaver also had a similar dilatation at the other end of the communicating artery.)

Statistics from the Cooperative Aneurysm Study are furnished by Kassell et al. (*Neurosurgery* 12:291–297, 1983). Only 8% of aneurysms in 1,092 patients were 15–30 mm. Most ruptured aneurysms are less than 10 mm in diameter when seen in angiograms. Those that are 5–7 mm and that have not ruptured should be operated on, and smaller ones should be followed with angiography intervals of one to two years. Piepgras (commenting) believes decision to operate should take into account not only the size but also the location and complexity of the aneurysm, the age and medical condition of the patient, and the expertise of the individual surgeon.

Endovascular occlusion was used in 15% of the 309 giant aneurysms that form the base for the collaborative effort of the French-speaking Neurosurgical Society. The study was published as supplement 1 to volume 30 of *Neurochi-*

*rurgie,* 1984. M. Sindou and Y. Keravel (with 14 collaborators using data from 25 neurosurgical services from Europe, Africa, and South America) describe the various therapeutic approaches; 54% of the aneurysms were attached directly and 31% by occlusion of the feeding vessel. In 48% of the cases, hemorrhage was the presenting sign; 47%, symptoms imitated a tumor; and 5% presented with thromboembolic phenomena. An English summary of this easy-to-read French monograph would have been valuable.—O.S.

---

**Cerebral Arteriovenous Malformations: Indications for and Results of Surgery, and the Role of Intravascular Techniques**
Alfred J. Luessenhop and Louis Rosa (Georgetown Univ.)
J. Neurosurg. 60:14–22, January 1984                                    25–13

---

The authors reviewed findings over a 20-year period in 450 patients with cerebral arteriovenous malformations (AVMs). The estimated natural risks of death and morbidity from each hemorrhage are 10% and 30%, respectively. Direct surgery was carried out in 90 patients. Hypotension now is routinely induced during resection of an AVM. Loupe magnification usually suffices. Lesions as large as 2 cm can be coagulated in situ, whereas larger lesions of the frontal or temporal lobes and cerebellar hemispheres are removed by bloc resection. The most commonly used technique is marginal resection, which requires establishing a plane adjacent to the bulk of the AVM or very close to it at sites where the margins become more diffuse. About half of the recently treated patients have had staged resections. Intravascular techniques used in more than 200 patients are based on the use of flow-directed, barium-impregnated Silastic emboli. Routine presurgical embolization no longer is carried out because it seems not to reduce operative difficulties. Embolization alone is used in older patients with large AVMs and progressive neurologic deterioration, as well as in younger patients who are inoperable.

Mortality and morbidity in patients with smaller AVMs have been lower than estimated. None of 74 such patients died, and only 3 experienced morbidity from the procedure. Seven of 16 patients with grade III lesions (4–6 cm) had morbidity, and 2 died. One death occurred in a patient who had recent hemorrhage, and the other resulted from severe circulatory breakthrough.

Excision of cerebral AVMs that are 4 cm or smaller is nearly always indicated; however, in patients with larger lesions, the surgical risk probably exceeds the natural risk in most circumstances after the fourth to fifth decade of life. Early or mild neurologic dysfunction from a large hemispheric AVM usually is not in itself an indication for surgery, nor is the presence of seizures or incipient focal neurologic dysfunction without other complicating factors a proper surgical indication. Intravascular methods may come to be used chiefly to convert large inoperable AVMs to operable ones.

▶ In the next article in the same issue of the *Journal of Neurosurgery,* Stein discusses 25 malformations that involved the medical aspect of the cerebral hemispheres. By the criteria of Luessenhop and Rosa, these would be considered grades I and II lesions, and hence should be operable. The position of the lesions, however, makes them more than usually difficult. Results were good or excellent in 22 cases; 2 had fair outcome; 1 had a poor result, but none died.

Viñuela, from London, Ontario, reported to the 31st Annual Meeting of the Italian Neurosurgical Society in Rome in 1982 (*Acta Neurochir.* [*Wien*] 69:154, 1983) the results of treatment of 64 patients with cerebral arteriovenous malformations with embolization using embolization with isobutyl-*S*-cyanoacrylate. Complete obliteration was achieved in 8 of 45 patients who did not have resection after embolization. There were 3 deaths due to hemorrhage which took place during embolization. Two cases of gluing of the balloon catheter were encountered; this did not appear to cause any adverse effects. Seven patients had hemianopia or quadrantanopia predicted before embolization. Five patients had residual motor weakness; the symptoms were considered moderate or severe in two of them, but both had had large malformations in eloquent areas.

In four cases described by Viñuela et al. (*AJNR* 4:1233–1238, 1983) embolization with cyanoacrylate produced incomplete occlusion, but there was progressive thrombosis thereafter so that late follow up in two cases showed complete obliteration of the malformation. The authors warn that the thrombosis may extend into draining veins and induce obstruction to cerebrospinal fluid circulation.

At the same meeting (*Acta Neurochir.* [*Wien*] 69:153, 1983) Steiner (from Stockholm) reported results in 175 patients treated with the intersecting beam technique of the $^{60}$Co gamma unit of Leksell. Optimum dose was delivered to the entire malformation in 120 of the patients. The general result was a progressive decrease in size and eventual obliteration of the malformation after single doses of 30–50 Gy (3,000–5,000 rad). More malformations were obliterated after two years than after one. Rebleeding occurred in 4.5% of the entire series; in the optimally treated patients the rate was only 1.6%.

Gelfoam is easy to use as an embolization material for arteriovenous malformations and other lesions. It is quickly degraded in the body and permits recanalization. Polyvinyl alcohol foam is effectively permanent, for it takes months or years to be absorbed. Its high coefficient of friction (compared with gelatin foam, for instance) makes it prone to blockage of the catheter. A synergistic mixture of the two has been prepared by Horton et al. (*Am. J. Neuroradiol.* 4:143–147, 1983). Gelfoam powder is stirred with contrast material in such a way as to form a slurry which has the consistency of mucilage. It is then mixed with polyvinyl alcohol particles of the desired size. In a different mixture, microparticles of the alcohol foam, much smaller than the ordinary particles, are mixed with particles of Gelfoam made by cutting the foam. After animal experiments showed the occluding possibilities of the mixtures, they were used in patients with dural, pial, and facial arteriovenous malformations, as well as somatic malformations. A total of 14 patients were treated. As a preoperative adjunct to surgery, the mixture permits a planned stabilization interval between embolization and surgery without concern that the occlusion and additional thrombosis will be resorbed. Solid occlusion occurs long enough to kill tissue. The presence of internal elastic lamina is a constant finding. The value of the mixture is such that the authors recommend its use for trial by the therapist; the additional time required to prepare the combination is more than rapid by the ease of its introduction and use.

Acting on the assumption that incomplete removal of arteriovenous malformations might be followed by postoperative bleeding, Hassler et al. (*Neurochirugia* [*Stuttg.*] 26:146–148, 1983) have routinely performed postoperative angiography under the same anesthetic as that used for operation. One incompletely removed angioma was not involved with postoperative bleeding, yet postoperative bleeding has occurred in patients with apparently complete removal of the malformation. There were immediate hemodynamic changes in diameter of large vessels, but decreases in the diameter of the internal carotid arteries were accompanied by filling of vascular territories not previously injected. It was found that there was an increased risk of postoperative bleeding and brain swelling in patients with long feeding vessels (e.g., parietal lobe malformations), which are visible for longer than 10 seconds in the angiogram. Localized postoperative swelling occurred in 4 of 25 patients, and in 3 of these, the entire hemisphere was involved. In a few patients with angiography after 8–17 days, stagnating vessels were no longer found. Alterations in hemodynamics occur during operation; with progressive exclusion of the angioma, hemostasis of small pial vessels in the borderline between angioma and brain becomes more difficult. This tendency was related to blood pressure, and it ceased with artificial hypotension.

Fasano (Univ. of Turin) reported to the Third Annual Meeting of the American Society for Laser Medicine and Surgery that satisfactory results could be obtained with lasers in treating arteriovenous malformations. No postoperative deficits resulted from use of the neodymium-yttrium-aluminum-garnet (Nd:YAG) laser in two patients with brain stem malformations. Other reports from this meeting concerned small, superficial, or deep-seated AVMs in critical areas. New studies relate to progressive thrombosis of the bulk of the AVM with the ND:YAG laser. See also the article by Fasano in *Neurosurgery* (11:754–760, 1982).

A rare occurrence of thrombosis of an aneurysm of the vein of Galen has been noted by Di Rocco et al. (*Eur. Neurol.* 22:293–299, 1983). Increased head size led to cerebral angiography at age 4 months in their patient. The parents refused operation. The boy's head continued to grow, and there were retardation and mild right hemiparesis. At age 9 years, the child was comatose following severe headache and right-sided seizures with loss of consciousness. The head was 54 cm in circumference, with a mild right hemiparesis. Repeat angiography revealed hydrocephalus, but no aneurysm was visualized although a CT scan had shown a small opacity with calcification in the vicinity of the original massive vascular dilatation. A ventriculoperitoneal shunt was placed, with improvement in clinical status; and six months later, only a mild right hemiparesis persisted.

In place of making decisions about arteriovenous malformations on the basis of recent cases, memories of outcomes, etc., Iansek, Elstein and Balla (*Lancet* 1:1132–1135, 1983) have turned to decision analysis. Based on available statistics, they have analyzed the risks of operation and of no-operation in cases of arteriovenous malformation that has or has not bled. For natural history, they estimate the annual hemorrhage rate at 1%, and over a 20-year cumulative period, 18%. If the malformation bleeds, immediate death will follow in 14%, and 20% will have a significant morbidity. With surgical therapy, they assume that a patient with arteriovenous malformation which had never bled will die in 10% of cases, and another 27% will have significant morbidity. If the malformation has bled, mortality from operation is 8% and morbidity, 23%. Based on mathematical considerations of these data, the authors conclude that the best management for a malformation that has not bled is a conservative one. They do not believe the risks and outcomes vary appreciably for operation under varying conditions—that is, the rates would not vary appreciably for a young patient with a small superficial malformation in a silent area!

The usual dictum is, I believe, that the indications for operation on an arteriovenous malformation that has not bled should include intractable headache or intractable seizures. These matters were not considered in this analysis, and hence it seems to me that the authors are really not facing reality. In the case report used as an example of iatrogenic neurologic deficit, the patient involved was 28 years of age and had had seizures two years earlier, which were well controlled with phenytoin. Operation was done after several recent patients had emerged intact from surgery for malformations of this sort. I do not think that most experienced neurovascular surgeons would have operated on this patient.—O.S.

---

**Intracranial Cavernous Hemangiomas: Neuroradiologic Review of 36 Operated Cases**
Mario Savoiardo, Liliana Strada, and Angelo Passerini (Istituto Neurologico, Milan, Italy)
AJNR 4:945–950, July–August 1983                                    25–14

---

Cavernous hemangiomas of the brain are well-circumscribed vascular malformations composed of thin-walled sinusoidal spaces lined with endothelium, but lacking elastic membranes, muscular tissue, and intervening nervous parenchyma. Although they often remain undiagnosed, these lesions are the second most common cerebral vascular malformation after arteriovenous malformations (AVMs). The authors reviewed findings in 20 males and 16 females aged 14 months to 61 years with histologically verified intracranial cavernous hemangiomas. The most common clinical presentation was epilepsy (25 patients), usually focal (21). Focal neurologic signs were present in 12 patients. At time of surgery, the average duration of symptoms was 4.3 years (maximum, 27 years). Skull films were available in all 36 patients, radionuclide studies in 19, pneumoencephalograms in 17, and computed tomographic (CT) studies in 18. Angiography was performed (carotid or vertebral or both) in 35 patients. Of the supratentorial cavernous hemangiomas, 14 were in the left hemisphere and 18 in the right hemisphere without preferred localization. One lesion was extradural, and in three instances the lesions were in the posterior fossa.

Skull films showed fine granular or coarse calcifications in three patients, and sellar changes consistent with increased intracranial pressure were found in three others. Results of radionuclide brain scans were positive in 17 of 19 examinations; the negative scan results occurred in the presence of two small lesions less than 2 cm in diameter. Findings on pneumoencephalography were abnormal in 11 of 17 patients; the location of the cavernous hemangioma was usually indicated by mass effect on the ventricular system. Angiography results were normal in 7 of 35 patients. In 13 patients vessel displacement was mild or moderate. In eight others, the pathologic findings were limited to an avascular area visible in the capillary phase. In seven lesions, pathologic circulation was seen usually as a faint capillary blush or early draining veins. The lesion was seen on CT in 17 of 18 patients. Calcifications not seen in plain films were noted in five patients. In five a mass effect was present, markedly so in two instances. In some instances, differentiation was made easier by patchy vascularity in external carotid angiograms, which was different from that seen typically in meningiomas. In seven patients a poorly defined hypodensity surrounding the lesion was considered consistent with edema or gliosis.

Thus, the most frequent angiographic findings in the presence of cavernous hemangioma are a mild mass effect and an avascular area in the parenchymatous phase. In addition to detecting the lesion in 17 of 18 patients, CT also demonstrated asymptomatic vascular malformations in one. There are no pathognomonic features of cavernous hemangiomas, but the most common CT findings are slightly hyperdense areas with enhancement after intravenous injection of contrast medium, without a significant mass effect; CT was superior to angiography in defining the exact boundaries of the lesions. Although CT has largely replaced radionuclide brain study, the latter is recommended as a complementary investigation. The combination of a clinical history of focal epilepsy with CT and angiographic findings should suggest the diagnosis of cavernous hemangioma. In all patients with spontaneous hematoma and negative results on angiography, CT should be repeated after a long interval to exclude the presence of a cavernous hemangioma or other cryptic vascular malformation.

---

### Bragg-Peak Proton-Beam Therapy for Arteriovenous Malformations of the Brain

Raymond N. Kjellberg, Tetsu Hanamura, Kenneth R. Davis, Susan L. Lyons, and Raymond D. Adams (Massachusetts Genl. Hosp., Boston)
N. Engl. J. Med. 309:269–274, Aug. 4, 1983                    25–15

The authors reviewed the results of stereotactic Bragg-peak proton-beam therapy in 74 patients treated for arteriovenous malformations in 1965–1978. The mean patient age was 31 years. Malformations were exclusively supratentorial in a large majority of patients. Hemorrhage or a seizure were the usual presenting features. The patients were generally considered unsuitable for craniotomy with excision or embolization because of the location or size of the lesions or the operative risk. Treatment was delivered using local anesthesia in a single session. Doses producing necrosis were sometimes deliberately used in small malformations in silent areas of the brain, but were avoided in lesions involving motor, speech, or visual projections or other neurologically active structures.

Two deaths from bleeding occurred in the first year after treatment, but there were no subsequent disabling or lethal hemorrhages. Seizures, headaches, and progressive neurologic deficits were arrested or improved in most cases on follow-up for 2–16 years after treatment. Eight patients had craniotomy for excision of residual lesions. Five shunt procedures were done after proton-beam therapy. No patient has died of procedure-related causes. No angiographic evidence of worsening of a lesion after treatment was obtained. Pathologic studies in three cases showed a decrease or occlusion of the lumens of nearly all the vessels.

Protection from death due to bleeding appears to develop gradually in a period of one to two years following proton-beam treatment of intracranial arteriovenous malformations. The treatment appears to be associated with low risk and is especially useful for treating malformations that are unsuited to other treatment methods. Further treatment may be indicated two years or longer after presentation.

▶ The use of the proton-beam for treatment of certain arteriovenous malformations of the brain emphasizes again the current dilemma in American medicine: who shall have access to expensive and scarce therapy? I do not have any panacea; it may be necessary to create a board that would evaluate and create priorities for such treatment. One additional source for proton-beam therapy could be the accelerator in the suburbs of Chicago. Just why it can't be adapted for this purpose is unclear to those of us not involved in the protracted negotiations.—O.S.

---

**The Surgical Approach to Arteriovenous Malformations of the Lateral and Sigmoid Dural Sinuses**
Thoralf M. Sundt, Jr., and David G. Piepgras (Mayo Found.)
J. Neurosurg. 59:32–39, July 1983.                                     25–16

---

The authors reviewed the surgical treatment of 27 patients seen in 1973–1982 with arteriovenous malformations (AVMs) of the lateral sinus. Excluding an infant, the mean patient age was 54 years. Five patients had been operated on previously. Papilledema was a common presenting finding. The most common symptom was pulsatile tinnitus. All patients had angiography preoperatively.

TECHNIQUE.—The operative approach is illustrated in Figure 25–2. Preparations must be made for major blood loss. Two dural incisions are made paralleling the long axis of the lateral sinus and are enlarged by secondary incisions vertical to them before an attempt is made to resect the AVM. The chief source of bleeding at the epicenter of the AVM is the petrous bone itself. The sigmoid sinus is opened and occluded with Surgicel, but need not be resected. Bridging veins that are red with blood draining the AVM may be divided; black bridging veins, such as the vein of Labbé, must be resected. The dura is replaced with a homologous dural graft or a piece of fascia lata.

Two patients died; both had previously been operated on with incom-

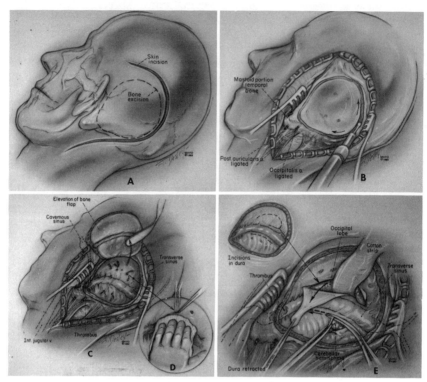

**Fig 25–2.**—**A**, skin incision and area of bone to be excised. **B**, bone plate is elevated with use of air drill held at a 30-degree angle to prevent perforation of dura. Area of osteotomy is gradually increased peripherally around margin of bone plate until dura is just barely visible through thin layer of cortical bone. Bone plate is then elevated with use of periosteal elevator. **C** and **D**, after removal of bone plate, possible profuse dural bleeding can be controlled with bipolar coagulation of bleeding points; large piece of Gelfoam is placed over entire expanse of exposed dura and is held in place with uniform digital compression. Margins of dura are then gradually exposed as packing is retracted and bleeding points are coagulated individually. **E**, preparations are made for excision of lateral sinus by opening dura above and below lateral sinus with incisions that parallel long axis of sinus. *(Continued.)*

plete removal or obliteration of the AVM at attempted embolization. One was an infant with a truly congenital AVM; the other cases are considered to have lesions evolving after earlier thrombosis of a dural sinus. Twenty-two surviving patients had excellent results, and 1 had a good outcome. The two poor results were due to blindness that preceded the operation. No recurrences of symptoms, other than transient bruits in two early cases, were noted. Two patients had venous infarctions postoperatively.

An attempt should be made to remove an AVM of the lateral dural sinus as completely as possible at the initial operation. The operating microscope has not been especially helpful because of the size of the operative field, but magnification loupes are useful. Embolization through the external carotid artery may be a definitive approach in cases with

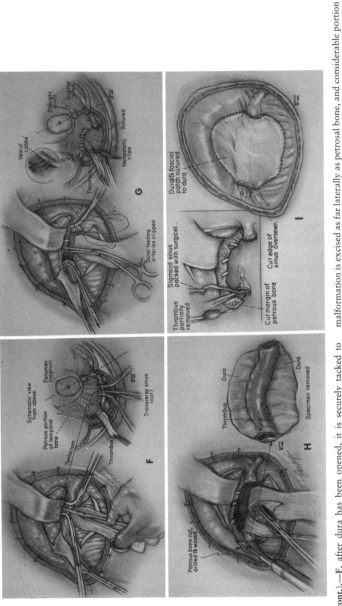

**Fig 25–2 (cont.).—F,** after dura has been opened, it is securely tacked to margins of craniotomy with multiple closely placed dural tacking sutures. Sinus then is incised between two hemostats occluding sinus proximally and distally. **G,** medial portion of sinus is closed with running dural suture. Lateral portion of sinus containing arteriovenous malformation is elevated from wound with hemostat and excised from tentorium. Major bleeding points on tentorium are best controlled with hemostatic clips. If vein of Labbé is large, it may be possible to save it by carrying incision directly into sinus itself and then closing sinus with running suture so that vein can drain into superior petrosal sinus. **H,** arteriovenous malformation is excised as far laterally as petrosal bone, and considerable portion of petrosal bone is removed with high-speed air drill. Bleeding can be profuse but is controlled with cauterization of bone with use of cutting current of Bovie coagulator and bone wax. Examination of excised specimen will often reveal thrombus in situ. **I,** after excision of lateral sinus at point of junction with sigmoid sinus, sigmoid sinus is packed with Surgicel and then closed with running suture to dural or fascial patch. (Courtesy of Sundt, T.M., Jr., and Piepgras, D.G.: J. Neurosurg. 59:32–39, July 1983.)

exclusively external carotid feeders, but in some cases it may give only transient improvement and ultimately compound the problem.

▶ Aside from the intrinsic subject, this article is valuable for indicating the acquired nature of these dural arteriovenous malformations, and for the advice that when the dura mater is involved in an increased blood flow the surgeon would do well to make the bone flap with an air drill instead of the usual craniotome or Gigli saw techniques to avoid tearing the vascular dura or sinus. When the dural vessels are similarly involved in a vascular meningioma, the same advice may well be followed.

Enlarged torcular and transverse sinuses as well as bilateral vascular malformations of the occipital and suboccipital dura mater were found in a macrocephalic child, aged 23 months, studied by Albright et al. (*Neurosurgery* 13:129–135, 1983). Gelfoam and polyvinyl alcohol foam mixtures were embolized into the middle meningeal and occipital arteries before excising the involved dura mater. Ten months later, return of bruit in the head led to angiography, which showed recanalization. Embolization with isobutyl cyanoacrylate was carried out without attempt to treat pial malformations. The authors considered these to be congenital developmental malformations (see article abstracted above for a different opinion). The discussors of this case history were concerned with relationships between venous pressure and cerebrospinal fluid absorption and with treatment of the steal phenomenon.—O.S.

---

**Spinal Cord Arteriovenous Malformations With Significant Intramedullary Components**
Philip Cogen and Bennett M. Stein (Columbia-Presbyterian Med. Center, New York)
J. Neurosurg. 59:471–478, September 1983                                      25–17

---

Arteriovenous malformations constitute 3%–4% of spinal cord masses. They occur chiefly in the thoracolumbar region and are much more frequent in males (Fig 25–3). From 10% to 15% of cases have both intramedullary and extramedullary components. The authors reviewed experience with 17 spinal cord arteriovenous malformations resected by a single surgeon. Six patients had malformations with a significant intramedullary component.

The six patients with partially intramedullary malformations were aged 9–55 years. Five lesions were in the thoracolumbar region, and one was cervical. Three patients with patent venous aneurysms associated with the component within the spinal cord presented with subarachnoid bleeding. The three without hemorrhage had thrombosed venous aneurysms that presumably led to rapid neurologic deterioration. Myelography documented the lesion in all cases, and angiography was helpful in defining the intramedullary component or patent venous aneurysm. All patients presented with rapid neurologic deterioration. All had microsurgical resection of the malformation. Pain was often worse after operation than it had been before, and it was persistent, but all patients except one had significant

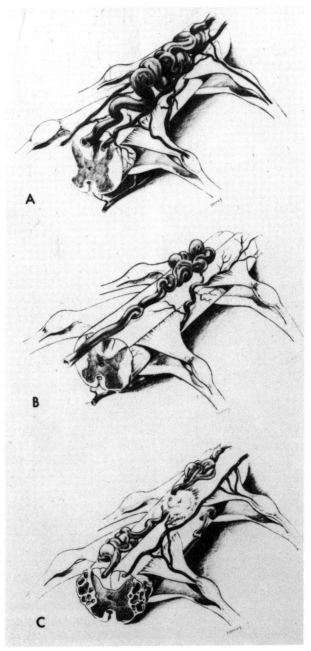

**Fig 25–3.**—Three major types of spinal arteriovenous malformations. **A,** tortuous extensive coiled and enlarged veins fed by numerous small arteries at multiple levels. **B,** an arteriovenous shunt in a nidus form consisting of two or more major feeders to a coil of arterialized veins. **C,** a cuirass of abnormal vessels involving the spinal cord. There is both intramedullary and extramedullary extension. (Courtesy of Cogen, P., and Stein, B.M.: J. Neurosurg. 59:471–478, September 1983.)

neurologic improvement after surgery. Improvement persisted during follow-up for as long as eight years after surgery.

These spinal cord arteriovenous malformations with intramedullary components all were associated with venous aneurysms, some of which were thrombosed. Active lesions that were not extensively thrombosed were supplied mainly by branches of the anterior spinal artery and drained via abnormal veins both dorsal and ventral to the cord. Radical resection of these lesions has given gratifying results, although they remain the potentially most dangerous vascular lesions of the spinal cord.

▶ A nicely illustrated article on "Treatment of Vascular Malformations of the Spinal Cord" by Riche et al. (*Surgical Rounds* April:60–75, 1984) summarizes the experience at l'Hôpital Lariboisière in Paris with patients treated jointly by the neurosurgical and neuroradiological services since 1976. These 126 malformations included 45 intramedullary and mixed lesions, 17 extramedullary fistulae supplied by spinal arteries, and 64 dural fistulae drained by medullary veins. Embolization alone or combined with operation and operation alone may be effective, depending on the type of lesion and the ease of determination of the feeding vessels. Solid particles are preferred to nonsolid ones; cyanoacrylate is not used for medullary arteries, and balloons are used for large arteries following directly into a macroshunt.

In the case demonstrated by Levy et al. (*AJNR* 4:1217–1218, 1983) digital subtraction angiography by arterial injection revealed the feeding vessels after myelography had shown serpiginous vessels from C7 to T5. This subtraction technique offers promise in decreasing the risks of large-volume routine spinal angiography.

Intraarterial digital subtraction angiography appears to be better than intravenous subtraction angiography for demonstration of arteriovenous malformations of the cord, according to Doppman et al. (*AJNR* 4:1081–1085, 1983). Nevertheless, in the current state of equipment and knowledge, supplemental selective arteriography (instead of the simpler injection into the aorta) is still needed to demonstrate additional small feeders and the normal vascular anatomy.—O.S.

---

**Treatment of 20 Direct Carotid-Cavernous Fistulas**
F. L. M. Peeters (Univ. of Amsterdam)
Diagn. Imaging 52:127–136, March–June 1983                25–18

The author reviewed the management of direct carotid-cavernous fistulas in 20 patients using a detachable balloon catheter. The fistula was post-traumatic in 17 cases and developed from rupture of an intracavernous carotid aneurysm in 3 cases. A puncture site in the common carotid artery was dilated with a catheter tip for insertion of a cannula into the internal carotid and placement of the balloon catheter into the cavernous sinus. An attempt was made to prevent development of a false aneurysm by introducing slightly more silicone into the balloon than was needed to occlude the fistula. A risk of temporarily stenosing the carotid artery was involved.

The fistula was closed with one or more balloons while leaving the carotid artery patent in 15 cases; in 3 other cases the fistula was closed but patency of the internal carotid was not maintained. Exophthalmus and bruit resolved after closure of the fistula. One patient had a transient oculomotor nerve palsy, and one had a persistent abducens palsy. In one case introduction of the balloon was prevented by a narrow fistula neck. Another patient required an emergency Hamby operation after the balloon ruptured. This involved intracranial ligation of the internal carotid artery, embolization by a muscle fragment, and, finally, ligation of the cervical carotid.

The excellent results obtained when balloon closure of a carotid-cavernous fistula is successful warrant its use as the initial measure in cases of direct carotid-cavernous fistula.

▶ In the patient with posttraumatic carotid-cavernous fistula described by Leipzig and Mullan (*J. Neurosurg.* 59:524–528, 1983), the metrizamide-filled balloon used to obliterate the fistula was visualized periodically by radiographs. It remained filled for at least two weeks. Use of this contrast material permits safe visualization of the detachable balloon catheter, which should remain inflated for about a week to ensure fibrous attachment to the vascular wall and thus prevent intraarterial migration or failure to occlude the fistula.

On the basis of follow-up from 13 months to 9 years 8 months Nukui et al. (*Neurol. Med. Chir.* [*Tokyo*] 23:789–796, 1983) believe that the best treatment for spontaneous carotid-cavernous fistulas is conservative (except for those with a very high shunt rate). Regression of symptoms for more than six months without reappearance was seen in 17 cases, and marked improvement was noted in another. In four cases, the interval between appearance and disappearance of symptoms was within six months; between six months and one year in four cases; between one and two years in four cases; and in six, more than two years.

In the woman, 34, who spontaneously developed an internal carotid-cavernous sinus fistula, angiogram done five months earlier (because of focal motor seizures) had shown an aneurysm of the carotid artery in the cavernous portion just beyond the petrous bone. There was no trauma. Lesoin et al. (*Acta Neurochir.* [*Wien*] 70:53–58, 1984) discuss the genesis of fistulas of nontraumatic type and point out that weakness of the wall may also be due to arteriosclerosis, syphilis, endocarditis, or arteritis.—O.S.

---

**Hypertensive Putaminal Hemorrhage: Treatment and Results—Is Surgical Treatment Superior to Conservative One?**
Shiro Waga and Yoshisuke Yamamoto (Mie Univ., Japan)
Stroke 14:480–485, July–August 1983                    25–19

---

The proper management of patients with hypertensive putamil hemorrhage (HPH) remains controversial. The authors reviewed data on 74 patients who, between 1977 and 1980, had HPH and were followed up for at least six months after treatment. Eighteen patients admitted in 1977 had surgical treatment. Fifty-six patients admitted from 1978 to 1980, had conservative treatment, which included intensive supportive care and treatment for increased intracranial pressure and cerebral edema. The groups were similar in average age. Seventy percent were admitted within 24 hours of the onset of the ictus.

Mortality after surgical treatment was 28% in this series, and mortality in the conservatively treated group was 14%. The difference was significant. Thirty-four percent of patients were working full time or living independently without disability six months after conservative treatment, and 26% had only minimal disability. Eight percent of patients were totally disabled. Only 23% of surgically treated patients returned to full-time work or an independent life without disability; another 8% had minimal disability. Forty-six percent were partially disabled, and 8% of the group were totally disabled. Fifteen percent were dead at the time of follow-up.

Surgery is not better than conservative treatment in the management of HPH. The clinical state at admission and the prognosis are worse in patients with larger hemorrhages, and surgery does not alter this situation. The size and extent of hemorrhage correlate with the neurologic grade at the time of admission.

▶ Let the reader take heed! Only 5 of the 18 "surgical" patients were in neurologic grades I and II (alert, confused, or somnolent), whereas 8 were in grade IV and V (semicoma to deep coma). In the "conservative" group, 35 (60%) of 56 patients were in the lower two grades, whereas 11 (20%) were in the higher grades. Taking only the first three grades, none of the 10 surgical patients died, and 1 of the 45 conservatively treated patients died. The conclusion concerning mortality *should* be: Surgery should be avoided in patients with putaminal hemorrhage who are in grades IV and V.

The number of surgical patients in the better neurologic grades is too small to be able to compare their disabilities with those in the nonoperated group. Missing from this study are data on the disability status (not the consciousness status) of patients before and after operation and the side of the hemorrhage, which might from the beginning prejudice the ultimate outcome of disability. The authors clearly do not equate "conservative" treatment with doing nothing; I wonder if the earlier surgical patients had the same kind of attention to raised intracranial pressure, edema, and hypertension. This was not a properly randomized series.

By far the most common locus for spontaneous intracerebral hemorrhages described in 96 cases by Pertuiset and colleagues (*Rev. Neurol.* [*Paris*] 139:359–366, 1983) was the central gray nuclei (43 cases). The inner part (internal capsule) was involved in 18, the external capsular area in 19, and both in 6. Lobar hemorrhages (26) involved frontal (7), temporal (9), occipital (6), and parietal lobes (4). Multilobar hemorrhages occurred in 17; there were 4 in the cerebellum and 6 in the brainstem. Circumscribed hemorrhages (60) contrasted with irregular forms (27) mainly in the medial structures. The latter are especially notable for the depressed state of consciousness compared with outer gray structures and lobar hemorrhages.

The patients with depressed consciousness were intubated, had mechanical respirators, cinemet, and decadron; but mannitol (25% solution of 2 gm/kg) was not given unless there was evidence of herniation, and then primarily as a prelude to operation. Clonidine was given intramuscularly or intravenously to stabilize the arterial blood pressure. Tracheobronchial and urinary cultures were carried out at least every two days, leading to antibiotic therapy in most cases.

External ventricular drainage was used for primary relief of pressure followed by direct exposure of intracerebral clot (after preliminary aspiration through the dura mater to prevent cerebral herniation). All patients in grade IV (coma with brain stem involvement) died. Those in grade I (well oriented with or without neurologic signs) and grade II (somewhat obtunded with or without neurologic signs) did well and could be treated conservatively; if after two weeks they had persistent motor, sensory, or psychic defect, they could have evacuation of the clot (via bone flap). It is in those of grade III (coma, without useful responses to pain, with or without neurologic deficit) that prognosis can be helped; those with lobar hemorrhages should have clots removed before the sixth hour. (The authors have not done this, since their patients did not arrive so soon; they refer to the apparent benefits reported by the Japanese neurosurgeons). The authors waited for four or five days before removal of the clot by bone flap, since the operation is easier after this delay. In such patients, simple aspiration of liquid collections of blood may be tried.

There is no established criterion for deciding whether patients should be treated medically or surgically after intracerebral hemorrhage, according to Sakai and colleagues (in: Meyer, J. S., et al., (eds.): *Cerebral Vascular Disease,* vol. 4. Amsterdam, Excerpta Medica, 1983, pp. 96–99). Medical treatment was given to 42 patients with putaminal hemorrhage confirmed by computed tomographic (CT) scan. Glycerol 10% was given intravenously in 41; 19 patients died within 2.3 ± 1.1 days. Of 33 survivors, 20 were able to function independently and 13 were dependent on aids to daily living. Computer analysis of some 54 categories (age, history of hypertension, level of consciousness, time for evolution of signs, CT, blood sugar level, etc.) and multidimensional quantification indicated clear separation of those who would or would not survive. Differentiation between good and fair prognosis (independent of or dependent on aids to daily living) was not so perfect. Main discriminators were CT classification (size and extension of hematoma), signs of herniation, level of consciousness, early aggravation of signs and symptoms, age, blood pressure, and blood sugar level. If similar analysis were done on patients who received surgical treatment, it might be possible to give better indications for operation.

Thalamic hematomas occurred in about 21% of hypertensive intracerebral hemorrhages seen by Kagawa (in Mizukami, M. et al. (eds.): *Hypertensive Intracerebral Hemorrhage,* New York, Raven Press, 1983, pp. 225–231). Early experience with direct removal of such clots were disappointing. Now, the author believes, small thalamic hematomas should not be operated on for grades I and II (localized, alert or drowsy patient with or without minimal neurologic deficits; drowsy, thalamocapsular type, without acutely increased intracranial pressure). For stuporous patients with increased pressure from thalamocapsular hemorrhage (grade III) or those with early signs of herniation or subthalamomidbrain bleeding (grade IV) one may try wash-out therapy with continuous ventricular drainage using antifibrinolytic agents. Only conservative therapy is indicated for grade V patients (comatose, with ventricular blood cast), since fatal outcome is inevitable, regardless of treatment.

According to Kwak et al. (*Stroke* 14:493–500, 1983), spontaneous thalamic hemorrhages constitute between 20% and 35% of all cerebral hemorrhages. In their series of 29 cases studied in the acute stage, recovery was poorer in older patients (not statistically more than a trend). There was no correlation of recovery with side of hemorrhage. State of consciousness was a relevant factor; those with retained consciousness were most apt to survive. The authors refer to a 3–3–9 scale of estimating consciousness based on a Japanese article (from the proceedings of the Third Conference of Surgical Treatment of Stroke in 1976) by Ohta et al. and give an outline of this in their own article. Three grades are established and scored, and in each grade three levels of responsiveness are noted; the lower the number, the more nearly normal is the patient (e.g., grade I includes patients who are awake without needed stimulus, and subgroup 1 implies the patient is seemingly alert; grade III includes patients who cannot be aroused with any forceful mechanical stimulus, and subgroup 3 is not responsive to anything except with some changes in respiratory rhythm. Bilateral Babinski signs carry poor prognosis. Better outcomes occur with lateral basal hemorrhages than with those involving the entire thalamus. Volumes larger than 10 ml portend a grave outcome. When the diameter of the blood clot is less than 25 mm, outlook is much better than with larger ones, which exceed the confines of the thalamus. Ventricular penetration need not carry a poorer prognosis, but basically the degree of ventricular penetration and secondary hydrocephalus seem to be of prognostic value. Deviations of the third ventricle by more than 2 mm tend to imply poor prognosis. Ventricular drainage appears to be of some value in treating the patients with secondary hydrocephalus, and if needed for more than 7–10 days, it should be converted into a ventriculoperitoneal shunt.

Analysis of the outcome of 74 patients with spontaneous intracerebral hemorrhage by Bolander et al. (*Acta Neurochir.* [*Wien*] 67:19–28, 1983) indicates no difference in late results between those operated and those treated without operation, although in general those with surgical evacuation of hematoma were worse—but had had larger hemorrhages. Mortality, however, favored the surgical group. It appears that considerable prognostic information can be obtained from the CT scan: when there is a large hemorrhage, a bad prognosis is indicated by obliteration of the basal cisterns, dislocation of the ventricular system, and especially dilatation of the contralateral ventricle; surgery may be of value by virtue of the lower mortality as compared with patients treated conservatively.

Retrospective study of 138 patients with intracerebral hemorrhage indicates to Sluga et al. (*Nervenarzt* 54:181–185, 1983) that there is a considerable divergence in virtually all characteristics conventionally ascribed to these bloody collections since the advent of CT. Early mortality had dropped from 63% to

28%; lobar hemorrhages are more common, but localizations in the basal ganglia are less frequent. The latter location shows fewer massive bleedings and more collections in just one or two nuclear areas. Hypertension is still the most common cause, and diabetes and hyperlipemia are now more commonly found. The total number of intracerebral hemorrhages found has increased since the advent of CT scanning.

An investigation of hemorrhage produced in cats by injection of blood indicates that little edema occurs unless hypertension is added. More edema is produced, according to Ishii et al. (in Mizukami, M. et al. (eds.): *Hypertensive Intracerebral Hemorrhage.* New York Raven Press, 1983, pp. 11–17), if craniotomy is added. Later, more edema developed even after the hematoma was removed. Intense staining of white matter with Evan's blue dye (a marker for the edema) occurred even in areas remote from the surgical site. Tissue pressure gradients take longer to dissipate when craniectomy has been done. The authors raise some question as to the benefit of early surgery for hypertensive intracranial hemorrhage, and they conclude that for acute hemorrhages with hypertension, control of hypertension is the most important first step. If surgery must be done, they advise avoidance, if possible, of decompressive craniotomy.—O.S.

---

**Long-Term Evaluation of Ultraearly Operation for Hypertensive Intracerebral Hemorrhage in 100 Cases**
Mitsuo Kaneko, Keisei Tanaka, Tsutomu Shimada, Kengo Sato, and Kenichi Uemura (Hamamatsu Univ., Shizuoka, Japan)
J. Neurosurg. 58:838–842, June 1983                                      25–20

---

The authors evaluated early operation in cases of hypertensive intracerebral bleeding for the following reasons: hematoma probably reaches maximal size within 30 minutes; enlargement can occur suddenly on coughing or straining; and cerebral edema develops after seven to eight hours. Review was made of data on 63 male and 37 female patients having operation within seven hours of putaminal bleeding. All patients had hypertensive or primary intracerebral hemorrhage. The age peak was in the sixth decade. Surgery was done in patients with obvious hemiplegia and altered consciousness who had Glasgow Coma Scale scores of 6–12. Most patients had a hematoma of more than 20–30 ml with a midline shift of more than 5 mm on computed tomography (CT). Sixty patients were operated on within three hours of the onset of symptoms. Angiography was done only when a specific disorder such as aneurysm was suspected.

Both transsylvian and transtemporal approaches have been used. The goal is to identify the ruptured stump of the bleeding lenticulostriate branch and securely coagulate it without damaging the main trunk. Fifteen patients were fully recovered six months after operation, and 35 others were independent at home. There were only nine fatal and vegetative cases. Complications were less frequent than in conservatively managed patients or those having delayed operation. Twelve patients deteriorated subsequently because of recurrent intracerebral bleeding, and 10 of them died; control of hypertension was inadequate in 8 of these cases. Fifty-eight patients ultimately had useful recovery on follow-up for as long as 10 years.

Surgery within hours of hypertensive putaminal hemorrhage can be done through a small craniotomy with easy hemostasis. The level of consciousness is the most useful indication for surgery. More than 80% of the present patients had useful functional recovery six months postoperatively, and more than half had such recovery on long-term follow-up.

▶ Emphasis should be placed on the lateral basal (putaminal) location of the hemorrhage, with operation done before edema becomes marked. These 100 early cases were selected from 139 who had early or late operation and from a total of 238 cases of putaminal hemorrhage. Cryptic vascular lesions were excluded, the authors say; however, after 1977 angiography was done only when aneurysm or arteriovenous malformations were suspected, and before 1977 angiograms were done on all patients. The CT scans are relied upon for all cases now. Comparison with earlier statistics is impeded by the disparity between the figures of "ultimate useful recovery rate" of 58% in this group of 100 patients followed for as long as 10 years, and the rate of 83% ambulatory cases (groups 1, 2, and 3) at six months.

The consecutive cases of intracerebral hemorrhage not due to trauma or to ruptured arterial anomalies collected by Gärde et al. (*Eur. Neurol.* 22:161–172, 1983) amounted to 100, all examined by CT. Almost half had volumes estimated at less than 10 ml, and the authors think most of these would have escaped diagnosis without CT scanning. There were 64 men and 36 women, aged 33–86 years (mean, 63 years). Locations were lobar in 29, central white matter in 21, thalamus in 17, lentiform nucleus in 15, cerebellum in 12, and pons and caudate 3 cases each. The hemorrhages of more than 20 ml were almost all lobar or central; the ones in the basal ganglia were almost all less than 20 ml. Decreasing consciousness and the location and size of the hematoma were general indications for operation, which was carried out in 36 patients, usually in the first three days after the onset. Onset was usually acute, but six patients had a protracted onset ranging from several days to a week. Arterial hypertension was noted in 59%, especially in those with hemorrhage in the basal ganglia. The authors believe that the results of treatment (which was conservative in two thirds of the patients) cannot be compared with groups studied before the advent of CT. Continued hemorrhage was not noted in any of these cases, and consequently the authors found no reason to operate on patients who were alert or in a slightly lowered state of consciousness.

The authors believe that hemorrhages in lentiform nucleus and caudate are benign and need no operation and that thalamic hemorrhages are not accessible (a statement disagreed with by some more radical neurosurgeons who used stereotactic or ultrasonic approaches). The chief determinant of outcome is level of consciousness, regardless of size of hemorrhage or location. The mortality in this series of hemorrhages was 37%; 35% returned to work, and 6% required institutional care. The mortality of patients operated on was 53%, but is should be remembered that the operations were done primarily in those who were sickest and had deeper grades of coma.—O.S.

---

**Acute Cerebellar Hemorrhage with Brain Stem Compression in Contrast With Benign Cerebellar Hemorrhage**
D. Chin and P. Charney (Royal Adelaide Hosp., Australia)
Surg. Neurol. 19:406–409, May 1983                                    25–21

Acute cerebellar hemorrhage is being increasingly operated on, but the operative mortality remains very high. The authors describe two cases of acute cerebellar hemorrhage with brain stem compression in patients who recovered after emergency evacuation. Cerebellar hemorrhage was diagnosed in 29 of 240 patients seen in 1974–1980 with intracranial hemorrhage, excluding aneurysmal bleeding; 26 cases were confirmed by computed tomography (CT) or at autopsy.

Hypertension was present in 60% of the confirmed cases. The overall mortality was 62%. Eight patients were comatose on admission or within the first 12 hours, and the others had some degree of impaired consciousness. Two of the comatose patients were those who recovered after emergency evacuation of the hematoma. The others died within 24 hours. Four of 10 deaths of noncomatose patients were due to unrelated causes. All three CT studies of comatose patients showed cerebellar hemorrhage and some degree of hydrocephalus. At autopsy the other five comatose patients all had evidence of ventricular dilatation and tentorial herniation. All 10 patients who survived had positive CT studies; one had delayed evacuation, and 7 patients were treated conservatively with follow-up CT. Five patients in all had evacuation of the hematoma; two of them died due to unrelated causes. Six of the 10 noncomatose patients who died were incorrectly diagnosed, 3 of them despite CT examination.

Computed tomography has helped distinguish this disorder from both primary pontine hemorrhage and cerebral hemorrhage due to ruptured aneurysm. Emergency evacuation of the hematoma can be lifesaving in cases of acute cerebellar hemorrhage. Patients who are not comatose at admission and who are correctly diagnosed have had a relatively benign course. Emergency suboccipital craniectomy is indicated only in patients with a large hemorrhage and hydrocephalus on CT or in patients who deteriorate and have early signs of brain stem compression.

▶ In two fatal cases of cerebellar hemorrhage, extravasation of contrast material during vertebral angiography was encountered by Ito and Nakajima ("Surgical Treatment of Acute Cerebellar Hemorrhage," in Misukami, M. et al. (eds.): *Hypertensive Intracerebral Hemorrhage*. New York, Raven Press, 1983, pp. 215–223). In a 10-year period, they encountered 43 patients with cerebellar hemorrhage; 20 had clot evacuation via suboccipital craniectomy, 5 had ventricular drainage, and 2 had decompression alone. Overall mortality with clot evacuation was 20%. In severely symptomatic cerebellar hemorrhage, emergency operation is required if the clot is more than 4.1 cm in diameter or if there is rapid deterioration of consciousness (with a volume of 30 ml) commencing more than six hours after onset. Two thirds of such patients recover fully. Even milder symptoms with clots of 2.8–4 cm in diameter should lead to operation, especially if there is deterioration of consciousness or increasing cerebellar signs plus evidence for acute hydrocephalus or tonsillar or upward tentorial herniation. Immediate CT examination in the first six hours after onset, plus careful observation of neurologic changes should provide reliable indicators for the need to evacuate cerebellar hemorrhage.

Of all hemorrhages in the brain, 10% are in the cerebellum; they are usually in patients older than age 40 and are usually accompaniments of arterial hypertension. Severe headache, vomiting, and vertigo with imbalance are the somewhat stereotyped presentations, according to Labauge et al. (*Rev. Neurol.* [*Paris*] 139:193–204, 1983). They have reviewed 28 personal and 189 published cases. In acute and subacute instances, consciousness is rapidly impaired, and death is certain if there is no relief of pressure. Computed tomography is needed for accurate diagnosis and demonstration of effect on other structures. Surgical evacuation with or without ventricular drainage has beneficial results if done at a timely occasion and if the state of consciousness is favorable. Brain herniation is always possible, and the possibility of vascular malformation must always be held in mind. The authors believe there is a dangerous size (diameter of 3 cm), above which obstructive hydrocephalus occurs and below which it may be possible to have conservative therapy with repeated CT scans to follow the course of the disorder. These cases, more than the others, deserve angiography to ensure the absence of vascular malformations which might induce consideration of operation.

In a series of 1,033 patients with primary intracerebral hemorrhage, Nakajima (*Stroke* 14:485–493, 1983) found 60 (5.8%) with pontine hemorrhage; 49 were male and 11 were female. Ages ranged from 33 to 77 (mean, 51.1 years). Only 17 patients survived. Autopsy rate was 88.4% of the 43 who died. About 75% of the patients had preexisting arterial hypertension, and this was not related to survival. Among the neurologic findings were ocular bobbing, syndromes of the medial longitudinal fasciculus, skew ocular deviation, hyperthermia, gastrointestinal bleeding, Horner's syndrome, and neurogenic bladder. In 8 of the 17 survivors, visual hallucinations were noted (not hitherto related to pontine hemorrhages). In 21 of the 24 patients coming to autopsy, the hematoma extended into the fourth ventricle, and in 4, it broke through to the clivus. Downward extension into the medulla occurred only once. In one specimen a ruptured microaneurysm was found at the edge of the hemorrhage.—O.S.

---

**Spinal Subdural Hematoma: A Review**
N.A. Russell and B. G. Benoit
Surg. Neurol. 20:133–137, April 1983                                        25–22

---

The authors reviewed 58 reported cases of spinal subdural hematoma seen at Ottawa Civic Hospital; enough data for analysis were available in

50 of these patients. Women predominated in a ratio of 2.1 : 1. The average patient age was 41 years. The thoracic and thoracolumbar regions were involved most often. Major spinal trauma was infrequent. Coagulation abnormalities caused bleeding in 19 cases. Lumbar puncture was a factor in 11 of these cases and caused hemorrhage in 7 others. Severe back pain localized to the spine was a prominent presenting feature; it usually was accompanied by radicular pain. Sensorimotor impairment of varying degrees ensued. Eight patients, six of whom had had major spinal injuries, had immediate and total paralysis. Ten patients had a protracted course. In nine cases the hematoma was found only at autopsy.

Myelography showed a total block in 20 of 26 cases and a partial block in the other 6 cases. Thirty-one cases were classified as acute, 5 as subacute, and 10 as chronic. Thirty-six patients underwent laminectomy and evacuation of the clot; reoperation was necessary in two cases. Ten patients recovered completely and six incompletely. Seventeen of the 20 who did not recover were completely paraplegic preoperatively, and 3 were paraparetic. Two patients died of unreported causes early in the postoperative period.

The source of bleeding in spinal subdural hematoma is difficult to determine. Myelography is the diagnostic procedure of choice. Prompt removal of the hematoma is indicated. The prognosis is good if the diagnosis is made before irreversible cord changes have taken place. The lesion should be considered in patients with signs of progressive cord compression when a cause is not readily apparent, especially in patients with bleeding disorders or those on anticoagulant therapy and especially if a lumbar puncture has recently been done.

▶ Two cases of spontaneous spinal epidural hematoma are reported by Twerdy et al. (*Nervenarzt* 55:96–98, 1984). One involved a woman, 30, with sudden severe thoracic pain and progressing paraparesis, which led to myelography and to removal of a hematoma in the epidural space from T8 to T12. No cause for the bleeding was found. The other case occurred in a man, 68, who was receiving anticoagulants because of vascular insufficiency in the legs. He had severe pain, and in a few hours a cauda equina syndrome developed; but investigation was not done for two weeks. Computed tomography showed a lesion compressing the cauda from a posterior direction, from L1 to L5. Removal of this partially organized, partially liquid epidural hematoma was followed by neurologic recovery. The authors decry delay in operation in patients who have sudden onset of paraparesis even when the cause is uncertain.—O.S.

# 26 Vascular Occlusions

▶ ↓ In a review on asymptomatic carotid bruits (*Vascular Disease Therapy,* July–August: 39–49, 1983), W. S. Fields reemphasizes the justification for carotid endarterectomy which requires operative morbidity and mortality not to exceed the risk of subsequent stroke. The corollary is that operations for asymptomatic bruit (itself an indication of systemic vascular disease) are reasonable only when the outcome of endarterectomy for symptomatic disease has been good. Whether operation for asymptomatic bruit is proper really awaits prospective results in patients randomly allocated to surgical or nonsurgical treatment. Fields opines that therapy aimed at preventing platelet aggregation is beneficial in patients with transient ischemic attacks; aspirin is most often used.

Three papers presented at the 11th Salzburg Conference were published in *Cerebral Vascular Disease,* vol. 4 (Meyer, J. S., et al. [eds.] Amsterdam, Excerpta Medica, 1983. Eschwege et al. (pp. 118–121) (Paris) found significant reduction in fatal and nonfatal cerebral infarction in a double-blind study of 604 patients with ischemic events by using 1 gm of aspirin per day; no additional benefit came from adding dipyridamole 225 mg/day. There was no difference in effectiveness with sex. There was also a significant decrease in myocardial infarction rates.

Armani and co-workers (ibid. pp. 122–130) from Genoa, Italy, reported better results with 500 mg of aspirin every 72 hours than with 1 gm/day in a group of 40 patients with transient ischemic episodes and minor strokes.

The doses of aspirin used by Boysen et al. (ibid. pp. 131–133) in treating 18 women and 24 men ranged from 50 to 1,000 mg/day in the first 14 patients, declining to 25–50 mg/day in later ones. In 75% of the patients, the daily requirement to inhibit platelet aggregation was 50 mg or less; the highest dose, in two patients, was 125 mg/day.—O.S.

---

**1,009 Consecutive Carotid Endarterectomies Using Local Anesthesia, EEG, and Selective Shunting With Pruitt-Inahara Carotid Shunt**
J. Crayton Pruitt (Univ. of South Florida)
Contemp. Surg. 23:49–58, September 1983                                  26–1

---

The author reviewed the results of carotid endarterectomies done using cervical block anesthesia, EEG control, and selective shunting with an internal T-shunt. The 1,009 cases represented about one third of all carotid endarterectomies done at this institution in the past two decades. The Pruitt-Inahara T-shunt was used if a patient became confused, or was unable to speak clearly or to move the contralateral extremities on command; if the EEG showed slowing or suppression of brain wave activity indicative of ischemia; or if backbleeding from the internal carotid artery was not pulsatile.

▶ The T-shunt is 30 cm long; the proximal end, which goes into the common carotid artery, has a balloon which holds as much as 2 ml of saline. The balloon on the distal end of the shunt, which goes into the internal carotid artery, holds only 0.5 ml of saline. The "T" portion communicates with the main lumen and allows flow and pressure measurements, angiography, or instillation of heparin solution. An occlusion catheter was used in the internal carotid when an internal shunt was not placed. The superior thyroid artery was found to be an important source of collateral circulation at certain stages of the operation.

Ten strokes and eight transient neurologic deficits occurred. Eight other patients had transient ischemic attacks that resolved within 24 hours. Three patients died of acute myocardial infarction. The T-shunt was used in 353 cases. It was easily inserted with a little practice. The balloon shunt is considered less traumatic than other types of shunt. It is very advantageous when dealing with a plaque that extends high in the internal carotid artery. Occasionally, the "T" part of the shunt is useful for flushing out debris from an ulceration. The smaller arteriotomy required permits a shorter procedure and helps prevent restenosis.

Safer carotid endarterectomy now is possible with the use of local cervical block anesthesia with EEG monitoring, observation of the back-flow pressure from the internal carotid artery, and selective use of the Pruitt-Inahara T-shunt as indicated.

The divergence of opinion concerning the utility of shunts during carotid endarterectomy continues. Voegele et al. (*Am. Surg.* 5:197:234–237, 1983) concluded from their retrospective study of 323 patients that shunting could not be relied upon to decrease the risk of neurologic deficit. Bilateral staged endarterectomies were done under general endotracheal anesthesia and systemic heparinization. Shunting was done in 485 operations and was not done in 161 (depending on routine preferences of the surgeons involved). There were 30 (4.6%) neurologic events in 29 patients, with a mortality of 1.5%. The shunted group had 27 of the neurologic deficits, whereas only 3 occurred in the non-shunted group. The authors believe that results may be superior if shunts are not used for endarterectomies!

Carotid arterial back pressure and EEG changes were noted after clamping during carotid endarterectomy during a study of 100 patients (Ricotta et al.: *Ann. Surg.* 198:642–645, 1983). Shunts were inserted in the 15% of patients who showed EEG changes after a trial of clamping. Back pressures were significantly lower in those who needed shunts, and these roughly correlated with the EEG changes. The only patient with a back pressure of more than 40 mm Hg had had a recent mild stroke. None of the patients in this series of 100 awoke with a neurologic deficit. The authors believe the EEG is more discriminating for shunt insertion than is back pressure, although a pressure of more than 40 mm Hg is safe in those without recent stroke.

Information obtained from experiments on dogs by Ercius et al. (*J. Neurosurg.* 58:708–713, 1983) indicates that although systemic heparinization is necessary during carotid endarterectomy, it is best to wait for 10 minutes after operation before reversal with protamine. This interval can be shown to be critical for the formation of mural thrombus; after 10 minutes, there is a well-established fibrin-free platelet monolayer over the endarterectomized surface.

Given the high prevalence of symptomatic coronary arterial disease in patients considered for carotid endarterectomy, the surgeon cannot reject out of hand every patient with cardiac symptoms. O'Donnell et al. (*Ann. Surg.* 198:705–712, 1983) reviewed 531 cases of endarterectomy with an overall mortality of 0.9% and a 2.5% incidence of myocardial infarction in spite of the prevalence (66%) of coronary artery disease in the group. Only 23% of the myocardial infarcts led to fatality. Analysis of experience at the Cleveland Clinic indicates to this group that routine coronary arteriography should not be used as a screening method before carotid endarterectomy. The combination of endarterectomy and coronary bypass surgery was reserved for patients with crescendo or decubitus angina with symptomatic carotid disease or asymptomatic carotid disease with high risk (e.g., ipsilateral stenosis and contralateral occlusion, bilateral stenosis, or unilateral high-grade stenosis). Most of the patients with both coronary and carotid disease had endarterectomy alone or bypass coronary surgery staged to follow the carotid surgery. The authors emphasize the values of "cardiac method of anesthesia" even for carotid endarterectomy: slow induction, atraumatic intubation, balanced narcotic maintenance avoiding myocardial depression, with assessment of left ventricular function during operation by Swan-Ganz catheter. Electroencephalography is continually used to monitor cerebral perfusion, and hypertension monitored with the Swan-Ganz catheter is promptly controlled with intravenous nitroprusside.

Transient ischemic attacks were noted in 29 of 42 patients who were found to have coexistent carotid and coronary artery disease in a review undertaken by Emery et al. (*Arch. Surg.* 118:1035–1038, 1983). Angina pectoris was found in 33 patients, congestive heart failure in 6 (and both heart failure and angina in 2); 1 patient had primarily a positive exercise test. Three coronary vessels were involved in 32 patients, and in 17 the left main occlusion was greater than 50%; others had one- or two-vessel disease. Asymptomatic carotid bruits were present in 13 patients. Carotid stenoses greater than 70% were proved by angiography in 38 patients, and ulcerated plaques in 2 others. Two had no angiography. The usual procedure was to expose the carotid artery and sternotomy at the same time. The endarterectomy was carried out first, with shunt if the individual surgeon felt the need. After closure of the arterial incision, the patient was put on cardiopulmonary bypass, and the coronary vascularization was carried out with reversed saphenous vein grafts (mammary artery was used in one patient). Two (5%) patients died; there were no strokes or perioperative myocardial infarctions. One patient had postoperative headache, two had weakness of one upper extremity, and one had transient facial weakness. The authors believe the primary morbidity and mortality of the combined operation to lie chiefly in the cardiac status. Cerebral protection is offered by doing the carotid endarterectomy first. Two teams should be used in doing this "simultaneous" combined operation, with intensive monitoring of cardiac and cerebral function.—O.S.

## Is Siphon Disease Important in Predicting Outcome of Carotid Endarterectomy

Ghislaine O. Roederer, Yves E. Langlois, Anthony R. W. Chan, Paul M. Chikos, Brian L. Thiele, and D. Eugene Strandness, Jr

Arch. Surg. 118:1177–1181, October 1983          26–2

The internal carotid artery is divided into an extracranial portion, extending from the bifurcation to the base of the skull, and an intracranial one, the siphon. The latter runs from the external opening of the carotid canal to the circle of Willis and consists of the petrous, cavernous, and intradural segments. Atherosclerosis is much more prevalent in the carotid bulb than in the siphon, but with substantially different pathologies. The relationship between the prevalence of atherosclerosis at the carotid bifurcation and in the siphon and that between the severity of siphon disease and recurrent symptoms after endarterectomy was studied.

Twenty-three female and 118 male patients (mean age, 62.5 years) underwent endarterectomy. Eight had staged bilateral procedures, providing a total of 149 endarterectomized sides. Lesions identified in angiograms of the carotid bifurcation and in the siphon were rated as smooth or ulcerated (irregular). Follow-up after endarterectomy ranged from one day to 56 months (mean, 22.3 months), with data available on 125 patients (133 endarterectomized sides).

In 281 of 282 sides with arteriographic confirmation, disease was present in the carotid bulb; in 58% of the cases, plaque had reduced the diameter by at least 50%. Most lesions (73%) were potentially the source of emboli. Prevalence of siphon disease was lower; most segments with lesions had diameters reduced by 20%–49%, with plaques smooth in 65% of the cases. The degree of carotid bulb disease was not predictive of that in the siphon. No correlation was found between severity of siphon disease and the presence of focal symptoms; the same proportion (40%) of symptomatic sides was found for all categories of siphon disease.

Both the rates of recurrent focal symptoms (10%) and of recurrent stroke (4%) on the sides undergoing endarterectomy were in agreement with other studies. Of 18 patients with symptoms recurring ipsilateral to the procedure, only 2 had high-grade lesions in the siphon. The distribution and surface structure of siphon disease were comparable on all the endarterectomized sides, independent of recurrent focal symptoms. Endarterectomy on the side of a severe siphon lesion showed an ipsilateral recurrent symptoms risk of 13%, somewhat less than when the siphon had mild or no disease. Therefore, these data do not support the hypothesis that patients operated on with a severe lesion in the siphon are at a greater risk of recurrent symptoms.

▶ Wasserman et al. (*Arch. Surg.* 118:1161–1163, 1983) studied patients suspected of carotid artery disease with ultrasonic imaging, oculoplethysmography, and ocular pneumoplethysmography, and they compared relative accuracy with contrast angiography. They believe the ultrasonic imaging and the pneumoplethysmography together provide accurate anatomic and hemodynamic information useful in evaluation of carotid occlusive disease. They believe that an asymptomatic patient with occlusive diagnosis need not be subjected to angiography, and a symptomatic patient with occlusion diagnosed by noninvasive methods may also be spared angiography, apparently because operation would need to be done anyhow. For stenoses, the noninvasive methods are not so accurate as to obviate angiography. I don't believe I would depend on these methods to make an ultimate decision for operation, for I believe it is imperative to know what is going on in the head, with second occlusions, aneurysms, tumors, collaterals, etc. The noninvasive methods may well be used to follow asymptomatic patients with bruit, for instance, or postoperative cases, with avoidance of risk. Whether digital subtraction angiography will make the elaborate noninvasive techniques obsolete remains to be seen.—O.S.

---

**Durability of Carotid Endarterectomy**
William H. Baker, Andrew C. Hayes, Debbie Mahler, and Fred N. Littooy (Loyola Univ. Med. Center, Maywood, Ill.)
Surgery 94:112–115, July 1983                                                26–3

---

Carotid endarterectomy has produced satisfactory clinical results in patients with carotid stenosis and transient ischemic attacks, but the long-term outcome has not been well documented. The authors used repeated noninvasive testing to follow patients after endarterectomy. Supraorbital Doppler examination, oculoplethysmography, carotid phonoangiography and, in later cases, spectral analysis of the carotid Doppler velocities were utilized after a total of 193 carotid endarterectomies. A total of 158 studies were initially done within three months of operation, and 35 were done three months or longer after surgery.

Twenty-four of the arteries were considered abnormal on the basis of the first postoperative noninvasive testing. Four of these were symptomatic. Of the 133 patients with normal initial findings who were reevaluated after a mean of 23 months, 18 were found to have become abnormal. Ten of these arteries had greater than 75% stenosis, and 8 had 50%–75% stenosis. Five of the eight vessels studied by contrast examination were abnormal and underwent reoperation. Only two patients had symptoms related to the abnormal test findings.

These findings suggest that carotid endarterectomy is a reasonably durable procedure. Recurrent stenosis was detected in 10% of the serially tested patients in this study. Other series also suggest that significant stenosis occurs in 10% or fewer cases. Carotid restenosis appears to be due to myointimal fibroplasia, or to atherosclerosis if it occurs more than two years after operation. The risk of restenosis makes long-term follow-up after carotid endarterectomy essential. The authors have begun a study (using noninvasive methods, including digital subtraction angiography) of patients who have evidence of stenosis.

▶ Saletta and Baker have modified their technique for removal of clots in the internal carotid artery (*Am. Surg.* 49:238–240, 1983). The external and common carotid arteries are clamped, but the internal carotid is not. Opening is made and back pressure in the internal carotid forces the thrombus retrogradely through the arteriotomy. After extraction of the thrombus, an occluding finger controls back bleeding until the internal carotid is encircled and clamped. The authors end with the statment, "In general, operation upon the chronic total [internal carotid artery] occlusion is discouraged."—O.S.

### Neurologic Deficit After Carotid Endarterectomy: Pathogenesis and Management

David Rosenthal, William D. Zeichner, Pano A. Lamis, and Paul E. Stanton, Jr. (Georgia Baptist Med. Center, Atlanta)
Surgery 94:776–780, November 1983                    26–4

The etiology of postoperative neurologic deficits is controversial, having been attributed to temporary cerebral ischemia during carotid occlusion or to reperfusion or technical error, both of which result in thromboembolic events.

From 1975 through 1982, 768 patients underwent 818 carotid endarterectomies (CEs). Indications included transient ischemic attacks (399 patients), vertebrobasilar insufficiency (174), postreversible ischemic neurologic deficit or poststroke (129), amaurosis fugax (58), prophylactic CE or asymptomatic bruit (50), and stroke in evolution (8). Patients were divided into three groups: 318 had CE performed with a shunt (CE-shunt), 274 had CE without a shunt (CE-no-shunt), and 226 had CE monitored by EEG surveillance (CE-EEG). There were 499 male and 269 female patients, aged 40–81 (mean age, 62). A history consistent with coronary artery disease was present in 510 (66%) patients, and hypertension was present in 468 (61%), diabetes mellitus in 276 (36%), and abnormal lipid profiles in 307 (40%).

Transient deficits occurred in nine patients in the CE-shunt group (2.8%), while permanent deficits occurred in five patients (1.6%). Transient deficits occurred in 8 (2.9%) of the CE-no-shunt group and permanent deficits in 6 (2.2%). Transient deficits occurred in five member (2.2%) of the CE-EEG group and permanent deficits in four (1.8%). Overall, 22 patients had transient postoperative deficits, and 15 had permanent deficits. There was no significant statistical difference in the incidence of postoperative neurologic deficits among the groups. Of 22 patients with transient deficits, 16 had ulcerated plaque disease; so did 7 of the 15 patients who had a postoperative stroke. Of 12 patients with immediate profound postoperative deficits, emergency reoperation revealed a patent CE site in 5 patients and a thrombosed carotid artery in 7. Postoperative deficits included neurologic dysfunction disappearing within 24 hours, those resolving within 3 weeks, and fixed nonprogressive strokes.

Patients with ulcerated plaque disease appear to be more susceptible to an embolic event during CE (where intraluminal cellular debris is not adherent within the ulcer bed) than are patients with calcific high-grade obstructive lesions. Of the 37 patients with a postoperative deficit, 11 had intracranial occlusive disease (stenoses at the siphon or the circle of Willis). Severe intracranial disease previously has been shown to place patients at high risk for postoperative complications. While extracranial carotid and vertebral artery occlusive disease may indicate severity of cerebrovascular insufficiency, intracranial occlusive disease appears to be the limiting factor in cerebral ischemia during carotid cross-clamping. When intraoperative EEG monitoring is not performed in cases of severe intracranial or extra-cranial occlusive disease, an intraluminal shunt should be used.

Since the incidence of postoperative neurologic deficits when CE was performed with a shunt, without a shunt, or under EEG surveillance did not differ, inadequate cerebral collateral flow during CE could not be indicted as the causative factor. Technical errors that result in carotid thrombosis or cerebral emboli therefore account for most of the neurologic deficits after CE. Patients with a minimal, focal postoperative neurologic deficit will improve without intervention, and supportive observation is sufficient management in these patients. However, in cases of severe post-operative deficit the prompt use of arteriography is indicated, permitting appropriate operation when indicated.

▶ Monitoring during carotid endarterectomy remains a controversial matter. It is usually proposed as a means of determining which patient should have an intraoperative shunt, but would not seem to have much value when a shunt is routinely placed. Whittemore et al. (*Ann. Surg.* 197:707–713, 1983) cite opin-ions that indicate that shunt placement does not prevent difficulties with main-taining blood flow. Monitoring by EEG can not only indicate which patients need shunting but also can indicate whether the shunt is working properly during operation. It appeared to be especially useful in maintaining safe blood supply to the brain in a series of 69 in whom endarterectomy was done at the same occasion as open heart surgery. Only one patient had a fixed neurologic deficit, and two had transient ones. The four fatalities in this series were at-tributed to cardiac surgical procedures.

Long-latency somatosensory evoked potentials were used during carotid en-darterectomy by Jacobs et al. (*Am. Surg.* 49:338–344, 1983). The only stroke in this series of 25 patients was in one who developed electrical unresponsive-ness on one side; one other patient had bilateral loss of potentials for four minutes of clamping of the left internal carotid artery (the right one being al-ready totally occluded), but he regained potentials after the clamp was re-moved, and was neurologically intact at the end of the operation. Changes in the various peaks of the evoked potentials demonstrate lesser degrees of vas-cular insufficiency with no permanent damage. The authors believe that intra-luminal shunting is not needed in unilateral disease, but is needed in the pres-ence of contralateral occlusion or stenosis.—O.S.

---

**Cranial and Cervical Nerve Damage Associated With Carotid Endarterec-tomy**

T. C. B. Dehn and G. W. Taylor (St. Bartholomew's Hosp. Med. College, Lon-don)

Br. J. Surg. 70:365–368, June 1983                                                    26–5

As the incidence of stroke after carotid endarterectomy has diminished, minor local neurologic deficits assume greater importance.

Of the 40 patients who underwent carotid endarterectomy, 3 had bilateral surgery, for a total of 43 operations. Indications for surgery were transient ischemic attacks (19 carotid cases), ischemic attacks with a previous stroke (9 cases), and completed stroke (9 cases); 6 cases were asymptomatic. There were 31 male and 9 female patients, aged 39–81 (mean, 53.1 ± 16.8). None of the patients exhibited cutaneous or cranial nerve deficit preoperatively; vocal cord examinations were also normal.

Postoperatively, cutaneous nerve damage involving the greater auricular nerve (26 patients at one week postoperatively, 22 at six weeks, and 20 at six months) or the transverse cervical nerve (30 patients at one week, 27 at six weeks, and 16 at six months), or both (22 patients at one week, 16 at six weeks, and 10 at six months) was observed. The vagus nerve and its branches were also affected. One week postoperatively, 16 patients complained of hoarseness (11 had an immobile vocal cord ipsilateral to the endarterectomy); at six weeks, 3 patients had regained both voice and vocal cord function; at six months, 8 patients still had vocal abnormalities. Transient hypoglossal nerve lesions producing difficulty in deglutition and articulation were seen in two patients who recovered fully within five and eight weeks, respectively.

Damage to the auricular nerve may be diminished if, at the time of surgery, the incision is curved toward the mastoid process. However, lesion of the transverse cervical nerves is frequently unavoidable, producing anesthesia over the anterior triangle. Damage to the superior laryngeal nerve leads to cricothyroid muscle paralysis, with tiring of the voice and inability to reach high pitches. Two patients complained of this; however, indirect laryngoscopy did not show the affected cord to be lax. The fibers of the recurrent laryngeal nerve are likely to be injured owing to direct vagal nerve trauma during retraction or diathermy. Bipolar cautery should be used to achieve hemostasis in close proximity to the vagal trunk.

Unrecognized damage to either the superior laryngeal nerve or the external branch could account for the symptoms of intermittent voice changes in patients with apparently normal vocal cords. Injury to the hypoglossal nerve during endarterectomy is well documented; it is more commonly due to overzealous retraction than to division of the nerve trunk, especially in patients with a high carotid bifurcation. Patients undergoing carotid endarterectomy should be informed of possible transient voice changes, as well as loss of cutaneous sensation which may persist for several months.

▶ In a three-year period at the Cleveland Clinic, 535 endarterectomies were done in 517 patients; 133 had specific examination for neural function before and after endarterectomy by members of the Department of Peripheral Vascular Surgery. Cranial nerves were injured in 74 (14.3%) patients; 1 patient had three nerves injured, 8 had two nerves injured, and the other 65 had only one nerve damaged. The recurrent laryngeal was injured in 31 patients, hypoglossal in 30, marginal mandibular nerve in 11, and superior laryngeal in 7. The rarity of problems with the vagus nerve in radical neck dissections is ascribed to the wide mobilization of that nerve, and such mobilization is advised for exposure in endarterectomy. Atraumatic mobilization is also easily accomplished for the hypoglossal nerve, which crosses the internal carotid variably in different patients. If necessary, the descendens can be transected, along with elective ligation of hypoglossal veins. If the superior laryngeal nerve is identified where it lies adjacent to the superior laryngeal nerve, it is not likely to be injured. Avoidance of use of self-retaining retractors for the upper cutaneous flap helps avoid injury to the marginal mandibular nerve.

In 158 patients with carotid endarterectomy studied by Massey et al. (*Stroke* 15:157–159, 1984), there were 24 (15.1%) who developed "peripheral cranial nerve palsies." The extracranial portion of the hypoglossal nerve was involved in 13 patients, cervical branch of the facial nerve in 5, and the recurrent branch of the vagus nerve in 8. Residual defect was present at one year in two of the patients with facial nerve and in four with hypoglossal nerve involvement. "Be careful out there."

Schmidt et al. (*J. Neurol.* 230:131–135, 1984) found cranial nerve injury in 14 of 102 patients with carotid artery reconstructions. In nine patients, the ipsilateral hypoglossal nerve was injured, the marginal mandibular nerve in three, and the recurrent laryngeal nerve in 4; in two patients, two nerves were injured. The hypoglossal nerve recovered in 2–52 weeks. The authors note that although cranial nerve palsies are usually mild, their occurrence may lead to delay of contralateral carotid reconstruction lest bilateral hypoglossal palsy, even temporary, occur. This is a disorder that can cause upper airway obstruction, marked difficulty in swallowing, and dysarthria. In severe cases, tracheostomy may be necessary.—O.S.

---

**Local Fibrinolysis in Subtotal Stenosis of the Middle Cerebral Artery**
H. Zeumer, E. B. Ringelstein, M. Hassel, and K. Poeck (Aachen, Federal Republic of Germany)
Dtsch. Med. Wochenschr. 108:1103–1105, June 15, 1983                    26–6

---

Although lesions of the middle cerebral artery are not life-threatening, the indication for therapy must be determined following strict criteria. Arteries blocked by a thrombus or embolus branch from the immediate occlusion of the basal cerebral artery into the cerebral parenchyma. Collaterals or residual flow beyond a subtotal stenosis can maintain a considerable share of residual function. However, the clinically progressive course of apoplexy proves that this stage is labile and temporary, and that the functional disturbance increases until it finally stabilizes at a defective level.

Recanalization or an intracranial-extracranial bypass may serve the peripheral area of the infarct territory in which functional metabolism is broken down, but structural metabolism is still intact. Therefore indications for fibrinolysis are that the definitive defect must be restricted and that there is a large area which is only functionally impaired or not impaired at all. Early studies showed the lack of effectiveness of injections of streptokinase into the internal carotid artery. Only since the use of a floating balloon microcatheter has success followed. The first patient so treated had a right-sided trifurcation occlusion of the middle cerebral artery. However, overly high doses of streptokinase caused a hemorrhaging swelling leading to a defect which most likely would have occurred even without fibrinolysis. In a second patient, recanalization and clinical improvement were established. However, a new embolus occurred which negated any success. One case is featured in the following report.

Woman, 60, had fluctuating neurologic and neurophysiologic symptoms. Small infarcts were evident. At this time neither a complete hemiplegia nor a global aphasia could be observed. These clinical factors combined with a subtotal stenosis in a short segment of the middle cerebral artery just before the trifurcation were decisive indications for proceeding with fibrinolysis via a floating balloon catheter. A dose of 10,000 IU of streptokinase was sufficient to achieve a partial canalization. A late control angiography showed lysis occurring after canalization, which was ascribed to accumulation of enough activating streptokinase complex in the thrombus to continue the proteolytic process after the injection.

The authors emphasize that it is useless to perform local fibrinolysis by injection into the internal carotid artery because the justified safe dose of streptokinase is not concentrated enough to affect the clot. Fibrinolysis via a floating balloon catheter can be recommended only in the early stages of progressive apoplexy.

▶ Gagliardi et al. (*Neurosurgery* 12:636–639, 1983) have done emergency angiography for demonstrating the cause of acute hemiplegia with aphasia in four patients. Having found occlusion of the middle cerebral artery, the surgeons then did embolectomy with microsurgical technique. Two patients did well; one died, and the fourth had a poor result neurologically and died on day 48 from purulent pleuritis. The authors agree that the results have not been conclusive and that further clinical trials are needed. In as much as the natural history of such lesions is unknown, it seems unlikely that such case reports as these will elucidate the problem. I am particularly critical because of the lack of a four-vessel study, for such angiograms (instead of just left-carotid injections) may indeed show collateral flow from other vessels (e.g., anterior and posterior cerebral vessels), which might well explain improvement with or without operation—and certainly it does occur!

Caution is the watchword for the initial investigations into the use of transluminal angioplasty of the carotid artery in the neck. Bockenheimer and Matthias (*AJNR* 4:791–792, 1983) show pictures of the enlargement of the lumen of the carotid artery by the balloon expansion technique. Platelet suppressive therapy was instituted beforehand; intraarterial heparin was given immediately after catheterization and for two days thereafter. Two patients were successfully treated without complication; the balloon (3.5 cm in length and 6 mm in diameter) was manually filled with contrast material to inflate it against the stenotic artery. In one patient, hemiparesis occurred 20 minutes later; recovery was complete after 20 hours.

The criteria suggested by Wiggli and Gratzl (ibid. 4:793–795, 1983) include the presence of stenosis of length not more than 10 mm and the absence of gross mural calcification (as seen in computed tomographic scan); patients selected should be considered if they lack collaterals sufficient to protect the brain during endarterectomy, if they are at high risk for general anesthesia due to cardiovascular disease, or if a short-term effect might be considered sufficient. Follow-up evaluation should include clinical assessment, Doppler sonography, and angiography about six weeks after angioplasty. During the successful dilatation of one internal carotid artery, and of a stenotic common carotid artery in a different patient, heparinization was continued during and for two days after the dilatation. the dilatation was undertaken three times in each of the two cases, for a total of 3 minutes and 2.5 minutes respectively; total occlusion times was 15–25 seconds, with 20–30 seconds between dilatations.

Successful angioplastic dilatation of stenotic external carotid arteries has been carried out in eight external arteries in seven patients; in one patient, the guide wire could not be passed through the stenotic area. When manipulation spasm occurred, it was successfully treated with intraarterial papaverine, according to J. J. Vitek (ibid. 7:798–799, 1983). Benefits are derived from making the source of blood for a superficial temporal anstomosis more secure or from increasing the collaterals from external to internal carotid artery.—O.S.

---

**The Treatment of Cerebral Ischemia by External Carotid Artery Revascularization**
James J. Schuler, D. Preston Flanigan, James R. DeBord, Timothy J. Ryan, John J. Castronuovo, and Leonardo T. Lim (Univ. of Illinois)
Arch. Surg. 118:567–572, May 1983                                           26–7

---

The external carotid artery is an important source of collateral flow to the intracerebral circulation when the internal carotid is chronically occluded, and extracranial-intracranial (EC-IC) microvascular bypasses have become accepted in selected cases of cerebrovascular disease. The authors performed external carotid revascularization in 13 patients with internal carotid occlusion and ipsilateral external carotid stenosis or ulcerative plaques or both. The 12 men and 1 woman had a mean age of 63 years. External carotid endarterectomy was done in 10 cases, and a subclavian-to-external carotid artery bypass in 3. Surgery was done without shunts under normotensive, normocapnic general anesthesia. Ten patients had oculopneumoplethysmography both before and after surgery.

There were no complications or deaths during surgery. No late strokes occurred during the follow-up of 12 patients for a mean of 20 months. Two late deaths were due to myocardial infarction. One patient required an EC-IC bypass after endarterectomy because symptoms persisted. Nine of the other 11 patients had immediate, complete relief of symptoms, but 1 had a recurrence due to progressive disease and required an EC-IC bypass. Two other patients had substantial but incomplete relief of symptoms after endarterectomy and declined a bypass procedure. Oculoplethysmography confirmed improvement on the side that was operated on. All evaluable arteriograms showed filling of the distal internal carotid artery in the area of the carotid siphon by periorbital collateral vessels.

External carotid revascularization is a low-risk means of completely relieving symptoms of cerebral ischemia in selected cases; EC-IC bypass for symptoms of external carotid stenosis should be reserved for patients who are not helped by endarterectomy. No angiographic or oculoplethysmographic criteria are available to reliably predict the need for EC-IC bypass after external carotid revascularization.

▶ "Chronic internal carotid artery occlusion" plus ipsilateral stenosis or ulceration of the external carotid in symptomatic patients were the prerequisites for the external carotid endarterectomy or subclavian-to-external carotid artery bypass in these patients. Shunts were not used, which raises the question of how the ipsilateral hemisphere was supplied with blood during the procedure; if this was done from the opposite side, then why were the patients symptomatic before operation? The problem of visualization of the internal carotid in the head via collaterals from the external carotid is discussed, but again without reference to intracranial collaterals (including those from the vertebrobasilar system, well known to be adequate in some patients with bilateral internal carotid artery occlusion). Very possibly, study of patients with occlusive carotid disease with dynamic computed tomography or by xenon blood flow techniques might give incisive data on selection of patients for endarterectomy of any vessel leading to the brain.—O.S.

---

**Indications and Results of Extra- Intracranial Arterial Bypasses**
Susan Engel and Heber Ferraz (Univ. of Vienna)
Int. Surg. 68:197–200, July–September 1983                    26–8

---

The authors reviewed the results of superficial temporal artery–middle cerebral artery (STA-MCA) extracranial-intracranial arterial bypass surgery in 410 patients seen in 1975–1982. Men predominated in a ratio of 3:1; the median age was 49 years. Surgery was done for transient ischemic attacks in 23% of cases, prolonged reversible neurologic deficit (PRIND) in 14%, progressive stroke in 5%, and completed stroke in 58%. Internal carotid artery occlusion was present in nearly 60% of patients. Selection of patients for surgery was based on the history and physical findings, serial angiography, computed tomographic (CT) scan, and regional cerebral blood flow.

All but 2% of bypasses in patients with transient ischemic attacks were patent, and 93% of patients improved after operation; however, 2% had further attacks and 4% died. Improvement occurred in 74% of the PRIND group, while 15% of patients were unchanged. The patency rate was 97%. Fifty-eight percent of patients with progressive stroke improved, and 9% became worse after operation. Eighty-two percent of the vessels were patent. In the group with completed stroke, 64% of patients improved and 5% became worse. Ninety percent of vessels were angiographically patent. Motor deficits improved in two thirds of patients with completed stroke, and sensory deficits in 60%. Speech impairment showed improvement in more than half the patients. More than two thirds had less impairment of intellectual function after operation. The operative mortality was 1%, the postoperative mortality 4%, and the late mortality 12%. Late mortality from cerebrovascular causes was 3.5%.

These long-term results indicate encouraging relief from neurologic symptoms or protection from the development of completed strokes in a significant number of patients having STA-MCA extracranial-intracranial arterial bypass surgery. The procedure is useful even in patients with completed stroke, but not in those with long-standing neurologic deficits. Mortality and morbidity have been low.

▶ Based on an experience covering 10 years of performing extracranial-intracranial anastomoses in the treatment of cerebral ischemia, Deruty (*Neurochirurgie* 29:175–190, 1983) concludes there is no good way of comparing his surgical series of 85 cases and the natural history of the cerebrovascular atheromatous disease because of the small numbers of patients and the difference in pathologic lesions between surgical and medical patients. The best indication for operation is reversible ischemia or mild stroke with angiographic evidence of complete occlusion on one side and contralateral carotid atheromatous disease. The aim of surgery is therapeutic (to suppress repeated ischemic episodes and improve the situation at the time of operation) and also prophylactic (protection against subsequent ipsilateral infarction, contralateral infarction, or low-perfusion syndrome). Deruty believes middle cerebral artery stenosis or occlusion is probably not a good indication, since the results have not been very good; the stenotic artery becomes occluded in 75% of cases. By pass surgery should be accepted in cases of intracranial carotid or siphon stenosis only if the stenosis is very tight. Those with a low-perfusion syndrome should probably be operated on as soon as the disorder is diagnosed. Although bypass surgery will not help patients with completed stroke to recover, it should be done when there are lesions of the opposite carotid artery to diminish risk of further generalized ischemia (all this in the presence of an occluded carotid on one side).

In this series, there were three operative deaths; an ipsilateral infarction occurred in one case in the reversible ischemia group and in one case in the mild stroke group. A subsequent contralateral infarction occurred in one of the reversible ischemia group and in one of the mild stroke group. Ten patients died in the follow-up period owing to cardiac disease (4), cerebrovascular disease (1), pulmonary embolism (1), cancer (3), and trauma (1).

Maira and co-workers from Rome discuss failure of extracranial-intracranial arterial anastomosis (in Meyer, et al. [eds.]: *Cerebral Vascular Disease*, vol. 4. Amsterdam, Excerpta Medica, 1983, pp. 169–176). In one case, EC-IC bypass was done in a man, 52, with small temporal infarct after total occlusion of left internal carotid. Flow studies showed impairment, so bypass was made. Unusual cortical hyperemia was found; when bypass was finished, small hemorrhages began. After this happened on repeated closure and opening of bypass, the latter was abandoned. In a second case, a 60-year-old man with mild left cerebral dysfunction was found to have decreased flow on the left, and this side was fed only from the right. When EC-IC bypass was made, it functioned well; the patient's condition became worse, and repeat angiogram showed that the left was no longer being aided by the right side, and blood flow was less than before. When angiography was repeated closing the bypass percutaneously, the flow was improved, and the right side again fed the left. After the bypass was narrowed, the flow improved and so did the patient's symptoms.

Vascular injury can be produced by the Biemer temporary clips used in carrying out cerebral vascularization procedures. Modification in clip design to prevent such notches shown in posteroperative angiograms is advocated by Fein et al. (*Neurosurgery* 13:520–522, 1983).

Intraluminal dilatation of a markedly stenotic innominate artery was carried out by Garrido and Garafola (*Neurosurgery* 13:581–583, 1983) in a man, 72, who also had bilateral internal carotid artery occlusions, which had produced some permanent dysphasia and right-sided weakness, as well as transient episodes of numbness of the left upper extremity, He was doing well six months after the dilatation and staged bypasses from external carotid to middle cerebral arteries on both sides.—O.S.

---

**Short Vein Grafts for Cerebral Revascularization**
John R. Little, Anthony J. Furlan, and Bernadine Bryerton (Cleveland Clinic)
J. Neurosurg. 59:384–388, September 1983                                26–9

---

The authors reviewed experience with use of a short saphenous vein bypass graft for cerebral revascularization in 20 patients who had 21 bypasses for symptomatic atherosclerotic occlusive disease. A 5–10-cm saphenous vein graft (SVG) extended from the superficial temporal artery (STA) trunk anterior to the ear in 19 bypasses and from the occipital artery just behind the mastoid process to the posterior temporal or angular branch of the middle cerebral artery in two cases. End-to-side anastomosis of the vein graft to the cortical artery was followed by connection to the STA trunk or occipital artery. The ipsilateral carotid system was assessed two weeks and one to six months after operation by either conventional or intravenous digital subtraction angiography.

Ninety percent of the bypasses were patent two weeks after operation. The mean SVG diameter in the 17 patients having late postoperative studies was 4 mm. Two of four patients with SVG occlusion had substantial resolution of a severe inaccessible internal carotid stenosis at late follow-up. Late conventional angiograms showed filling of multiple major branches of the middle cerebral artery branches through the SVG in 90% of cases. The STA trunk or proximal occipital artery was consistently enlarged. No patient had recurrent transient ischemic attacks on follow-up. A patient with severe internal carotid stenosis had a small cerebral infarction three days postoperatively, despite a widely patent SVG, and eventually recovered completely. Autopsy of a patient who died of renal failure seven months after surgery showed a widely patent SVG with mild fibrosis in the wall of the vein.

Cerebral revascularization with short saphenous vein grafts may be a useful primary procedure or an alternative when a scalp artery cannot be used for any reason. The effect of a short SVG on the cerebral circulation may be more favorable than that of the conventional bypass procedure. A relatively large-caliber bypass is immediately established. Preoperative carotid arterial stenosis has improved after operation in a few cases.

---

**Acute Obstructive Hydrocephalus Caused by Cerebellar Infarction: Treatment Alternatives**
Norman H. Horwitz (George Washington Univ.) and Carol Ludolph (Washington Hosp. Center, Washington, D.C.)
Surg. Neurol. 20:13–19, July 1983                                        26–10

---

Acute obstructive hydrocephalus and associated brain stem compression require immediate treatment. In cases of nontraumatic cerebellar infarction with swelling, the chief finding is ischemic or hemorrhagic infarction with tissue softening and swelling, usually due to thrombosis caused by embolism or atherosclerotic plaque. Control of the cerebellar swelling will relieve the obstruction of the fourth ventricle and posterior aqueduct.

The surgical case mortality for 81 reported cases was 21%. No particular advantage can be found in ventriculostomy with or without permanent shunting, ventriculostomy and craniectomy used together, or craniectomy. It seems likely that there is not a permanent need for cerebrospinal fluid shunting. Some patients who were reported to improve after ventriculostomy might not have required cerebellar surgery. The quality of survival after craniectomy has been good.

The authors recommend immediate intubation (to reduce the $Pa_{CO_2}$ to at least 35 torr) and intravenous steroid and mannitol when a patient has vertigo that progresses to stupor or coma and when computed tomography shows a hypodense mass lesion of the cerebellum and internal hydrocephalus. If the state of consciousness does not improve promptly, ventriculostomy and external ventricular drainage are recommended. Shunting is done later if clamping or elevation of the emptying pressure of the ventriculostomy tube is followed by clinical regression. If improvement does not occur within a few hours after ventricular decompression, suboccipital craniectomy should be done with resection of necrotic cerebellar tissue. Temporary improvement after external ventricular drainage suggests the need for direct cerebellar decompression.

---

**The Surgical Management of Vertebrobasilar Insufficiency**
R. A. de los Reyes, J. I. Ausman, F. G. Diaz, H. Pak, J. E. Pearce, and M. Dujovny (Henry Ford Hosp., Detroit)
Acta Neurochir. (Wien) 68:203–216, 1983                                26–11

---

Vertebrobasilar insufficiency can result from structural lesions anywhere along the vertebrobasilar system. Modern angiographic and microsurgical methods have made this system increasingly accessible to surgical treatment. The most common causative lesions appear to be atherosclerotic stenosis and occlusion in the posterior circulation. The diagnosis is based on a history of transient ischemia involving the brain stem, cerebellum, and/or occipital cortex. Dizziness alone is not interpreted as indicating vertebrobasilar insufficiency unless accompanied by transient symptoms of specific involvement of cranial nerves, cerebellum, or visual cortex. Computed tomography is a useful adjunct, but angiography remains the definitive procedure. About a third of patients have cerebral infarction. Only anticoagulation among various medical measures has consistently reduced the occurrence of infarction.

Stenotic lesions at the vertebral origin or of the proximal subclavian artery are best managed by vertebral-to-common carotid artery transposition. Eleven of 12 such operations have produced a patent shunt, and 9 patients have had relief of symptoms. Where stenosis in the intraforaminal part of the vertebral artery results from a plaque or from compression by cervical spondylosis, osteophytes and scar tissue can be removed, or the stenosis bypassed or treated by endarterectomy. Stenoses in the third part of the vertebral artery can either be bypassed or attacked directly by microsurgical endarterectomy. An occipital-to-anterior inferior cerebellar artery anastomosis was used by Ausman et al. for stenosis between the posterior and anterior inferior arteries. Midbasilar stenosis has been managed by a superficial temporal-to-proximal superior cerebellar artery anastomosis. Overall mortality in 40 cases has been 5%, ranging from zero in cases of vertebral origin to 12% for occipital artery–to–posterior-inferior cerebral artery anastomosis. No patient has had vertebrobasilar infarction following surgery.

Angiography seems warranted in patients with clinical evidence of vertebrobasilar insufficiency. In this study, permanent complications of vertebral angiography occurred in 3.4% of the patients. The morbidity and mortality of surgery probably will decline as more experience is gained.

▶ At the May 1984 meeting of the newly formed Society of Neurovascular Surgeons in Chicago there were several reports concerning operations for stenosis at the vertebral artery origin. Dr. Morris (Baylor Univ.) reported that best results occur with patch graft enlargement without endarterectomy. Patula (Univ. of Missouri) believes transposition of vertebral artery to the common carotid artery is technically the easiest procedure and the most effective way of dealing with this problem. Ansell (Univ. of Texas, San Antonio) finds success with the use of prosthetic material to bypass obstruction of the proximal vertebral artery.

On the other hand, Kojima et al. (*Surg. Neurol.* 20:481–486, 1983) find direct operations on the vertebral artery for correction of vertebrobasilar insufficiency not to be satisfactory. They report the successful use, apparently for the first time, of the superior thyroid artery to bypass constriction of the vertebral artery at its origin.

A cooperative study by vascular surgeons and neurosurgeons from Paris (Laurian et al.: *Sem. Hop. Paris* 60:547–552, 1984) reviews 11 cases of distal revascularization of the extracranial vertebral artery above C2 (7 instances of extensive atheromatous stenotic or occlusive disease, 3 cases of dissecting aneurysm, and 1 instance of malformed vertebral artery). Venous grafting at C1–2 (above C1 in one instance) was carried out with satisfactory results and without postoperative neurologic problems. The situation with regard to lesions under the clavicle and proximal vertebral artery is not so clear-cut.

Evaluation of 34 patients with vertebrobasilar insufficiency was carried out by Ausman and Diaz (*Otolaryngol. Head Neck Surg.* 92:102–108, 1984). Residual strokes were found in 12, while 22 had transient episodes of insufficiency. Local vertebral endarterectomy at the C1 level was carried out in four. Seven had anastomosis of the occipital artery to the posterior inferior cerebellar artery; three had occipital anastomosis to the anterior inferior cerebellar artery. Anastomosis of the superficial artery to the superior cerebellar artery was done in 20 patients for stenosis or occlusion of the vertebrobasilar junction or mid-basilar occlusive lesions. The connections were patent in 26 of 27 patients. Although early surgical morbidity is high, it is only transient (meningitis, cerebrospinal fluid leaks, temporal lobe swelling, and seizures). Two patients died (one of congestive heart failure and one of brain stem infarction). Long-term morbidity included a Brown-Séquard syndrome, Wallenberg's syndrome, and one patient who had the "locked-in" syndrome remained in that condition after operation. Complete resolution of the symptoms occurred in 26 patients, and 3 have minor residual dizziness. The authors contend that the surgical approach of the vertebrobasilar area can lead to ultimate recovery of most patients.

On the other hand, Karnik et al. (*Wien. Klin. Wochnschr.* 96:26–30, 1984) report a case of acute thrombosis of the basilar artery producing hemiplegia and brain stem symptoms in a woman aged 28. An angiography catheter was placed in the vertebral artery, and infusion of streptokinase, followed by urokinase, led to complete reopening of the vessel and marked improvement in neurologic symptoms. The authors suggest further trials of such thrombolytic therapy in acute thrombosis of the basilar artery.—O.S.

---

## Treatment of Moyamoya Disease by Temporal Muscle Graft "Encephalo-Myo-Synangiosis"

Shigekazu Takeuchi, Tadashi Tsuchida, Keishi Kobayashi, Mitsunori Fukuda, Ryoji Ishii, Ryuichi Tanaka, and Jusuke Ito (Niigata Univ., Japan)
Child's Brain 10:1–15, 1983                                                                          26–12

---

Moyamoya disease is an occlusive cerebrovascular disorder of unknown etiology characterized by progressive narrowing or occlusion of the internal carotids, bilateral abnormal vascular networks in the basal ganglia region, leptomeningeal anastomoses, and multiple transdural external-internal carotid anastomoses. Children are more often affected than are adults. The authors performed temporal muscle graft surgery in 10 children aged 7–16 years with moyamoya disease; all had ischemic cerebrovascular features without intracranial bleeding. Eight children had encephalo-myo-synangiosis (EMS) only, and two had superficial temporal-middle cerebral artery anastomosis as well. Cerebral blood flow was measured before and after surgery by the radioxenon inhalation method.

Technique.—The temporal muscle is detached from the skull. After craniotomy, the dura mater is opened, with care taken to avoid cutting the main branches of the meningeal artery. Part of the periosteum and fascia is stripped from the inner surface of the muscle. The temporal muscle is placed over the arachnoid membrane of the cortex and sutured to the dura. Rongeuring the lower part of the bone flap prevents compression and constriction of the temporal muscle pedicle. The bone flap is then replaced and fastened to the cranium; the scalp is closed in two layers. To avoid compression of the brain, only the deep layer of the muscle is used, when possible.

Transient ischemic attacks ceased in four of seven children and became less frequent in the others. Limb paresis resolved in one child and improved in two. Some improvement was obtained in all cases, and three children had an excellent outcome. The seven others had slight neurologic deficits or less frequent ischemic attacks postoperatively. Postoperative carotid angiography showed prominent filling of the middle cerebral arteries, mainly via the deep temporal arteries, in most of the children. The full-scale IQ at follow-up was improved significantly in two children, but had deteriorated in one. Performance IQ was better in five and unchanged in five. Verbal IQ improved in one child and deteriorated in two. Hemispheric blood flow increased significantly in half of the children. Complications included a subcutaneous abscess and sensory aphasia lasting for eight months.

The pathogenesis of moyamoya disease remains to be established. The present results indicate that EMS is a reasonable procedure for increasing extracranial and intracranial collateral circulation in children with this disease.

▶ Takeuchi (*Neurol. Med. Chir.* [*Tokyo*] 23:711–719, 1983) has studied surface filling of human cerebral cortex (outer aspect of gyrus) at the time of enceph-alo-myo-synangiosis in patients with moyamoya disease. Delay in arterial filling after carotid arterial injection of fluorescein was marked in 7 of 15 hemispheres studied. Nevertheless, surface filling was noted after intravenous injection of the dye. Heterogeneous patterns of epicerebral microcirculation are thought to be due to the multiple collateral pathways and extensive occlusions of main arteries in moyamoya disease. Takeuchi (ibid. 23:720–728, 1983) has also used the $^{133}$Xe inhalation technique to study blood flow in normal subjects and in patients before and after encephalo-myo-synangiosis and/or superficial temporal-middle cerebral bypass. There was a gradual increase in regional blood flow in 9 of 12 patients beginning three months after surgery. This was much more apparent in children than adults.

A remarkable paper has appeared in *Surgical Neurology* (20:318–322, 1983) by Lesoin and co-workers from the Regional Hospital in Lille, France. Thirty cases of encephaloarteriosynangiosis [sic] have been done for cerebral isch-emia. This new operation involves isolating as long as possible a length of the superficial temporal or occipital arteries (5–10 cm may be available); a linear craniectomy is done, the dura mater incised and its edges coagulated, the artery is laid on the cerebral cortex *without doing any arterial anastomoses*, and a careful musculoaponeurotic closure is done to hold the artery in place. In-creased diastolic pulsations in Doppler studies have started about 10 days later, and have progressively increased for a year. Arteriography was possible in 20 patients (the others refused), and in 16 of these there was cerebral revascularization from the scalp artery! The effectiveness of the operation remains to be determined. The new operation appears superior to superficial temporal artery–middle cerebral artery bypass anastomosis in cases of middle cerebral stenosis or thrombosis, intracranial carotid stenosis, and thrombosis of the internal carotid artery with good collateral circulation. Both before and after operation, the patients were treated with "nicergoline (Sermion:Specia)" (whatever that may be).—O.S.

# 27 Pain

▶ ↓ I hope that the talk on pain by C. Miller Fisher, given at the meeting of the Congress of Neurological Surgeons in Chicago on October 31, 1983, is soon published. It deals with many aspects of the pain problem, starting with the causation of pain. He doubted that there was proof that the pain of cancer, even cancer infiltrating into the brachial and sciatic plexuses, is really of nerve origin; most cancer pain is from extraneural sources (e.g., bone pain).

One way of dealing with pain is by giving morphine intrathecally, intraventricularly, or epidurally. The following short references may illuminate the state of current thinking in this field.

When peridural catheter instillation for injection of morphine failed to maintain a passageway, a ventricular Holter apparatus was implanted in eight patients with intractable pain due to cancer by the neurosurgical service in Montpellier, France. Experiences with these cases are reported by Roquefeuil et al. (*Neurochirurgie* 29:135–141, 1983). Excellent analgesia was obtained without respiratory depression, and very small amounts of morphine were needed (less than 1 mg per day in three cases!). In four of the cases, the morphine was administered by the patient from a reservoir bag worn around the neck, and connected to the ventricular apparatus by a catheter entering under the skin of the neck and tunneled up to the ventricular catheter. Appropriate valves were inserted to prevent accidental injection. This ventricular injection system offers the opportunity to block the painful impulses regardless of where they have their origin.

The benefits of intraventricular administration of morphine in patients with intractable pain of neoplastic origin are described by Roquefeuil et al. (*Surg. Neurol.* 21:155–158, 1984). In four patients, injection was made into a reservoir under the scalp; in the other four, the intraventricular catheter was connected to a sterile nonpyrogenic collecting bag by way of a one-way Cordis valve unit. The bag was placed at the clavicular level and was used for injection by the patient by opening a clamp, permitting 50 μg of morphine to be released from the bag wherein the morphine solution in saline had been placed. There was a gratifying absence of respiratory depression although myotic pupils, vomiting, and other annoyances were noted. The authors advocate peridural morphine administration as the first route of administration in cancer patients; intrathecal morphine released into the lumbar subarachnoid space is particularly useful when there is pelvic pain. The intraventricular system is advised when the other two techniques are no longer effective.

Lobato et al. (*J. Neurosurg.* 59:627–633, 1983) used morphine injected into an Ommaya reservoir emptying into a lateral ventricle for satisfactory control of intractable pain from cancer in 17 terminal patients. Preliminary injection into the cisterna magna (0.5–0.75 mg of morphine) or lumbar theca (0.5–1 mg) was used to assess analgesic effect and possible risks. Doses put into the reservoir ranged from 0.25 mg every 12–48 hours to 1 mg/24 hours to 0.75 mg/72 hours. Some tolerance was noted, so doses at the end of the period were as high as 2 mg every 3 hours, but most were in the range of 0.5 mg every 12–24 hours. Side effects included pruritis, urinary retention, disorientation, and hallucinations—all of which subsided without discontinuing the medication. Infection in one patient necessitated removal of the reservoir.

Excellent postoperative pain relief was achieved in patients after laminectomy by injection of 2–6 mg of morphine sulfate solution (in nonbacteriostatic water) epidurally by a catheter inserted at the time of operation (Schmidek and Cutler: *Neurosurgery* 13:37–39, 1983). The catheter passed out of the incision directly and was capped at its end affixed to the anterior chest wall for easy access for injection. When the patient was free of pain without use of morphine for 24 hours, the catheter was removed (usually two to five days after operation). No complications of note have been encountered.

Twenty-five patients had similar epidural injection of morphine in the series reported by Ray and Bagley (ibid. 13:388–393, 1983). They compared the results with 25 similar patients receiving oral and parenteral narcotics. The epidural dosages were more effective in promoting comfort, and there were fewer side effects such as nausea and lassitude. Doses of morphine given every 12–24 hours were only 1.0–2.5 mg. The tube for injection was placed under the uppermost exposed lamina and threaded upward to the T10 or T11 level. It was led out of the intact skin lateral to the upper end of the operative incision through a needle puncture, and, with its cap, was attached to the anterior chest wall. No complications have been encountered. An epilogue describes a variant procedure in which a single dose of epidural morphine was given (with no indwelling catheter), followed by oral dexamethasone for 72 hours after operation. In more extensive operations, the catheter technique appears superior.

Epidural morphine is no longer used for treatment of pain by Barron and Strong (*Pain* 18:279–285, 1984) because it is hydrophilic, and the route of administration is not totally reliable. They now use intrathecal diamorphine (0.005–0.015 mg/kg) in the control of postoperative pain following total hip replacement and spinal surgery. The upper limit for a single dose is 1 mg. Headache is reduced by use of a 25-gauge needle for injection intrathecally.

Stereotactic chemical hypophysectomy (with ethanol) has been used by Levin et al. (*J. Neurosurg.* 59:1002–1006, 1983) to combat intractable pain from the thalamic pain syndrome with good results. Three patients (aged 62–69) have had relief for 19, 39, and 58 months. None had complete hypophysectomy, but all have remained on thyroid and hydrocortisone replacement therapy. It is of interest that no mention is made of the Italian originator of the concept of injecting alcohol to produce chemical hypophysectomy (which is done, however, for pain from carcinoma).—O.S.

---

## Alterations of Hypothalamopituitary Interaction and Pain Threshold Following Pituitary Neuroadenolysis: A Clinical investigation of the Mechanism of Cancer Pain Relief

Fumikazu Takeda, Takashi Fujii, Jiro Uki, Ryuji Tozawa, Yoshiaki Fuse, Yasuharu Kitani, and Tatsushi Fujita
Neurol. Med. Chir. (Tokyo) 23:551–560, July 1983                27–1

In 1977–1982 pituitary neuroadenolysis (NALP) was performed 136 times in 102 patients with intractable pain due to disseminated malignancy. Forty-three patients had hormone-dependent carcinomas. Televised fluoroscopy was used to guide the instillation of 1–2.4 ml of 100% ethanol through a nostril into the pituitary gland. Complete pain relief ultimately was achieved in 80% of patients, including 95% of those with hormone-dependent carcinomas. Relief was immediate in most instances and persisted for more than two years in some cases.

The degree of anterior pituitary suppression did not correlate closely with the outcome of NALP, and the same was true of posterior pituitary function. The cerebrospinal fluid (CSF) level of ACTH was abruptly elevated in patients with complete relief of pain but not in other patients. No significant increase in CSF endorphin levels was observed. The outcome could not be related to CSF levels of thyrotropin-releasing hormone or vasopressin following NALP. The duration of tourniquet tolerance in patients with complete relief of cancer pain was twice as great after NALP as before, but no such change was noted in other patients. Radiant heat dolorimetry showed no significant differences between these groups. Sensory decision theory analysis indicated an increased pain threshold and improved discriminability in patients with complete relief after NALP.

The immediacy of relief of cancer pain in some patients following NALP suggests that it is mediated through the CNS rather than endocrine factors. The exact role of peptides in pain sensation remains unclear, but the increases of some peptides in the CSF after NALP, along with suppressed pituitary function, may contribute to suppression of the mediation and perception of cancer pain through the C-fibers and the CNS.

---

## Dorsal Root Entry Zone Lesions (Nashold's Procedure) for Pain Relief Following Brachial Plexus Avulsion

D. G. T. Thomas and J. P. R. Sheehy (London)
J. Neurol. Neurosurg. Psychiatry 46:924–928, October 1983          27–2

---

Brachial plexus avulsion is a significant cause of intractable severe pain, especially in young motorcyclists. The authors produced dorsal root entry zone lesions to relieve pain in 19 patients with partial or complete brachial plexus avulsion, 15 of whom had had motorcycle accidents. Pain usually began within days of injury, but a two-year interval was noted in one case. Typically there was crushing or burning in the deafferentated extremity, which tended to be felt globally throughout the arm. There had been no sustained response to such procedures as stellate ganglion block, cordotomy, amputation, midbrain stimulation, and narcotic analgesics. Varying degrees of motor paralysis were present; a completely flail extremity was the most common finding. Myelography showed cord displacement, root avulsion, or pseudomeningocele formation in all cases.

Lesions were produced by thermocoagulation using a steel wire electrode inserted for 2 mm into the cord at the intermediolateral sulcus. Typically 20–24 lesions, spaced at 2-mm intervals, were required over the C5–T1 segments. Eleven patients had 75% or greater persisting relief of pain, and five others had 25%–75% relief. There often was a slight decrease in initial relief in the early postoperative months to a level that persisted. Six patients have been followed for longer than 18 months; three of them had a good response. Ten patients had some initial postoperative deterioration in motor or sensory function in the ipsilateral leg. One had a marked motor deficit. These changes resolved to some extent in all cases. All the patients were ambulatory at follow-up.

A large majority of these patients with severe, intractable pain from brachial plexus avulsion had significant, persistent pain relief from the placement of dorsal root entry zone lesions. Intraoperative monitoring or somatosensory evoked potentials might improve localization of the dorsal root entry zone and minimize damage to the adjacent long tracts.

▶ I realize the advantages of freedom from governmental interference quite well; my parents emigrated from Eastern Europe. Nevertheless, I cannot agree with the argument that freedom of choice dictates that motorcyclists should not be required by law to wear helmets to prevent some of the dreadful complications of their accidents. After all, the law requires that they have licenses to operate their vehicles safely, and those who need eyeglasses are required to wear them. If this route of control cannot be used, then I would suggest rigid application of a doctrine of participatory negligence in assaying financial damages when motorcycle riders are involved. And I wonder how impractical it might be for a neurosurgeon to hire a lawyer to sue an injured motorcyclist who has compounded his injury by not wearing a helmet, for depriving the physician of his civil rights by making him give emergency care for the head injury (often without payment of money) which might not have occurred without the negligence of the driver!

Apparently, lesions in the dorsal root entry zone are capable of interfering with the gray matter into which the pain fibers find their way. I presume that this end station for pain is also in fact the end station for the afferent fibers in the ventral roots, presumably the reason for the failure of dorsal rhizotomy to consistently relieve pain. Chung et al. (*Science* 222:934–935, 1983) provide the first physiologic data at the single-unit fiber level showing that ventral root afferent fibers can modify the activity of neurons in the dorsal horn. Latency measurements indicate that the fibers involved are probably unmyelinated; unlike the ventral afferents thought to be responsible for the failure of dorsal rhizotomy, these newly described fibers probably double back after looping into the ventral root and ultimately go into the dorsal root.—O.S.

---

**Neurosurgical Treatment of Nonmalignant Intractable Rectal Pain: Microsurgical Commissural Myelotomy With Carbon Dioxide Laser**
Robert A. Fink (Univ. of California, San Francisco)
Neurosurgery 14:64–65, January 1984                                  27–3

---

Neuroablative procedures for intractable midline pain have been limited by frequent side effects and disability caused by manipulation of adjacent normal structures. The author reports findings in a patient with pain from nonmalignant disease in whom the $CO_2$ laser was used to perform commissural myelotomy.

Woman, 67, experienced virtually continuous rectal pain that was not improved by surgery for a rectocele. As a result, she became addicted to narcotics. No significant psychiatric disorder was present. A large meningocele of the posterior sacrum was present, with herniation of nerve roots through the bone defect. Sacral rhizotomies failed to relieve the pain, and a ventriculoperitoneal shunt procedure and implantation of a morphine pump also were ineffective. The patient became severely depressed and attempted suicide. A laminectomy of T10 through L1 then was done to expose the conus medullaris, and the $CO_2$ laser was used to make a 4-cm midline incision in the spinal cord between the fasciculi gracili. Under the operating microscope, the crossing fibers of the anterior white commissure were easily identified as they were sectioned. No bleeding occurred during the procedure. Somatosensory evoked potentials remained intact. Rectal pain was absent immediately after the procedure. Existing lower limb weakness from poliomyelitis was slightly worse for several days. Pinprick sensation was absent below L4 bilaterally, and position sense in the left toes was slightly impaired. Cystometrography showed essentially normal function. Only mild rectal discomfort persisted, and the patient stopped using narcotics. She was fully functional seven months after the procedure.

The $CO_2$ laser offers a means of performing commissural myelotomy and other neuroablative procedures with much less morbidity. Improved surgical laser techniques may make it feasible to reevaluate older neuroablative procedures used for intractable pain that have been limited or abandoned because of high risk to other neural functions.

▶ Midline pelvic pain from cancer may respond to a small mechanical or radiofrequency lesion at the center of the spinal cord at the thoracolumbar junction or at C1, according to Gildenberg and Hirshberg (*J. Neurol. Neurosurg. Psychiatry* 47:94–96, 1984). The hypothesis on which this treatment is based is that there is a spinal cord pathway for pain in addition to the lateral spinothalamic tract and that this pathway ascends near the central canal of the spinal cord. Observations leading to this conclusion include relief of midline pain exceeding the amount of analgesia following standard lumbosacral commissural myelotomy. An alternative hypothesis is that the combination of inevitable damage to the dorsal funiculi in addition to that of the commissural fibers may so alter the normal time and space pattern of pain impulses as to elimination of the perception of the pain.—O.S.

---

**Bilateral Percutaneous Cervical Cordotomy: Immediate and Long-Term Results in 36 Patients With Neoplastic Disease**
Stefano Ischia, Aldo Luzzani, Alberto Ischia, and Gianfranco Maffezzoli (Univ. of Verona)
J. Neurol. Neurosurg. Psychiatry 47:141–147, 1984                    27–4

---

Bilateral percutaneous cervical cordotomy has many potential adverse effects, but it is indicated when bilateral pain due to neoplastic disease occurs that cannot be controlled by any other means. The authors reviewed findings in 36 patients with chronic bilateral pain from neoplastic disease who underwent bilateral percutaneous cervical cordotomy. Twenty-nine patients had surgery in two stages at intervals of one to two weeks in which radiofrequency diathermocoagulation was carried out using a traditional electrode bearing a fixed 3-mm exposed tip. Six patients had lesions made bilaterally at a single session with the Levin thermocouple-monitored cordotomy electrode. One patient had bilateral lesions made 22 months apart with both methods. Fluoroscopy and iophendylate myelography were used to guide lesion placement. Both motor and sensory stimulation were carried out as the lesion was made in an incremental manner. Contralateral pain was often not seen until after successful cordotomy for what appeared to be unilateral trunk pain.

Deep analgesia to pinprick was obtained in all patients but one, in whom hypalgesia occurred. Mortality during the first week was 11%. Weakness in the ipsilateral lower extremity occurred in 36% of the patients, but generally improved in time. One patient was paretic, but none was hemiplegic. Permanent sphincter disorder developed in 14 of 24 evaluable patients. Anal sphincter incontinence occurred in one. Thirteen patients had some degree of orthostatic hypotension. No patient had Ondine's syndrome of sleep apnea. Complete long-term pain relief was obtained in 47% of the patients and partial relief in another 12.5%.

Bilateral cervical cordotomy results in a fairly high mortality, caused mainly by sleep-induced apnea and cardiovascular collapse. Impaired sympathetic tone is usual after bilateral cordotomy. The absence of sleep apnea is ascribed to avoidance of reticulospinal fibers by proper placement of the needle tip close to the dentate ligament. Almost half of the present patients had complete relief of pain for the rest of their lives. An improved quality of life was apparent in patients in good general condition without cardiocirculatory problems. Bilateral percutaneous cervical cordotomy now is done in patients who have bilateral neoplastic pain and no strong evidence of deafferentation pain. Open cordotomy is no longer warranted.

▶ According to Batzdorf and Bentson (*J. Neurosurg.* 59:545–547, 1983), visualization of the spinal cord by lumbar subarachnoid injection of metrizamide (7 ml of solution containing iodine [250 mg/ml]) makes percutaneous cordotomy more reliable and easier than when air alone or air plus iophendylate are used. Lateral displacement of the cord by the cordotomy needle can be readily visualized, since the opaque material allows visualization in both lateral and anteroposterior projections. The lumbar technique was found to be superior to the lateral cervical puncture route for introduction of the metrizamide. No complications have been found in the four patients in whom the technique has so far been used. It does seem to me that it is useful to outline the dentate ligament for producing a target for the needle, but the visibility of anterior and posterior borders of the spinal cord would appear to reduce the importance of this landmark.—O.S.

**Spontaneous Saphenous Neuralgia**

Thomas G. Luerssen, Robert L. Campbell, Ray J. Defalque, and Robert M. Worth (Indiana Univ.)
Neurosurgery 13:238–241, September 1983                    27–5

Entrapment of the saphenous nerve in scar tissue is recognized by orthopedic surgeons as a complication of medial arthrotomy, and by vascular surgeons as a complication of procedures involving the saphenous vein. The authors encountered six patients with spontaneous saphenous neuropathy that responded well to surgical treatment. The nerve apparently is subject to compromise in the subsartorial canal where it crosses the femoral artery superficially and penetrates the roof of the canal. All the patients presented with medial knee and leg pain and exhibited tenderness over the subsartorial canal and sensory changes in the cutaneous distribution of one or both terminal branches of the saphenous nerve. The diagnosis was confirmed by saphenous nerve block, and all patients improved after external neurolysis. Three of the six required saphenous neurectomy because of recurrent symptoms. If neurectomy is necessary, the nerve is sectioned well proximal to the subsartorial canal.

Saphenous neuralgia should be considered in patients with medial lower extremity pain who have no other signs of lumbar radiculopathy or knee arthropathy. All the patients were seen after having had extensive studies for knee joint disease. All had pain localized to the medial aspect of the knee, radiating variably to the medial portion of the leg. Women seem to be affected more often than men. The disorder should be distinguished from the more common entrapment of the infrapatellar branch of the saphenous nerve. Saphenous neuralgia can be easily confirmed by anesthetic block of the saphenous nerve. Surgical decompression is considered when the symptoms are severe enough. External neurolysis is done initially, and recurrent symptoms are managed by saphenous neurectomy. No operative complications have occurred.

**Selective Percutaneous Thermolesions of the Ninth Cranial Nerve by Lateral Cervical Approach: Report of Eight Cases**
Giuseppe Salar, Carlo Ori, Vittrorio Baratto, Ivo Iob, and Salvatore Mingrino (Univ. of Padua)
Surg. Neurol. 20:276–279, October 1983                    27–6

A lateral cervical approach (Fig 27–1) rather than the anterior lateral approach was used for destruction of the ninth cranial nerve at the level of the glossopharyngeal or petrous ganglion in the jugular foramen. Percutaneous radiofrequency thermolesioning of the petrous ganglion under local anesthesia was used to treat glossopharyngeal neuralgia in eight patients. Three had essential glossopharyngeal neuralgia, and five had pain from oropharyngeal tumors. An electrode was inserted below the external auditory meatus in front of the mastoid to touch the styloid process; it was then retracted and angled posterior to the styloid. The tip was ultimately inserted 3.5–4 cm beneath the skin surface, and its position in the

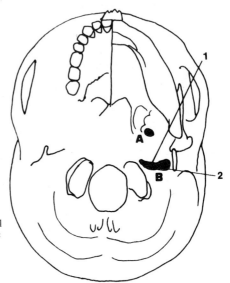

**Fig 27–1.**—Schematic diagram of the skull base: *1*, anterior lateral approach; and *2*, lateral cervical approach. (Courtesy of Salar, G., et al.: Surg. Neurol. 20:276–279, October, 1983.)

jugular foramen was confirmed radiographically before low-voltage stimulation was carried out. The thermal lesion was made with temperatures of 60–65 C for 1–2 minutes. The results were immediate and included disappearance of pain provoked by deglutition in patients with essential neuralgia and of acute attacks in others. Pain perception was reduced in the external acoustic meatus and auricular concha. All the patients were men, and the mean age was 56 years. Those with essential neuralgia did not benefit substantially from treatment with carbamazepine or phenytoin.

The immediate results were satisfactory in all cases. Slight continuous pain in the tonsillar region persisted in the cancer patients, but no major analgesics were requested. There were no persistent complications. The jugular vein was accidentally perforated in one case, but the needle was repositioned and no complication ensued. Transient vagal dysfunction occurred in three fourths of the cases. Only one patient, the first in the series, had a complete recurrence of pain. Two subsequent thermocoagulations gave good results for two to three months in this patient.

Radiofrequency thermocoagulation of the ninth cranial nerve is an effective treatment for essential neuralgia and is simpler and less traumatic than other operations in patients with cancer pain. No technical difficulties have been encountered, and there have been no permanent complications with the lateral cervical approach. Neoplastic masses at the skull base are avoided by this approach.

▶ Observed side effects of percutaneous radiofrequency thermocoagulation of the glossopharyngeal nerve include, according to Ori et al. (*Neurosurgery* 13:427–429, 1983), interference with swallowing and phonation and vocal cord paralysis. These signs of involvement of the vagal nerve have induced some to advocate restricting use of the technique to those with pain of malignant origin; others claim that vagal involvement is not necessary or likely with appropriate technique. Ori et al. encountered hypotension, bradycardia, asystole, syncope, and seizures in a patient, 34, who had radiofrequency thermocoagulation for glossopharyngeal neuralgia of idiopathic origin. After resuscitation of the patient, he was free of pain—and had no evidence of vagal involvement! The route for needle insertion was the same as that devised by Bonica for injection of local anesthesia at the jugular foramen. The exact mechanism for production of these side effects is discussed by the authors and by J. N. St. John in commenting on the case; no conclusion is reached that is satisfactory to me.

By using evoked potentials, Bennett and Jannetta (*Neurosurgery* 13:242–247, 1983) believe they can distinguish classic trigeminal neuralgia (significant increase of latency) from atypical neuralgia and other atypical face pains (no increase in latency). Their results support the view that atypical and classic trigeminal neuralgia syndromes are caused by different types of physiologic dysfunction, and the latter are associated with compression of the trigeminal nerve root.

A new percutaneous stereotactic rhizotomy electrode with a curved tip is considered to give a better procedure for trigeminal neuralgia by Tobler et al. (*Neurosurgery* 12:313–317, 1983). Thanks to the rotation of the needle, the tip can be placed so as to reduce undesirable side effects. Thus in 150 patients, masseter weakness has occurred in only 7.3% as compared with 24% in the series of 700 treated with a straight electrode. The proportion of excellent results has risen from 76% to 88% of patients. In comment, Nugent reports benefits from an angled cordotomy type of electrode, which is smaller and permits monitoring the location and extent of the lesion while the patient is awake, instead of putting the patient to sleep for the lesion making. This technique does not require temperature monitoring, but depends on patient responses in incremental lesions. Apfelbaum comments that the need to use stimulation to evoke a paroxysm of pain for proper localization of the needle tip is a drawback, but awakening the patient between lesions so that the extent can be monitored makes such procedures valid in the treatment of trigeminal neuralgia.

As Mullan and Lichtor (*J. Neurosurg.* 59:1007–1012, 1983) put it, percutaneous microcompression of the trigeminal ganglion for trigeminal neuralgia "is essentially a percutaneous simplification of the older Taarnhøj-Sheldon-Pudenz operation." It gives about the same relief from pain over a 4.5-year follow-up as alternative established procedures. Its advantages are freedom from discomfort, ease of performance, absence of associated mortality, and minimal morbidity rate. The no. 4 Fogarty catheter is inserted through a large bore needle through the foramen ovale and compresses the ganglion for five to seven minutes. Experience with 50 patients indicates the benefits to be obtained.—O.S.

# 28 Miscellaneous

**Monitoring Auditory Functions During Cranial Nerve Microvascular Decompression Operations by Direct Recording From the Eighth Nerve**
Aage R. Møller and Peter J. Jannetta (Univ. of Pittsburgh)
J. Neurosurg. 59:493–499, September 1983                                    28–1

Monitoring of auditory function is of great value in preventing auditory nerve damage during surgery in the cerebellopontine angle. Recording of brain stem auditory evoked potentials (BAEPs) does not provide information at the time of insult, and a gradual change in latency may not present as a meaningful pattern in the averaged response. The authors recorded directly from the auditory nerve in order to monitor nerve function without averaging. Compound action potentials are recorded continually from the time the nerve is exposed and during the entire microvascular decompression procedure. Teflon-coated silver wires are used. Tone bursts of 2,000 Hz and 1 or 5 msec are delivered through an earphone.

Direct eighth nerve recordings were used in 19 patients, 8 with hemifacial spasm and 6 with trigeminal neuralgia. Four patients had surgery for tinnitus and vertigo and one for facial palsy. In most cases, the compound action potentials changed very little during microvascular decompression, as did the latencies. Latencies of the main negative peak varied by less than 0.5 msec in 12 patients. Those with more marked changes were being treated for hemifacial spasm. When substantial change in latency was found during operation, prompt release of the cerebellar retractor was effective in restoring the potentials to normal. The pure-tone average increased 5–10 dB in five patients when tested four to eight days postoperatively and increased even more than that in two cases. Two patients with Meniere's disease could not be assessed, but they had no obvious change in their hearing. In two cases, the hearing threshold improved postoperatively. No patient had significant hearing loss as a result of the surgery. The greatest increase in the pure-tone average was 15 dB.

Direct recording of compound action potentials from the eighth nerve during microvascular decompression to relieve cranial nerve dysfunction provides immediate information and avoids the need for signal averaging. It also is a useful teaching tool. It is helpful to monitor the BAEP before the eighth nerve is exposed. Lateral-to-medial retraction of the cerebellum may be hazardous to eighth nerve function; rostral-to-caudal and caudal-to-rostral retraction is well tolerated.

▶ There is as yet no good explanation as to why hemifacial spasm begins in the orbicularis oculi or for the exact mechanism whereby compression appears to instigate it. Nevertheless, the fact is that decompression of the facial nerve by way of the posterior fossa is effective in relieving the spasms. Loeser and

Chen (*Neurosurgery* 13:141–146, 1983) found that 85% of their series of 20 patients had relief of symptoms, which is close to the overall improvement rate of 93% of cases reported in the literature. (These authors summarized 15 reports for a total of 433 cases, including the current ones; 88% were cured by one or two operations, 5% were improved, and 2% were treatment failures. There has been one death resulting from complications in the entire series; of the 341 cases with complications, 6% involved seventh-nerve dysfunction, and 13% involved eighth-nerve difficulties.

Neurovascular decompression for hemifacial spasm was done in 40 cases (31 women, 9 men) in a four-year period. The left side was involved in 24 and right in 15. One had bilateral facial spasms! In 38 of the cases reported by Goya et al. (*Neurol. Med. Chir.* [*Tokyo*] 23:651–658, 1983) vertebral angiography was done; in 12 there was projection of tortuous and elongated vertebral arteries into the cerebellopontine angle. At operation, the vessel causing the vascular compression was found to be the anterior inferior cerebellar artery in 25 patients, the vertebral artery in 8, and the posterior inferior cerebellar artery in 7. Using Jannetta's classification, the authors found that the results were excellent in 29 patients, good in 8, fair in 2, and poor in 1.

A rather remarkable article by three otologists (Martin et al: *Ann. Otolaryngol. Chir. Cervicofac.* 100:79–82, 1983) is worthy of mention. They list as treatments for facial hemispasm muscular resection (palpebral orbicularis) in isolated blepharospasm, and surgery of the facial nerve (alcohol injection, combing [peignage], neurotomies, and neurectomies). A new treatment—avulsion of the infraorbital (suborbital) nerve—is proposed for the treatment of recurrences (which are frequent). The procedure (done in two women) was undertaken after infiltration of the nerve gave relief. The hypothesis offered is one in which anastomoses between facial and trigeminal branches may be setting off reflex facial contractions which are eliminated by removing the infraorbital nerve. These anastomoses are well known and at times are responsible for incredible anomalous sequelae of facial nerve injury. In one instance quoted, total parotidectomy was not followed by facial weakness, but the performance of a retrogasserian neurotomy was followed by total facial paralysis. In another patient, complete evisceration of the internal auditory meatus in removal of an acoustic tumor led to no facial paralysis. Failure of section of the facial nerve to produce relief of spasm would appear to indicate that the facial nerve was not carrying the motor fibers to the face. Otherwise it is not possible to explain both the (more or less temporary) facial paralysis that follows combing of the nerve and the failure of facial nerve sections to cure the spasm. Avulsion of the infraorbital nerve would then be effective because it suppresses sensitivity of a very sensitive area and also destroys an aberrant motor innervation. The fact that vascular lesions and cholesteatomas can also produce authentic hemispasm does not invalidate the hypothesis, according to Martin and co-workers. The future will decide the value of the proposed treatment; its simplicity and lack of harm to the patient make it appealing. No specific reference is given to the work of Jannetta et al. in the text of the article, but the literature thereof is cited in the bibliography; Pulec's work on decompression of the facial nerve in its canal is given a few lines.

There would appear to be justification for using this infraorbital nerve avulsion technique in a patient who would prefer not to have a posterior fossa decompression (or whose medical status forbids it); the existence of trigeminal pathways for movement of the face is one that has raised an eyebrow in the past, but it appears to have some reality, rare though it may be.

Preoperative evaluation of patients for proposed decompression of the trigeminal or facial nerves could make diagnosis and technique more exact, according to Okamura et al. (*Neurol. Med. Chir.* [*Tokyo*] 23:776–782, 1983). They have made measurements in cadaver brains and in radiographs thereof to locate the optimal tomographic planes for angiotomography of vertebral arteries. Thus for the trigeminal root proximal zone, the center of the entry zone in the lateral view was 12 mm from the clivus and on a line crossing the external auditory canal and perpendicular to the anthropologic baseline. In the anteroposterior view, the most medial part was 16 mm from the midline.

Another technique for seeing the base of the brain at the clivus is described by Chakeres and Kapila (*Radiology* 149:709–715, 1983). This involves having the patient supine and the neck flexed, with gantry angled to parallel the clivus, 70 degrees to the anthropologic baseline. Either 1.5- or 5-mm sections (10–20 to complete the examination) are taken in patients who have had lumbar injections of 5–8 ml of metrizamide with 170 mg of iodine per milliliter for cisternography. Indications include neuromas of cranial nerves, brain stem and cerebellar tumors, Arnold-Chiari malformations, and lesions of the clivus, as well as tentorial and foramen magnum meningiomas.

In 46 patients (of 52 undergoing exploration of the posterior fossa for idiopathic trigeminal neuralgia), anatomical abnormalities were found by Richards et al. (*J. Neurol. Neurosurg. Psychiatry* 46:1098–1101, 1983). Most common was an arterial loop indenting or distorting the nerve at the root entry zone. In 25 patients, the vessel involved was the superior cerebellar artery. The operative procedure of choice is now considered to be microvascular decompression instead of root section, with percutaneous thermocoagulation of the ganglion or root in patients who are aged, unfit, or fearful of operation, and for those not concerned about sensory loss.

On the basis of review of 37 cases with follow-up, Barba and Alksne (*J. Neurosurg.* 60:104–107, 1984) conclude that microvascular decompression is a safe and effective operation for trigeminal neuralgia. Benefits were more likely in those who had had no prior operation (radiofrequency coagulation), which the authors believe should be reserved for older patients. The lateral position for access behind the mastoid process is excellent, and does not involve the hazards of the sitting position. The results of primary decompression are better than those after preliminary needle operation, and allow the patient to have relief without facial numbness.—O.S.

---

**The Middle Scalene Muscle and Its Contribution to the Thoracic Outlet Syndrome**
George I. Thomas, Thomas W. Jones, L. Stanton Stavney, and Dev R. Manhas (Providence Hosp., Seattle)
Am. J. Surg. 145:589–592, May 1983                                28–2

Various anatomical structures have been implicated in the cause of thoracic outlet syndrome without bony abnormality. Simple anterior scalenotomy has failed to consistently cure affected patients. The authors reviewed experience with 108 patients who had scalenotomy and first rib resection in 128 arms for thoracic outlet syndrome. Seventy-four percent of the patients were women. The average age was 31 years. Five procedures were reoperations for failed transaxillary surgery done elsewhere. As much as 90% of the first rib is removed by a supraclavicular approach, leaving the neck of the rib in place to avoid injuring the long thoracic nerve. The middle scalene muscle is clearly separated from the first rib by this procedure; it is removed as far back as the tubercle and neck of the first rib.

Good to excellent results were obtained in 83% of patients operated on in the period 1966–1976 and in 91% of those treated in the period 1976–1982. Four percent of the earlier patients failed to improve after operation. Two patients required reexcision of first rib segments. Several of the most recent 33 patients who were meticulously assessed for anatomical variations exhibited a very broad insertion of the middle scalene muscle anterior to and behind the anterior scalene muscle, in close approximation to the lower trunks of the brachial plexus. The so-called middle scalene band was similar to the sharp anterior medial edge of the middle scalene muscle in some cases. Fifty-eight percent of 29 arms reviewed in detail showed a significant contribution of the middle scalene muscle and its anterior edge to crowding of the interscalene triangle.

The middle scalene muscle seems to be involved in many cases of thoracic outlet syndrome. A supraclavicular operative approach is favored because of the ease of anatomical assessment and the minimal trauma to the rib.

▶ Neurosurgeons are involved with thoracic outlet syndromes in two ways: to aid in diagnosis and surgical treatment and to assay the occasional end result of overly vigorous approaches to the first rib via the transaxillary approach. Most of us are uncomfortable with a transaxillary operation, from lack of experience; many neurosurgeons are familiar with the supraclavicular region, through exposure of the plexus and section of the anterior scalene muscle. Now it seems likely that some neurosurgeons might consider section of the middle scalene muscle to help their patients who have symptoms of thoracic outlet syndrome. Parenthetically, the authors appear to believe that this is such a well-defined symptom complex that they did not need to describe it; I wish I could be as certain.

In a study of 21 patients with thoracic outlet syndrome, Coccia and Satiani (*Am. Fam. Physician* 29:121–126, 1984) give as reasonable indications for operation persistence of incapacitating symptoms, absence of associated cervical or neurologic disorders, and failure to respond to conservative therapy (exercises to strengthen shoulder girdle and ultrasound therapy). Operation in five of those who failed to respond to conservative treatment involved resection of the first rib by the transaxillary approach. One patient was treated by resection of a supraclavicular cervical rib. After 10 months, five patients were asymptomatic, and the sixth had minor residual symptoms. None of the 15 treated without surgery had an excellent result, and only half were partially relieved.

On the other hand, Batt et al. (*J. Chir.* [*Paris*] 120:687–691, 1983), having used the axillary approach 94 times between 1974 and 1980, were so discontented with the 10% postoperative complications and 19.5% poor or incomplete results that they have reverted to the supraclavicular route which they consider better, especially if the patient has neurologic disturbance.

Almost 98% of patients with thoracic outlet syndrome have symptoms of brachial plexus compression. Significant vascular compression is very rare, with arterial compression less frequent than venous. The 63 patients in the series reported by Sällströmand Gjöres (*Acta Chir. Scand.* 149:555–560, 1983) were selected as having the syndrome from a group of 410 suspected of compression. Bilateral symptoms were present in 30, and in 9 of these, symptoms were equally severe on both sides. Mean age was 37 (range 13–61), and women predominated (36:27). When symptoms persisted after three months of conservative management with physiotherapy, surgery was carried out. Altogether, 72 operations were done (9 bilateral), with transaxillary removal of the first rib in 70; in 2, supraclavicular removal of a cervical rib was done. In addition, after rib removal, excision of all bands was done, an essential part of operation for relief of symptoms. Some passed from neck of the first rib to the rib behind the scalene tubercle; some from the medial to the anterior scalene muscles; and one type was a minimal scalene muscle attaching to the first rib behind the scalene tubercle. Excellent results were reported in 64% and good results in 17%. Fair results were reported in 12%, and in 5 (7%) patients results were poor. In two of these the long thoracic nerve was injured; one had venous thrombosis, and the other was injured at reoperation for shortening the rib stump. Of the three other failures, cervical rhizopathy was found in two, and shoulder joint disturbance in the third.—O.S.

---

## Spinal Cord Stimulation in Peripheral Vascular Disease

R. C. Tallis, L. S. Illis, E. M. Sedgwick, C. Hardwidge, and J. S. Garfield
J. Neurol. Neurosurg. Psychiatry 46:478–484, June 1983                28–3

---

Observations of increased cutaneous blood flow in patients having spinal cord stimulation for chronic neurologic disorders led to its use in patients with severe arterial disease. The authors evaluated epidural cord stimulation in 10 patients with marked intractable symptoms of angiographically proved peripheral arterial disease. All had disabling symptoms that had failed to respond to conventional surgical and medical measures. Four patients had given up smoking. Cutaneous blood flow was measured by the radioxenon clearance technique, as was muscle blood flow in muscle at rest and on exercise. Stimulation of the spinal cord using percutaneously inserted epidural electrodes used square-wave pulses of 200 μsec, 8 mA, and about 33 Hz. Transcutaneous stimulation over the lumbar spine also was evaluated in eight cases.

Three of five patients with severe rest pain obtained complete or very marked relief, and 1 of 2 with moderate rest pain in the leg had complete relief. One of two evaluable patients with indolent ulcers had healing. Four patients had a striking increase in claudication distance, and two others improved moderately. Four patients had no benefit from spinal cord stimulation. No patient responded to transcutaneous stimulation. Bicycle exercise endurance increased insignificantly with epidural cord stimulation. Cutaneous blood flow increased significantly, as did muscle blood flow at rest. The increase in muscle blood flow on exercise was insignificant. Improved blood flow was apparent only in those patients with good clinical responses to epidural cord stimulation. The same was true of exercise tolerance.

Epidural stimulation of the spinal cord can produce clinical improvement in association with increased cutaneous blood flow in patients with severely symptomatic peripheral arterial disease who are unresponsive to conventional surgical and medical methods. The effect probably is due to antidromic stimulation of the central processes of the first-order sensory neurons, and it may be mediated by release of prostaglandins, as well as indirectly by pain relief.

---

**Iatrogenic Lesions of the Spinal Accessory Nerve: Microsurgical Repair**
L. Sedel and Y. Abols (Hôpital Saint-Louis, Paris)
Presse Med. 12:1711–1713, June 25, 1983                                    28–4

---

Even a cursory review of legal actions brought against surgeons quickly reveals the high frequency of malpractice suits involving injury to the spinal accessory nerve during cervical lymph node biopsy. The striking contrast between the benign nature of the procedure and the severity of functional impairment resulting from trapezius paralysis easily explains the justified discontent of such patients, particularly because they generally had not been apprised of the risk involved. These considerations led the authors to report their experience with eight such patients, three men and five women, ranging in age from 18 to 71 years. All had undergone a minor procedure involving the posterior triangle of the neck: lymph node biopsy (four patients) or excision of a tuberculous lymph node (two), of a cyst (one), or of an angioma (one). In four patients the paralysis was obvious upon awakening, leaving no doubt as to etiology; however, in the other four the symptoms were noted only several days or weeks after the procedure. Pain, atrophy of the trapezius, and drooping and limited abduction of the shoulder were the principal signs. An electromyogram confirmed the diagnosis in all patients. Microsurgical repair involved primary suture, neurolysis, or grafts using the external saphenous nerve. Of seven patients followed up for an average of 14 months, three recovered completely; three had satisfactory but incomplete recovery; and one did not recover.

The small size and superficial location of the external branch of the spinal nerve easily explain its vulnerability when cervical lymph node biopsy is performed. However, these lesions need not cause irreversible trauma, and repair should be attempted whenever technically possible because the chances for successfully limiting or even reversing the handicap are good.

▶ H. Millesi and J. K. Terzis were two members of a committee set up by the

International Society of Reconstructive Microsurgery to consider problems of terminology in peripheral nerve surgery. Their report appears in the new journal *Microsurgery* (4:51, 1983). They include a table of nerve repair procedures that could be used as a protocol sheet which could lead to accumulation of data to improve the reporting of results of various techniques in nerve surgery. Incidentally, the term used by the committee to describe opposition of nerve ends with special attention to bringing together properly aligned fascicles of fibers is *coaption.* The term *anastomosis* should be restricted to microvascular repairs, "as it implies communication between two vessels." In fact, the word has a long and honorable history of use in general surgery to put together portions of the intestinal tract, for its derivation from the Greek includes *ana* (up) and *stoma* (mouth, opening).

The subtitle of an article in *Science* (221:538–539, 1983) reads, "A new method of reconnecting peripheral nerves virtually ensures that they will grow back correctly." This sounded so intriguing that it led me to read the three articles by de Medinaceli et al. that appeared in *Experimental Neurology* (81:459–468, 469–487, 488–496, 1983). In the last article the authors say, "We believe that overlooking physical and chemical damage to the fibers renders illusory the most precise surgical reunions, because this leaves a large interposition of dead or dying tissues. Negligible to the eye, the scar that ensues is large relative to the size of the axons, and promotes wandering, branching, and misdirection of the sprouts. In the peripheral nervous system, the scar does not actually arrest axonal regrowth but instead disrupts the repair effort by disorganizing routing of the growing fibers."

In an attempt to mitigate these adverse effects, the investigators froze the cut nerve, soaked it in a solution that resembles the interior of a cell (containing sodium chloride and potassium chloride, but also containing chlorpromazine and polyvinyl alcohol) and cut the nerve end with a vibrating razor blade to avoid crushing the nerve fibers. The cut ends were then held together with a rubber device. Apparently the method works very well for the cut sciatic nerves of rats. Nonhuman primates are next.—O.S.

## Operative Management of Selected Brachial Plexus Lesions
David G. Kline and Donald J. Judice (Louisiana State Univ.)
J. Neurosurg. 58:631–649, May 1983                                                    28–5

Controversy continues regarding the value of surgery for brachial plexus lesions. The authors reviewed experience gained over 12 years with 171 patients having severe brachial plexus lesions who were followed up for at least 1½ years. The average age was 36 years; only seven patients were children. Selection for operation and the timing of surgery were aided by categorizing each brachial plexus element as completely or incompletely injured, and as in continuity or not in continuity. A delay of surgery for several months is recommended for most lesions in continuity. Lacerations causing loss of continuity are best repaired primarily if the injury is a sharp one. The predominant level of involvement was roots to trunks in 72 of the present cases, divisions to cords in 43, and cords to nerves in 56.

Of 282 gunshot-wounded and stretch-injured elements, 210 of which were considered clinically complete, 63 were spared resection because of the finding of nerve action potentials at testing during surgery. Fifty-seven recovered function with neurolysis alone. The 120 resected elements were confirmed as neurotmetic by both electrical study during surgery and histologic examination. Acceptable results were obtained in 16 of 24 suture procedures, 43 of 89 grafts, and all 7 split repairs. Fourteen of 18 lacerated elements with lost continuity recovered after primary repair. Grafts often were necessary where secondary repair was done, and only half of 37 elements so managed recovered function. Seventeen elements with complete loss were in continuity, and 6 of them were found to be regenerating and were not resected.

Surgery is worthwhile in selected cases of brachial plexus injury. Many benign tumors can be removed without significant functional loss using surgical loupes or the operating microscope and repeated action potential recording. End-to-end repair is preferred when resection is necessary, but the use of grafts often is required. The only serious complication in the present series was embolization from a repaired axillary artery in a patient previously operated on, requiring below-the-shoulder amputation.

▶ The term *split repairs* refers to the following: a partially damaged nerve or trunk is split so that the part found to conduct electrical impulses is left alone, and the nonconducting portion is repaired, using grafts from the sural or antebrachial cutaneous nerves.—O.S.

The purpose of reporting a series of 25 patients operated on for brachial plexus lesions was, according to Stevens et al. (*Surg. Neurol* 19:334–345, 1983), to show that the brachial plexus can be anastomosed and reconstructed to improve function without producing additional neurologic deficits. Anastomosis was done in 14 patients, clavicular decompression in 2, and neurolysis in 9 by Dr. MacCarty over the period from 1946 to 1978. No patient was explored immediately; those with open wounds were explored when the wound permitted, and the rest when there had been no improvement after three months following the injury. Lesions in continuity that did not respond to electric stimulation distally or proximally were treated by anastomosis. Evidence of nerve regeneration was observed in 93% of those so treated. Anastomosis of medial cord or of median and ulnar nerves did not help most of the patients with such lesions. Intraoperative nerve stimulation with visualization of action potentials was not available for these operations. Delayed compression of the neural structures by clavicular irregularities after fracture were well suited to operation (removal of clavicle, decompression of nerves). In civilian practice, it is difficult for a neurosurgeon to gain the experience needed to explore usefully the brachial plexus, especially when scarring has distorted relationships. In experienced hands, the benefits of exploration and treatment of brachial plexus injuries outweigh the risks.—O.S.

---

**Subdural Effusions Reappearing After Shunts in Patients With Nontumoral Stenosis of the Aqueduct**

T. Kuurne, A. Servo, and M. Porras (Helsinki University Central Hosp.)
Acta Neurochir. (Wien) 67:127–134, 1983                    28–6

---

Patients with nonneoplastic aqueductal stenosis and clinical findings resembling those of normal-pressure hydrocephalus are managed by shunting. The authors report data on three such patients in whom progressive symptoms developed a few months after shunting, despite initially correct opening pressures. The patients presented with considerable lateral and third ventricular enlargement on computed tomography (CT), and findings of aqueductal stenosis on metrizamide ventriculography, with persistence of a narrow passage to the fourth ventricle. A Spitz-Holter ventriculoauricular shunt was successfully placed in all cases, but headache when the patients were upright developed in about four months, and CT showed bilateral subdural effusions 1–5 cm thick in all three patients. The effusions were evacuated, two shunts were revised and one closed. However, symptoms of increased intracranial pressure were present a month later, and CT showed enlarged cerebral ventricles. The effusions had disappeared. The two open shunts had opening pressures of 20 and 36 cm $H_2O$, respectively. These valves were replaced with ones having opening pressures of 6 and 8 cm $H_2O$, and the on-off device of the third valve was reopened.

Symptoms due to ventricular collapse and subdural effusion developed about four months after shunt surgery in these cases despite careful preoperative pressure recording and individualization of the opening pressure of the shunt valve. A clinical check and CT should be done about three months after shunt surgery in patients with initially large supratentorial cerebral ventricles and an Evans index exceeding 0.40. Intraventricular pressure recording should be carried out in these patients at the time of initial surgery in order to select the correct opening pressure of the shunt valve before inserting the shunt.

▶ The Evans index is the ratio of the width of the ventricles (at the level of the caudate nuclei) to the transverse diameter of the brain at the same level.— O.S.

## Long-Term Results of Conventional Surgical Treatment for Epilepsy: Delayed Recurrence After a Period of 10 Years

J. E. Paillas, H. Gastaut, R. Sedan, and M. Bureau (Hôpital de la Timone, Marseilles, France)

Surg. Neurol. 20:189–193, September 1983                28–7

Results of surgical treatment for epilepsy were reviewed in 44 patients initially treated more than 10 years earlier. Thirty-seven patients were operated on only once and were followed up at 11–26 years. Seven patients had a recurrence within five years and required a second operation, and they were followed for 11–17 years after reoperation. All the patients were free of seizures after their last operation, and 32 of them had been persistently seizure free for 15–27 years. Nine patients had recurrent seizures in the 11th year, and three others after 14–19 years. Except for one patient who was reoperated on for recurrent seizures after 10 years without them, all had rare seizures that were adequately controlled medically.

Eight of the patients reoperated on had severe behavioral disorder in addition to seizures. Nearly two thirds of the patients who were recovered for more than 10 years presently work regularly, and half have achieved social acceptance. Surgery on the right side yielded better long-term results than did operations on the left side because of inadequate resections on the left in patients with temporal epilepsy. All but 3 of 17 patients whose lesion was attributed to dystocia had lasting recovery. Most patients with long-delayed relapse had had temporal lobectomy for psychomotor seizures, with involvement of the supra-Sylvian areas.

The long-term results of surgery for epilepsy appear to be more enduring if the epileptogenic areas are completely excised. In some cases, secondary maturation of a minor epileptogenic focus that is initially masked by a major irritative lesion or a new epileptogenic scar of surgical origin will cause seizures after initial operation. All except one of the very late recurrences in the present series were adequately treated medically.

▶ This series includes five hemispherectomies (four right and one left); all patients had lasting relief of their seizures, but one had to have a shunt put in for hydrocephalus 23 years after operation and thereafter died of meningitis.

An interesting exchange of letters to the Editor of *Annals of Neurology* (13:580–581, 1983) deals with the varied opinions available concerning the propriety of basing patient selection for operation for epilepsy on scalp electrode recordings. Zifkin and Ehrenberg urge that extensive testing be continued and that ictal and interictal scalp and sphenoidal electrode recordings be the cornerstone of the investigation. Implantation of depth electrodes is not essential for all patients. Spencer et al. believe that depth electrode studies are currently essential. Engel et al. believe that depth electrodes are not always needed if other techniques are consistent in their indications of the focal origin of the seizures; they are especially impressed with the use of positron computed tomography to indicate the pathologic area by demonstrating a zone of hypometabolism.

Rasmussen has written an intriguing article on characteristics of a pure culture of frontal lobe epilepsy (*Epilepsia* 24:482–493, 1983). At the Montreal Neurological Institute, between 1930 and 1971, frontal cortical excisions were carried out in 239 patients with nonneoplastic epileptogenic lesions. Twenty patients have had no seizures for at least five years, and another 20 have been seizure-free after a few seizures in the immediate postoperative period. The median follow-up of these 40 patients has been 14 years. Meningocerebral cicatrix was found in 24 cases, gliosis in 12, and porencephalic cyst in 3; 1 patient had a hamartoma. Of particular interest (and concern) is the finding that some patients have postoperative spiking in the EEG, yet in some patients this may indicate transient seizures with subsequent freedom, and in others there may be no seizures at all. Excisions ranged from excision of the anterior third or half of a frontal lobe, to complete frontal lobectomy, to excision of only convexity of the frontal lobe. As is true in seizure-free temporal lobe operations, there is need for improving accuracy of evaluation of those zones beyond the actual damaged brain that may still be epileptogenic, as well as some guide as to how much of the surrounding brain needs to be removed.

Rasmussen hopes that improved and sophisticated EEG techniques may improve selection of surgical candidates and help to tailor the procedure to the individual patient who had medically refractory focal epilepsy.

The difficult problem of locating the focus of refractory seizures has been attacked recently by Theodore and colleagues (*Ann. Neurol.* 14:429–437, 1983). Scalp EEG and positron emission tomography were used simultaneously in 20 patients with complex partial seizures and normal computed tomography. Using fluorodeoxyglucose 18, the authors found a hypometabolic lesion in 16 patients; these same areas had hypermetabolism during seizures, which occurred in 3 of the patients during their positron emission studies.

Epidural recordings were used for localization of seizure focus in 100 cases studied by Goldring and Gregorie (*J. Neurosurg.* 60:457–466, 1984). For temporal lobe epilepsy, an epidural array is put in place by way of a low temporal craniectomy. For sensorimotor epilepsy, a formal flap is turned, the brain is stimulated electrically, and sensory evoked potentials are used to identify the sensorimotor region. The dura mater is sewed back, and a large array of epidural electrodes is put in place for extraoperative monitoring of spontaneous seizures, usually easily found because the prime consideration for operation is inability to control seizures with medication. Of the 100 patients, 72 underwent resection of an epileptogenic focus. Follow-up for more than one year in 57 patients reveals 64% good results in the 28 adults and 62% good results in the 29 children. Epidural recordings instead of depth electrode tracings were made in 20 with temporal lobe seizures. In 15, seizure focus excision was carried out; all had definite cerebral pathology by histologic study. In 11, epidural recordings distinguished medial from lateral foci. The 48-electrode array for the hemispheral recordings permits a wide range of combinations for recordings, and ease of electronic switching shortens time for recording. The ability to substitute epidural for depth electrodes for temporal lobe cases similarly has enhanced the results of operating in these patients.

Most neurosurgeons do not have the opportunity to carry out the detailed neurophysiologic investigations of localization of sensory function in the brain described by Van Buren (*J. Neurosurg.* 59:119–130, 1983). During the course of 134 craniotomies under local anesthesia, electrical stimulation evoked from the precentral region sensory responses that were apt to be sensation of movement and specific sensation; however, stimulation from the postcentral region was apt to be more crude, i.e., sensation that was not likely to be experienced in a particular normal situation. Sensory responses for the trunk and extremities are almost entirely contralateral to the side of brain stimulation, whereas for the orofacial areas, almost a fourth were either ipsilateral or bilateral. Most of the responses allocated to the second sensory area arise from stimulation inferior and anterior to the terminus of the central sulcus—between it and the Sylvian fissure—and most of these are contralateral.

Van Buren hypothesizes that the "highest level" or "consciousness" appears to be in the striatum, which appears to be capable of sensorimotor modulation and selective direction of motor responses with access to material acquired in the past. "This capability would appear to define, in part, consciousness itself."—O.S.

**Forebrain Commissurotomy for Epilepsy: Review of 20 Consecutive Cases**
R. E. Harbaugh, D. H. Wilson, A. G. Reeves, and M. S. Gazzaniga
Acta Neurochir. (Wien) 68:263–275, 1983                                    28–8

The authors reviewed the results of division of the forebrain commissures in 20 patients seen in the past decade at Dartmouth-Hitchcock Med. Center, Hanover, N.H. The patients had intractable generalized, generalized and partial, or partial seizures. A "complete" commissurotomy was done in the first three cases, and a "frontal" commissurotomy in the next five, with section of one fornix, the anterior commissure, and the rostral half of the corpus callosum. Because of the high morbidity of those procedures, including one death, "central" commissurotomy now is done, with division of only the corpus callosum and underlying hippocampal commissure. Six patients have had this operation in a single stage and another six in two stages, a month apart. All the patients had been incapacitated by seizures for at least four years despite aggressive medical management.

Five of the 19 patients followed up have had excellent results, with three or fewer seizures a year. Anticonvulsants have been stopped in two of these cases. Eleven other patients had more than a 50% reduction in seizures and a change to a less debilitating type of seizure. Two patients had fair results, and one was unimproved. Seven patients had postoperative complications, but these have been fewer with the use of a central commissurotomy. Ten of the 12 patients having this procedure had excellent or good results. None of them have had neurologic injury apart from the subtle deficits produced by commissurotomy and the reversible changes of the acute disconnection syndrome.

Forebrain commissurotomy is effective in controlling intractable seizures in selected patients who are incapacitated despite vigorous medical measures and who are not candidates for resection of an epileptogenic focus. Patients with obvious unilateral hemispheric injury and those with atonic seizures have done well after commissurotomy, but those who are severely retarded have benefited the least. A two-stage procedure with division of only the corpus callosum and underlying hippocampal commissure appears to be effective and relatively safe.

▶ The surgical technique used for the 18-year-old epileptic youth described by Sussman et al. (*J. Neurosurg.* 59:514–519, 1983) consisted of section of the corpus callosum and hippocampal commissure but not the anterior commissure. The third ventricle was not entered. There was transient decrease in blood flow in the frontal regions, and it is to this that the authors ascribe the mutism that followed operation—and lasted for 16 months except for eight brief one-sentence outbursts of speech. Intellectual testing showed marked IQ changes preoperatively (mild to moderate mental retardation). Retardation was aggravated after operation, but IQ scores gradually improved to at least preoperative levels by 24 months after operation. This particular patient lacked speech or vocalization for about five minutes after each hemisphere was depressed with 100 mg of amobarbital injected into the internal carotid artery. The authors consider it possible that the mutism resulted from severing interhemispheric connections in a person who required both hemispheres for speech production.

---

**Selective Posterior Rhizotomy for Treatment of Spasticity**
Lauri V. Laitinen, Stefan Nilsson, and Axel R. Fugl-Meyer (Umeå Univ., Sweden)
J. Neurosurg. 58:895–899, June 1983                                         28–9

Fasano et al., in 1976, described a modification of Foerster's posterior rhizotomy based on electrical stimulation of the posterior roots. In the present study, a similar technique was used to treat nine spastic patients, six of whom had spastic paraplegia from multiple sclerosis. The others had cerebral hemorrhage, cord injury, and unspecified myelopathy as the causes of spasticity. The patients with multiple sclerosis had a mean age of 39 years, and had been ill for a mean of 16 years. All the patients had some sensory deficit in the affected extremities, and four had pain in the legs. The fascicles of the posterior T12–S1 roots, or the C6–C8 roots in the patient with arm spasticity, were stimulated electrically under general anesthesia. The 60%–80% of fascicles that responded to the 60-Hz, 1–6-V stimuli with tonic muscle jerks were cut.

No serious complications occurred. Eight patients were satisfied with the outcome, but one had erroneously expected that intention tremor of the arms would be relieved. Spasticity was abolished in four cases and much diminished in five. No patient had flaccidity that impaired rehabilitation. Spasticity did not return during follow-up for as long as 26 months after surgery. Two of six patients who had been functionally paraplegic before surgery learned to walk using crutches and splints. Two patients with painful muscle spasms have remained free of pain, and the deafferentation type of pain in two patients was temporarily relieved. Two patients reported very slight deterioration in pinprick sensation in the area corresponding to the rhizotomy. No patient had worsening of multiple sclerosis following rhizotomy.

Partial selective posterior rhizotomy consistently relieves spasticity without producing significant sensory deterioration. Better results can be expected in the leg than in the upper extremity. Long-term physiotherapy is necessary to obtain optimal results from the procedure. There is no evidence that surgery, general anesthesia, or both cause acute exacerbations of multiple sclerosis.

▶ When spasticity in paraplegic or quadriplegic patients persists in spite of trials on baclofen, dantrolene, or diazepam, Herz et al. (*Spine* 8:729–732, 1983) have turned to percutaneous radiofrequency foraminal rhizotomies. Under fluoroscopic control and local anesthesia (when needed), 12-gauge spinal needles are placed into the intervertebral foramina, usually from T12–L1 through L5–S1. Through each, a radiofrequency probe is placed until a maximal motor response is obtained by electrical stimulation. A lesion is then made at each locus. Complete flaccidity was achieved in 73%; reduction in spasticity sufficient to be of some value was obtained in another 21%. Recurrence of spasticity occurred in 40% of the patients and yielded to repetition of the procedure in all but one elderly patient. Hemothorax occurred in one patient early in the series. Selective spasticity (e.g., quadriceps) can be treated by selective radiofrequency rhizotomy.

An excellent article on surgical posterior rhizotomies for the treatment of pain by Sindou and Goutelle has appeared in *Advances and Technical Standards in Neurosurgery,* vol. 10 (Krayenbühl, H. [ed.]; New York, Springer-Verlag, 1983). Intradural and extradural rhizotomies and ganglionectomy are described in detail, including Sindou's selective posterior rhizotomy, which is useful for treatment of spasticity as well as for pain. The similarity of the incision of the nociceptive fibers as they pass into the cord to the operation on the dorsal root entry zone described by Nashold is worthy of further investigation.

A nice essay on the pathophysiology of spasticity appeared in *Triangle:* Sandoz Journal of Medical Science (22:165–174, 1983). Two possible mechanisms are considered: abnormal descending control of a normal spinal cord, and plastic changes at the spinal level, such as collateral sprouting. The role of changes in the muscles is also discussed, with reference to recent proposals that these may be responsible for clinical signs of spasticity!—O.S.

# Subject Index

## A

Abdominal
  complications of ventriculoperitoneal
    shunts, 298
Abscess
  brain, 366 ff.
    clinical stages on CT scans, 366
    evacuation of, open, 369
Absence seizures (see Seizures, absence)
Acoustic
  nerve tumor, gas-CT cisternography in,
    244
  neurinoma, stereotactic radiosurgery in,
    385
Acquired immune deficiency syndrome
  encephalitis and, Toxoplasma, in
    Haitians, 147
  neurological complications of, 189
Adenoma
  pituitary, preoperative vascular studies
    in, 391
Age
  cerebral blood flow and cerebrovascular
    $CO_2$ reactivity in stroke and, 62
  multiple sclerosis and, 165
Aging
  normal, and cerebral vasomotor
    responses during oxygen inhalation,
    90
AIDS (see Acquired immune deficiency
    syndrome)
Air
  embolism prevention with positive end-
    expiratory pressure, 272
Akinesia
  psychic, with bilateral lesions of basal
    ganglia, 131
Alcohol
  syndrome, fetal, 73
  withdrawal seizures, antiepileptic drugs
    in, 113
Alcoholism
  images, impairments, interventions, 157
Aldose reductase inhibitor
  in diabetic neuropathy, painful, 182
Alexia
  without agraphia, in composer, 42
Allergic
  neuritis, plasma exchange in (in rabbit),
    183
Allergy
  food, and migraines, 135
Allogeneic skull disks
  in craniotomy, 279

Alzheimer's disease
  genetic aspects and associated clinical
    disorders, 86
  tomography in, 88 ff.
    computed, and ventricular size, 89
    positron emission, 88
Alzheimer type
  of senile dementia, 85
Amaurosis fugax
  arteriography in, 177
γ-Aminobutyric acid
  in epilepsy, refractory, 96
Amnesic syndrome
  after hypoxic ischemic injury, 38
Amphetamine
  oral, and intracerebral hemorrhage, 161
Amyotrophic lateral sclerosis
  syndromes, relation to Creutzfeldt-
    Jakob disease, 87
Anastomosis
  primary, in aneurysm of petrous portion
    of internal carotid, 426
Anesthesia
  hemodilution, in children, 271
  local, in carotid endarterectomy, 465
Aneurysm, 420 ff.
  carotid artery
    giant, transvascular treatment of, 426
    internal, petrous portion,
      management of, 426
  cerebral, surgery of
    mannitol in, 269
    prevention of symptomatic vasospasm
      and, 420
  ophthalmic artery, 424
  rebleeding, 421
  rupture (see Rupture, aneurysm)
  surgery
    early, causes of unfavorable outcome,
      415
    ultrasound during, real-time, 427
  vertebral artery, giant, transvascular
    treatment of, 428
Angiography, 240 ff.
  cerebral, complications of, 240
  digital subtraction
    in cerebrovascular disease diagnosis,
      23
    with intravenous injection, 242
Antibiotics
  prophylactic, and postoperative
    infections, 339
Anticholinergic therapy
  in dystonia, 128
Anticonvulsant
  syndrome, fetal (in rat), 93

# Index to Authors

# TO ORDER: DETACH AND MAIL

Please enter my subscription to the periodical(s) checked below:
(To order by phone, call toll-free **800-621-9262**. In IL, call collect **312-726-9746.**)

| | PRACTITIONER | INSTITUTION | RESIDENTS |
|---|---|---|---|
| Current Problems in Surgery® | ☐ $45.00 | ☐ $60.00 | ☐ $25.00 |
| Current Problems in Pediatrics® | ☐ 37.50 | ☐ 60.00 | ☐ 25.00 |
| Current Problems in Cancer | ☐ 47.00 | ☐ 60.00 | ☐ 25.00 |
| Current Problems in Cardiology® | ☐ 47.00 | ☐ 60.00 | ☐ 25.00 |
| Current Problems in Ob/Gyn. | ☐ 42.50 | ☐ 60.00 | ☐ 25.00 |
| Current Problems in Diag. Radiology® | ☐ 39.00 | ☐ 60.00 | ☐ 25.00 |
| Disease-a-Month® | ☐ 35.00 | ☐ 55.00 | ☐ 25.00 |

Binder ☐ $6.95 (each year)

Illinois and Tennessee residents will be billed appropriate state sales tax. Prices in Canada slightly higher but billed in Canadian funds. International prices, also slightly higher. A small additional charge will be made for postage and handling. All prices quoted are subject to change.

NAME _____ ACCT. NO. _____
(Please print including middle initial)

ADDRESS _____

CITY _____ STATE _____ ZIP _____

Printed in U.S.A.                                                                                    PAYB

**YEAR BOOK MEDICAL PUBLISHERS • 35 EAST WACKER DRIVE • CHICAGO, ILLINOIS 60601**